W9-BNU-335

Handbook of Kidney
Transplantation

Handbook of Kidney Transplantation

Second Edition

Edited by
Gabriel M. Danovitch, M.D.

Professor of Clinical Medicine, University of California,
Los Angeles, UCLA School of Medicine; Medical Director,
Kidney Transplant Program, UCLA Medical Center, Los Angeles

Little, Brown and Company

Boston   New York   Toronto   London

Library of Congress Cataloging-in-Publication Data

Handbook of kidney transplantation / edited by Gabriel M. Danovitch. –
– 2nd ed.
    p.   cm.
  Includes bibliographical references and index.
  ISBN 0–316–17276–6
  1. Kidneys--Transplantation. I. Danovitch, Gabriel M.
  [DNLM: 1. Kidney Transplantation.   WJ 368 H236 1996]
RD575.H25 1996
617.4'610592—dc20
DNLM/DLC
for Library of Congress   90-10790
                                             CIP

Printed in the United States of America
RRD-VA

10 9 8 7 6 5 4 3 2

Cover: Schematic diagram of the structure of a representative class I MHC molecule (HLA-A2). The α_1 and α_2 domains form a peptide-binding site with the binding groove, which faces the T cell receptor at the top (see Chaps. 2 and 3). (This remarkable structure is described in detail by PJ Bjorkman, MA Saper, B Samraoni et al. Structure of the human class I histocompatibility antigen, HLA-A2. *Nature* 329:506–512, 1987. Reprinted with permission.)

Editorial: Jo-Ann T. Strangis, Kristin Odmark
Production Services: Silverchair Science + Communications
Copyeditor: Dana L. Tackett
Indexer: Elizabeth Willingham

For Nava, my "emotionally related" spouse,
and for our "1-haplotype–matched" children,
Itai, Roy, and Yaël

Contents

Preface

The 4 years that have elapsed since publication of the first edition of *Handbook of Kidney Transplantation* have seen dramatic progress in the world of organ transplantation. Much has been learned about the immunobiology of the alloimmune response, the mechanism of action of immunosuppressive agents, and the pathophysiology of acute and chronic rejection. Potent new immunosuppressive agents are being developed and tested in clinical trials and introduced into clinical practice.

Yet this progress is clouded by frustration. The demand for cadaveric organs grows inexorably, while the supply remains essentially stagnant. Patients wait months and sometimes years for organs and may deteriorate or die in the process. Though new immunosuppressive agents may have a favorable impact on the early post-transplant course, their impact on the development of chronic graft failure remains unproved. Attempts to expand the donor supply may lead to the acceptance of organs for transplantation whose long-term function may be limited.

The high success rates for transplantation, while gratifying in themselves, have brought with them unanticipated dilemmas and challenges. The limited armamentarium of immunosuppressive agents that was available in the 1980s was extremely effective, with the result that it is becoming increasingly difficult to prove unambiguously the additional benefit of new therapeutic approaches. Large-scale, prolonged, multicenter clinical trials are often required. The transplant community needs the wisdom to reap the benefits of new agents and protocols without awakening the all-too-familiar enemies, opportunistic infection and cancer, that continue to lurk in the shadows of immunosuppression. The prolific efforts made to ensure the equity of the transplantation endeavor for all our patients must not be distorted by the financial constraints that are intrinsic to our times.

This edition of the *Handbook of Kidney Transplantation*, like its predecessor, is designed to make this rapidly changing world of kidney transplantation fully accessible to those privileged to serve our long-suffering patients with end-stage kidney disease.

G. M. D.

Contributing Authors

William J. C. Amend Jr., M.D.
Professor of Clinical Medicine and Surgery,
University of California, San Francisco, School of Medicine,
San Francisco

Zoran L. Barbaric, M.D.
Professor of Radiological Sciences, University of California,
Los Angeles, UCLA School of Medicine; Chief, Abdominal
Imaging Division, UCLA Medical Center, Los Angeles

Arthur H. Cohen, M.D.
Professor of Pathology and Medicine, University of
California, Los Angeles, UCLA School of Medicine; Attending
Pathologist, Cedars Sinai Medical Center, Los Angeles

Gabriel M. Danovitch, M.D.
Professor of Clinical Medicine, University of California,
Los Angeles, UCLA School of Medicine; Medical Director,
Kidney Transplant Program, UCLA Medical Center,
Los Angeles

Robert B. Ettenger, M.D.
Professor of Pediatrics and Head, Division of Pediatric
Nephrology, and Vice Chairman for Clinical Affairs,
University of California, Los Angeles, UCLA School of
Medicine; Director, Pediatric Renal Transplant Program,
and Director, UCLA Histocompatibility Laboratory, UCLA
Medical Center, Los Angeles

William G. Goodman, M.D.
Professor of Radiology and Medicine, University of
California, Los Angeles, UCLA School of Medicine;
Associate Director, Dialysis Program, UCLA Medical Center,
Los Angeles

Simin Goral, M.D.
Clinical Instructor in Medicine, Division of Nephrology,
Vanderbilt University School of Medicine, Nashville,
Tennessee

J. Harold Helderman, M.D.
Professor of Medicine, Microbiology, and Immunology,
Vanderbilt University School of Medicine; Medical Director,
Vanderbilt Transplant Center, Nashville, Tennessee

Carl K. Hoh, M.D.
Assistant Professor of Molecular and Medical Pharmacology
and Radiological Sciences, University of California, Los
Angeles, UCLA School of Medicine; Nuclear Medicine
Residency Director, UCLA Medical Center, Los Angeles

Curtis D. Holt, Pharm.D.
Assistant Clinical Professor of Pharmacy, University of
California, San Francisco, School of Pharmacy; Transplant
Pharmacy Specialist, UCLA Medical Center, Los Angeles

Steven Katznelson, M.D.
Assistant Professor of Medicine, University of California,
Davis, School of Medicine; Medical Director, Kidney and
Pancreas Transplantation, University of California, Davis,
Medical Center, Sacramento, California

Bernard M. Kubak, M.D., Ph.D.
Assistant Clinical Professor of Infectious Diseases,
University of California, Los Angeles, UCLA School of
Medicine

Mary M. Meyer, M.D.
Assistant Professor of Medicine, Division of Nephrology and
Hypertension and Division of Pulmonary and Critical Care
Medicine, Oregon Health Sciences University School of
Medicine; Medical Director, Lung Transplantation and
Plasmapheresis, University Hospital, Portland, Oregon

Cynthia C. Nast, M.D.
Associate Professor of Pathology, University of California,
Los Angeles, UCLA School of Medicine; Associate
Pathologist, Cedars Sinai Medical Center, Los Angeles

Allen R. Nissenson, M.D.
Professor of Medicine, University of California, Los Angeles,
UCLA School of Medicine; Director, Dialysis Program,
UCLA Medical Center, Los Angeles

Douglas J. Norman, M.D.
Professor of Medicine, Oregon Health Sciences University
School of Medicine; Director, Transplantation Medicine,
University Hospital, Portland, Oregon

John D. Pirsch, M.D.
Associate Professor of Medicine and Surgery, University of
Wisconsin Medical School; Transplant Physician,
Departments of Medicine and Surgery, University of
Wisconsin Hospital and Clinics, Madison

Nagesh Ragavendra, M.D.
Professor of Radiological Sciences, University of California,
Los Angeles, UCLA School of Medicine; Chief, Ultrasound
Section, UCLA Medical Center, Los Angeles

J. Thomas Rosenthal, M.D.
Professor of Surgery, Division of Urology, University of
California, Los Angeles, UCLA School of Medicine; Surgical
Director, Renal Transplantation, UCLA Medical Center,
Los Angeles

Leslie Steven Rothenberg, J.D.
Associate Professor of Clinical Medicine, University of California, Los Angeles, UCLA School of Medicine; Director, Program in Medical Ethics, UCLA Medical Center, Los Angeles

Hans W. Sollinger, M.D., Ph.D.
Professor of Surgery and Pathology, University of Wisconsin Medical School; Chairman, Division of Organ Transplantation, University of Wisconsin Hospital and Clinics, Madison

Thomas B. Strouse, M.D.
Assistant Clinical Professor of Psychiatry, University of California, Los Angeles, UCLA School of Medicine; Director, Psychosocial Services, Cedars-Sinai Comprehensive Cancer Center, Los Angeles

Paul I. Terasaki, Ph.D.
Professor of Surgery, University of California, Los Angeles, UCLA School of Medicine; Director, Tissue Typing Laboratory, UCLA Medical Center, Los Angeles

Stephen J. Tomlanovich, M.D.
Associate Professor of Clinical Medicine, University of California, San Francisco, School of Medicine

Flavio Vincenti, M.D.
Professor of Clinical Medicine, American University of Beirut, Lebanon; Professor of Clinical Medicine, University of California, San Francisco, School of Medicine

Susan E. Weil, R.D., C.S.
Renal Dietitian, Dialysis and Renal Transplant Programs, UCLA Medical Center, Los Angeles

Alan H. Wilkinson, M.D., M.R.C.P.
Clinical Professor of Medicine, Division of Nephrology, University of California, Los Angeles, UCLA School of Medicine; Medical Director, Kidney and Pancreas Transplantation, UCLA Medical Center, Los Angeles

Deane L. Wolcott, M.D
Associate Clinical Professor of Psychiatry and Biobehavioral Sciences, University of California, Los Angeles, UCLA School of Medicine; Director, Psychosocial Services, Comprehensive Cancer Centers Inc., Los Angeles

Peter Zimmerman, M.D.
Assistant Professor of Radiological Sciences, University of California, Los Angeles, UCLA School of Medicine; Staff Radiologist, West Los Angeles Veterans Affairs Medical Center, Los Angeles

Handbook of Kidney Transplantation

Notice

The indications and dosages of all drugs in this book have been recommended in the medical literature and conform to the practices of the general medical community. The medications described do not necessarily have specific approval by the Food and Drug Administration for use in the diseases and dosages for which they are recommended. The package insert for each drug should be consulted for use and dosage as approved by the FDA. Because standards for usage change, it is advisable to keep abreast of revised recommendations, particularly those concerning new drugs.

1

Options for Patients with End-Stage Renal Disease

William G. Goodman and Allen R. Nissenson

Since the mid-nineteenth century, when Richard Bright described his experience with patients dying of renal failure, until the late 1960s, little hope was available for patients afflicted with end-stage renal disease (ESRD). A few kidney transplants had been performed, and a small number of patients were being maintained on chronic dialysis. The following decade saw a rapid expansion in the availability of ESRD care throughout the medically developed world; in the United States, the passage of Medicare entitlement legislation to pay for chronic dialysis and transplantation was a major stimulus for this expansion.

Despite a tremendous increase in knowledge and skill in the management of ESRD patients, such individuals, particularly those treated by dialysis, remain unwell. Impaired quality of life, dependence on others, poor rehabilitation, and depressed sexual function all contribute to the physical and emotional disabilities that may persist even in well-dialyzed ESRD patients. This is not surprising because the most efficient hemodialysis technique used today provides only 10–12% of the small solute removal of two normal kidneys and considerably less removal of larger solutes. Kidney transplantation offers the greatest potential for the full return of a healthy, productive life.

DEMOGRAPHICS OF THE END-STAGE RENAL DISEASE POPULATION

United States

Each year, the United States Renal Data System (USRDS), based at the University of Michigan, provides a report describing the demographics of the U.S. ESRD population. The 1995 report is based on data available as of December 1993. At that time, approximately 160,000 patients were receiving maintenance dialysis in the United States (Table 1-1). This number is increasing at a rate of 8–10% per year and is expected to be considerably greater than 200,000 by the year 2000. The average age of the dialysis population is also increasing; nearly 50% of the patients are over the age of 65. Men slightly outnumber women, and approximately one-fourth of the dialysis population is black. Diabetic nephropathy remains the most common cause of ESRD. Compared with other countries, the United States more commonly accepts dialysis patients who are older and more likely to have diabetes. In addition, patients accepted for dialysis in the United States now have more comorbid factors (e.g., atherosclerotic heart disease, cerebrovascular disease, peripheral vascular disease, cancer, chronic obstructive pulmonary disease) than did those accepted in the early 1980s. This trend to treat older, sicker patients and more diabetics in part accounts for the gradual worsening outcome reported for U.S. dialysis patients over the past 10 years. A similar trend is found in the population seeking transplantation (see Chap. 6).

Table 1-1. Demographics of the end-stage renal disease population in the United States (percentage of new patients in 1992)

Demographic	Percentage
Age (yrs)	
<20	1.5
20–44	18.5
45–64	33.6
65–74	28.2
≥ 75	18.1
Sex	
Male	53.4
Female	46.6
Race	
Black	29.0
White	66.4
Asian	2.2
Native American	1.5
Cause of end-stage renal disease	
Diabetic nephropathy	36.2
Hypertensive nephrosclerosis	29.7
Glomerulonephritis	11.0
Cystic kidney disease	2.8
Other*	20.3

* Nearly 10% of ESRD patients have a failed transplant.
Source: LYC Agodoa, PW Eggers. Renal replacement therapy in the United States: Data from the United States Renal Data System. *Am J Kidney Dis* 25:119, 1995.

While the number of dialysis patients is steadily increasing, the number of cadaveric kidney transplants has remained essentially stable, at approximately 8,000 per year for the last 4 years. There has been a modest increase in the number of live transplants, which are now performed at a rate of nearly 3,000 per year. As a result of this widening discrepancy, the number of patients awaiting cadaveric kidney transplants is inexorably increasing and is over 31,000 as of early 1996. The gap between supply and demand is illustrated graphically in Fig. 1-1 and is reflected in the distressing increase in the average waiting time for a cadaveric transplant, often measured in years (see Chap. 3).

Worldwide

Compared with the United States, most other countries have a lower incidence of treated ESRD (Fig. 1-2). In part, this reflects the high incidence of ESRD in blacks in the United States, but additional factors, such as rationing of dialysis for the elderly in some countries, also play a role. There are currently no age restrictions for dialysis in the United States, a fact that contributes to the steady increase in the age of the dialysis population. The choice of treatment modality also varies worldwide. Whereas some countries, such as the United Kingdom, Australia, and Canada, heavily use home dialysis modalities, others, such as Japan, rarely use these forms of treatment. Age is clearly an important factor for patient selection in many countries. Transplantation rates also vary among industrial-

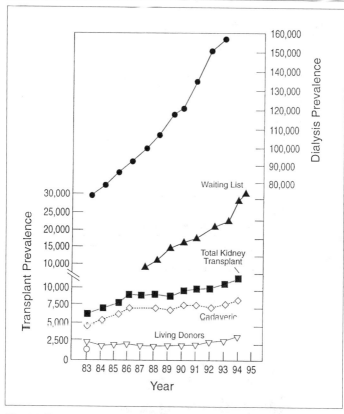

Fig. 1-1. Comparative numbers of patients on dialysis and awaiting and receiving kidney transplants in the United States between 1985 and 1995. (From LYC Agodoa, PW Eggers. Renal replacement therapy in the United States: Data from the United States Renal Data System. *Am J Kidney Dis* 25:119, 1995.)

ized countries, with notably low rates in Italy, Israel, and Japan (Fig. 1 3). Legal and cultural acceptance of brain death criteria (see Chaps. 5 and 16) are critical determinants of national rates of cadaveric transplants.

TREATMENT OPTIONS FOR END-STAGE RENAL DISEASE

Dialysis

Hemodialysis

Hemodialysis can be performed either in medical facilities specifically designed for this purpose or in the patient's home. Hemodialysis requires the creation of a permanent vascular access, preferably an autologous arteriovenous fistula, although synthetic graft arteriovenous fistulas are increasingly used, particularly in elderly and diabetic patients whose native blood vessels may be inadequate. When

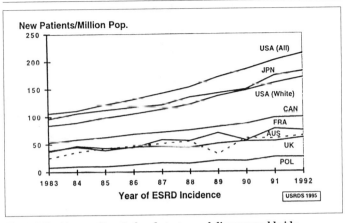

Fig. 1-2. Incidence of treated end-stage renal disease worldwide (1983–1992) expressed per million population for Australia, Canada, Japan, United States, and selected European countries. (From LYC Agodoa, PW Eggers. Renal replacement therapy in the United States: Data from the United States Renal Data System. *Am J Kidney Dis* 25:119, 1995.)

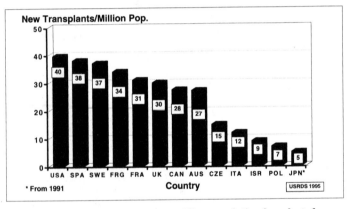

Fig. 1-3. Kidney transplant rate per million population for selected countries as of 1992. (From LYC Agodoa, PW Eggers. Renal replacement therapy in the United States: Data from the United States Renal Data System. *Am J Kidney Dis* 25:119, 1995.)

performed in a dialysis facility, treatments range from 2 to 4 hours, usually three times a week. During the dialysis, solutes are removed by diffusion across a semipermeable membrane. The majority of such membranes are cellulosic, and they provide highly efficient small solute removal, with urea clearances of 150–200 ml/minute easily achievable. As solute molecular weight rises, however, dialysis efficiency falls dramatically. Thus, the clearance of a molecule such as vitamin B_{12} (molecular weight = 1,350 daltons) rarely exceeds 40–60 ml/minute. Fluid removal is achieved by adjusting the transmembrane pressure across the dialyzer, usually by generating negative pressure in the dialysate compartment. Modern hemodialysis machines have volumetrically controlled ultrafiltration systems that ensure accurate, programmable fluid removal during the treatment. The procedure is generally well-tolerated, although ultrafiltration is at times associated with hypotension, nausea, and muscle cramps. Vascular access failure from repeated needle punctures and the need for intermittent heparinization to prevent clotting in the extracorporeal circuit are additional concerns. Finally, the intermittent nature of this therapy may contribute to postdialysis fatigue and malaise. For highly motivated patients with an appropriate living environment and an assistant (usually a spouse), hemodialysis can be carried out at home, freeing the patient from the need to come to a dialysis center and maintain a rigid treatment schedule.

Peritoneal Dialysis

Peritoneal dialysis is a widely practiced alternative ESRD treatment modality that exploits the fluid and solute transport characteristics of the peritoneum. It can be performed as either **continuous ambulatory peritoneal dialysis (CAPD)** or **continuous cycling peritoneal dialysis (CCPD).** Access to the peritoneal cavity is achieved surgically by placing a Silastic **Tenckhoff** catheter through the abdominal wall. Surgery is done several weeks before starting treatment; patients are subsequently trained to perform the dialysis procedure, which consists of instilling 1,500–3,000 ml of peritoneal dialysate into the abdomen by gravity, letting the fluid dwell 4–6 hours, and then draining and discarding it. During the dwell period, solute removal and fluid ultrafiltration take place.

Solute removal occurs by diffusion down a concentration gradient, with the peritoneum acting as a semipermeable membrane. The efficiency of removal of small solutes is relatively low compared with that of hemodialysis, whereas large solute clearance is greater. Ultrafiltration is achieved by osmotic water movement in response to the high osmolality induced by hypertonic dialysis solutions containing high concentrations of dextrose, ranging from 1.50–4.25%. The low rates of solute removal are offset by performing peritoneal dialysis 24 hours a day, 7 days a week. With CAPD, continuous dialysis is accomplished by exchanging the peritoneal fluid three, four, or five times daily, with the last exchange done at bedtime. With CCPD, a cycling device automatically exchanges predetermined volumes of dialysate three, four, or five times during the night; a final exchange is done in the morning before the patient disconnects from the cycling machine, providing a final dwell volume that remains in the abdomen during the day.

Peritoneal dialysis has some advantages over hemodialysis, including maintenance of steady-state blood chemistries, a higher hematocrit, and better blood pressure control. In addition, this form of self-dialysis promotes patient independence. The major complication of peritoneal dialysis is peritonitis, which occurs with a mean frequency of one episode per patient per year. Although these infections are generally not severe, they are a nuisance and can lead to scarring of the peritoneal cavity and to the loss of the peritoneum as an effective dialysis membrane. Gram-positive organisms such as *Staphylococcus epidermidis* are usually responsible for peritonitis, but gram-negative infections and fungal infections may also occur.

With few exceptions, there are no particular medical advantages of hemodialysis compared with peritoneal dialysis. Both treat uremia in a roughly equivalent manner (Table 1-2). Modality selection

Table 1-2. Comparison of hemodialysis and peritoneal dialysis

	Hemodialysis	Peritoneal dialysis
Advantages	Short treatment time Highly efficient for small solute removal Socialization occurs in the dialysis center	Steady-state chemistries Higher hematocrit Better blood pressure control Dialysate source of nutrition Intraperitoneal insulin Self-care form of therapy Highly efficient for large solute removal Liberalization of diet
Disadvantages	Need for heparin Need for vascular access Hypotension with fluid removal Poor blood pressure control Need to follow diet and treatment schedule	Peritonitis Obesity Hypertriglyceridemia Malnutrition Hernia formation Back pain

should primarily take into account life-style and other psychosocial issues. Home dialysis provides the opportunity for substantial independence and rehabilitation but may be stressful on the home helper and family members and may not be appropriate in some family settings. The socialization provided by in-center dialysis may be advantageous for an older, single patient with few friends or family members for support.

Technical Advances

There have been significant advances in the treatment of dialysis patients over the past decade that have made the procedure less onerous for the patients and have permitted significant improvements in their quality of life.

High-Efficiency Hemodialysis. A variation of standard hemodialysis, high-efficiency hemodialysis uses synthetic membranes that are more permeable to carry out the dialysis process. The result is a more rapid treatment and therefore a shorter dialysis time for an equivalent amount of small solute removal. This approach is growing in popularity, particularly among patients. However, it requires more expensive synthetic membrane dialyzers and more sophisticated dialysis delivery and monitoring systems to precisely control fluid removal. The long-term outcome for patients treated in this way is not known, and there is some concern that uremia may begin to appear after some months or years of therapy. Nevertheless, high-efficiency hemodialysis has improved the quality of life for some patients by decreasing the amount of time they spend on dialysis.

Bicarbonate Dialysis. For many years, hemodialysis solutions have contained acetate as the alkalinizing buffer to correct the metabolic acidosis of chronic renal failure. During dialysis, the acetate is metabolized, and bicarbonate is generated. The use of acetate, however, was often associated with unpleasant intradialytic symptoms such as hypotension, nausea, vomiting, and muscle cramps. More recently, dialysate solutions containing bicarbonate have been introduced and have been found to lead to better correction of chronic metabolic acidosis and a concomitant reduction in associated side effects.

Y-Set Dialysis Tubing. CAPD has traditionally been performed by manually changing bags of dialysate several times daily, either by inserting a spike connector into a fresh dialysate bag or by using a Luer-Lok connection system. CCPD involves a spike attachment to each of several dialysis bags and an additional connection and disconnection daily from the CCPD cycling machine. Most studies have shown a decreased peritonitis rate in CCPD compared to CAPD, probably because there are fewer opportunities for touch contamination with CCPD. Recently, a new concept—the Y-set, "flush-before-fill" system—was introduced, in which a small amount of fresh dialysate flushes the tubing system (sometimes with a disinfectant added) after the connection is made, removing the possibility of bacteria entering the system by touch contamination. Peritonitis rates of one episode every 24–60 months have been reported using this system. Such a dramatic decrease in peritonitis rates should permit long-term peritoneal dialysis to be performed on a greater number of patients.

Recombinant Erythropoietin. Approximately 90% of patients on hemodialysis and more than 50% of patients on peritoneal dialysis have anemia, often with hematocrit values below 30%. Uremic anemia contributes to many of the symptoms associated with chronic renal failure, including weakness, lethargy, depression, decreasing mental acuity, poor appetite, and impaired sexual function. The anemia is caused by the relative lack of erythropoietin, a glycoprotein normally produced in the kidneys. With the development of recombinant human erythropoietin ("epo"), the anemia of kidney failure can be corrected in more than 95% of treated patients. As a result, patients have more energy, improved appetite, increased sexual function, better mental capacity, and more normal skin color. Although anemia clearly does not cause all of the symptoms seen in uremic patients, its correction greatly improves their sense of well-being and potential for an active life. Consequently, the relative attractiveness of transplantation may be diminished for some patients.

Technique Success. One measure of the effectiveness of an ESRD treatment modality is technique success—that is, how many patients remain on the chosen modality over time. Patients on peritoneal dialysis, both diabetics and nondiabetics, are more likely to change modality than are those on hemodialysis. Choices may vary by country; in Canada there is a small difference in technique success that favors hemodialysis, whereas in the United States there is a three- to five-fold difference favoring hemodialysis. Most patients switch from peritoneal dialysis to hemodialysis because of recurrent peritonitis and catheter exit site or tunnel infections. Technique success for peritoneal dialysis is expected to improve with the wider application of new technology such as Y-set dialysis tubing.

Long-Term Complications

As the survival rate for patients on dialysis improves, a number of debilitating complications of long-standing uremia or dialysis may become apparent even in well-rehabilitated and compliant patients. The development or the potential for the development of these complications may have an impact on the medical indications for transplantation and on the patient's decision to choose transplantation.

Renal Osteodystrophy. Secondary hyperparathyroidism develops in many ESRD patients. Several factors, including hyperphosphatemia, decreased gastrointestinal calcium absorption, bone insensitivity to parathyroid hormone (PTH), low 1,25 vitamin D levels, and progressive parathyroid gland hyperplasia, contribute to this disorder. Dialysis itself, calcium and vitamin D supplementation, and adequate control of serum phosphorus levels may help, but the majority of ESRD patients will have some degree of hyperparathyroidism. In severely affected patients, bone pain, fractures, hypercalcemia, and visceral and vascular calcifications may develop.

In the past, some patients developed osteomalacia or adynamic lesions of the bone due to aluminum accumulation, conditions that manifested clinically as fractures and bone pain. The source of the aluminum in most cases was aluminum-based phosphate-binding antacids administered to control the serum phosphate level. The adynamic lesion of renal osteodystrophy has also been recognized without bone aluminum deposition; in these cases, hypercalcemia may develop without marked elevations of PTH levels. Adynamic renal osteodystrophy is somewhat more common in patients undergoing peritoneal dialysis than in patients undergoing hemodialysis. The impact of transplantation on uremic bone disease is discussed in Chap. 9.

Amyloidosis. Patients with long-standing renal failure, including those on dialysis, may develop a unique form of amyloidosis in which the amyloid is composed of $beta_2$-microglobulin, a protein that is present on the surface of all cells. As it is released into the circulation, it is normally freely filtered by the glomeruli and metabolized in the proximal renal tubules. In renal failure, $beta_2$-microglobulin accumulates in plasma and eventually precipitates as amyloid in tissues. It has a particular propensity for the carpal tunnels and other articular and bony structures. Severe, deforming joint disease usually begins to appear after 5 or more years of chronic renal failure; the clinical course is progressive. Deposits of amyloid can be documented in the majority of patients undergoing hemodialysis for more than 8 years.

It has been suggested that blood-membrane interactions during hemodialysis, particularly when cellulosic membranes are used, accelerate the progression of amyloid by stimulating increased $beta_2$-microglobulin production. Amyloid deposition also occurs in peritoneal dialysis patients, so blood-membrane contact is certainly not essential for its development. At present, only symptomatic relief is available.

Acquired Cystic Disease. Patients with chronic renal failure of any cause may develop acquired cystic disease in their kidneys after

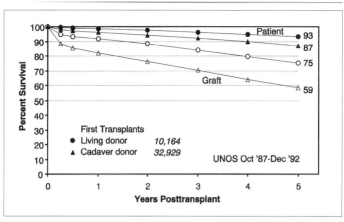

Fig. 1-4. Patient and graft survival in a group of more than 40,000 first kidney transplant recipients transplanted between October 1987 and December 1992 and reported to the United Network for Organ Sharing as of June 1995.

several years. This condition is characterized by multiple, usually bilateral, renal cysts in small, contracted kidneys and is thus distinct from adult polycystic kidney disease. The cysts may become infected, bleed, cause pain, or undergo malignant transformation. They have been seen in both long-term hemodialysis and peritoneal dialysis patients and may be a source of significant morbidity. Acquired cysts may remain a source of complications in transplant recipients.

Other complications of long-term dialysis may occur. They include uremic cardiomyopathy, accelerated atherosclerosis, peripheral neuropathy with muscle atrophy, dialysis ascites, and dialysis encephalopathy or aluminum-related dialysis dementia. These morbidity-producing disorders may improve, sometimes dramatically, after successful transplantation.

Transplantation

The relative prevalence of the major ESRD treatment options over the last decade in the United States is shown in Fig. 1-1. Cadaveric transplantation accounts for approximately 75% of kidney transplants in the United States. A critical shortage of donor organs is the major limitation to expanding this modality (see Chap. 3). Live-related transplants (organs from living donors who are close biological relatives of the patient) and a small number of live, unrelated transplants account for the remainder. The use of renal transplantation varies considerably among patient groups. Transplant rates are lower in older patients, who represent a relative high-risk group (see Chap. 5). Transplant rates tend to be lower in black ESRD patients largely because of biological reasons that tend to restrict access to cadaveric organs (see Chap. 3).

Figure 1-4 provides data on overall patient and graft survival in the United States for recipients of a first kidney transplant. Mean 1-year graft survival for all types of live donor transplants is greater than 90% and is greater than 80% for all match grades of cadaveric transplants. These results are discussed in more detail in Chap. 3. Results for both cadaveric and live-related transplantation have improved steadily since the early 1980s following the introduction of cyclosporine-based immunosuppression.

PATIENT SURVIVAL
Difficulties with Data Analysis

To help select the most appropriate option in a particular clinical setting, clinicians and patients are understandably interested in the comparative survival with different ESRD modalities. Such comparisons are difficult, since data in the literature often do not reflect the fact that patients change modalities frequently and that the characteristics of patients selected for each modality may differ substantially when therapy is begun. For dialysis patients, a number of comorbid factors may adversely affect survival, including age and the presence of diabetes, coronary artery disease, chronic obstructive pulmonary disease, or cancer. In addition, blacks have a better survival rate with ESRD than nonblacks, and certain renal diagnoses, such as amyloidosis, multiple myeloma, and renal cell cancer, are associated with a poor prognosis. Nutritional status, reflected by albumin and pre-albumin levels, is being increasingly recognized as an important predictor of survival on dialysis (see Chap. 17). If these factors are not considered, accurate modality comparisons cannot be made. Another problem with survival data in the United States is that most data are obtained from Health Care Financing Administration (HCFA) records. The patient's initial 90 days on dialysis are not included in these records. It has been suggested that up to 25% of patients on dialysis die during the first 90 days.

Comparison of Treatment Modalities

Most of the data comparing the survival rates of patients treated with hemodialysis, CAPD, and cadaveric kidney transplantation suggest that a patient's health before treatment, rather than the treatment modality itself, is the most important factor that determines survival. There does, however, appear to be a reduction in the relative risk of mortality in dialysis patients who subsequently receive a transplant rather than remain on dialysis. This survival benefit is more marked for live-related transplantation than for cadaveric transplantation and can be detected within the first post-transplant year despite the increased mortality associated with the surgical procedure itself and the initiation of immunosuppression (Fig. 1-5).

Cost of Therapy

The annual cost of medical care for patients undergoing chronic dialysis in the United States is estimated at $50,000. The cost associated with the first post-transplant year is nearly $100,000. After the first post-transplant year, the cost of care is less for transplant recipients than for dialysis patients despite the fact that the annual drug costs of cyclosporine-based immunosuppressive therapy is nearly $10,000. The mean cumulative cost of dialysis and transplantation is approximately the same after 4 years of therapy. Thereafter, there is a cost benefit to successful transplantation.

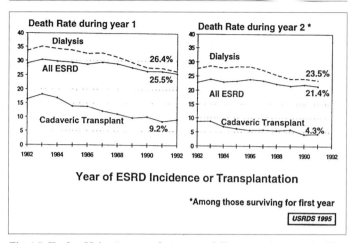

Fig. 1-5. Kaplan Meier 1-year end-stage renal disease patient survival by modality and year of incidence or transplantation from 1980 to 1990. Starting at day 91 following certification for end-stage renal disease for dialysis patients and censored at first transplant, and at the day of transplant for transplanted patients. Adjusted for age, race, gender, and diagnosis. (From LYC Agodoa, PW Eggers. Renal replacement therapy in the United States: Data from the United States Renal Data System. *Am J Kidney Dis* **25:119–133, 1995.)**

Survival by Diagnosis

When the most common causes of kidney disease are analyzed using a Cox proportional hazards model, only diabetes mellitus has an adverse effect on patient survival. Other common etiologies of renal failure do not significantly affect survival. The survival rate of patients with ESRD caused by other less common diseases such as collagen vascular disease and the vasculitides is generally similar to that seen in nondiabetics with more common causes of ESRD. Not surprisingly, systemic and renal malignancies confer a poorer prognosis.

Quality of Life

Although survival is similar in matched patients treated with dialysis or cadaveric kidney transplantation, much attention has been focused on the quality of life achievable with these modalities. Most studies demonstrate that the quality of life of patients on peritoneal dialysis exceeds that of patients on hemodialysis when the latter is done in a dialysis center. Home hemodialysis patients reportedly have a high quality of life, although selection factors, such as the level of patient motivation and the patient's overall health status at the beginning of treatment, make it difficult to attribute this higher quality of life to the modality itself.

Most dialysis patients choose the transplantation option in the hope of improving their quality of life and, indeed, successful renal transplantation recipients consistently report a better quality of life than do dialysis patients, including both peritoneal dialysis and home hemodialysis patients. Life satisfaction, well-being, psychological affect, and return to work are significantly better in transplant recipients than in dialysis patients, although the benefits tend not to be as great in recipients of cadaveric transplants. Transplantation may correct or improve some complications of uremia that are typically not fully reversed by dialysis; these include anemia, peripheral neuropathy, autonomic neuropathy, and sexual dysfunction (see Chap. 9). The quality of life following live-related transplantation compares favorably to that seen in the general population.

INITIATION OF END-STAGE RENAL DISEASE THERAPY

Most patients with progressive renal failure become symptomatic and require ESRD treatment with either dialysis or transplantation when the glomerular filtration rate (GFR) falls to 5 ml/minute. Hemodialysis or peritoneal dialysis access placement should be planned far enough in advance so that treatment can be initiated when needed. Since permanent vascular access for hemodialysis requires 4–12 weeks to adequately "mature," placement is usually undertaken when the GFR reaches 10 ml/minute. For peritoneal dialysis, peritoneal catheter placement can be delayed until dialysis is more imminent, since only 2–4 weeks' waiting time is needed before the access can be used. The decision to start dialysis is a clinical one and should be based not only on the plasma values for creatinine, blood urea nitrogen, and electrolytes, but also on an assessment of the degree of uremic symptomatology. Outcome on dialysis is better for patients who start "early" rather than "late."

Patients with diabetic nephropathy often become symptomatic at a lower serum creatinine level and a higher GFR than do other patients with ESRD. Generally speaking, vascular access for hemodialysis in diabetic patients should be placed when the GFR is 15–20 ml/minute, and dialysis should be initiated when the GFR falls to 10–15 ml/minute.

In the past, it was customary to withhold kidney transplantation until after a patient had begun dialysis. High rates of graft failure justified such a policy, and the initiation of dialysis under the circumstances of a failed transplant was a severe psychological stress for some patients. The excellent current graft survival rates make such a policy inappropriate. An increasing number of patients are receiving kidney transplants before starting dialysis, and it is reasonable to begin patient education and evaluation for transplantation 6–12 months before the initiation of dialysis is anticipated (see Chap. 6). The avoidance of the expense and morbidity of placing dialysis access is an added benefit of such a policy. Predialysis ESRD patients who are placed on the cadaveric transplant list or prepared for live-related transplantation should be warned explicitly not to delay dialysis if it becomes necessary before a kidney becomes available; this avoids a "race against time" that can be dangerous and emotionally stressful for patients and caregivers alike.

SELECTED READINGS

Agodoa LYC, Eggers PW. Renal replacement therapy in the United States: Data from the United States Renal Data System. *Am J Kidney Dis* 25:119, 1995.

Chugh KS, Jha V. Differences in the care of ESRD patients worldwide: Required resources and future outlook. *Kidney Int* 48:S7, 1995.

Evans RW. Quality of life assessment and the treatment of end-stage renal disease. *Transplant Rev* 4:28, 1990.

Hakim RM, Lazarus JM. Initiation of dialysis. *J Am Soc Nephrol* 6:1319, 1995.

Holley JL, McCauley C, Doherty B et al. Patients' views in the choice of renal transplant. *Kidney Int* 49:494, 1996.

Ifudu O, Paul H, Mayers JD et al. Pervasive failed rehabilitation in center-based maintenance hemodialysis patients. *Am J Kidney Dis* 23:394, 1994.

Nissenson AR, Fine RN (eds). *Dialysis Therapy* (2nd ed). Philadelphia: Hanley & Belfus, 1993.

Nissenson AR, Port FK. Outcome of end-stage renal disease in patients with rare causes of renal failure. III. Systemic/vascular disorders. *Q J Med* New Series 74, 273:63, 1990.

Port FK, Nissenson AR. Outcome of end-stage renal disease in patients with rare causes of renal failure. II. Renal or systemic neoplasms. *Q J Med* New Series 73, 272:1161, 1989.

2

Transplantation Immunobiology

J. Harold Helderman and Simin Goral

Renal transplantation is the preferred mode of renal replacement therapy for virtually all patients with end-stage renal disease. Despite the increasing success of renal transplantation over the past 10 years, acute transplant rejection and chronic transplant rejection still remain major problems. During the past decade, new discoveries have led to a better understanding of transplant immunobiology, out of which have come a number of novel immunosuppressive regimens.

The following is a brief glossary of the terminology used by transplant immunologists to describe the cells and tissues encountered in the transplant setting.

Transplantation of one's own tissue to another site is called an **autologous graft** (or **autograft**). A graft transplanted between two genetically identical individuals is called an **isogeneic** or **syngeneic graft** (or **syngraft**). A graft transplanted between two genetically different individuals of the same species is called an **allogeneic graft** (or **allograft**). A graft transplanted between members of different species is called a **xenogeneic graft** (or **xenograft**). The antigens that are recognized as foreign on allografts are called **alloantigens**, whereas those recognized as foreign on xenografts are called **xenoantigens**. The lymphocytes that recognize and respond to the alloantigens or xenoantigens are called **alloreactive** or **xenoreactive lymphocytes**, respectively.

MAJOR HISTOCOMPATIBILITY COMPLEX

Human Leukocyte Antigens

After several unique discoveries in organ transplantation, it has become clear that rejection and acceptance of a transplant are inherited characteristics. There is an array of inherited proteins on cell surfaces that contribute to transplant rejection. The genes that encode for these proteins, the so-called **histocompatibility genes,** are located on different chromosomes in each species. The histocompatibility genes are responsible for the graft's being recognized as similar to one's own tissues or as foreign. Because of its central role in antigen recognition and transplantation immunobiology, this group of genes has been defined as the **major histocompatibility complex (MHC)**. The incompatibility of the MHC antigens between a donor and a recipient of an allograft leads to graft rejection.

Although discovered and named for the capacity to induce graft rejection, the principal immunologic function of the MHC gene product is to present antigens as fragments of foreign proteins, forming complexes that can be recognized by T lymphocytes through specific antigen receptors. In each individual, these antigen receptors are specific for foreign antigens recognized in the context of MHC molecules. Because MHC molecules are membrane-associated, antigen-specific T lymphocytes can recognize fragments of the antigens only when they are bound to the surfaces of other cells that bear the MHC molecule. These cells that bear MHC molecules present the antigen to T cells. Mature T cells recognize and react to foreign antigens but do not react to self-proteins, since during the ontogeny of the immune system, self-reactive T lymphocytes are removed in the thymus by a variety of processes including **clonal deletion**, which permits **self-tolerance** (see the section on tolerance).

The MHC is a complex of genes found in all vertebrates and in humans has been located on the short arm of chromosome 6. The MHC genes in humans encode polymorphic cell surface molecules, alloantigens known as **human leukocyte antigens** (**HLAs**). The polymorphism of HLAs involves specific hypervariable regions of the molecule and contributes both to self-recognition and to antigen binding. HLA gene products are inherited in a mendelian codominant fashion. At least six separate genes are involved in the HLA system; phenotypically each one is represented by two codominant alleles, one from the paternal gamete and the other one from the maternal gamete. Developed in the gamete during meiosis and located on a single strand of parental chromosome, alleles of the HLA system comprise a **haplotype** unless a crossover has occurred (see Chap. 3). HLAs have been divided into two general types—**class I** and **class II**—according to their cellular distribution, chemical and crystallographic structure (Fig. 2-1), and immunologic function.

Class I Antigens

HLA class I antigens (HLA-A, -B, and -C) are found on virtually all cell surfaces, although the concentration of these molecules varies widely. These molecules are composed of one highly polymorphic MIIC-encoded polypeptide chain designated alpha (heavy) and a monomorphic chain, beta$_2$-microglobulin, encoded by genes on chromosome 15 (see Figs. 2-1 and 2-2). The beta chain interacts noncovalently with the heavy chain and has no direct attachment to the cell. The aminoterminus portion of the heavy chain that extends into the extracellular space is composed of three domains: alpha$_1$, alpha$_2$, and alpha$_3$. The alpha$_1$ and alpha$_2$ domains interact to form the sides of a cleft (or groove), with a floor formed by strands of beta-pleated sheets. The cleft is the site where foreign proteins bind to MHC molecules for presentation to T cells. The size of the cleft is too small to bind an intact globular protein; therefore, native globular proteins need to be processed into smaller fragments that can bind to MHC molecules. The amino acid residues located in the groove are highly variable, which determines the specificity of peptide binding and T cell antigen recognition. Both class I and class II molecules bind foreign protein antigens and form complexes that are recognized by antigen-specific T lymphocytes. Class I molecules function as immunorecognition sites for endogenously synthesized foreign proteins such as viral proteins and tumor antigens. Antigens associated with class I molecules are recognized by cytotoxic CD8+ T lymphocytes. The nonpolymorphic alpha$_3$ region contains the binding sites for CD8+ T cells, which enhances the affinity of the antigen-bearing MHC with the T cell antigen receptor (see the section on T cell receptor/CD3 complex).

Class II Antigens

In contrast to class I antigens, class II antigens (HLA-DR, -DP, and -DQ) have a more restricted cell distribution, as they are generally expressed by **antigen-presenting cells** (**APCs**), such as B monocytes, macrophages, dendritic cells of lymphoid organs, renal mesan-

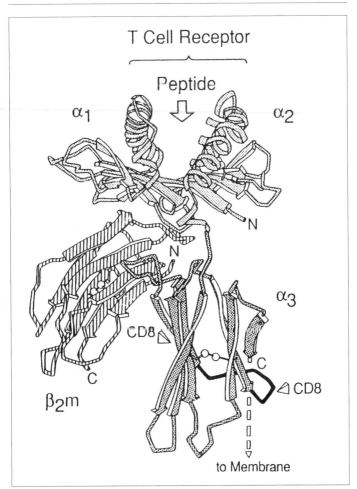

Fig. 2-1. Schematic diagram of the structure of a representative class I major histocompatibility complex molecule (HLA-A2). The alpha$_1$ and alpha$_2$ domains form a peptide binding site with the binding groove that faces the T cell receptor at the top. (Reprinted with permission from PJ Bjorkman, MA Saper, B Samraoni et al. Structure of the human class I histocompatibility antigen, HLA-A2. *Nature* **329**:506, 1987.)

gial cells, Kupffer's cells, and alveolar type 2 lining cells, and certain other elements of the immune system, such as lymphocytes and thymic epithelial cells. A subset of activated T lymphocytes may also express class II molecules. All parenchymal cells of the germline retain the genes for class II molecules. Engagement of the appropriate promoter sequences at the five prime (5') end of the coding start site by inflammatory cytokines such as **interferon-gamma (IFN-γ)** can initiate coding for the synthesis of the class II protein.

Class II genes are composed of two MHC-encoded and noncovalently associated polymorphic chains (alpha and beta chains) (see

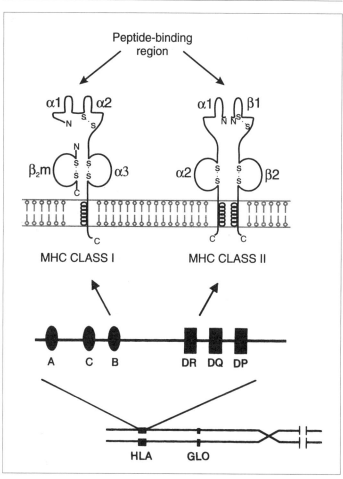

Fig. 2-2. The lower half of the figure depicts the major histocompatibility complex class I and class II genes on the short arm of chromosome 6. The upper half is a schematic diagram of the class I and class I molecules, which are the transmembrane glycoprotein products of these genes. (N = amino terminus of the polypeptide chains; C= carboxy terminus of the polypeptide chains; S..S = intrachain disulfide bonds.)

Fig. 2-2). Each alpha and beta chain is composed of two extracellular domains (alpha₁ and alpha₂ and beta₁ and beta₂). Similar to class I molecules, x-ray crystallography reveals a spatial configuration of helices surrounding beta-pleated sheets, into which are embedded antigen-binding grooves or clefts. For class II molecules, there are two separate grooves, in contrast to the single groove for class I, formed by domains of alpha₁ and beta₁, which permit binding of peptide fragments of about 12 amino acids in length rather than the nine for class I.

Class II molecules play a central role in the initiation of the immune response to transplantation antigens. Recognition of foreign class II molecules activates helper CD4+ T lymphocytes, which begins the process of clonal expansion and also supports cytotoxic T cell clonal expansion by stimulating the CD4+ lymphocyte generation of regulatory cytokines. Additionally, the class II region of the MHC contains genes such as **transporter in antigen processing (TAP) 1** and 2 genes, necessary for the assembly of peptide fragments with the MHC and for ultimate surface expression of class I MHC molecules.

Both class I and class II antigens play essential roles in the recognition of nominal, nontransplantation antigens by the immune system. Receptors on the cells that are responsible for initial recognition of antigens recognize not only some piece of the molecular structure of the antigen, but also surface proteins, which are self-identifying molecules. Certain antigens are preferentially recognized in association with class I antigens, whereas other antigens are recognized in association with class II antigens. This role of self-identification by the MHC is the essence of its immunoregulatory function. In rejection, allogeneic class I and class II molecules become the targets for the efferent responses of the immune system.

Minor Histocompatibility Antigens

The observations of rejection of skin grafts between MHC-identical mice and the development of severe **graft-versus-host disease** in bone marrow transplantation between MHC identical siblings imply the existence of structures other than MHC that can be recognized by T cells to activate the immune response. As many as 20 gene regions, so-called **minor loci**, encoded by a large number of chromosomes, are thought to function as **minor histocompatibility antigens (MiHAs)**. There is compelling evidence that MiHAs are small endogenous peptides that occupy the antigen-binding site of self-MHC molecules and can trigger T cell responses between MHC identical individuals. Whereas MHC antigens can be recognized by both B and T lymphocytes, responses to MiHAs appear to be strictly T cell–mediated and therefore **MHC-restricted**. MHC restriction is the most fundamental characteristic of MiHA recognition. Most MiHAs are processed and presented to recipient T cells in association with either donor MHC or self-MHC molecules. The MiHAs become important for initiating rejections in patients receiving allografts from living-related donors matched for the entire HLA. Only for transplants between identical twins, for whom one can establish identity at both major and minor gene regions, can one dispense with the need for immunosuppression.

ALLOGENEIC RECOGNITION

The recognition of transplantation antigens by T cells is referred to as **allorecognition** or **alloresponse** and is determined by the inheritance of codominant MHC genes. Because of the resemblance of a foreign MHC molecule to an MHC molecule bound to a foreign peptide, this recognition of a foreign MHC molecule is actually a cross-reaction of a T cell receptor that recognizes a self-MHC molecule bound to a foreign peptide. As many as 2% of the host peripheral blood lymphocytes are capable of recognizing and responding to a single foreign MHC molecule. The reason for strong allograft rejection is the presence of this high frequency of T cells reactive with allogeneic MHC molecules. The principal target of the immune response to the graft is the MHC molecule itself, and T cell recognition of allo-MHC is the major event that triggers rejection.

There are at least two distinct pathways of allorecognition. In the **direct pathway**, T cell receptors directly recognize intact allo-MHC molecules with or without relevant antigen fragments carried in the groove of the MHC structure on the surface of donor target cells. This pathway accounts for the generation of a primary cytotoxic CD8+ T cell response and thus plays the dominant role in early allograft rejection. In the **indirect pathway** of allorecognition, CD4+ helper T cell receptors recognize donor MHC allopeptides after processing and presentation by self-APCs. The donor MHC may be shed from the surface of parenchymal cells of the graft into the circulation to be engulfed by APCs, processed, and presented by self-MHC, or phagocytic cells may encounter the donor MHC in the graft itself, where processing can be accomplished. In any case, recipient APCs internalize the exogenous foreign proteins shed from the graft and process the peptides for presentation (in the context of self-HLA) to T cells, thereby providing the requisite signal for lymphocyte activation. Recent observations suggest that the indirect pathway enhances acute rejection and is predominant for chronic rejection. Once the antigen-specific T cell receptor on the surface of the helper T cell is triggered, a series of intracellular events is initiated, culminating in the synthesis of an array of new molecules targeted to the nucleus, the cytosol, the cell membrane, and the external milieu.

T Cell Receptor/CD3 Complex

T cells express protein receptors that specifically bind the peptide-MHC complexes. The **T cell receptor (TCR)** is a heterodimer that consists of two polypeptide chains, alpha and beta chains, linked to each other by disulfide bonds (Fig. 2-3). Both chains have variable (V) and constant (C) regions. The C-terminal end of the V region is encoded by a joining (J) segment gene, and, in the beta chain only, a diversity (D) segment gene. The V regions of these TCR proteins are responsible for antigen binding. The structure and the genes encoding TCR molecules with V, D, J, and C regions are similar to those of immunoglobulins (Ig). Both TCR and Ig are members of a family of molecules called the **Ig superfamily**.

Although the TCR allows T cells to recognize antigen-MHC complexes, the cell-surface expression of TCR molecules and the initiation of intracellular signaling depend on a complex of additional peptides known as the CD3 complex (see Fig. 2-3). The CD3 complex consists of at least five peptide chains—γ, δ, ε, ζ, and η chains—which noncovalently bind to each other and are closely arrayed in the membrane alongside the TCR (see Fig. 2-3). This relationship is necessary for surface expression and the function of both TCR and CD3 proteins. When the TCR binds the antigen, there is a conformational change in CD3 that activates intracellular signal pathways, including tyrosine kinase, thus transferring the activating signals to the cytoplasm of the T cell. This antigen-driven signal transduced by the TCR-CD3 complex is called **signal one** and is essential *but not sufficient alone* for the activation of T cells. A **second signal**, antigen-independent,

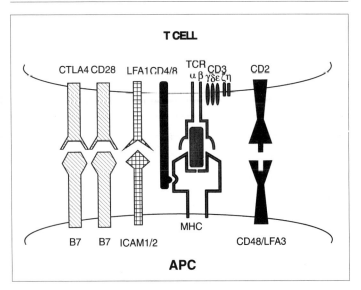

Fig. 2-3. T cell receptor/CD3 antigen complex with accessory molecules binding to a major histocompatibility complex containing a peptide in its groove

must be provided through additional so-called **accessory molecules**. The provision of signals through the TCR alone indeed leads to clonal and antigen-specific **anergy**, which can be defined as unresponsiveness to a subsequent antigenic challenge rather than activation. T cells receiving signal one without signal two not only do not activate, but are refractory to activation even when all necessary activation elements are later presented.

Accessory Molecules

Accessory molecules, nonpolymorphic membrane proteins that can serve as cell surface markers, are often involved in adhesion reactions and are identical on all T cells of a species. Accessory molecules play at least three roles in the alloimmune response: (1) Accessory molecules on T cells stabilize the interaction between cytotoxic T cells and the target cell by binding their specific ligands on the surfaces of target cells, an essential step in the cytotoxic effector response; (2) accessory molecules provide the nonantigen-driven second signal for T cell activation and play a direct role in signal transduction; (3) **adhesion molecules** enhance antigen recognition by increasing the affinity between the TCR and the MHC-bearing antigen.

CD4 and CD8 molecules, expressed as T cell surface proteins, are accessory molecules that enhance the interaction between the TCR and APCs through the MHC. By binding class II MHC molecules, the CD4 molecule facilitates TCR-CD3 complex–mediated signal transduction and assists the actions of class II–restricted T cells. Similarly, the CD8 molecule binds to class I MHC molecules and stabilizes the interaction of the class I MHC–restricted T cell with a target cell mediating signal transduction. CD4/CD8+ TCR-CD3 proteins function together in initiating the signals for T cell activation. It has been shown that monoclonal antibodies against CD4 or CD8 molecules inhibit T cell activation and thus are important potential targets for immunosuppression.

Several other T cell membrane proteins, including CD2, CD28, lymphocyte function-associated antigen-1 (LFA-1), and very late activation molecules (VLA), also affect T cell activation. These proteins belong to a family of cell adhesion molecules: the **integrin superfamily**. By binding to its ligand LFA-3, CD2 serves as an intercellular adhesion molecule. In addition, evidence suggests that the CD2-LFA-3 interaction may provide a costimulatory signal to T cell activation and proliferation. Recent studies support the primacy for CD28 binding to its ligand B7 for transplantation allorecognition and through the provision of a strong second signal for T cell activation. The binding of B7 to CD28 is also important for the delivery of costimulatory signals that are necessary for full activation of T cells. LFA-1 is a cell surface protein that is expressed on all bone marrow–derived cells and mediates a potent stimulatory signal for T cell activation. Intercellular adhesion molecule-1 (ICAM-1) and -2 (ICAM-2) are specific ligands for LFA-1. ICAM-1 is expressed on both hematopoietic and nonhematopoietic cells, including endothelial cells, keratinocytes, and fibroblasts. It has been demonstrated that anti-LFA-1 monoclonal antibody can be used in HLA-mismatched bone marrow transplantation in order to prevent rejection. The VLA molecules VLA-4, VLA-5, and VLA-6 are expressed on resting T cells. These molecules interact with their extracellular matrix ligands (fibronectin and laminin) and provide additional signals to T cells. VLA-4 also interacts with vascular cell adhesion molecule-1 (VCAM-1) and mediates the binding of lymphocytes to endothelium at inflammatory sites. There are several additional cell surface proteins, such as CD44, Thy-1, and CD45, that also transduce signals for T cell activation on binding their ligands.

T CELL ACTIVATION

T cells require at least two different signals to be activated. The first signal is initiated by the binding of the alloantigen or the processed antigen presented by self-MHC to the TCR/CD3 complex. The second signal for T cell activation is provided by the interaction between a number of accessory molecule-ligand pairs on APCs and on T cells, such as that between the CD28 molecule on the T lymphocyte with its ligand B7 on the surface of the APC. On specific ligand binding, a signal is delivered that will act synergistically with TCR-induced signals to produce T cell activation. These dual signals trigger the CD4+ T cell to activate the cytokine interleukin-2 (IL-2) and IL-2 receptor gene expression, leading to induction of the expression of other cytokines, which permits the entire cascade of T cell activation to proceed, leading to cell division. If a TCR is triggered without an accompanying second signal, the cell is driven into an anergic state in which it is not only inactivated, but also becomes refractory to the full range of activating signals.

Within minutes of stimulation, T cells leave the quiescent phase of cell division (G0). The specific events of this activated cell are described in terms of the synthesis and the cell content of RNA, DNA, and protein concentrations that culminate in the attainment of new molecules targeted for the cell surface, called **activation**

markers, for the cytosol, for the nucleus, and for the external milieu. In the first phase of the cell cycle (G1a), T cells begin to transcribe and express cellular proto-oncogenes, such as c-*myc*, c-*myb*, c-*fos*, and c-*jun*, and the genes for IL-2 and its receptor. The products of the cellular proto-oncogenes, c-*fos* and c-*jun*, are believed to function within the nucleus to regulate cell growth, including transcriptional regulation of the IL-2 gene, whereas c-*myc* and c-*myb* regulate DNA synthesis required for ultimate mitosis and cell division. The binding of IL-2 to its receptor propels the cell into the G1b phase, in which an array of proinflammatory cytokines and additional cell surface receptors, such as that for transferrin, are synthesized. Eventually, the cell enters the S phase of the cell cycle, doubles its DNA content, arranges its chromosomes along a spindle pattern, and undergoes a mitotic division in a process called **postantigenic differentiation**, which leads to **clonal expansion**. The net result of the clonal expansion of both helper (CD4+) and CD8+ T cells is the development of **cytotoxic T lymphocytes** (**CTL**s), which act as **effector** cells capable of inducing graft rejection (see the section on acute rejection).

The events that initiate and regulate the activation of T cells can be understood at the single cell level as a series of events that begins with antigen recognition and leads to the synthesis of various **second messengers** that activate the promoter sequences of the crucial genes involved in the synthesis of the regulatory molecules capable of driving the activated lymphocyte through the activation cascade (Fig. 2 1). Following alloantigen recognition, the antigen-specific TCR permits the passage of signals into the cell. The immediate effect is the appearance of newly phosphorylated tyrosine residues on a number of proteins mediated by phosphotyrosine kinase. Phosphorylation of tyrosine residues activates an enzyme called phosphatidylinositol phospholipase Cγ1 (PI-PLC-γ), which, in turn, catalyzes the breakdown of a plasma membrane phospholipid called phosphatidylinositol 4,5-biphosphate, leading to the signaling events such as second messengers, inositol 1,4,5 triphosphate (IP3) and diacylglycerol (DAG). IP3 stimulates the release of ionized calcium from intracellular stores. DAG, in the presence of increased cytoplasmic calcium, activates protein kinase C (PKC) on binding to it. PKC activation leads to the synthesis of nuclear regulatory elements such as the proto-oncogenes c-*fos* and c-*jun*. Cytoplasmic calcium forms a complex with the calcium-dependent regulatory protein called calmodulin. These calcium-calmodulin complexes activate other kinase and phosphatases, including **calcineurin**. Calcineurin, a calcium-calmodulin–dependent phosphatase, plays a key role in the activation of factors required for IL-2 gene transcription. As a consequence of this enzyme activation, the activated form of a molecule called **nuclear factor of activated T cells (NF-AT)** is generated by dephosphorylation of a cytosolic precursor. Increased calcium promotes the dephosphorylation of NF-AT by calcineurin and allows NF-AT to migrate from the cytoplasm to the nucleus. In the nucleus, NF-AT binds cooperatively with c-*fos* and c-*jun*, products of cellular proto-oncogenes, to the distal NF-AT binding sites in the promoter sequence of the IL-2 gene and enhances transcription of this gene. C-*fos* and c-*jun* stabilize the binding of NF-AT to DNA. After synthesis, IL-2 functions as an **autacoid** by binding to its own receptor on helper T cells, providing an internal signal for completion of the lymphocyte activation cascade. The

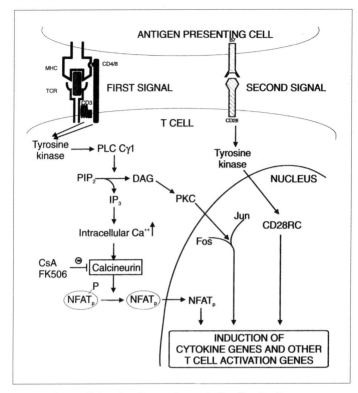

Fig. 2-4. Intracellular signaling pathways in T cell activation.

immunosuppressive agents cyclosporine and tacrolimus (FK506) inhibit the phosphatase activity of calcineurin when they bind to their immunophilin-binding proteins in the cytosol, leading to the inhibition of IL-2 gene transcription (see Chap. 4).

Cytokines

Cytokines are soluble, antigen-nonspecific proteins that are synthesized in response to antigenic stimuli by several different cell types, including monocytes and T cells, especially CD4+ T lymphocytes. They initiate their action by binding to their specific receptors on the surface of the target cells. The same cell that secretes the cytokine may be the target cell (**autocrine** action). A nearby cell (**paracrine** action) or a distant cell may also be stimulated by cytokines (**endocrine** action). The molecular weights of cytokines vary between 15,000 and 25,000 daltons. They induce both humoral and cellular responses, including activation, proliferation, and differentiation of T cells, B cells, macrophages, and hematopoietic cells, by binding to high-affinity receptors on target cells (Table 2-1). Cytokines increase MHC expression, target cell injury, and inflammation involving neutrophils and platelets. Cytokines also augment the expression of cellular adhesion molecules on endothelial and

Table 2-1. Cytokines in transplant immunology

Cytokine	Cell source	Cell target	Primary action
Interleukin-2	T cells	T cells NK cells B cells	Growth, cytokine production Growth, ↑ cytolytic function Growth, ↑ antibody synthesis
Interleukin-4	CD4+ cells, mast cells	T cells	Growth
Transforming growth factor-beta	T cells, macrophages	Macrophages T cells	Inhibit activation Inhibit activation and maturation
Gamma-interferon	T cells, NK cells	Macrophages Macrophages Endothelial cells NK cells	Inhibit activation Activation Activation Activation ↑ Class I and class II MHC expression
Interleukin-10	T cells	Macrophages B cells	Inhibit function Stimulation
Interleukin-12	T cells, B cells, NK cells, monocytes	NK cells T cells	Stimulation Stimulate differentiation
Interleukin-1	Macrophages, T cells, epithelial and endothelial cells	Macrophages Vascular endothelium Liver and hypothalamus	↑ Acute phase reactants Inflammation Fever
Tumor necrosis factor	Macrophages, T cells, NK cells, mast cells	Vascular endothelium Neutrophils Macrophages Liver and hypothalamus	↑ Expression of adhesion molecules Inflammation Fever
Interleukin-6	Macrophages, vascular endothelial cells, fibroblasts, T cells	Liver B cells	↑ Acute phase reactants (fibrogen) Growth, stimulate differentiation

MHC = major histocompatibility complex; NK = natural killer.

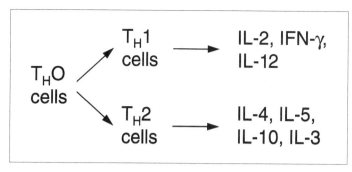

Fig. 2-5. Subsets of helper T lymphocytes.

epithelial cells of the graft and facilitate natural killer (NK) and macrophage-mediated cytotoxicity. These proteins usually influence the synthesis and the action of other cytokines. Cytokines can also play inhibitory roles to downregulate the immune response. The balance between stimulatory and inhibitory cytokines sets the vigor of any given immune response to an antigen.

Because of the fact that there are a large number of cytokines with similar, often interchangeable functions, there is a degree of promiscuity and redundancy to these systems. A pattern of response emerges in which one set of cytokines is generally involved with the enhancement of antibody responses to an antigen and may downregulate cellular response (**TH2 cytokines**, synthesized by the TH2 subset of lymphocytes), and one set of cytokines is generally involved with the enhancement of cellular immune responses (**TH1 cytokines**, a product of the TH1 subset of lymphocytes) (Fig. 2-5). In the initiation of an immune response, several cytokines, such as **tumor necrosis factor (TNF)** and **IFN-γ**, direct the maturation of the lymphocyte pool to favor the TH1 subset of cells that elaborate IL2, IFN-γ, and IL-12. The anti-inflammatory cytokines, such as **transforming growth factor-beta (TGF-β)**, direct the maturation process of the TH2 cytokines IL-4 and IL-10, which dampens the cellular response to alloantigen. During rejection, all of these cytokines are found in the graft, but in states of tolerance, the TH1 cytokines are reduced and TH2 are enhanced, suggesting a causal relationship.

The cytokines play additional roles in the alloresponse in addition to their roles in the maturation of specific T cell subsets and in the balance between the cellular and humoral arms of immunity. As discussed in the section on lymphocyte action, IL-2 plays a pivotal role in regulating T cell activation by providing the signals needed to complete the activation program of both helper and cytotoxic T cells and by stimulating the synthesis of the proto-oncogenes needed for DNA synthesis and clonal expansion. T cell activation, however, can occur in the absence of IL-2. In animals with targeted deletion of the IL-2 gene (**IL-2 "knockout" mice**), acute rejection can still occur with the functions of IL-2 substituted by other cytokines. This is an example of the **redundancy** that is a frequent feature of the immune response.

IFN-γ, in addition to its subset maturational role, regulates the quantitative expression of MHC class I and class II molecules on cells for which these molecules initiate the alloresponse and are tar-

Table 2-2. Classification of transplant rejection

Form	Pathogenesis	Histopathology	Therapy
Hyperacute	Preformed, IgG, anti-HLA class I	Ischemic necrosis, thrombosis	No successful treatment; prevention with crossmatch
Acute	Cellular and humoral immune response	Tubulitis, vasculitis, lymphocytic infiltrates	Steroids, antilymphocyte antibodies
Chronic	Alloantigen dependent and alloantigen independent	Interstitial fibrosis, tubular atrophy, glomerular sclerosis	No effective treatment

HLA = human leukocyte antigen.

gets for the effector responses to transplants. Lastly, the cytokines may play a purely inflammatory role as mediators of the constitutional responses to transplantation antigens. IL-2, TNF, and IL-6 are responsible for the fever, myalgias, arthralgias, and capillary leak syndrome that lead to edema, and swelling of the graft often perceived as graft tenderness during the rejection response.

FORMS OF ALLOGRAFT REJECTION

Renal graft rejection can be defined as a series of events in which the graft is recognized as nonself. This process involves the participation of both local and systemic immune responses involving CD4+ T lymphocytes, CD8+ T lymphocytes, B cells, natural killer cells, macrophages, and cytokines; the establishment of a local inflammatory injury; induction of MHC expression; and eventually deterioration of renal function and necrosis of the transplanted tissue. Rejection can be classified as hyperacute, acute, or chronic on the basis of etiologic, clinical, and pathologic parameters (Table 2-2).

Hyperacute Rejection

Hyperacute rejection occurs within minutes to hours after the vascular clamps to the transplanted organ are released. This dramatic event is caused by preformed, cytotoxic, anti-HLA class I (IgG isotope) or anti–ABO blood group antibodies (IgM isotope) in the recipient. These antibodies bind to the endothelial surfaces of the arterioles on the graft, activate complement, and lead to severe vascular injury, including thrombosis and obliteration of the graft vasculature. The endothelial cells are stimulated to secrete von Willebrand factor, which mediates platelet adhesion and aggregation. Complement activation initiates the coagulation cascade and the generation of multiple inflammatory mediators. Eventually, transplanted tissue suffers irreversible ischemic damage. The current ABO-matching policy has largely eliminated hyperacute rejection by anti–ABO antibodies (see Chap. 3). Hyperacute rejection is mediated by antibodies against alloantigens that have appeared in response to previous exposure to alloantigens through blood transfusions, prior transplantations, or multiple pregnancies. Pathologic findings show fibrinoid necrosis of the vessel walls, fibrin thrombus formation, margination of neutrophils, and ischemic necrosis. The graft may become flaccid or cyanotic and hard, then even rupture within minutes after revascularization.

There is no successful treatment at the present time for hyperacute rejection. It can be prevented by testing recipients for the presence of the preformed, cytotoxic antibodies that react with the cells of the donor in a sensitive test called a **crossmatch** (see Chap. 3).

Accelerated Acute Rejection

Rejection occurring within a few days after transplantation (between 24 hours to 4 days post-transplant) is called accelerated acute rejection. It occurs when the recipient has been sensitized by prior interactions with graft antigen, generally by prior transplants but also by transfusions, and is thought to represent an immunologic memory response to prior sensitization. The recipient develops rejection in a rapid fashion. This event has also been seen after donor-specific transfusions in recipients of kidneys from living-related donors. This type of rejection may represent a combination of cellular and antibody-mediated injury. The cellular infiltration may not be as intense as with acute rejection. This serious event may be difficult to control with current immunosuppressive regimens and may contribute to early graft loss.

Acute Rejection

Acute rejection, which generally occurs days to weeks after surgery, is a systemic inflammatory disorder that in its full-blown manifestation may be associated with multiple constitutional symptoms, including fever, chills, myalgias, and arthralgias. Many of these symptoms are manifestations of cytokine release (e.g., TNF, IL-1); expression of IL-2 and IFN-γ has been shown to increase *prior* to the development of the typical interstitial infiltrate. Acute rejection is described in clinical and pathologic detail in Chaps. 8 and 12. In this era of potent immunosuppressive agents, the constitutional inflammatory signs and symptoms are often masked, and only renal physiologic derangements may be present. Acute rejection should be diagnosed immediately in order to initiate the appropriate treatment and prevent irreversible damage.

About 90% of acute rejections are predominantly cellular-mediated and are more easily reversed with appropriate treatment than those rejections in which antigraft antibodies are the predominant effectors. Evidence suggests that CD4+ T cells are important for the initiation of rejection, and CD8+ T cells are critical at the later stages. CTLs and natural killer cells contain powerful cytolytic granules of the **effector molecules**, **granzymes** and **perforins**. Granule exocytosis releases these molecules, which cause membrane damage and induce **programmed cell death (apoptosis).**

Five to 10% of the rejection episodes are mediated by humoral immune response and are more difficult to reverse. Participation of donor-specific IgG antibodies against endothelial cell alloantigens activate complement and lead to vascular injury in the graft. Perivascular infiltration with T cells, natural killer cells, and mononuclear cells and tubulitis accompanied by vasculitis on biopsy are defining features of acute rejection. In severe forms, vascular occlusion and interstitial hemorrhage may be seen (see Chap. 12).

Chronic Rejection

Chronic rejection is characterized by glomerular sclerosis, tubular atrophy, splitting of the glomerular basement membrane, and interstitial fibrosis. It occurs slowly over months to years and leads to progressive loss of renal function. The pathogenesis of chronic rejection is not fully understood but both immune (**alloantigen dependent**) and nonimmune (**alloantigen independent**) mechanisms are important (see Chap. 9). The healing process after repeated bouts of acute rejection, chronic graft injury by delayed type hypersensitivity response, chronic ischemia, and the role of immunosuppressive drugs such as cyclosporine have all been proposed as stimuli for the ubiquitous fibrosis. Unfortunately, this form of scarring injury has been resistant to current rejection therapies.

Cytomegalovirus and Rejection

Infection with cytomegalovirus (CMV) has been implicated in the development of both acute and chronic allograft rejection; late acute rejection has been ascribed to clinically covert CMV infection. CMV infection promotes a generalized immune response in a similar fashion to rejection. It has been shown that CMV upregulates MHC class I molecules and the various adhesion molecules. In the kidney, ICAM-1 expression is upregulated as a direct effect of the virus on CMV-infected proximal tubular epithelial cells or through activation of lymphocytes and the mononuclear cell release of IFN-γ. In a study of heart transplant recipients with CMV infection, persistent expression of VCAM-1 on capillary endothelial cells was reported. CMV infection was found to be associated with mild generalized lymphoid activation and intense ICAM-1 expression on hepatocytes in liver transplant patients. It has also been demonstrated that MHC class II antigens, which are no longer detectable in the graft after successful transplantation, are upregulated by CMV via IFN-γ release by activated T cells. Moreover, CMV encodes a molecule similar to MHC class I antigens, whereas a homology exists between the immediate-early region protein of CMV and the beta chain of the class II HLA-DR antigen that can cause a cross-reaction. Acute CMV infection induces antiendothelial cell antibodies, which may be risk factors for acute and chronic rejection. CMV has been associated with subendothelial inflammation of heart allograft vascular structures in rat models and humans. During active CMV infection, changes similar to rejection may be seen in transplant biopsies.

Prolonged or repeated courses of antilymphocyte preparations increase the risk of the disease, often by activating latent virus. Because of the morbidity of CMV infection and the association between CMV infection and rejection, different protocols for prophylaxis of CMV infection have been developed, including CMV hyperimmune globulin and high-dose oral acyclovir, interferon, and ganciclovir (see Chap. 10). Despite recent improvements in immunosuppressive and antiviral therapies, little is known about the impact of CMV prophylaxis on the development of rejection.

TOLERANCE

Immunologic tolerance can be described as an antigen-induced block in the development or differentiation of lymphocytes specific for the inducing antigen only. During lymphocyte ontogeny, the immune system eliminates autoreactive clones of lymphocytes and preserves the clones that can recognize foreign antigens in the context of self. In this process, the entire repertoire of response to be displayed by the mature individual is established. Self-tolerance is thus initiated during development in the thymus and maintained in the periphery.

The induction of human tolerance to defined foreign antigens while maintaining completely intact all the rest of the immune repertoire continues to be the dream of the transplant scientist and clinician. In defined animal models or experiments of nature, tolerance to transplantation antigens has been induced or encountered. Tolerance is induced in the thymus and can be global (**central tolerance**) or can be either maintained or even developed by mature lymphocytes populating lymphoid tissue (**peripheral tolerance**).

Introduction of antigen during ontogeny into the thymus at an appropriate point of T cell maturation leads to a similar clonal deletion for that defined antigen as for autoreactive clones. Such tolerance can be complete, or it may need to be maintained in the periphery. Introduction of antigen into the thymus after lymphocyte development may also culminate in tolerance to a defined antigen. An important contribution of an intact peripheral immune system is required, since immunosuppressant therapy can either reverse or block such tolerance development. In experimental settings, the creation of central tolerance leads to the acceptance of foreign lymphoid cells that can cocirculate unscathed in the host, a condition called **chimerism**. It has been suggested that the persistence of chimerism, even with a scant number of cells, called **microchimerism**, not only marks the tolerant state but also is mechanistically important in the maintenance of the tolerance in the periphery. Chimeric states can be introduced into the mature immune system with the provision of donor hematopoietic cells in the setting of immunosuppressant conditioning, often by forms of radiation. Total body irradiation has often been used to permit marrow or stem cell transplantation, leading to chimerism in experimental models. This technique has been limited in clinical medicine by the development of often fatal graft-versus-host disease (GVHD). **Total lymphoid irradiation (TLI)** involves radiation of the immune organs and the spleen and was developed for the treatment of Hodgkin's disease. It may permit chimerism and tolerance without GVHD in rodents and lower mammals, a promise not yet met in human biology. More recently, protocols have been developed to induce chimerism by using antilymphocyte antibody conditioning at the time of provision of donor antigen through directed donor cell transfusions or by "minimal" radiation conditioning and marrow reconstitution with both donor and recipient marrow elements.

The fact that the immune system can be manipulated to tolerate transplanted tissues without immunosuppressive drugs encourages the continued research for the induction of transplantation tolerance. It is clear that the continued presence of alloantigen either on the graft or as chimerism of cells is necessary for the maintenance of tolerance. T cells of donor origin that suppress the immune response, so-called **veto cells**, have been identified as the mediators in several models when protocols employing polyclonal T cell antibody–conditioned bone marrow have been used. Trials to induce specific T cell tolerance are in progress using peptides derived from polymorphic regions of donor MHC molecules. **CTLA4-Ig** is a fusion protein that blocks the CD28-mediated costimulatory signal and prevents the interaction between graft B7 molecules and recipient CD28 molecules (see Fig. 2-3). Other monoclonal antibodies directed against adhesion molecules and cytokines are being developed.

Despite the advances in our understanding of tolerance, clinical tolerance induction remains as one of the major unanswered challenges in transplantation.

XENOGENEIC TRANSPLANTATION

Transplantation of organs from other mammals to humans might solve the current problem of the clinical organ-donor shortage. Because of differences in the primary immune mechanisms culminating in graft destruction, xenografts are separated into those between closely related species, such as between chimpanzee or baboon and humans, called **concordant xenografts**, and those between distant species, such as swine to humans, called **discordant xenografts**.

The major discriminating feature of discordant xenogeneic transplantation is hyperacute rejection secondary to the presence of preformed, xenoreactive **"natural" antibodies** and **complement activation**. Many individuals develop natural antibodies that are directed against carbohydrate determinants of other species, including anti–alpha-galactose (important in swine-to-human transplantation), antiphosphatidylcholine antibodies, and isohemagglutinins. These antibodies bind to the endothelial cells of the xenograft and activate the complement cascade. Complement activation depends on the combination of species. Transplant between primates and pigs triggers the antibody-dependent, classic pathway. In contrast, in transplantation between guinea pigs and rats, complement activation occurs via the alternative pathway. This type of rejection cannot be controlled with the current immunosuppressive regimens. Natural antibodies are rare between concordant species, and an accelerated cellular rejection response, thought to be related to either heightened indirect antigen presentation or to more vigorous CD4+ delayed-type hypersensitivity response, characterizes the unique aspects of concordant xenotransplantation. Once the unique aspects of xenotransplant are overcome, the transplanter must then confound the conventional rejection pathways. Tolerance induction, organ or column absorption, and transgeneic presentation of complement inhibitor proteins are techniques being studied to overcome xenogeneic barriers to successful engraftment. Until they become clinically applicable, the most practical way to permit xenotransplantation may be to **immunoisolate** the xenogeneic tissue in capsules as membranes. Early trials of immunoisolated pancreatic islets show promise (see Chap. 13).

SELECTED READINGS

Goral S, Helderman JH. Cytomegalovirus and rejection. *Transplant Proc* 26(Suppl):5, 1994.

Hall BM. Tolerance and specific unresponsiveness in organ transplantation. *Immunol Allergy Clin North Am* 9:61, 1989.

Helderman JH. Principles and Practices of Renal Transplant Rejection. In F Jacobson, G Striker, S Klahr (eds), *The Principles and Practices of Nephrology* (2nd ed). St Louis: Mosby-Year Book, 1995. Pp 811–821.

Hricik DE, Almawi W, Strom TB. Trends in the use of glucocorticosteroids in renal transplantation. *Transplantation* 57:979, 1994.

Krensky AM, Clayberger C. Transplantation immunology. *Pediatr Clin North Am* 41:819, 1994.

Moller E. Cell interactions and cytokines in transplantation immunity. *Transplant Proc* 27:24, 1995.

Pavlakis M, Lipman M, Strom TB. Intragraft expression of T-cell activation genes in human renal allograft rejection. *Kidney Int* 49:57, 1996.

Pearson TC, Alexander DZ, Winn KJ et al. Transplantation tolerance induced by CTLA4-Ig. *Transplantation* 57:1701, 1994.

Rao A. NF-ATp: A transcription factor required for the co-ordinate induction of several cytokine genes. *Immunol Today* 15:274, 1994.

Remuzzi G, Perico N, Carpenter CB et al. The thymic way to transplantation tolerance. *J Am Soc Nephrol* 5:1639, 1995.

Rukavina D, Balen-Marunic S, Rubesa G et al. Perforin expression in peripheral blood lymphocytes in rejecting and tolerant kidney transplant recipients. *Transplantation* 61:285, 1996.

Sayegh MH, Krensky MH. Novel immunotherapeutic strategies using MHC derived peptides. *Kidney Int* 49:513, 1996.

Sayegh MH, Watschinger B, Carpenter CB. Mechanisms of T cell recognition of alloantigen. *Transplantation* 57:1295, 1994.

Tremblay N, Fontaine P, Perreault C. T lymphocyte responses to multiple minor histocompatibility antigens generate both self-major histocompatibility complex-restricted and cross-reactive cytotoxic T lymphocytes. *Transplantation* 58:59, 1994.

Wilson JL, Proud G, Forsythe JLR et al. Renal allograft rejection. *Transplantation* 59:91, 1995.

3

Histocompatibility Testing, Crossmatching, and Allocation of Cadaveric Kidney Transplants

Steven Katznelson, Paul I. Terasaki, and
Gabriel M. Danovitch

The major histocompatibility complex (MHC) is a group of cell surface antigens that define the "foreign" nature, or allogeneity, of transplanted organs and tissues. They provide the major, though not sole, inhibition to transplantation. This chapter deals with the structure of the MHC, its genetic determinants, techniques for its identification, its relevance to the results of clinical transplantation, and its role in public policy decisions regarding the allocation of donor organs.

THE HUMAN MAJOR HISTOCOMPATIBILITY COMPLEX

Nomenclature

The human MHC complex, known as the human leukocyte antigen (HLA) system, is encoded for by a series of genes located on the short arm of chromosome 6 (see Chap. 2, Fig. 2-1). The concentration of the HLA genes in one defined area of the chromosome allows these genes to be inherited as a packet, or **haplotype.** Each individual inherits a haplotype of HLA genes from each parent, which are inherited concomitantly and together make up the individual **HLA profile.**

The HLAs can be divided into two different classes based on their structure and cellular distribution. **Class I** molecules are named **HLA-A, -B,** and **-C; class II** molecules are named **HLA-DP, -DQ,** and **-DR**. In clinical transplantation, it is the A, B, and DR antigens that are the most important. The remarkable degree of polymorphism of these antigens accounts for the great difficulty in tissue matching, as opposed to the ease of matching for the relatively nonpolymorphic red cell antigens that determine blood types.

There has been a marked increase in the number of known HLA specificities due to the recent development of new molecular biology techniques (see the section on DNA typing). As shown in Table 3-1, most of the earlier known specificities have been split into several subtypes. For example, it is now known that HLA-A2 is composed of 12 subtypes.

Names for each of the specificities, or **splits,** have been omitted from this simplified table but can be obtained from the World Health Organization (WHO) Nomenclature Report. Although this high level of sophistication is useful in HLA paternity testing and in the identification of individuals, too many specificities make matching for transplantation almost impossible. Presumably, they are important in bone marrow transplants, which often fail when matched for the broader specificities. However, the more significant issue for kidney transplants is whether it is practical to match for so many HLA specificities.

Structure of Human Leukocyte Antigens

Class I antigens (A, B, and C) consist of a unique heavy chain of 45,000 daltons that has three globular domains (termed $alpha_1$, $alpha_2$, and $alpha_3$) (see Fig. 2-1). The $alpha_3$ domain is associated with $beta_2$-microglobulin that is not MHC encoded. Class I antigens are expressed on all nucleated cells. Class II antigens (DR, DP, and DQ) consist of two peptides—a heavy, longer alpha chain (35,000 daltons) and a lighter, shorter beta chain (31,000 daltons). Both chains have two globular domains. Class II antigens are not expressed on all cells but are found on all B and activated T lymphocytes, monocytes, dendritic cells, glomerular endothelium, and renal tubular cells and capillaries.

Alloantigenic sites occur at the $alpha_1$ and $alpha_2$ domains of the class I molecule and at the external domain of the beta chain of class II molecules. Some determinants, called **public antigens,** are shared by many antigens. Unique specificities are known as **private antigens** or splits. Between the highly polymorphic globular class I $alpha_1$ and $alpha_2$ domains and the two class II alpha and beta domains is a groove in which antigenic peptides may lie (see Chap. 2, Fig. 2-4). The interaction between the polymorphic area and the peptide with the T cell receptor of the helper T cells is vital to the initiation of the immune response (see Chap. 2). The MHC not only functions as an alloantigen but also as a vehicle to present foreign antigen to helper T cells.

Inheritance of Human Leukocyte Antigens

Each parental chromosome 6 provides a haplotype, or a linked set of MHC genes, to its offspring (Fig. 3-1). Parental chromosomes also provide other histocompatibility determinants that are not yet identified. Haplotypes are usually inherited intact from each parent, although in approximately 2% of offspring, crossover is seen between the A and B locus, resulting in a **recombination.** A child typically carries one representative antigen from each of the class I and class II loci of each parent. A child is, by definition, a 1-haplotype match to each parent unless recombination has occurred.

Inheritance of haplotypes occurs in a mendelian fashion. Siblings may share both parental haplotypes (**2-haplotype match**), one parental haplotype (**1-haplotype match**), or no haplotypes (**0-haplotype match**). In the latter case, unidentified loci may still be shared.

Human Leukocyte Antigen Phenotypes and Genotypes

Consider an individual with the following HLA profile or phenotype:

A1,A24; B8,B44; DR3,DR15

From this phenotypic information alone it is not possible to identify haplotypes, since it is not known from which parent each specificity was inherited.

Consider another individual:

A1,A3; B7,B8; DR3,DR2

If this individual is the parent or sibling of the first, it becomes possible to identify the shared haplotype or genotype of the family as A1,B8,DR3. The first individual also has an unshared haplo-

Table 3-1. Recognized human leukocyte antigen specificities

A		B*		C		DR*	
Number of splits	Specificity	Number of splits	Specificity	Number of splits	Specificity	Number of splits	Specificity
2	A1	5	B7	2	Cw1	6	DR1
17	A2	2	B8	3	Cw2	11	DR2
2	A3	3	B13	3	Cw3	6	DR3
2	A11	2	B14				
		2	B15	2	Cw4	22	DR4
1	A23	2	B18	1	Cw5	1	DR7
6	A24	10	B27	1	Cw6	14	DR8
1	A25	10	B35	4	Cw7	2	DR9
4	A26	1	B37	3	Cw8	1	DR10
2	A29	2	B38(16)			22	DR11(5)
5	A30	10	B39	4	Cw12	5	DR12(5)
2	A31	8	B40	1	Cw13	19	DR13(6)
1	A32	2	B41	3	Cw14	18	DR14(6)
3	A33	1	B42			5	DR15(2)
2	A34	6	B44(12)	5	Cw15	6	DR16(2)
2	A36	1	B45(12)	3	Cw16	2	DR17(3)
1	A43	1	B46			2	DR18(3)
1	A66	1	B47	1	Cw17	5	DR51
2	A66	2	B48			4	DR52
3	A68	1	B49(21)			5	DR53
1	A69	1	B50(21)				
1	A74	5	B51(5)				
1	A80						

2	B52(5)
1	B53
1	B54(22)
2	B55(22)
2	B56(22)
3	B57(17)
2	B58(17)
1	B59
2	B60(40)
2	B61(40)
8	B62(15)
2	B63(15)
1	B64(14)
1	B65(14)
2	B67
1	B70
1	B71(70)
1	B72(70)
1	B73
1	B75(15)
3	B76(15)
1	B77(15)
1	B78

*The numbers in parentheses represent prior designations.

Source: Data modified from JG Bodmer, SGF Marsh, ED Albert et al. Nomenclature for factors of the HLA system, 1994. *Hum Immunol* 41:1, 1994.

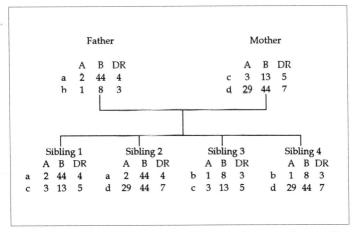

Fig. 3-1. Inheritance of haplotypes and human leukocyte antigen profile in four theoretical siblings. Sibling 1 is a 1-haplotype match to sibling 2 and 3 and a 0-haplotype match to sibling 4. The individual haplotypes are labeled a, b, c, and d.

type A24,B44,DR15, and the second individual an unshared haplotype A3,B7,DR2. These haplotypes may appear in the other parent or siblings.

If these two individuals are not related, it is not possible to identify the haplotypes, nor can it be presumed that other nonidentified loci are shared. Thus, in cadaveric transplantation, the haplotypes are unknown, and only the **"matching"** of individual determinants can be identified. The two individuals whose HLA phenotypes are listed would be called a 3-antigen match or a 3-antigen mismatch (see the section on matches and mismatches). Sharing of unidentified loci is serendipitous.

The improved results of live-related transplantation versus cadaveric transplantation (see the section on the impact of HLA matching on results of transplantation) are due, in part, to the shared whole haplotype and other unidentified loci. In the tissue typing example noted above, the statistical chances of successful transplantations will be better if the two individuals are a 1-haplotype sibling pair or a parent/child pair than if one individual is a 3-antigen–matched cadaveric donor. Similarly, 2-haplotype live-related transplants have graft survival rates that are higher than 6-antigen–matched cadaveric transplants. Even 0-haplotype–matched related transplants will do better than mismatched cadaveric transplants, due partly to the shared unidentified loci and partly to the excellent condition of the organ at the time of transplantation. The lower success rates of matched cadaveric transplants may also be due to the lesser likelihood of tissue typing errors influencing the choice of related donors.

Identical and Fraternal Twins

The differentiation between identical twins and 2-haplotype–matched fraternal twins may not be obvious, since their HLA phenotypes and genotypes are the same and physical appearance is unreliable. The differentiation is important, since the recipient of a transplant from an identical twin requires no immunosuppression because the procedure is immunologically equivalent to an autotransplant. Two-haplotype–matched siblings, whether they are fraternal twins or not, differ in their unidentified loci, and immunosuppression is required.

The absolute means of differentiation requires the observation of a single placenta and amniotic sac at birth. Such information, however, may be unavailable or unreliable. A small skin graft can be performed from the potential twin donor to the recipient; the graft will be rejected if the twins are fraternal. For practical purposes, it is best to perform extended blood typing. The genetic determinants of blood types (e.g., rhesus factor [Rh], MN) are dispersed throughout the genome, and their identity between identical twins obviates the necessity for immunosuppression.

Linkage Disequilibrium

As noted above, it is not possible to identify haplotypes from the phenotypic HLA typing information alone. There is a tendency, however, within racial or ethnic groups, for certain HLA determinants to be inherited together (e.g., HLA-A1,B8 and HLA-A2,B44 in whites). This phenomenon is known as **linkage disequilibrium** and is the basis of inheritance of haplotypes within racial groups.

Matches and Mismatches

It is not always possible to identify two HLA specificities of each HLA locus. Consider the HLA phenotype for the following two unrelated individuals:

1. A2 —   B27, B13   DR3, DR4
2. A2, A3   B7, B14   DR3 —

The absence of the second A as well as a DR specificity could be due either to failure to identify a yet undefined specificity or to the inheritance of the same specificity (A2 and DR3 in these cases) from both parents (homozygous). These two individuals could thus be described as a 1-A, 1-DR match, a terminology that does not take into account the unidentified loci. If individual 1 were a donor for individual 2, it would be more precise to describe the combination as a 0-A,2-B,1-DR mismatch. If individual 2 were a donor for individual 1, the combination would be a 1-A,2-B,0-DR mismatch.

TISSUE TYPING TECHNIQUES

The lymphocyte is the tissue generally used for tissue typing because it has been found to express the histocompatibility antigens in the greatest concentration. Technically, this cell has been the easiest to handle in vitro. In general, the basic principles of typing tissue are the same as those for typing red cells in that antigens present on the surface of the cell are detected by antibodies. Whereas the agglutination reaction is used to distinguish ABO and Rh types, the cytotoxicity reaction involving antibody and complement is used for HLA types. The cell is defined as being of that "type" when a specific antibody reacts with the cell. Testing for class I specificities is performed on peripheral blood lymphocytes or T lymphocytes. Class II typing requires the use of B lymphocytes.

Microlymphocytotoxicity Test

The microlymphocytotoxicity test is the most commonly used assay for the detection of class I antigens (Fig. 3-2). Lymphocytes from the person to be typed treated with carboxyfluorescein diacetate (CFDA), a fluorescent dye, are tested against a panel of antisera defining each of the HLA types. After the addition of rabbit complement and further incubation, quench (hemoglobin or India ink) with ethidium bromide is added, and the test is read using a fluorescence microscope.

Reagents

The serum of pregnant women and monoclonal antibodies are the primary sources for the antibodies used in tissue typing. Maternal antibodies are produced against the foreign antigens present in the fetus, which are inherited from the father. Massive screening programs are required to identify and select reagent-grade antisera that are highly specific for an HLA antigen and that have a high titer so that the cytotoxic reactivity is not lost under suboptimal conditions. Monoclonal antibodies specific for HLA antigens are produced from a single hybridoma and provide a highly specific, stable, high-titer reagent for typing.

Isolation of Lymphocytes

Immunomagnetic beads coated with monoclonal antibodies (MoAbs) provide the simplest method for the selective separation of lymphocytes from whole blood or a suspension of mononuclear cells (Fig. 3-3A). Anti–T cell or anti–B cell monoclonal antibodies are used to coat the immunomagnetic beads. When mixed with a blood sample, the target cells adhere to the beads, and the remaining cells in the supernatant may be removed to another tube or discarded. The target cells may be used on the beads or "detached" from the beads.

Another simple method for cell isolation uses a monoclonal antibody/complement cocktail called Lympho-Kwik (Fig. 3-3B). The reagent contains complement, a density gradient medium, and MoAbs against the cells that are to be eliminated from the suspension. When unseparated white cells are added to Lympho-Kwik and incubated, red cells, granulocytes, and platelets are lysed. After centrifugation, purified lymphocytes are deposited on the bottom of the tube, and the fragments of the other cells remain in the supernatant. The main advantage to this technique is that the isolation of lymphocytes takes place in one tube, thus eliminating the possibility of switching samples.

Procedure

The steps involved in standard testing for HLA are illustrated in Fig. 3-2. The standardized conditions were set at a National Institutes of Health (NIH) meeting; consequently, the test is often referred to as the **"NIH test."** Lymphocytes isolated from blood are added to tissue typing trays containing typing reagents. Although any type of anticoagulated blood can be used, citrated blood has been found to be the best for long-distance transport of blood samples. Lymphoycctes are purified from blood as described above. After incubation with the antibodies, rabbit complement is added, and the tray is incubated for another hour. Complement kills cells that react with the antibody. In a two-color fluorescence assay, the viable cells appear green when read with a fluorescence microscope, and the dead cells appear red.

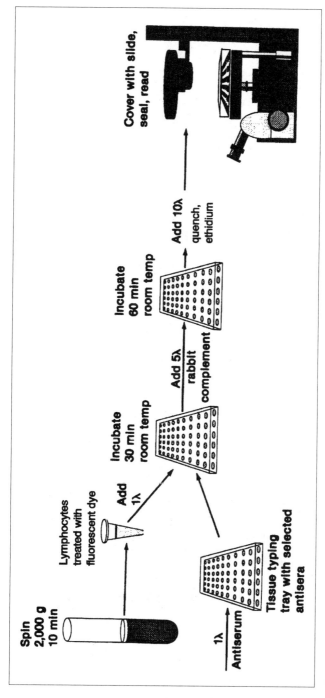

Fig. 3-2. Stages in the standard microlymphocytotoxicity test.

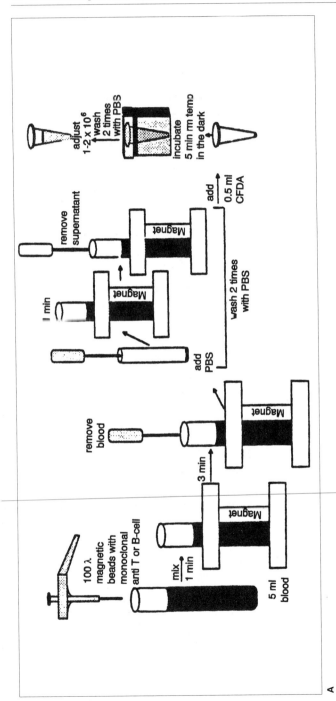

A

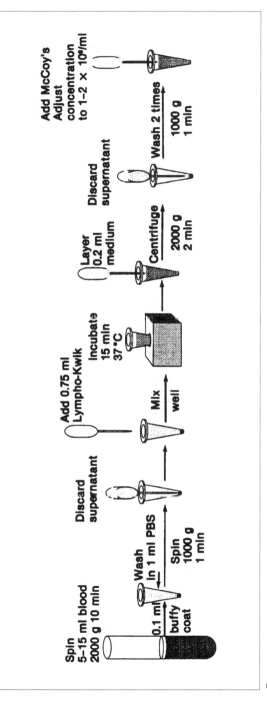

Fig. 3-3. Stages in the magnetic bead isolation technique (A) and the Lympho-Kwik isolation technique (B) for isolation of lymphocytes.

B

The reactions are scored using a rough scale to facilitate the estimation of cell killing based on the change in viability between the negative control and the test wells. A negative reaction is scored as a 1, a probable negative as a 2, and a weak positive as a 4. If the majority of cells are killed, the score is a 6; if all the cells are killed, the score is an 8. Results are analyzed and typing is assigned based on the specificity of the antisera producing the positive reactions (scores).

Mixed Lymphocyte Culture

When lymphocytes from one individual are mixed in culture with those of an unrelated individual, both groups of cells proliferate. This phenomenon is the basis of the mixed lymphocyte culture (MLC), or reaction (MLR), and is determined by mismatching at the class II loci. The test can be used for typing of class II loci. It has been largely superseded by the serologic tests described above and by DNA typing described below.

DNA Typing

It is now possible to type individuals by DNA-based rather than conventional serologic methods. At present, methods have been worked out for class II specificities, but methods for class I are just now becoming available. In general, two basic methods used are site-specific oligonucleotide probes (SSOP) and sequence-specific primers (SSP). SSOP is based on first amplifying by locus-specific primers using the polymerase chain reaction (PCR), then detecting the adherence of specific oligonucleotide probes tagged with radioactive or enzymatic markers. SSP depends on DNA amplification by specific primers and detection usually by gel electrophoresis. Several commercial kits are available for class II typing.

DNA typing has been advocated for kidney transplants, since typing of more difficult specificities can be more precise. For example, HLA-DR6 has been a troublesome specificity for many years, since antisera to it could not be obtained. We now know that HLA-DR6 is composed of 30 split specificities of HLA-DR13 and HLA-DR14. Monoclonal antibodies have been produced to various split specificities; however, no single antibody could be made to DR6 because no single epitope actually exists for it. According to nomenclature convention, all splits currently included in DR13 and DR14 are considered to be DR6. Generally, DNA typing has been favored for making this distinction. For the most part, the concordance of DNA and serologic typing for class II has been high for the broad specificities, but DNA is clearly the superior method for the split specificities.

DNA Typing and Matching for Kidney Transplants

The capability of DNA typing of identifying so many specificities has left the transplant community with a difficult dilemma. As seen in Table 3-1, to provide for good matches using all the known specificities, it would be necessary to match 48 A locus, 96 B locus, and 118 DR locus specificities. As a result, too few patients will match.

It is already difficult to find matched donors, even with the current use of broad specificities. Despite the use of known broad specificities and national sharing for a waiting pool of 31,000 kidney transplant recipients, it has been estimated that, even in ideal circumstances, only 20% of the recipients could obtain 0-A,-B,-DR mismatched transplants. Thus, our knowledge of HLA specificities has exceeded the practical capability of using them for matching cadaver donors for organ transplants. Fortunately, it appears that many patients with mismatches still have grafts that function well. This suggests that there are "immunogenic" and "nonimmunogenic" splits. It may be possible to reduce the number of known specificities to a practical list relevant for organ sharing.

DNA typing is an important reference method for confirming problematic tissue typing. For routine kidney transplant donor and recipient testing, serologic typing is probably sufficient. Efforts to reduce the number of specificities still further are detailed in the next section.

Cross-Reacting Groups Matching

Efforts are being made to decrease the number of antigens used for matching in order to obtain more matched patients within smaller local pools and to offer more kidneys to minority candidates. With extensive splitting of the HLA types, racial groups are more distinctly separated. On the other hand, combining broad specificities into even broader **cross-reacting groups** (CREG) tends to group individuals together, regardless of their racial background. The CREG groups are based on the concept that certain common **epitopes** (antigen-binding sites) are shared among the specificities. The groups have been based on common amino acid residues in the molecular composition of each specificity. Matching for the CREG groups has resulted in excellent graft survival, with larger numbers of patients achieving "good" matching in relatively small local pools. Thus, in addition to national sharing of 0-A,-B,-DR mismatched grafts, tissue typing can be used at the local level to identify a larger proportion of well-matched grafts.

An equally important consequence of the CREG matching concept is the more equitable distribution of kidneys to black patients. The higher incidence of kidney failure among blacks coupled with a lower donation rate has resulted in blacks having to wait longer than whites for a transplant. CREG matching produces more equitable distribution, since CREG groups have a more similar frequency between races than the split specificities.

CROSSMATCHING WITH T AND B LYMPHOCYTES

The lymphocyte crossmatch serves to detect preformed HLA antibodies in the serum of the transplant recipient directed against the lymphocytes of the proposed donor. It is the transplantation equivalent of the blood group crossmatch for blood transfusion. The consequences of proceeding with either transplantation or transfusion against a positive crossmatch are similar. The former produces red cell lysis and a transfusion reaction; the latter produces hyperacute rejection. Assiduous attention to pretransplant lymphocyte crossmatching has virtually eliminated hyperacute rejection as a clinical threat.

The Pretransplant Crossmatch

The lymphocyte crossmatch is a routine pretransplant screening test. Using the previously described NIH test, the potential donor's lymphocytes serve as the target cells for the patient's serum.

A **false-positive crossmatch** may be produced by antibodies that are typically more reactive at cold temperatures. In general, these antibodies are immunoglobulin M (IgM) **"autoantibodies,"** or more properly non-HLA antibodies, and thus irrelevant to transplantation. They are particularly common in patients suffering from systemic lupus erythematosus. These antibodies often produce false-positive results at colder temperatures, and by incubating at 37°C, most of the non-HLA antibodies are excluded. However, the most effective way to ensure that a reaction is produced by HLA antibodies rather than by autoantibodies is to treat the serum with a reducing agent such as dithiothreitol (DTT). IgM antibodies are inactivated by DTT so that if a positive reaction is still obtained, the reaction can be generally attributed to antibodies against HLA. The effect of DTT treatment of the serum depends on the non-HLA antibodies being IgM, which is the case more than 90% of the time. Nevertheless, the possibility that rare IgM HLA antibodies might produce hyperacute rejections must be kept in mind.

Panel Reactive Antibodies

To determine whether a patient is likely to have a positive cross-match against a donor at the time of transplantation, the microlymphocytotoxicity test can be used to screen for preformed anti-HLA **cytotoxic antibodies.** The patient's serum is incubated with B and T cells from a panel of donors selected to represent the HLA specificities. Complement is added and cell lysis detected as noted previously. The results are usually expressed as the percent of panel cells that show positive antibody activity.

The anti-HLA antibodies that are detected are thus called **panel reactive antibodies (PRAs).** The most important PRAs are those directed against T cells. The importance of antibodies to B cells remains controversial.

The higher a patient's percentage of PRAs, the more difficult it is to find a crossmatch-negative kidney. Simplistically, the finding of 60% T antibodies suggests that 60% of pretransplant crossmatches will be positive, since the panel used for testing is representative of the general population and hence donor population. Patients with levels of PRAs of 80% or more may wait years for their transplants. Such patients comprise more than 10% of the national pool awaiting cadaveric kidney transplants.

Patients awaiting transplantation should have their PRA levels checked at regular intervals. This allows for an ongoing assessment of their chances of a positive crossmatch, and the stored sera can also be used to screen potential cadaveric donors. In a patient with low or absent PRAs and without a recent blood transfusion, a negative screening crossmatch with recently obtained serum (within a month or 6 weeks) sometimes can be used in lieu of a fresh crossmatch. Sera of patients with high levels of PRAs can be placed on special trays to facilitate crossmatching against a large number of potential donors.

The most potent sources of high levels of PRAs are prior blood transfusions, pregnancy and parturition, and a rejected prior transplant. The widespread use of erythropoietin in chronic dialysis patients and the subsequent reduction in transfusion requirements may allow the high levels of PRAs to fall, thus enhancing the chances of a negative crossmatch.

Sensitive Crossmatching Techniques

To increase the sensitivity of the standard crossmatch, newer techniques have been developed in an attempt to detect antibodies that may be missed in the microlymphocytotoxicity reaction. Although the final place in clinical transplantation for these sensitive cross-matching techniques has not yet been well-defined, their clear benefit is to match donor kidneys to the best possible recipient, thus providing the best chance of long graft survival. This is especially important given the limited donor pool. Transplant patients with a positive flow cytometry or antiglobulin crossmatch (see below) have a statistically significant lower graft survival.

Flow Cytometry Crossmatch

The flow cytometry crossmatch test (FCXM or FACs) uses a flow cytometer (Fig. 3-4). The patient's serum is mixed with lymphocytes from the donor and then incubated with monoclonal mouse anti–T and anti–B antibody conjugated with phycoerythrin and an anti-human IgG antibody conjugated with fluorescein. With a flow cytometer, the T and B cells that stain red can be gated, making the amount of green fluorescence proportional to the concentration of anti–T cell and anti–B cell antibodies present in the serum. T and B cell flow cytometry crossmatches are usually performed separately, although new techniques involving three-color staining allow for the assays to be performed together.

The flow cytometry crossmatch is useful in detecting very low levels of circulating antibodies. Positive-flow cytometry crossmatches have been associated with a high rate of early acute rejection episodes and a reduced 1-year graft survival rate. Although false-positives may be a limitation of this procedure, the T cell FCXM is an excellent tool for improving early function. The T cell FCXM may be particularly useful in the pretransplant evaluation of sensitized and retransplant recipients and as a determinant in choosing the optimum living donor. Although the T cell FCXM has been used successfully as described above, the role of the B cell FCXM is still being debated. Most studies have shown that a positive B cell FCXM, when associated with a negative T cell FCXM, does not increase the risk of early rejection or graft loss. However, B cell FCXM results that are strongly positive may be associated with high titers of anti–DR antibodies and may predict poor graft outcome.

Antiglobulin Crossmatch

To increase the sensitivity of the standard crossmatch test, antiglobulin is added, followed by complement and the same steps as the standard procedure. The serum must be completely washed off before the addition of the antiglobulin reagent, since any free IgG will neutralize the reagent. The wash method consists of washing the serum off before adding the complement. Often serum is anticomplementary, and this maneuver aids in circumventing this problem.

IMPACT OF HUMAN LEUKOCYTE MATCHING ON TRANSPLANTATION

Cadaveric and Live Donor Transplants

The overall impact of matching for MHC antigens on the long- and short-term results of kidney transplantation can be illustrated by comparing the results of 2-haplotype, 1-haplotype, and cadaveric transplants. Figure 3-5 is based on the results of nearly 30,000 transplants performed between 1988 and 1992 and reported to the **United Network for Organ Sharing (UNOS).** When plotted on

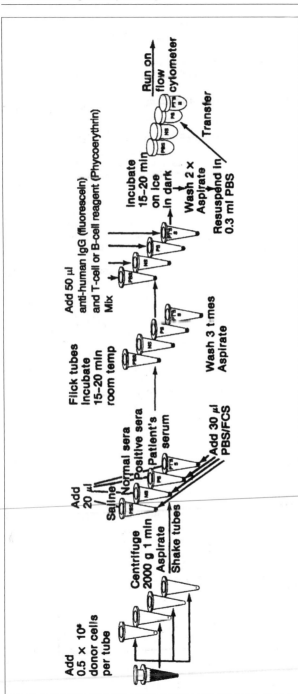

Fig. 3-4. The flow cytometry crossmatch.

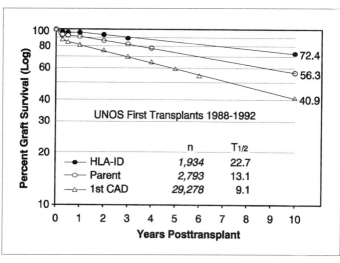

Fig. 3-5. Rate of graft loss for first kidneys transplanted between 1988 and 1992 and reported to the United Network for Organ Sharing. Note the difference in estimated half-life (T½) depending on the source of the kidney. All sibling transplants reported here are 2-haplotype matches or human leukocyte antigen–identical (HLA-ID). Parents are, by definition, 1-haplotype matches.

a log scale, the loss of transplants after the first post-transplant year proceeds at a precise linear rate. Kidney transplants from 2-haplotype–matched siblings provide grafts not only with the highest survival rates, but also the lowest long-term loss. The second highest rate of graft survival is noted in parental donor transplants in which donor and recipient have one haplotype in common. The lowest graft survival is found in transplants from cadaveric donors. In recent years, with the advent of cyclosporine, the 1-year graft survival of these three transplant categories has become similar. Their long-term graft survival, however, is markedly different. The loss rate is best expressed in terms of **half-life.** 2-haplotype–matched sibling donor (HLA-identical) transplants have a half-life of 22.7 years, 1-haplotype–matched donor kidneys have a half-life of 13.1 years, and cadaveric kidneys have a half-life of 9.1 years.

When the long-term effect is considered, 10-year graft survival can be predicted by extrapolation of the lines on a log scale. The 10-year graft survival of cadaveric donor transplants may be as low as 40%. Since most of the transplants performed today are from cadaveric donors, it is imperative that the problem of chronic long-term loss be solved. As shown in Fig. 3-6, the graft survival rates at 1 year have steadily improved through 1992; however, the long-term loss rate has remained constant. In fact, evidence is available that the long-term loss rate of cadaveric donor grafts has remained largely unchanged for the past 25 years. Improvements in immunosuppressive therapy have contributed to higher graft survival rates such that, in the cyclosporine era, 1-year live-related graft survival rates of greater than 90% and cadaveric graft survival rates of 80% have become routine. Some centers report nearly 100% graft survival

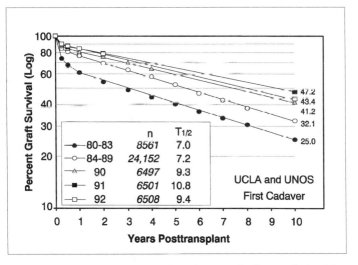

Fig. 3-6. After the first post-transplant (Tx) year, the linear relationship between graft survival and year(s) of the first cadaveric transplants did not significantly change between 1980 and 1992, indicating that the long-term cadaveric donor loss rate has not changed over time.

rates for live-related transplants and 90% graft survival for cadaveric transplants. These excellent early results, however, have had no recognizable impact on the long-term loss rate.

Most of the benefit of live-related transplants compared to cadaveric transplants was once thought to be a reflection of their better matching. The graft survival rate for living-unrelated donor grafts, however, approaches the long-term survival of 1-haplotype–matched living-related donor grafts. Most of the unrelated donors are spouses who, though presumably emotionally well-matched, are not HLA-matched. This observation underscores the beneficial effect of transplanting kidneys from excellent donors despite poor HLA-matching, since live donor kidneys are almost always in better condition at the time of transplant than cadaveric kidneys.

Matching for Cadaveric Transplants

One of the most effective ways in which the long-term loss rate could be improved is evident from Fig. 3-5. When the HLA chromosomes were matched, there was a half-life of 20 years, compared with 9.1 years when, in cadaveric transplants, both HLA chromosomes were mismatched. Thus, HLA matching has a very strong effect on the long-term loss rate. As shown in Fig. 3-7, patients with 0-A,-B,-DR mismatches (see the section on matches and mismatches) had the highest graft survival and the longest half-life, compared with patients with increasing numbers of HLA mismatches. Although the difference in graft survival at 1 year is relatively small, the long-term outcome is strongly influenced by the incompatibilities. The extrapolated 10-year graft survival differed by almost 30 percentage points. This type of evidence suggests that HLA matching is important in obtaining transplants that survive for many years.

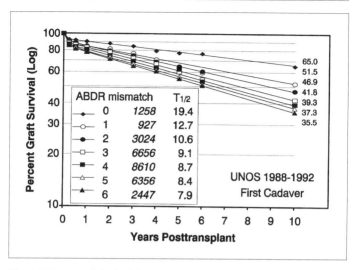

Fig. 3-7. Impact of -A, -B, -DR mismatches on early and late graft survival of more than 28,000 first cadaveric transplants reported to the United Network for Organ Sharing from 1988 to 1992.

Six-Antigen Match Program

In 1987, all the transplant centers in the United States mutually agreed to first match every kidney donor with the national patient pool, and if a patient with a six-antigen match (or 0-A,-B,-DR mismatch) was found, the kidney would be shipped to that recipient. As of 1992, more than 1,200 kidneys have been shipped through this program. The 1-year graft survival rate was 90%, and the 2-year survival was 87%, which was significantly higher than the 81% 1-year and the 76% 2-year graft survival of the control transplants (Fig. 3-8). Most important, the projected 5-year graft survival is markedly different for the six-antigen–matched (or 0-A,-B,-DR mismatched) transplants as compared to the controls. The projected half-life for these shared kidneys is 19.4 years, which is similar to the 20-year half life for 2-haplotype–matched sibling donors.

Second Transplants

For patients receiving second cadaveric transplants, a similar benefit of matching can be shown. Overall, survival rates of second transplants are 5–10% lower than for first transplants. Recipients of second cadaveric transplants whose first transplant functioned for more than a year, however, may have a chance of success not significantly different than for first cadaveric transplant recipients. If the first transplant was lost within the first 3 months, however, the 1-year graft survival is lower than 70%. This second transplant phenomenon provides a powerful incentive for the optimization of first transplant results.

HLA matching may be more important in second and multiple grafts than in first grafts. Sensitization may occur after a failed allograft, making a regraft more difficult. Repeat mismatches for HLA-

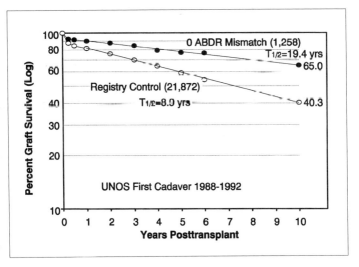

Fig. 3-8. Improved short- and long-term graft survival for six-antigen–matched (0-A, -B, -DR mismatched) kidneys shared through the United Network for Organ Sharing.

DR are deleterious to second grafts, whereas repeat mismatches for HLA-A and -B are not. Thus, some authors have suggested that repeat HLA-DR mismatches should be avoided in subsequent transplants. The overall degree of HLA-A, -B, and -DR mismatching correlates well with second and multiple allograft outcomes.

Transfusion Effect

In the mid-1970s it was recognized that patients who had received random blood transfusions had a greater chance of long-term graft function, with their 1-year graft survival rate being 10–15% better than that of nontransfused patients. This transfusion effect was cumulative, although most of the benefit was achieved with a single transfusion. The recognition of the benefit of transfusions led most programs to institute transfusion protocols whereby patients were transfused with bank blood prior to being placed on the transplant waiting list.

The mechanism of the benefit of transfusion has not been fully explained. Many patients develop cytotoxic antibodies that limit their donor options but may also exclude potentially incompatible donors. The transfusions may reduce the number of cytotoxic T cell precursors and induce suppressor cell mechanisms, producing a degree of nonspecific tolerance (see Chap. 2).

It is fortunate that the popularity of pretransplant transfusion protocols largely predated the human immunodeficiency virus (HIV) epidemic. With the advent of cyclosporine, the benefit of transfusions has been more difficult to demonstrate. Some transplant programs still prefer that their patients receive one or two transfusions prior to placement on the cadaveric list. The antipathy toward pretransplant transfusions is understandable because of the fear of HIV infection, hepatitis, and the induction of high levels of PRAs.

Center Effect

Not all transplant centers report similar results, and overall transplant statistics are a conglomerate of results from centers with discrepant experiences. Numerous factors independent of immunosuppressive protocols or tissue typing may determine why a given center may have results better than another center or better than general experience. Results tend to be unfavorably influenced by a high proportion of older and younger patients, diabetics, blacks, retransplanted patients, and patients with high levels of PRAs. The size of a center does not seem to have an impact on results. The center "effect" refers to the differences in results among transplant centers.

Awareness of these factors is important in analyzing data from single-center reports, particularly when such data suggest benefits of therapeutic maneuvers or organ distribution criteria.

KIDNEY ALLOCATION AND DISTRIBUTION

In the ideal situation, all end-stage renal failure patients awaiting transplants would receive a well-matched organ after a short waiting time. In the United States as of 1996, more than 160,000 patients were on chronic dialysis. More than 31,000 of them were awaiting cadaveric transplants, which were being performed nationwide at a rate of about 8,300 annually. The length of the wait for an organ can vary from several months to several years, and 3–4% of patients die before a kidney becomes available.

In 1984, to address problems of inadequate supply and equitable distribution, the U.S. Congress passed the **National Organ Transplant Act,** which, among other things, provides for the establishment and operation of an **Organ Procurement and Transplantation Network (OPTN).** In 1986, UNOS was awarded the contract to develop the OPTN and to this day operates the national OPTN. The mandate to UNOS includes the improvement of cadaveric organ procurement and distribution and the development of an equitable system for access to and sharing of renal and extrarenal organs.

To operate this system, the country is divided into organ procurement regions and areas with regional **organ procurement organizations (OPOs)** operating according to agreed distribution and sharing criteria.

Distribution by ABO Blood Groups

The ABO blood group antigens behave as strong transplantation antigens, and transplantation across ABO barriers usually leads to rapid hyperacute rejection. In principle, the same criteria determine kidney distribution according to ABO as do blood transfusions with group O (the universal donor) and group AB (the universal recipient). The disproportionate increase in type O recipients who are waiting for kidney transplants (Table 3-2) mandates that blood group identity rather than blood group compatibility determine distribution of type O kidneys; type A kidneys are sometimes given to type AB recipients. In live-related transplantation, ABO compatibility is adequate.

Attempts have been made to overcome blood group barriers with plasmapheresis, blood group antibody immunoabsorption, and

Table 3-2. Percent distribution of ABO blood groups according to ethnic groups and patients on the transplant waiting list*

Blood group	White	Black	Native American	Asian	Waiting list
O	45	49	79	40	52
A	40	27	16	28	29
B	11	20	4	27	17
AB	4	4	<1	5	2
Total number					31,045

*Waiting list is compiled by the United Network for Organ Sharing research department as of January 1996.
Source: Data modified from RH Walker (ed). *Technical Manual of the American Association of Blood Banks* (11th ed). Bethesda, MD: American Association of Blood Banks, 1993. P 204.

intense immunosuppression. For the present, such techniques should be regarded as experimental, and the ABO rules must be followed compulsively in kidney distribution.

The distribution of ABO groups among different ethnic groups and potential kidney transplant recipients is noted in Table 3-2. If all ethnic groups contributed equally to the donor pool and all ethnic groups suffered end-stage renal disease in direct proportion to their frequency in the general population and equally among blood groups, then waiting times for the different ethnic groups and blood group categories would be the same. In fact, whites contribute disproportionately to the donor pool, blacks contribute disproportionately to the recipient pool, and kidney disease is more common in blacks. Overall, blood group O and B patients wait the longest for transplants.

Distribution by Human Leukocyte Matching and Waiting Time

The importance of matching in determining graft outcome is well established. The extent to which matching should determine kidney distribution remains controversial. Were matching to be given absolute priority in kidney distribution, the whole country would represent a single donor and recipient pool. Such a policy has been widely accepted for six-antigen–matched kidneys with great success. Less well-matched kidneys are presently not shared nationally, although regional sharing programs are in place in many parts of the country.

To ensure that kidneys are allocated equitably, a **"point system"** has been proposed, adapted, and recommended for use throughout the United States (Table 3-3). Most points are allocated for highly matched kidneys, with a stepwise decrement in points for less well-matched kidneys. Points are also given for time spent waiting for a kidney, for a negative crossmatch in patients with PRA levels of greater than 79%, and for young children, in whom a prolonged wait for a kidney can have a catastrophic impact on growth and development (see Chap. 14). The point system is under constant review to ensure that it remains equitable; local OPOs may obtain modifications or **variances** in the system to reflect local needs. The kidney distribution point system differs from that used for the distribution of heart and liver transplants. Generally no points are given to

Table 3-3. United Network for Organ Sharing (UNOS) system for allocation of cadaveric kidneys as of January 1996

Time waiting[a]	1 point for longest waiting period in a blood group category; fraction of a point for relative position on the list; additional 0.5 point for each additional year of waiting time		
Quality of human leuko-cyte antigen match		0-A, -B, -DR	Mismatch[b]
	7 points	1-B, -DR	Mismatch
	5 points	0-B, -DR	Mismatch
	2 points	2-B, -DR	Mismatch
Panel reactive antibody	4 points for >79% and negative crossmatch		
Pediatric recipient	3 points for age 0–11 years		
	2 points for age 11–17 years		

[a]Defined from the time a patient is activated on the UNOS computer.
[b]All 0-A, -B, -DR mismatched organs are involved in the national mandatory sharing program (see text).

reflect the medical status of the patients, and there is no **"urgent need"** category, though some OPOs have introduced variances for this purpose. The absence of medical status points reflects the fact that livers and hearts are "life-saving" organs, whereas kidney transplants improve the life of patients requiring dialysis.

Transplantation in Racial Minorities

The role of race in the success of kidney transplantation has been the subject of considerable debate. In the United States, allograft survival in black recipients tends to be approximately 10% less than for white recipients, although this experience is not uniform among transplant centers. Several factors have been proposed to explain the lower survival of black recipients, including (1) a transplant center effect, (2) noncompliance and socioeconomic factors, (3) the prevalence of hypertension in blacks, (4) evidence of stronger immune responsiveness, and (5) racial differences in cyclosporine metabolism.

Some studies also report that black patients wait longer for cadaveric kidneys than do white patients. Differences in the frequencies of ABO blood groups (see Table 3-2) and of HLA determinants (see the section on linkage disequilibrium), as well as cultural and socioeconomic factors, may affect the rate of transplantation. Racial minorities have tended to be more likely to refuse to allow the use of cadaveric organs of their relatives. As a result, whites are represented disproportionately in the organ donor pool—a phenomenon that may favor white recipients when kidneys are allocated according to the blood group and tissue matching (see the section on kidney allocation and distribution). Efforts to encourage organ donation among minorities may help redress inequalities of allocation.

Nephron Dosing

Though immunologic rejection of incompatible transplants has always been regarded as the major cause of transplant failures, it has become clear that there are also important nonimmunologic contributions to graft loss. Factors similar to those described to account for the deterioration of function of chronically diseased native kidneys are likely to be relevant to renal allografts. It has been shown that when there is a discrepancy between the anticipated size of the kidney and the weight of the patient, the long-term survival of the kidney is diminished. For instance, heavier patients and patients with greater body mass and surface area have a somewhat lower graft survival rate, kidneys from very young donors and old donors have a lower graft survival, and male into female kidneys do better than the converse. These observations are consistent with the concept that the relative "dose" of transplanted nephrons is an important determinant of function. One explanation for the higher graft survival of kidneys from unrelated living donors compared with better matched cadaveric donors is that kidneys from cadaver donors suffer inevitable damage consequent on the sudden death of the donor, thus decreasing the number of functioning nephrons transplanted.

Clinical trials will be necessary to determine if the nephron dose concept is valid, in which case it would be logical to take into account size discrepancies in organ distribution or even to transplant two kidneys in some circumstances.

SELECTED READINGS

Bodmer JG, Marsh SGE, Albert ED et al. Nomenclature for factors of the HLA system, 1994. *Hum Immunol* 41:1, 1994.

Brenner BM, Cohen RA, Milford EL. In renal transplantation one size may not fit all. *J Am Soc Nephrol* 3:162, 1992.

Feldman H, Fazio I, Roth D et al. Recipient body size and cadaveric renal allograft survival. J Am Soc Nephrol 7:151, 1996.

Gaston RS, Ayres I, Dooley LG, Diethelm AG. Racial equity in renal transplantation—the disparate impact of HLA-based allocation. *JAMA* 270:1352, 1993.

Hirata M, Terasaki PI. Regrafts. In PI Terasaki, JM Cecka (eds), *Clinical Transplants 1994*. Los Angeles: UCLA Tissue Typing Laboratory, 1995. Pp 419–433.

Lau M, Terasaki PI, Park MS. International Cell Exchange, 1994. In PI Terasaki, JM Cecka (eds), *Clinical Transplants 1994*. Los Angeles: UCLA Tissue Typing Laboratory, 1995. Pp 467–488.

Lazda VA. Identification of patients at risk for inferior renal allograft outcome by a strongly positive B cell flow cytometry crossmatch. *Transplantation* 57:964, 1994.

Ogura K, Terasaki PI, Johnson C et al. The significance of a positive flow cytometry crossmatch test in primary kidney transplantation. *Transplantation* 56:294, 1994.

Opelz G, Mytilineos J, Scherer S et al. Analysis of HLA-DR matching in DNA-typed cadaver kidney transplants. *Transplantation* 55:782, 1993.

Rodey GE, Fuller TC. Public epitopes and the antigenic structure of the HLA molecules. *CRC Crit Rev Immunol* 7:229, 1987.

Takemoto S, Terasaki PI, Gjertson DW, Cecka JM. Equitable allocation of HLA compatible kidneys for local pools and for minorities. *N Engl J Med* 331:760, 1994.

Terasaki PI, Cecka JM, Gjertson DW et al. High survival rates from spousal and living unrelated donors. *N Engl J Med* 33:333, 1995.

4

Immunosuppressive Medications and Protocols for Kidney Transplantation

Gabriel M. Danovitch

The excellent results of kidney and other solid organ transplants that led to widespread acceptance of these procedures in the 1980s were achieved with a relatively limited therapeutic armamentarium. This consisted of only four major drugs or drug groups: corticosteroids, azathioprine, cyclosporine, and the monoclonal and polyclonal antibodies. Part I of this chapter reviews each of these drugs, emphasizing cyclosporine and the antibody preparations, which are the least familiar to medical practitioners. Part II reviews the features of a new generation of immunosuppressive agents, some of which have been introduced into clinical practice and some of which have not yet crossed the clinical threshold. Protocol guidelines for combination therapy are discussed in Part III.

Part I: Conventional Immunosuppressive Agents

CYCLOSPORINE

Cyclosporine (available in two forms—**Sandimmune** and the newer microemulsion **Neoral**) is a small cyclic polypeptide of fungal origin. It consists of 11 amino acids and has a molecular weight of 1,203. It is neutral and insoluble in water but soluble in organic solvents and lipids. The amino acids at positions 11, 1, 2, and 3 form the active immunosuppressive site, and the cyclic structure of the drug is necessary for its immunosuppressive effect.

Mechanism of Action

Cyclosporine differs from its predecessor immunosuppressor drugs by virtue of its selective inhibition of the immune response. It does not inhibit neutrophilic phagocytic activity as do corticosteroids, nor is it myelosuppressive as azathioprine is. Cell surface events and antigen recognition also remain intact (see Chap. 2). The immunosuppressive effect of cyclosporine depends on the formation of a complex with its cytoplasmic receptor protein **cyclophilin** (see Chap. 2, Fig. 2-4). This complex binds with **calcineurin**, whose normal function is to act as a phosphatase that dephosphorylates certain nuclear regulatory proteins (e.g., **nuclear factor of activated T cells**) and hence facilitates their passage through the nuclear membrane. Inhibition of calcineurin thereby impairs the expression of several critical T cell activation genes, including those for interleukin-2 (IL-2) and its receptor and the proto-oncogenes H-*ras* and c-*myc*. The importance of these factors in T cell activation is discussed in more detail in Chap. 2. Cyclosporine also enhances the expression of **transforming growth factor-beta (TGF-β)**, which also inhibits IL-2 and the generation of cytotoxic T lymphocytes, and may be implicated in the development of the interstitial fibrosis, which is an important feature of cyclosporine toxicity (see the section on cyclosporine's side effects). The mechanism of action of cyclosporine is very similar to that of tacrolimus (see the section on tacrolimus and Plate 1).

Patients receiving successful cyclosporine-based immunosuppression maintain a degree of immune responsiveness that is still sufficient to maintain host defenses. This relative immunosuppression may be a reflection of the fact that at therapeutic levels of cyclosporine, calcineurin activity is reduced by only approximately 50%, permitting strong signals to trigger cytokine expression and generate an effective immune response. The degree of inhibition of calcineurin may be at the fulcrum of the delicate balance that exists between over- and underimmunosuppression.

Pharmacokinetics

Oral cyclosporine is currently available in two forms: a 100 mg/ml solution that is drawn up by the patient into a graduated syringe and dispensed into orange juice or milk, or 25-mg and 100-mg soft gelatin capsules. Patients usually prefer the convenience of the capsule. The absorption of Sandimmune cyclosporine from the GI tract is incomplete and variable. The time to peak concentration is variable but averages 4 hours. A substantial proportion of transplant patients exhibit a second peak. Compared to IV infusion, the bioavailability of the orally administered drug is in the range of 30–45%. Conversion between the oral and IV forms of the drug perioperatively requires a 3:1 dose ratio. Bioavailability of oral cyclosporine increases with time, possibly due to improved absorption by the previously uremic GI tract. As a result, the amount of cyclosporine required to achieve a given blood level tends to fall with time and typically reaches a steady level within 4–8 weeks. Oral absorption is bile-dependent and may be unreliable in patients with diabetic gastroparesis, diarrhea, biliary diversion, cholestasis, and malabsorption. Eating tends to enhance the absorption of cyclosporine.

Neoral is a formulation of cyclosporine that incorporates the drug in a microemulsion. Studies in humans suggest improved bioavailability and less variability in cyclosporine pharmacokinetics with this formulation compared with Sandimmune. Peak cyclosporine levels are higher, and the trough concentration correlates better with the systemic exposure, as reflected by the **area under the curve** (**AUC;** see below). The improved GI absorption of the microemulsion and lesser dependence on bile for absorption may reduce the necessity for IV cyclosporine administration. The microemulsion may be particularly useful for patients with impaired GI absorption. There may be a reduction of up to 15% in the incidence of acute rejection with the microemulsion, and the dose required to achieve an equivalent trough level may be reduced by approximately 10%. Double-blinded studies are in progress in the United States and Europe to determine if the new formulation offers measurable clinical advantages.

Distribution and Metabolism

In the blood, one-third of absorbed and infused cyclosporine is found in plasma, bound primarily to lipoproteins. Most of the remaining drug is bound to erythrocytes. Whole blood drug levels (see the section on drug monitoring) will thus typically be threefold higher than plasma levels. The binding of cyclosporine to lipoproteins may be important in the transfer of the drug through plasma membranes, and the toxic effects of cyclosporine may be exaggerated by low cholesterol levels and reduced by high cholesterol levels. Cyclosporine is found in higher concentrations in the liver, fat, and pancreas than in blood and other tissues.

The parent drug has a half-life of approximately 8 hours and is metabolized to at least 25 metabolites by the cytochrome P450 IIIA found in the GI and liver microsomal enzyme system. GI metabolism produces a so-called first-pass metabolism of cyclosporine, and the heterogeneity in intestinal cytochrome P450 IIIA gene expression may explain some of the wide interpatient variability in cyclosporine kinetics. The most important site of metabolism is in the liver. Some of the metabolites may have immunosuppressive and nephrotoxic potential, and the plasma levels of the most important metabolite, M17, may be similar to that of the parent compound. The ratio of circulating cyclosporines to the parent compound is approximately 3:1. Cyclosporine is excreted in the bile, with minimal renal excretion such that drug doses do not need to be modified in the presence of kidney dysfunction. Cyclosporine is not significantly dialyzed and can be administered during dialysis treatment without dose adjustment. The pharmacokinetic parameters of cyclosporine may vary among patient groups, and these variations may have clinical consequences. For example, cyclosporine clearance is higher in children and in black transplant recipients, both of whom may require relatively larger doses and short dosage intervals. Longer dosage intervals may be required in older patients and in the presence of liver disease.

Cyclosporine Monitoring

The measurement of cyclosporine levels is an intrinsic part of the management of transplant patients because of the variation in its metabolism in individual patients and from patient to patient. There is also a relationship, albeit an inconsistent one, between blood levels of the drug and episodes of rejection and toxicity. Cyclosporine level monitoring is the source of much confusion because of the various assays available and the option of using different matrices (i.e., plasma or whole blood) for its measurement.

The trough level of cyclosporine rather than the peak level is measured (drawn immediately preceding the next dose) because its timing is more consistent and it may correlate better with toxic complications. More sophisticated techniques of monitoring have been suggested whereby a pharmacokinetic profile is constructed to calculate the AUC, which reflects the bioavailability of the drug and may theoretically allow for more precise and individualized patient management. Although attractive, these techniques have not proved popular because of their cost and inconvenience. Most centers continue to rely on trough levels.

Cyclosporine concentrations can be measured in serum, plasma, or whole blood. Whole blood levels are used in most centers because the plasma levels are temperature-dependent. The clinician cannot begin to assess the significance of a cyclosporine level without knowing what kind of assay is being used. The **high-performance**

liquid chromatography assay (HPLC) is the most specific method for measuring unmetabolized parent cyclosporine. HPLC, however, is expensive, difficult to run, and may vary between centers. The **INCSTAR** technique employs a cyclosporine parent-compound–specific **radioimmunoassay (RIA)** and produces values similar to the HPLC. The Abbot **TDx fluorescence polarization assay (FPIA)** has become popular and widely used because it is a rapid, technically simple, consistent assay. Two forms of this assay are available; it is very important to differentiate between them. The **polyclonal assay** employs antisera that measure both parent compound and metabolites; the **monoclonal assay** employs an antiserum that is designed to be parent-compound–specific (in fact, it overestimates the HPLC value by up to 25% in kidney transplant recipients). A monoclonal **enzyme immunoassay (EMIT)** is probably more specific than the monoclonal TDx assay but is not yet available in the United States. Target cyclosporine levels are discussed in the section on immunosuppressive protocols.

Drug Interactions

The interaction of cyclosporine with many commonly used drugs demands constant attention to drug regimens and cognizance of potential interactions. New drugs should be introduced with care, and patients should be warned to consult physicians familiar with cyclosporine before considering new pharmacologic therapy.

Drugs That Decrease Cyclosporine Concentration by Induction of P450 Activity

Antituberculous Drugs. Both **rifampin** and **isoniazid (INH)** markedly reduce cyclosporine levels, and it may be difficult to achieve therapeutic levels of cyclosporine in patients on rifampin, whose use should be avoided if at all possible. INH can be used with careful drug-level monitoring and dosage adjustment and is the preferred drug for tuberculosis prophylaxis if this proves essential (see Chap. 10).

Anticonvulsants. Barbiturates reduce cyclosporine levels to such an extent that their concomitant use with cyclosporine may not be possible. **Phenytoin** reduces levels but should be used with care. The average requirement for cyclosporine is approximately doubled in patients receiving phenytoin. **Carbamazepine** may also decrease cyclosporine levels, but the effect is less pronounced. Benzodiazepines and valproic acid do not affect cyclosporine levels, but the latter drug has been associated with hepatotoxicity. Patients who are receiving anticonvulsants prior to transplantation should have a neurologic assessment with a view to discontinuing them where possible.

Antibiotics. Nafcillin, IV trimethoprim, IV sulfadimidine, imipenem, and cephalosporins have been described to reduce cyclosporine levels in isolated reports. Their use requires careful monitoring.

Prolonged Use. If prolonged use of a drug that induces P450 activity is required, addition of a drug that inhibits or competes with the P450 system (e.g., diltiazem, fluconazole) may facilitate the achievement of therapeutic cyclosporine levels.

Drugs That Increase Cyclosporine Levels by Inhibition of P450 or by Competition for Its Pathways

Calcium Channel Blockers. **Verapamil, diltiazem,** and **nicardipine** may significantly increase cyclosporine levels. Other renal and hemodynamic effects of these drugs may justify their use as adjuncts to the immunosuppressive regimen. Their use may safely permit a reduction in the cyclosporine dose of up to 40%. Careful monitoring of drug levels is required when these calcium channel blockers are used for the management of hypertension or heart disease, and patients should be specifically warned that changing the dosage of these drugs is equivalent to changing the dosage of cyclosporine. Brand name and generic forms of these drugs (Cardizem and Dilacor are both forms of diltiazem) may have a different impact on cyclosporine levels. Calcium channel blockers of the dihydropyrimine group (e.g., nifedipine, isradipine, amlodipine, felodipine) have similar hemodynamic effects but have minimal impact on cyclosporine levels.

Antifungal Agents. **Ketoconazole, fluconazole,** and **itraconazole** markedly elevate cyclosporine levels. The interaction of cyclosporine with ketoconazole is a particularly potent one, which may permit a safe reduction in the cyclosporine dose of up to 80%. The combined use of ketoconazole with cyclosporine has been proposed as a cost-saving measure. Great care must be taken when stopping and starting these antifungals. An important interaction between ketoconazole and histamine blockers also has been described. The effective reabsorption of ketoconazole from the GI tract requires acidic gastric contents, and the addition of an H_2-receptor antagonist may reduce its absorption and thus indirectly produce a clinically significant fall in cyclosporine levels.

Antibiotics. **Erythromycin,** even in low doses, may increase cyclosporine levels and induce episodes of graft dysfunction both by impairing cyclosporine metabolism and increasing its oral absorption. Other macrolide antibiotics (e.g., josamycin, ponsinomycin) may also increase cyclosporine levels. Since erythromycin is prescribed so ubiquitously, physicians, dentists, and patients should be warned about this interaction.

Histamine Blockers. There are conflicting reports regarding the use of cimetidine, ranitidine, and omeprazole with cyclosporine. Cimetidine was initially reported to increase cyclosporine levels, but this effect has not been substantiated. These drugs may increase creatinine levels without reducing the glomerular filtration rate (GFR) by suppressing proximal tubular creatinine secretion. There may be increased hepatotoxicity when ranitidine and cyclosporine are used in combination. The interaction between H_2-receptor antagonists and ketoconazole has been noted above (see the section on antifungals).

Hormones. Corticosteroids in high and low doses may increase cyclosporine levels by decreasing the clearance of cyclosporine metabolites. This effect may be particularly pronounced during "pulse" steroid therapy and may suggest a confusing picture of nephrotoxicity. In this circumstance, it is the cyclosporine levels as measured by nonspecific assay that rise and not levels of the parent compound so that dose modification may not be required. Oral contraceptives, anabolic steroids, testosterone, and norethisterone may also increase cyclosporine levels.

Drugs That May Exaggerate Cyclosporine Nephrotoxicity

Any potentially nephrotoxic drug should be used with caution in combination with cyclosporine, since the vasoconstrictive effect of the drug tends to potentiate other nephrotoxic mechanisms. Well-substantiated enhanced renal impairment has been described when cyclosporine has been used in combination with **amphotericin** and **aminoglycosides**, and renal impairment may occur earlier than anticipated. **Nonsteroidal anti-inflammatory drugs** should be avoided if at all possible. Cyclosporine may potentiate the hemodynamic renal dysfunction seen with **enalapril** and other angiotensin-converting enzyme inhibitors. **Metoclopramide** may increase cyclosporine levels by increasing its intestinal reabsorption. A syndrome of diarrhea, hepatopathy, and renal dysfunction has been ascribed to the interaction between cyclosporine and **colchicine**, particularly when given to patients with familial Mediterranean fever. Occasional cases of enhanced cyclosporine nephrotoxicity have been described when the drug has been used in combination with ciprofloxacin and trimethoprim-sulfamethoxazole.

Lipid-Lowering Agents

Cholestyramine may interfere with cyclosporine absorption from the GI tract. The HMGCoase inhibitor **lovastatin** has been implicated in several cases of acute renal failure. When used in full doses in combination with cyclosporine, lovastatin may cause rhabdomyolysis with elevated creatine phosphokinase levels and acute renal failure. Myopathy alone has been observed in 30% of recipients of the lovastatin-cyclosporine combination, with symptoms of muscle pain and tenderness developing 6 weeks to 16 months following commencement of therapy. The myopathic syndrome has not been observed when lovastatin is used in a daily dose of 20 mg or less. Even this dose should be used with caution, however, and patients should be made aware of the potential interaction. The newer HMGCoase inhibitors pravastatin and simvastatin have not been described to produce this interaction.

Side Effects
Nephrotoxicity

Nephrotoxicity is the most important side effect of cyclosporine use and is the major "thorn in the side" of this remarkable drug. It is probably not coincidental that the two most powerful immunosuppressants in clinical practice, cyclosporine and tacrolimus (see the section on new immunosuppressant agents), have similar modes of immunosuppressant action and similar clinical and pathologic patterns of nephrotoxicity. Theories linking the mechanism of immunosuppression and nephrotoxicity are discussed below. The term cyclosporine nephrotoxicity is often used loosely, and it is important to note that the term encompasses several distinct, overlapping syndromes (Table 4-1) produced by both functional and morphologic changes within the allograft.

Table 4-1. Syndromes of cyclosporine nephrotoxicity

Exaggeration of early post-transplant graft dysfunction
Acute reversible decrease in GFR
Acute microvascular disease
Chronic nonprogressive decrease in GFR
Chronic progressive decrease in GFR
Hypertension and electrolyte abnormalities
    Hyperkalemia
    Hypomagnesemia
    Hyperchloremic acidosis
    Hyperuricemia

GFR = glomerular filtration rate.

Functional Decrease in Renal Blood Flow and Filtration Rate.
Cyclosporine produces a dose-related, reversible renal vasoconstriction that particularly affects the afferent arteriole (Fig. 4-1). The glomerular capillary ultrafiltration coefficient (Kf) also falls, possibly due to increased mesangial cell contractility. The picture is reminiscent of "prerenal" dysfunction, and in the acute phase, tubular function is intact.

The normal regulation of the glomerular microcirculation depends on a balance between calcium-mediated vasoconstriction offset by vasodilatatory eicosinoids. Cyclosporine vasoconstriction is due, at least in part, to the alteration of arachidonic acid metabolism in favor of the vasoconstrictor thromboxane. Cyclosporine is also a potential inducer of the powerful vasoconstrictor endothelin, and circulating endothelin levels are elevated in its presence. Cyclosporine-induced changes in glomerular hemodynamics can be reversed by specific endothelin inhibitors and by antiendothelin antibodies. Cyclosporine also impairs the endothelial production of vasodilatatory nitric oxide.

Cyclosporine-induced renal vasoconstriction may manifest itself clinically as delayed recovery of early malfunctioning grafts or as transient, reversible, dose-dependent and blood level–dependent elevation in serum creatinine concentration that may be difficult to distinguish from other causes of graft dysfunction. Vasoconstriction may be a reversible component of chronic cyclosporine toxicity, which may amplify the functional severity of the chronic histologic changes seen with prolonged use. The vasoconstriction also helps account for the hypertension and tendency for sodium retention that are so frequent with cyclosporine.

Chronic Interstitial Fibrosis. Interstitial fibrosis, which may be patchy or "striped" and associated with arteriolar lesions (see Chap. 12) is a frequent feature of long-term cyclosporine use. The capacity of this lesion to progress to end-stage renal failure, first described in recipients of cardiac transplants, together with the tendency of other chronic renal diseases to progress inexorably, initially led to fears that the great benefits of cyclosporine with respect to early graft function would be abrogated by progressive deterioration in function and graft loss. Fortunately, several long-term studies have shown that in the dose regimens currently employed, kidney function may remain stable, although often

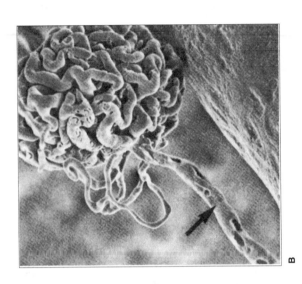

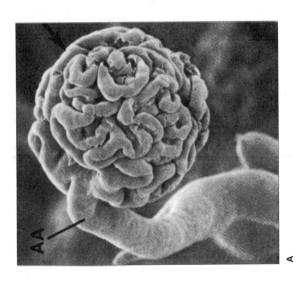

Fig. 4-1. Cyclosporine-induced afferent arteriolar vasoconstriction. A. Control rat showing afferent arteriole (AA) and glomerular tuft. B. Constricted afferent arteriole (arrow) and glomerular tuft after 14 days of cyclosporine at 50 mg/kg/day. (From J English et al. *Clin Res* 34:594A, 1986.)

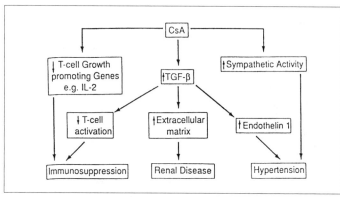

Fig. 4-2. Potential sequelae of cyclosporine-mediated augmentation of TGF-β expression. In this schema of events, the cyclosporine-associated increase in TGF-β expression is hypothesized to contribute to the following: immunosuppression (since TGF-β can prevent T cell activation and generation of cytotoxic T cells); renal interstitial fibrosis (since TGF-β can enhance extracellular matrix accumulation); and hypertension (since TGF-β can increase endothelin production by vascular smooth muscle cells). In this formulation, TGF-β represents the mechanistic link for the clinically desirable (immunosuppression) and deleterious (hypertension, fibrosis) consequences of cyclosporine use. (From A Khanna, B Li, KH Stenzel et al. Demonstration of a transforming growth factor β-dependent mechanism of inhibition of cell growth. *Transplantation* 57:577, 1994.)

impaired, for many years. The mechanism of cyclosporine-induced interstitial fibrosis remains poorly defined. Evidence from experimental models suggests that chronic nephropathy involves an angiotensin-dependent upregulation of molecules that are important in the scarring process, such as TGF-β and osteopontin. Cyclosporine has been shown to enhance the production of TGF-β in normal T cells (see the section on cyclosporine's mechanism of action), and this finding may provide the link between the immunosuppressive effects of cyclosporine and its nephrotoxicity (Fig. 4-2). Interstitial fibrosis may be a reflection of intense and prolonged vasoconstriction of the renal microcirculation. Cyclosporine may also impair the regenerative capacity of microvascular endothelial cells. The resulting chronic renal ischemia may enhance the synthesis and accumulation of extracellular matrix proteins in the interstitium.

Acute Microvascular Disease. Thrombotic microangiopathy (see Chap. 12 for pathology and Chap. 8 for clinical presentation and management) is an uncommon yet distinct form of cyclosporine vascular toxicity that may result from a direct toxic effect of cyclosporine on vascular endothelium, possibly by interfering with the generation of endothelial prostacyclin. It produces a syndrome reminiscent of the hemolytic uremic syndrome that is typically associated with a poor prognosis for graft survival. Clinically, it may be difficult to recognize and differentiate from acute vascular rejection.

Electrolyte Abnormalities.   Impaired sodium excretion is a reflection of the vasoconstrictive effect of cyclosporine and is not a manifestation of a tubular abnormality. Patients on long-term cyclosporine therapy tend to be hypertensive (see Chap. 9) and to retain fluid. Studies have shown activation of the renin-angiotensin-aldosterone system and suppression of atrial natriuretic factor, which results in attenuation of the natriuretic and diuretic response to an acute volume load. Mild **hyperkalemia** is very common and will occasionally require treatment, although it is rarely life-threatening as long as kidney function remains good. Hyperkalemia is often associated with a mild **hyperchloremic acidosis** with an intact capacity to excrete acid urine. The clinical picture is thus reminiscent of type IV renal tubular acidosis. Patients receiving cyclosporine may have an impaired capacity to excrete an acute potassium load, and there is evidence to suggest impaired production of aldosterone, an acquired impaired renal response to its action, and inhibition of cortical collecting duct potassium secretory channels. Hyperkalemia may be exaggerated by concomitant administration of beta blockers and angiotensin-converting enzyme inhibitors.

Cyclosporine is magnesuric, and **hypomagnesemia** is commonly concomitant with its use. In liver transplantation, hypomagnesemia may predispose patients to seizures, although this has not been observed in kidney allograft recipients. Magnesium supplements are often prescribed but may be ineffective due to a lowered renal magnesium threshold (see Chap. 17).

Methods of Amelioration.   The vexing issue of cyclosporine nephrotoxicity has spawned a variety of clinical and experimental approaches designed to modify the renal effects of the drug and particularly its capacity to produce vasoconstriction. Low-dose dopamine is used in some centers in the early postoperative period to "encourage" urine output. Various calcium channel blockers given both to the donor (see Chap. 5) and the recipient (see the section on adjunctive immunosuppressant agents) may reduce the incidence and severity of delayed graft function. Omega-3 fatty acids in the form of 6 g of fish oil each day were initially thought to increase renal blood flow and glomerular filtration rate (GFR) by reversing the cyclosporine-induced imbalance between the synthesis of vasodilator and vasoconstrictor prostaglandins, but long-term studies have shown no such benefit. The prostaglandin agonist misoprostol and thromboxane synthetase inhibitors may have a similar effect. Various protocol adjustments discussed later in this chapter may also be employed to minimize cyclosporine toxicity.

Nonrenal Cyclosporine Toxicity

Hepatotoxicity.   Episodes of hepatic dysfunction typically manifesting as subclinical, mild, self-limiting, dose-dependent elevations of serum aminotransferase levels with mild hyperbilirubinemia may occur in nearly half of all kidney transplant recipients on cyclosporine. Cyclosporine does not itself produce progressive liver disease; other diagnoses, most frequently one of the viral hepatitides, need to be considered when this occurs.

No specific hepatic histologic lesion has been described in humans, and the hyperbilirubinemia is a reflection of disturbed bile secretion rather than hepatocellular damage. In the presence of hepatic dysfunction, assays for the parent compound should be used in monitoring drug dosage. Cyclosporine therapy is associated with an increased incidence of **cholelithiasis** presumably due to an increased lithogenicity of cyclosporine-containing bile. Acute pancreatitis may occur in kidney transplant recipients but is not more common in those receiving cyclosporine.

Cosmetic Complications.   The cosmetic complications of cyclosporine, although not severe in a strict medical sense, must be treated seriously, particularly in women and adolescents, because of the misery they can produce and the temptation to resolve them through noncompliant behavior. Cosmetic complications are often exaggerated by concomitant use of corticosteroids.

Hypertrichosis in various degrees occurs in nearly all patients receiving cyclosporine and is particularly obvious in dark-haired girls and women. A coarsening of facial features is observed in children and young adults, with thickening of the skin and prominence of the brow. **Gingival hyperplasia** may develop and is exaggerated by poor dental hygiene and possibly by concomitant use of calcium channel blockers. Azithromycin, a macrolide antibiotic that does not affect cyclosporine metabolism, may reduce gingival hyperplasia. Gingivectomy may occasionally be indicated. Cosmetic complications tend to become less prominent with time. Sympathetic cosmetic counseling is required.

Hyperlipidemia and Glucose Intolerance.   Cyclosporine has been implicated as one of the various factors responsible for the generation of post-transplant hypercholesterolemia (see Chap. 9). The mechanism of this effect is not well-understood and may be related to abnormal low-density lipoprotein feedback control by the liver or to altered bile acid synthesis. Cyclosporine may also influence lipid metabolism by impairment of glucose tolerance through interference with the peripheral actions of insulin or by a direct toxic effect on pancreatic beta cells.

Neurologic Complications.   A spectrum of neurologic complications has been observed in patients receiving cyclosporine. Coarse **tremor** and dysesthesias are common and may be dose-related. More severe complications are uncommon in kidney recipients, although isolated seizures may occur in 1–2% of patients, and full-blown encephalopathy has been described. Patients receiving Neoral cyclosporine may complain of **headache** 1–2 hours after taking the drug, presumably due to high peak levels. Patients receiving cyclosporine may complain of **bone pain**.

Immunologic and Infectious Complications.   Despite cyclosporine's potency as an immunosuppressive agent, the incidence of infections and malignancy is not more common in patients receiving cyclosporine than in patients immunosuppressed with azathioprine alone, as long as it is prescribed within standard guidelines. The distribution of types of malignancies may be somewhat different (see Chap. 9), and bacterial and fungal infections may, in fact, be less common, possibly because of some intrinsic antifungal qualities of the drug and because of a diminished requirement for steroid use.

Hematologic Complications.   In vitro, cyclosporine increases adenosine diphosphate–induced platelet aggregation, thromboplastin generation, and factor VII activity. It also reduces production of endothelial prostacyclin. These findings may be causally related to the increased incidence of **thromboembolic events** that have been observed in cyclosporine-treated kidney transplant recipients. Renal artery and vein thrombosis and deep vein thrombosis have been described, although it may be difficult to clearly ascribe responsibility for these events to cyclosporine. Cyclosporine treatment may be associated with enhanced hemostasis and reduced thrombolysis in the early years following transplantation. All these factors may be related to the arteriolopathy commonly seen as part of chronic cyclosporine toxicity and the less common glomerular thrombi and hemolytic-uremic syndrome.

Hyperuricemia and Gout. Hyperuricemia, due to reduced renal uric acid clearance, is a common complication of cyclosporine therapy, particularly when diuretics are also employed. Episodes of gout have been reported in up to 7% of patients, and treatment requires great care. Nonsteroidal anti-inflammatory drugs should be avoided if at all possible. Allopurinol potentiates azathioprine myelosuppression (see the section on azathioprine); dose reduction and careful monitoring of the white blood cell count is required.

CORTICOSTEROIDS

Corticosteroids have commanded a central position in clinical transplantation since they were first used to treat rejection more than 30 years ago. Despite this long experience, there remains only a general consensus as to their best therapeutic use, and changing protocols often reflect both fear of prescribing them and fear of not prescribing them. It is hoped that the new generation of immunosuppressants will permit avoidance or withdrawal of corticosteroids for the majority of patients, although this point has not yet been reached.

The diffuse effects of corticosteroids on the body reflect the fact that most mammalian tissues have glucocorticoid receptors within the cell cytoplasm and can serve as targets for the effects of corticosteroids. The immunosuppressive actions of corticosteroids can be somewhat simplistically divided into their specific actions on macrophages and T cells and their broad, nonspecific immunosuppressant and anti-inflammatory actions.

Mechanism of Action

Blockade of Cytokine Gene Expression

Glucocorticoids exert their most important immunosuppressive effect by blocking the expression of several cytokine genes. They are hydrophobic and can diffuse intracellularly, where they bind to cytoplasmic receptors found in association with the 90-kDa heat shock protein. As a result, the heat shock protein becomes dissociated, and the steroid-receptor complex translocates to the nucleus, where it binds to DNA sequences referred to as **glucocorticoid response elements (GREs)**. GRE sequences have been found in the critical promoter regions of several cytokine genes, and it is presumed that the binding of the steroid-receptor complex to the GRE inhibits the transcription of cytokine genes.

Glucocorticoids inhibit the expression of IL-1, -2, -3, -6; tumor necrosis factor-alpha, and gamma-interferon. The blockade of IL-1 and IL-6 gene expression by antigen-presenting cells is particularly

Table 4-2. Side effects of corticosteroids

Cushingoid facies and habitus
Susceptibility to infection
Impaired wound healing
Growth suppression in children
Osteoporosis
Aseptic necrosis of bone
Cataracts
Glucose intolerance
Fluid retention and hypertension
Emotional lability and insomnia
Manic and depressive psychosis
Gastritis and peptic ulcer disease
Hyperlipidemia
Polyphagia and obesity
Acne

important, since these cytokines provide critical costimuli for IL-2 expression by activated T cells. Thus, IL-2 expression (the particular importance of which is discussed in Chap. 2) is blocked both directly and indirectly. IL-1 was previously called endogenous pyrogen and is responsible for the fever often associated with acute rejection. This fever typically resolves rapidly when high-dose corticosteroids are administered.

Nonspecific Immunosuppressive Effects

Glucocorticoids cause a lymphopenia that is due to the redistribution of lymphocytes from the vascular compartment back to lymphoid tissue. The migration of monocytes to sites of inflammation is also inhibited. Steroids block the synthesis, release, and action of series of chemotactants, permeability-increasing agents, and vasodilators, although these anti-inflammatory effects are a relatively minor aspect of their efficacy in the prevention and treatment of acute rejection. The total white cell count may rise several fold during high-dose steroid administration.

Complications

The ubiquitous complications of corticosteroids are familiar to medical practitioners and are not reviewed here in detail. Table 4-2 serves as a reminder of their major side effects. There is marked variation in individual response to these drugs, presumably due to the varied concentration of tissue steroid receptors and individual variations in prednisone metabolism. In the dose regimens currently prescribed, untoward complications can be minimized but not totally prevented. High-maintenance dose protocols of steroids sometimes used for collagen vascular disease and vasculitides are unnecessary and contraindicated in kidney transplantation.

Commonly Used Preparations

In clinical transplantation, steroids are used in several different ways: as a high-dose IV or oral **pulse** given over 3–5 days, as a steroid **cycle** with a gradually decreasing oral dose, or **taper,** over days or weeks, or as a steady low-dose daily or every-other-day **maintenance** regimen. Corticosteroid dosage is discussed in the protocol section.

Prednisolone, its 11-keto metabolite **prednisone**, and **methyl-prednisolone** (Solu-Medrol) are the corticosteroid preparations most commonly used in clinical transplantation. Prednisolone is the most active circulating immunosuppressive corticosteroid. Prednisone is the oral preparation usually used in the United States, whereas prednisolone is often preferred in Europe. Methylprednisolone is the most commonly used IV corticosteroid. These preparations have a half-life that is measured in hours, but their capacity to inhibit lymphokine production persists for 24 hours so that once-daily administration is adequate.

Corticosteroids are metabolized by hepatic microsomal enzyme systems. Drugs such as phenytoin, barbiturates, and rifampin, which induce these enzymes, may lower plasma prednisolone levels, whereas oral contraceptives and ketoconazole increase levels. Unfortunately, there is no readily available plasma prednisolone assay for clinical use, although empirical adjustments in dose may be advisable when potentially interacting drugs are administered.

AZATHIOPRINE

Azathioprine (Imuran) is an antimetabolite, an imidazole derivative of 6-mercaptopurine. It has been used in clinical transplantation for nearly 30 years. With the availability of cyclosporine, the role of azathioprine has been relegated to that of an adjunctive agent in most circumstances (see the section on protocol), and when the new generation of immunosuppressants are introduced, it is likely azathioprine use will be discontinued altogether.

Mode of Action

Azathioprine is a purine analogue that is incorporated into cellular DNA, where it inhibits purine nucleotide synthesis and interferes with the synthesis and metabolism of RNA. Unlike cyclosporine, it does not prevent gene activation, but it inhibits gene replication and consequent T cell activation.

Azathioprine is a broad myelocyte suppressant. It inhibits the proliferation of promyelocytes in the bone marrow, and as a result, it decreases the number of circulatory monocytes capable of differentiating into macrophages. Thus, it is a powerful inhibitor of the primary immune response and is valuable in preventing the onset of acute rejection. It is not effective in the therapy of rejection episodes themselves.

Side Effects

The most important side effects of azathioprine are hematologic (Table 4-3). Patients first receiving the drug, particularly in higher dosages (2 mg/kg or more), should have complete blood counts performed, including a platelet count, at least weekly during the first month of therapy and less frequently thereafter. Delayed hematologic suppression may occur. In the event of significant thrombocytopenia or leukopenia, the drug can be discontinued for long periods if the patient is also on cyclosporine without great danger of inducing acute rejection. If discontinuation for more than 2–3 days is

Table 4-3. Side effects of azathioprine

Bone marrow suppression
  Leukopenia
  Thrombocytopenia
  Macrocytic anemia
Susceptibility to infection
Susceptibility to neoplasia
Hepatotoxicity
Nausea and vomiting
Alopecia
Pancreatitis
Allopurinol interaction

required in a patient who is receiving the drug alone, the introduction of cyclosporine should be considered. It is not necessary to maintain a low white cell count for the drug to be an effective immunosuppressant. The white count should be monitored with particular care when corticosteroid dose is reduced or discontinued.

Azathioprine may occasionally cause hepatitis and cholestasis, which usually present as reversible elevations in transaminase and bilirubin levels. Azathioprine dose is usually reduced or stopped during episodes of significant hepatic dysfunction. Pancreatitis is a rare complication.

Azathioprine is converted to inactive 6-thiouric acid by xanthine oxidase. The inhibition of this enzyme by allopurinol demands that this drug combination be avoided or used with great care. When allopurinol is commenced, the azathioprine dose should be reduced to 25–50% of its initial level, and the white count and platelet count frequently monitored.

Dose and Administration

Approximately 50% of orally administered azathioprine is absorbed so that the IV dose is equivalent to half of the oral dose. Blood levels are not valuable clinically, since its effectiveness is not blood level–dependent. The drug is not significantly dialyzed or excreted by the kidney. Dose reduction is often practiced during kidney dysfunction, although it may not be necessary. When used as the primary immunosuppressant, the daily oral dose is 2–3 mg/kg. When used as adjunctive therapy with cyclosporine, the dose is 1–2 mg/kg.

MONOCLONAL AND POLYCLONAL ANTIBODIES

Various polyclonal antibodies—antilymphocyte globulin (ALG), antilymphoblast serum, and antithymocyte globulin (ATG)—have been available for use in clinical transplantation for more than 20 years. Currently, the only polyclonal antibody widely available in the United States is antithymocyte globulin (ATGAM). The monoclonal antibody muromonab-CD3 (Orthoclone OKT3—"OKT3") has been available for clinical use since 1987. Table 4-4 compares and contrasts them. Unfortunately, there have been few "head-to-head" comparisons between these drugs, although the overall impression is that their clinical effectiveness is similar when used for both rejection prophylaxis and treatment.

Table 4-4. Comparison of OKT3 and polyclonal antibodies (ATG, ALG, ALS)

Monoclonal	Polyclonal
Homogenous	Heterogenous
Consistent reactivity	Batch-to-batch variability
Smaller dose	Larger dose
Readily available	Irregularly available
Peripheral line administration	Central line administration
First-dose reactions	No first-dose reactions
Potential for monitoring	Not usually monitored
High repeat rejection rate	Low repeat rejection rate
Potential for second course	Rarely given twice
Potential for outpatient use	Inpatient use only
Antibody development	Potential for serum sickness
Lower cost*	Higher cost

ATG = antithymocyte globulin; ALG = antilymphocyte globulin; ALS = antilymphoblast serum.
*Particularly if administered in the outpatient setting.

OKT3

Monoclonal antibodies are produced by the hybridization of murine antibody–secreting B lymphocytes with a nonsecreting myeloma cell line whose neoplastic potential permits the secretion of antibody in perpetuity. A number of monoclonal antibodies have been produced that are active against different facets of the immune response. OKT3, directed against the CD3 antigen complex found on all mature human T cells, is currently the only commercially available monoclonal antibody for therapeutic use. It is a highly effective yet potentially toxic drug. Its introduction into clinical transplantation was the most important therapeutic advance since the advent of cyclosporine. It is most frequently used for the treatment of episodes of steroid-resistant rejection but may also be used with great effect as primary rejection treatment, for rejection prophylaxis, or for induction therapy in the immediate post-transplant period (see the section on protocols).

Mode of Action

OKT3 reacts only with human T cells. It is an IgG immunoglobulin that binds to one of the 20-kD subunits of the CD3 complex, an intrinsic part of the T cell receptor (see Chap. 2). The subsequent deactivation of the CD3 complex causes the T cell receptor to undergo endocytosis and be lost from the cell surface. The T cells become ineffectual, and within an hour they become opsonized and are removed from the circulation into the reticuloendothelial system. OKT3 also blocks the function of killer T cells in the allograft, which have an important role in generating the rejection response.

Concomitant with the initial depletion of CD3-positive cells, there is depletion of T cells with other surface markers (CD4, CD8, CD11). Within a few days, T cells reappear in the circulation that carry CD4, CD8, and CD11 markers but are devoid of CD3 and are hence ineffectual, or so-called **modulated**, cells (Fig. 4-3). CD3-positive functional cells may reappear later in the course of OKT3 and during a second course, possibly due to the production of neutralizing antibodies. The clinical importance of this reappearance is discussed below.

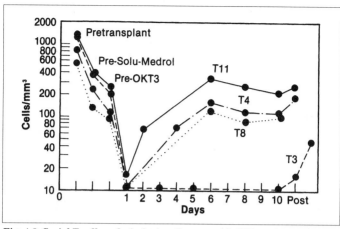

Fig. 4-3. Serial T cell analysis during therapy with OKT3. The fall in T cell count from pretransplant levels before the use of OKT3 is due to routine immunosuppression and high-dose steroids. Note the appearance of "modulated" cells a few days after commencement of OKT3.

Dosage and Administration

The standard dose of OKT3 is 5 mg given as an IV bolus through a Millipore filter. The standard course consists of a daily dose for 10 days, although shorter (5–7 days) or longer (14 days or more) courses are sometimes given. Protocols using lower doses of OKT3 may be just as effective but are less well-tested. OKT3 protocol recommendations are given in Table 4-5. The first few doses of OKT3 must be given in the hospital, preferably at an institution familiar with OKT3's use and side effects. The first dose can be safely administered intraoperatively as long as the protocol recommendations are adhered to. If the drug is well-tolerated, the course can be completed on an outpatient basis with substantial financial economy and patient convenience.

Monitoring

OKT3 monitoring refers to the repeated assessment of the effectiveness of the drug during a course because of the potential for the development of antibodies, which may abrogate its action and allow for the reappearance of potent CD3-positive T cells. Antibodies may be directed against the antibody site itself (**anti-idiotypic**), against the IgG protein subclass (**anti-isotypic**), and against the mouse protein of origin (**antimurine**).

During an effective course of OKT3, the percentage of CD3-positive T cells falls precipitously (see Fig. 4-3) within 24–48 hours, from approximately 60% to less than 5%. The fall may be somewhat slower in an effective second course. Failure of the CD3-positive percentage to fall or a fall followed by a rapid rise indicates the appearance of blocking antibodies. Measurement of CD3 cells is available as a routine laboratory test in sophisticated immunology laboratories. Measurement of OKT3 blood levels is not yet routinely available. OKT3 antibodies can be measured by a time-consuming enzyme-linked immunosorbent assay (ELISA) technique or by the more con-

Table 4-5. Protocol recommendations for OKT3 use

1. Before administration of first dose, patient should be edema-free and within 3% of dry weight and have negative chest x-ray.
2. Use high-dose diuretics, dialysis, or ultrafiltration alone to achieve euvolemia in a volume-overloaded patient.
3. Administer premedication 15–60 mins before first and second dose consisting of methylprednisolone, 5–8 mg/kg; diphenhydramine hydrochloride (Benadryl), 50 mg IV; and acetaminophen, 500 mg PO.
4. Before first and second dose, monitor vital signs every 15 mins for 2 hrs, then every 30 mins for 2 hrs.
5. Premedication is not required for remainder of the course; use acetaminophen prn for fever.
6. If OKT3 is stopped for more than one dose, repeat first-dose precautions.
7. Continue cyclosporine or azathioprine during the course, but not both.
8. If cyclosporine is continued, use half dose; return to full dose 2 days before completion of the course, and ensure therapeutic levels.
9. After first two doses, continue prednisone according to the protocol schedule.
10. During second course of OKT3, monitor CD3 levels at least twice weekly.
11. After the first two doses, encourage hydration in diuresing patients.

venient **Transtat OKT3 assay**. The clinical value of these assays has yet to be clearly defined.

During an initial course of OKT3, minimal CD3 monitoring is required, since it typically takes 2 weeks for antibody to develop. During retreatment, CD3 levels should be measured at least twice weekly. If CD3 levels are elevated, consideration should be given, depending on the overall clinical status of the patient, to doubling the OKT3 dose to overcome the antibody response. Two to 3 weeks following a course of OKT3 or before the next course, the presence of antibodies should be determined. A low-titer antibody response (<1 per 100) can be overcome by treatment. Such treatment, however, brings with it a significant risk of development of a high titer response that may abrogate the effectiveness of all mouse protein monoclonal antibodies. The concomitant use of a low dose of either cyclosporine or azathioprine during a course of OKT3 (see Table 4-5) serves to minimize the antibody response.

Side Effects

Significant, potentially life-threatening adverse reactions may occur during the first days of treatment with OKT3. These adverse reactions occur as the percentage of potent T cells plummet and a series of T cell–derived cytokines, including **tumor necrosis factor** (TNF), **IL-2**, and **gamma-interferon**, are released into the circulation. The term **cytokine release syndrome** has been used to describe the clinical events that follow. Immediate complement activation may also play an important etiologic role. The OKT3 administration protocol (see Table 4-5) is designed to minimize the severity of the syndrome. High-dose corticosteroids, indomethacin, anti-TNF antibodies, and pentoxifylline have also been reported to be effective. A double-blind, randomized study of pentoxifylline, however, showed no measurable benefit.

Fever and Chills

Following the first exposure to OKT3, nearly all patients become febrile, and many suffer rigors. The fever and rigors often occur "like clockwork" 45 minutes after the injection, but may be delayed for hours. By the second or third dose, the fever typically abates, although some patients remain febrile for several days or throughout the whole course. Patients being treated with OKT3 are all immunosuppressed by definition, so infectious causes of fever should always be considered. If the fever is prolonged for more than two to three doses, a fever workup should be performed. The development of fever later in the course of OKT3 after an afebrile period is particularly suggestive of a infectious etiology (with cytomegalovirus [CMV] infection at the top of the differential diagnosis) and demands careful consideration of the wisdom of continuing the course.

Pulmonary Edema

A rapidly developing, potentially life-threatening noncardiogenic pulmonary edema may occur after the first or second dose of OKT3 if the patient is not euvolemic, or very close to his or her dry weight at the time of injection. Even "dry" patients may wheeze and become dyspneic. Post-OKT3 pulmonary edema is a preventable syndrome as long as the precautions listed in Table 4-5 are adhered to compulsively. It should be remembered that clinical volume assessment is often unreliable, and patients may "hide" liters of fluid that are not clinically detectable. It is often wise and expeditious to dialyze or ultrafilter a patient before OKT3 administration to ensure that the required amount of fluid is removed.

Following the first doses of OKT3, the fluid restrictions can be relaxed. Patients may, in fact, become hypotensive and dehydrated because of fever, diarrhea, and prior fluid restriction. The decision to continue OKT3 in a hypotensive febrile patient may be a difficult one. In these circumstances, OKT3 can be continued safely as long as other causes of hypotension and fever are considered and ruled out and hydration is maintained.

Nephrotoxicity

Renal function, as judged by serum creatinine levels, may deteriorate during the early days of an OKT3 course; a previously nonoliguric patient may even require dialysis. This deterioration of function is typically transient and is followed by a brisk diuresis. It may even be a harbinger of a successful course, since it is presumably a manifestation of the hemodynamic abnormalities following cytokine release as the OKT3 takes its toll on the T cells. This transient nephrotoxicity probably accounts for the fact that the prophylactic use of OKT3 immediately post-transplant ("sequential" therapy) does not clearly reduce the frequency of delayed graft function as compared to postoperative cyclosporine use, although the length of the oliguric period may be reduced in sequential therapy (see below). Occasional cases of irreversible graft thrombosis have been described following OKT3 administration and may be due to OKT3-induced activation of the coagulation cascade.

Neurologic Complications

A spectrum of neurologic complications may occur during a course of OKT3, varying in severity from a commonly occurring mild headache to severe encephalopathy. The severe complications are more common when OKT3 is given for prophylaxis in patients with delayed graft function; diabetics may also be more susceptible.

The aseptic meningitis syndrome is self-limiting and typically resolves spontaneously without the necessity for discontinuing the OKT3 course. If a lumbar puncture is performed, a mild culture-negative leukocytosis with pleocytosis is often found. Clinicians may be more comfortable discontinuing the OKT3 for one or two doses while the results of lumbar puncture culture are awaited and the patient's clinical status is observed. Approximately one-third of patients with a diagnosis of aseptic meningitis have coexisting evidence of encephalopathy. OKT3 should be discontinued in severely encephalopathic patients.

Infection

Infection, most commonly with CMV, may be a late adverse sequela of OKT3 use. The frequency of infection varies with the number of courses of OKT3 and the overall amount of immunosuppression given. Some programs routinely employ CMV prophylaxis prior to or during a course of OKT3, with recipients of CMV-positive allografts representing a particularly high-risk population. Techniques of CMV prophylaxis are discussed in Chap. 10.

Rejection Recurrence

Episodes of rejection may occur after up to 60% of courses of OKT3. These episodes, which are typically mild, can usually be controlled by a low-dose prednisone pulse. They occur as potent CD3-positive T cells reappear in the circulation. At the completion of a course of OKT3, it is important to ensure that cyclosporine levels are in the high therapeutic range (see Table 4-5). It may be wise to routinely increase the steroid dose in the first 3–4 days following the course.

Post-Transplant Lymphoproliferative Disease

The development of lymphoma in transplant patients is a well-recognized, although infrequent, consequence of effective immunosuppression and is discussed in Chap. 9. Use of repeat courses of the OKT3 or polyclonal antibodies has been associated with a particularly fulminant and typically rapidly fatal B cell lymphoma that develops within the first few months post-transplant. Epstein-Barr virus (EBV) antibody–negative patients receiving a graft from an EBV-positive donor appear to be at greatest risk. Occasional cases respond to discontinuation of immunosuppression, high-dose acyclovir, and chemotherapy. The concomitant use of ganciclovir with OKT3 for prophylaxis against CMV infection (see Chap. 10) may reduce the incidence of EBV-related lymphomas.

POLYCLONAL ANTIBODIES

Polyclonal antibodies are produced by immunizing either horses or rabbits with human lymphoid tissue and then harvesting the resultant immune sera to obtain gamma globulin fractions. Attempts are then made to purify these fractions to eliminate unwanted antibodies, which are responsible for some of their side effects. The only widely available polyclonal antibody in the United States is **ATGAM.** Some centers manufacture their own antilymphocyte sera; the once popular Minnesota ALG (MALG) is no longer available. Polyclonal antibodies are effective agents for rejection prophylaxis in the early post-transplant period and for treatment of steroid-resistant rejection.

Mode of Action

The precise mechanism of action of the polyclonal antibodies is difficult to define, partly because of the diffuse nature of their effects. Following their administration, the total lymphocyte count falls. Lymphocytes, T cells in particular, are either lysed or cleared into the reticuloendothelial system, and their surface antigens may be masked by the antibody. Suppressor cells may be responsible for the prolonged immunosuppressive effect of these drugs and for the relative infrequency of episodes of rejection recurrence compared with OKT3.

Dose and Administration

Polyclonal antibodies are given in a dose of 10–20 mg/kg/day for 7–14 days. The antibodies are mixed in 500 ml of normal or half-normal saline and infused over 6 hours into a central vein or arteriovenous fistula. Use of a peripheral vein is often followed by vein thrombosis or thrombophlebitis.

To avoid allergic reactions, the patient should receive IV premedication consisting of methylprednisolone, 30 mg, and diphenhydramine hydrochloride (Benadryl), 50 mg, 30 minutes before injection. Acetaminophen should be given before and 4 hours after commencement of the infusion for fever control. Vital signs should be monitored every 15 minutes during the first hour of infusion and then hourly until the infusion is complete.

Thrombocytopenia (see the section on side effects) requires dose modification, with a half dose given for a platelet count of 50,000–100,000 cells/ml. Azathioprine should be discontinued during the course of treatment so as not to exacerbate thrombocytopenia. Cyclosporine can be omitted during the course or given in a low dose, and oral prednisone is replaced by the methylprednisolone given in the premedication.

Side Effects

Most of the side effects of polyclonal antibodies relate to the fact that large quantities of foreign protein are administered. Chills, fevers, and arthralgia are common, although the severe first-dose reactions seen with OKT3 do not occur. There have been occasional cases of anaphylaxis; a serum sickness–like illness may occur during a prolonged course.

The potency of preparation of polyclonal antibodies may vary somewhat from batch to batch. Unwanted antiplatelet and antileukocyte antibodies may cause thrombocytopenia and leukopenia, necessitating curtailment of drug dosage. The infectious complications are similar to those described for OKT3. The incidence and severity of CMV infection is clearly more common with all of these agents.

ADJUNCTIVE IMMUNOSUPPRESSIVE AGENTS

Calcium Channel Blockers

The inclusion of either diltiazem or verapamil in the standard immunosuppressive regimen has several potential advantages. In addition to their antihypertensive properties, both drugs may minimize cyclosporine-induced vasoconstriction and protect against ischemic graft injury and cyclosporine toxicity. Both drugs compete with cyclosporine for excretion by the P450 enzyme system, thus raising drug levels and permitting safe administration of lower doses of cyclosporine. Calcium channel blockers may also possess some intrinsic immunomodulatory activity of their own related to the role of cytosolic calcium levels or gene activation. The routine inclusion of calcium channel blockers to the post-transplant protocol may improve 1-year graft survival by 5–10%, with up to a 40% reduction in cyclosporine dosage.

Prostaglandin Analogues

Prostaglandins of the E and I series possess intrinsic immunosuppressive effects that have not been precisely defined. Prostaglandin E (PGE) also tends to attenuate the vasoconstrictive effect of cyclosporine and reduce kidney injury following ischemic insult. Misoprostol is an orally administered PGE analogue that has been shown in early clinical trials to reduce the incidence of acute rejection and improve graft function. Controlled trials of the related agent enisoprost showed no clinically significant benefit.

HMGCoA Reductase Inhibitors

Pravastatin is an HMGCoA reductase inhibitor (HCRI) that has been shown to safely lower cholesterol levels in transplant patients and to reduce the incidence of clinically severe rejection in cardiac transplant recipients. A similar beneficial effect has been observed in preliminary studies in kidney transplant recipients. The mechanism of this effect may be related to the capacity of HCRIs to suppress the cytotoxic activity of natural killer cells (see Chap. 2). HCRIs may have an important role in the post-transplant immunosuppressive regimen.

Part II: New Immunosuppressive Agents

When the history of organ transplantation is written, the 1990s will very likely be referred to as the decade of new immunosuppressive agents. More than a dozen promising new immunosuppressive candidates are at various stages of development, and the race for their introduction into clinical transplantation practice can be likened to an obstacle course. Some drugs have passed the finishing line (e.g., tacrolimus, mycophenolate mofetil), some have already faltered and fallen from current consideration (e.g., brequinar sodium, cyclosporine G), and some are still in the race with obstacles ahead (e.g., sirolimus, deoxyspergualin, and the new monoclonal antibodies).

The great success of organ transplantation that has been achieved in the 1990s with currently available agents is, paradoxically, making it exceedingly difficult (and enormously expensive) to prove the added benefit of new agents. In clinical trials of new agents, the use of the traditional marker of drug or protocol superiority—patient or graft survival—is often proving to be impractical; more easily achieved shorter termed endpoints are required. Examples of such alternative endpoints include reduced incidence of acute rejection episodes, improved renal function, and more cost-effective immunosuppression.

The mechanism of action of several of the agents reviewed below is discussed in Chap. 2 in the context of the immunobiology of transplant rejection.

CLINICAL TRIALS

Before any clinical trials can be performed with an investigational agent, an **investigational new drug application (IND)** has to be submitted to the **Federal Drug Administration (FDA)** or equivalent regulatory body outside of the United States. Approval of the IND is based on the evaluation of preclinical studies that suggest potential therapeutic benefits of a new agent and on the evaluation of studies in a variety of animals that suggest its safety.

Phase 1 clinical studies are performed in healthy human volunteers or patients to evaluate human metabolism, pharmacokinetics, dosage, safety, and, if possible, effectiveness. **Phase 2** includes controlled, open-labeled, clinical studies conducted to evaluate the effectiveness of the drug for a particular indication or indications and to determine common side effects and risks. Phase 2 studies of immunosuppressive drugs are often performed on relatively small groups of transplant patients who are often suffering from recurrent rejections and who are refractory to standard treatment. **Phase 3** studies are expanded trials based on preliminary evidence from the previous phases that suggest efficacy and safety. They typically involve large, usually multicentered, clinical trials that are randomized and, if possible, double-blinded. These studies serve to refine dosage, determine benefit, and further evaluate the overall risk-to-benefit ratio of the new drug. In organ transplantation, particular care has to be taken to ensure that any potential benefit of a new agent is not outweighed by the consequences of overimmunosuppression or by organ-specific toxicity. Successful completion of Phase 3 should provide an adequate basis for physician labeling and permit approval of the drug for its defined indications.

Any human use of an experimental drug is strictly governed by the predetermined rules of the experimental protocol under which the drug is administered. Patients must read, understand, and sign an informed consent form that clearly defines the nature of the experiment in which they are involved and its potential risks and benefits. They must also receive a copy of the **patient's bill of rights**, which clearly defines the nature of their commitment. The experimental protocol and consent form must have been approved by an **institutional review board (IRB)** or **human subjects protection committee (HSPC)**, and the medical staff administering the protocol must feel totally comfortable with it. Once a drug is licensed, it is often used "off label" for indications different from those precisely defined. Such use does not require a formal consent procedure, although it is wise to inform the patient that the drug is being given for an unapproved use.

TACROLIMUS

Tacrolimus (Prograf), formerly known as FK506, is a macrolide antibiotic compound isolated from *Streptomyces tsukabaensis*. Although it is biochemically distinct from cyclosporine, it shares many of cyclosporine's properties. It is at least tenfold more potent than cyclosporine on a weight basis.

Most of the clinical experience with tacrolimus has come from large clinical trials in liver transplant recipients, and the drug has been approved for use in liver transplantation based on the finding that it was at least as effective as cyclosporine in terms of patient and graft survival. In these studies, the incidence of episodes of acute rejection has been somewhat lower in the patients receiving tacrolimus, and the drug may have a steroid-sparing effect. The side effect profile of tacrolimus is very similar to that of cyclosporine, although tacrolimus may be more toxic (see the section on tacrolimus's side effects). Tacrolimus has not yet been approved for use in kidney transplantation, although it is being used "off label" in many kidney transplant programs, most frequently for the treatment of refractory rejection (see the section on immunosuppressive protocols). Phase III randomized clinical trials comparing tacrolimus to cyclosporine in kidney transplantation are in progress. Preliminary results of these studies appear very similar to the liver transplant studies. It is probably unnecessary to use azathioprine with tacrolimus. Some comparative features of cyclosporine and tacrolimus are reviewed in Table 4-6.

Mechanism of Action

Although tacrolimus is structurally unrelated to cyclosporine, its mode of action is very similar. Tacrolimus inhibits T cell function by impairing the release of IL-2 and other cytokines. Like cyclosporine, it binds to a specific intracytoplasmic binding protein (FKBP), and the combination of the drug and its binding protein block the action of calcineurin probably by impairing access to its phosphatase site (see Plate 1, the section on cyclosporine's mechanism of action, and Chap. 2). Tacrolimus and cyclosporine must not be administered simultaneously because of the potential for synergistic toxicities.

Pharmacokinetics

Tacrolimus is available in an IV and an oral formulation. It is absorbed primarily from the small bowel, and, as opposed to cyclosporine, its absorption is independent of bile salts. Because of the effectiveness and relative consistency of its absorption, it is rarely necessary to use the IV formulation, and, if necessary, the drug can be administered via a nasogastric tube. The recommended starting dose of tacrolimus is 0.15–0.30 mg/kg/day administered in a split dose each 12 hours. An ELISA assay is available in centers that use tacrolimus for liver transplantation. Target levels in whole blood are usually 10–20 ng/ml when the drug is first introduced; however, levels are usually allowed to fall during long-term use, and effective immunosuppression may occur below the level of detection of the currently available assay.

Tacrolimus is protein-bound and distributes in all major solid organs (but not in the cerebral spinal fluid). It is metabolized primarily by the liver P450 IIIA system and excreted through the biliary system. Renal excretion is negligible, and tacrolimus is not dialysable. Drug interactions described to date are quite similar to

Table 4-6. Some comparative features of cyclosporine and tacrolimus[a]

	Cyclosporine	Tacrolimus
Mode of action	Inhibition of calcineurin	Inhibition of calcineurin
Daily maintenance dose	~3–5 mg/kg	~0.15–0.3 mg/kg
Administration	PO and IV	PO and IV[b]
Absorption bile-dependent[c]	Sandimmune Yes Neoral No	No
Oral dose available (capsules)	100 mg; 25 mg	5 mg; 1 mg
Therapeutic drug levels (high-performance liquid chromatography assay)	100–400 ng/ml[d]	5–20 ng/ml
Drug interactions	Similar	Similar
Capacity to prevent rejection	+	++
Capacity to treat ongoing rejection	+	++
Necessity for azathioprine	±	–
Use with mycophenolate mofetil	+	Untested
Predisposition to infections	+	++
Nephrotoxic	+	+
Long-term stability of renal function	+	+?
Steroid-sparing	+	++
Hypertension and sodium retention	++	±
Pancreatic islet toxic	+	++
Neurotoxic	+	++
Cosmetic side effects	+	–
GI side effects	–	+
Hyperkalemia	+	+
Hypomagnesemia	+	+
Hypercholesterolemia	–	–

+ = known effect; ++ = effect more pronounced ;
± = effect inconsistent; – = no effect; +? = probable effect.
[a]Based on available literature and clinical experience.
[b]IV rarely needed because oral absorption is good.
[c]Independence of bile absorption is an advantage in liver transplantation.
[d]See Table 4-7.

those described with cyclosporine (see the section on cyclosporine's drug interactions)—for example, anticonvulsants reduce levels, and antifungals and calcium channel blockers increase levels.

Side Effects

The toxicity profile of tacrolimus is remarkably similar to that of cyclosporine (see Table 4-6). Tacrolimus is nephrotoxic and may produce acute, reversible deterioration in renal function as well as a chronic interstitial fibrosis that is essentially indistinguishable from that produced by cyclosporine (see Chap. 12). Tacrolimus causes less vasoconstriction than cyclosporine so that hypertension is less marked. A hemolytic-uremic syndrome has been described similar to that seen with cyclosporine. Hyperkalemia and hypomagnesemia are common.

Tacrolimus is neurotoxic; headaches, insomnia, parasthesias, pruritis, and a course tremor are common. Coma was described when the drug was first introduced but is rarely reported now. Both cyclosporine and tacrolimus are islet cell–toxic, although tacrolimus is probably more so (see Chap. 9). Nausea, vomiting, and diarrhea are common in patients receiving tacrolimus. Hirsutism and gingival hypertrophy, both bothersome complications of cyclosporine use, are relatively uncommon.

MYCOPHENOLATE MOFETIL

Mycophenolate mofetil (CellCept) (MMF), previously known as RS61443, is a promising new immunosuppressive drug that has been shown to be effective in a variety of experimental animal models of organ transplantation and in both open-labeled and double-blinded, randomized clinical trials in renal transplantation. The active compound is mycophenolic acid (MPA), a fermentation product of several *Penicillium* species; the mofetil moiety serves to markedly improve its oral bioavailability. MMF was approved for clinical use in mid-1995 for the prevention of acute allograft rejection. Its place in clinical transplantation will be largely determined by the final results of several pivotal clinical trials that are still in progress (see the section on clinical trials).

Mechanism of Action

MPA is a reversible inhibitor of the enzyme **inosine monophosphate dehydrogenase** (IMPDH). IMPDH is a critical, rate-limiting enzyme in the so-called "de novo" synthesis of purines and catalyzes the formation of guanosine nucleotides from inosine. Depletion of guanosine nucleotides by MPA has relatively selective antiproliferative effects on lymphocytes, since lymphocytes seem to rely on de novo purine synthesis more than other cell types that have a "salvage" pathway for production of guanosine nucleotides from guanine (Fig. 4-4).

MMF is thus a more selective antimetabolite. It differs radically in its mode of action from cyclosporine, tacrolimus, and sirolimus in that it does not affect cytokine production or the more proximal events following antigen recognition. It differs from azathioprine by virtue of its selective effect on lymphocytes. In vitro, MMF blocks the proliferation of T and B cells, inhibits antibody formation, and inhibits the generation of cytotoxic T cells. MMF also downregulates the expression of adhesion molecules on lymphocytes, thereby impairing their binding to vascular endothelial cells. The capacity of MMF to treat ongoing rejection (see the section on clinical trials) may be a reflection of its ability to inhibit the recruitment of mononuclear cells into rejection sites and the subsequent interaction of these cells with target cells.

Preclinical Studies

In preclinical studies in a variety of animal models of organ transplantation, MMF, usually in combination with cyclosporine or other immunosuppressants, has been shown to be effective in the prevention of rejection and in the treatment of ongoing rejection. MMF may also exert a preventive effect on the development and progression of proliferative arteriolopathy, a critical pathologic lesion in chronic rejection (see Chap. 12). If this finding proves relevant to

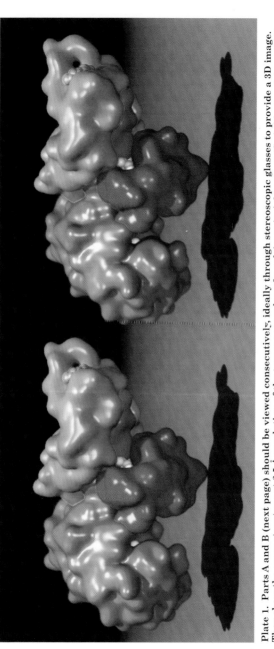

Plate 1. Parts A and B (next page) should be viewed consecutively, ideally through stereoscopic glasses to provide a 3D image. They show the x-ray structure at 2.5 Å resolution of the ternary complex of a calcineurin A fragment (CnA; blue), calcineurin B (CnB; green), tacrolimus-binding protein (FKBP; red), and tacrolimus (FK506; white). Note that the FKBP-FK506 complex does not directly contact the phosphatase active site on CnA that is more than 10 Å removed. Instead, the FKBP-FK506 complex is positioned so that it can inhibit the dephosphorylation of its substrates (e.g., nuclear factor of activated T cells [NFATpl) by physically hindering their approach to the active site. (The bound phosphate in the phosphatase active site of CnA is shown in yellow.) A. The solvent accessible surface of the ternary complex.

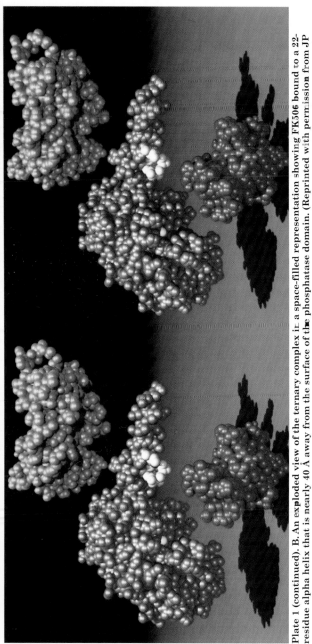

Plate 1 (continued). B. An exploded view of the ternary complex in a space-filled representation showing FK506 bound to a 22-residue alpha helix that is nearly 40 Å away from the surface of the phosphatase domain. (Reprinted with permission from JP Griffith, JL Kim, EE Kim et al. X-ray structure of calcineurin inhibited by the immunophilin-immunosuppressant FKBP12-FK506 complex. *Cell* 82:507, 1995.)

B

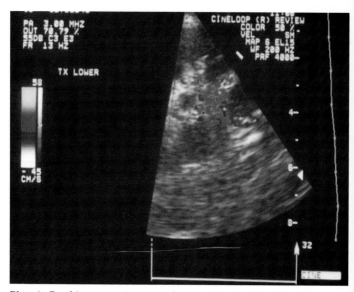

Plate 2. Postbiopsy arteriovenous fistula. Color Doppler image shows an area of random color assignment. Pulsed gate Doppler analysis revealed high-velocity, low-resistance arterial flow and arterialization of the venous waveform.

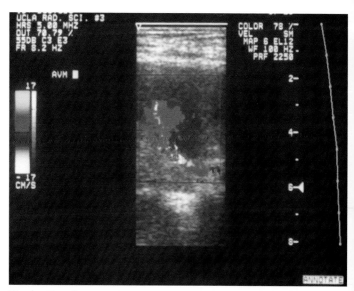

Plate 3. Pseudoaneurysm. Gray-scale image demonstrated a cystic lesion, and color Doppler image shows swirling internal flow.

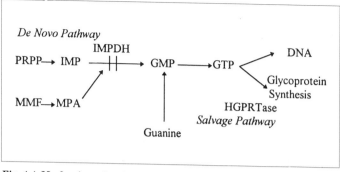

Fig. 4-4. Mechanism of action of mycophenolate mofetil by inhibition of "de novo" purine synthesis. (PRPP = 5-phosphoribosyl-1-phosphate; IMP = inosine monophosphate; MPA = mycophenolic acid; IMPDH = inosine monophosphate dehydrogenase; GMP = guanosine monophosphate; HGPRTase = hypoxanthine guanine phosphoribosyl transferase; GTP = guanosine triphosphate.)

human transplantation, it will make MMF unique among immunosuppressant drugs, none of which have had an impact on the development of chronic rejection to date.

Clinical Trials

Several clinical trials of MMF are in progress; the results of these trials will determine the eventual place of this drug in clinical transplantation. Results of the primary endpoints of the following two studies are available and permit a preliminary evaluation of the effectiveness and side effect profile of MMF.

Mycophenolate Mofetil Versus Corticosteroids for the Treatment of Refractory Renal Transplantation Rejection

A randomized, open-labeled, multicenter phase III trial compared the use of MMF in an oral dose of 1.5 g bid to a standardized steroid pulse for the treatment of refractory rejection occurring within 6 months of transplantation. "Refractory" was defined as biopsy-proven rejection occurring within 4 weeks of a course of an antilymphocytic preparation for a prior rejection. The primary endpoint of the study was designated to be patient loss or graft loss 6 months postenrollment.

The study was designed to determine if MMF would be of benefit to a group of patients believed to be at a particularly high risk of graft loss. At 6 months postenrollment, 14% of the patients receiving MMF had lost their grafts or died, compared with 26% in the patients receiving steroids. At 12 months, graft losses or death had occurred in 18% and 32%, respectively. Further episodes of rejection, use of OKT3, and pulse steroids were approximately halved in the MMF group. This study appears to establish MMF as a valuable option for the treatment of refractory rejection.

Mycophenolate Mofetil for the Prevention of Acute Rejection in Cadaveric Renal Allograft Recipients

The purpose of this randomized, double-blind, multicenter phase III study is to evaluate the efficacy of MMF for the prevention of acute

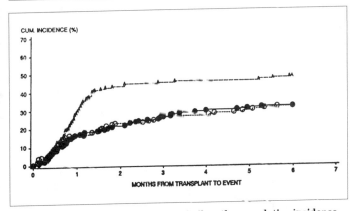

Fig. 4-5. Impact of mycophenolate mofetil on the cumulative incidence of biopsy-proven acute rejection episodes in the first 6 months post-transplant. (A = azathioprine group; O = mycophenolate mofetil, 1.0 g bid; • = mycophenolate mofetil, 1.5 g bid.) (From HW Sollinger for the U.S. Renal Transplant Mycophenolate Mofetil Study Group. Mycophenolate mofetil for the prevention of acute rejection in primary cadaveric renal allograft recipients. *Transplantation* 60:225, 1995.)

rejection episodes during the first 6 months following transplantation. The prevention of rejection rather than the improvement of graft or patient survival was chosen as the primary endpoint of the study because of the morbidity associated with these episodes and the relationship between acute rejection and the eventual development of chronic rejection. The study is the largest and most complex of its kind ever performed in solid organ transplantation.

The study compares two doses of MMF (1.0 g bid and 1.5 g bid) and azathioprine in combination with standard therapy with cyclosporine and prednisone. The study was placebo-controlled and blinded until all patients had reached the primary endpoint and in the United States involved 500 recipients of a first cadaveric transplant (very similar studies involving another 1,000 patients were performed in Europe, Canada, and Australia). Figure 4-5 illustrates the clear-cut benefit of MMF in that the incidence of acute rejection episodes or treatment failure was reduced from nearly 50% in the azathioprine group to 31% in both the MMF groups. Use of high-dose steroids and OKT3 was also markedly reduced in the MMF groups.

Although the primary endpoint of this pivotal study has been reached and analyzed, several critical secondary endpoints have not. Protocol kidney biopsies will be performed at 1 and 3 years post-transplant, and the evaluation of these biopsies, together with long-term follow-up of patient and graft survival and function, will permit an evaluation of the impact of MMF on the development chronic rejection.

Pharmacology and Toxicity

MMF is a generally well-tolerated and "user-friendly" compound. Orally administered MMF is rapidly absorbed and converted to MPA. Bioavailabilty of MMF in the capsule form is 90%, with a half-life of 12 hours. There is no unusual accumulation of MPA in hepatic or renal impairment, and neither MMF or MPA is dialyzed. It does not appear to be necessary to measure blood levels.

Extensive safety data are available from early trials of MMF in rheumatoid arthritis and from the large clinical trials reviewed above. The most common adverse events are related to the GI tract, with diarrhea occurring in approximately one-third of the patients, esophagitis and gastritis in approximately 5%, and GI hemorrhage in 4%. Most of these symptoms respond to transient reduction of drug dosage. The incidence of post-transplant infectious complications does not appear to be increased by MMF, with the exception of CMV invasive gastritis/esophagitis, which has been reported in approximately 10% of patients on MMF. This relatively high incidence may be a reflection of the increased attention paid to the upper GI tract with the resultant endoscopic procedures.

Despite the relatively specific action of MMF on lymphocytes, leukopenia and anemia occur with a frequency similar to that seen with azathioprine. The two drugs should not be administered concomitantly. No other drug interactions have been reported with notable frequency. The dose of cyclosporine need not be altered when it is administered with MMF. The incidence of lymphoproliferative disorders in all the various clinical trials of MMF is less than 1%, which is not different from that anticipated in an immunosuppressed transplant population. Nephrotoxicity, neurotoxicity, and hepatotoxicity have not been observed with MMF. Its safety in pregnancy has not yet been established.

SIROLIMUS

Mechanism of Action

Sirolimus (Rapamune), formerly known as rapamycin, is a macrolide antibiotic that is structurally related to tacrolimus. It has demonstrated potent antirejection activity, as well as the ability to prolong allograft survival in a number of animal models of organ transplantation. The immunosuppressive activity of sirolimus appears to be mediated through a mechanism distinct from that of tacrolimus and from that of cyclosporine. Like these two compounds, it binds to a cytoplasmic binding protein (the same one that binds tacrolimus, FKBP). The resultant sirolimus-FKBP ligand, however, does not block calcineurin (see Chap. 2 and the section on cyclosporine's mechanism of action), but rather engages a protein designated **rapamycin and FKBP target (RAFT)** and thereby impairs the capacity of cytokines to trigger T cells to enter the cell division cycle at the G1-to-S phase. Much still needs to be learned about this pathway. Since sirolimus occupies the same binding protein as tacrolimus, it impairs the action of tacrolimus; combined use of the drugs is contraindicated. Sirolimus may have a synergistic effect with cyclosporine.

Clinical Trials

Phase I studies have been conducted using an oral formulation of sirolimus administered to renal transplant recipients. The drug appeared to be relatively safe and well-tolerated. Preliminary evaluation of phase II studies suggest that sirolimus, when administered concomitantly with either full or reduced doses of cyclosporine, can markedly reduce the occurrence of rejection episodes, although not without toxicity. Blinded phase III trials will be required to fully assess the risk-to-benefit ratio of this compound.

OTHER EXPERIMENTAL IMMUNOSUPPRESSANTS

Deoxyspergualin

15-Deoxyspergualin trihydrochloride (BMY-42215-1) (DSG) is an antitumor antibiotic that has been found to facilitate organ acceptance in animal models and to have some potential clinical value in early phase I and II clinical trials. It has been approved for use in Japan for the treatment of acute rejection. Its precise mechanism of action has not yet been defined. The drug appears to be a poor inhibitor of lymphocyte proliferation and may interfere at a later point in the activation process that leads to the generation of antigen-specific cytotoxic T cells. Its mechanism of action is clearly different from the immunosuppressive agents in current clinical use.

The drug is typically administered as a slow IV infusion in a dose of 3–5 mg/kg/day over a 7- to 10-day period. Hypotension may occur during the infusion, and varying degrees of reversible myelosuppression have been described. The place of DSG in clinical transplantation will depend on the results of phase III clinical trials.

Mizoribine

Mizoribine, also of antibiotic origin, exerts its immunosuppressive effects as a metabolic antagonist of purine synthesis. When used alone, it is less powerful than cyclosporine or azathioprine. It is not marrow toxic, and in early clinical trials in Japan, it has been used synergistically with cyclosporine and prednisone with minimal side effects.

Cyclosporine OG-37-325

Cyclosporine OG-37-325 has a structure that is similar to the familiar cyclosporine A. Its action is also very similar. The story of the development of cyclosporine OG is an instructive one. Phase I and II clinical trials suggested that this form of cyclosporine might be more potent and less nephrotoxic than cyclosporine A. In blinded phase III trials, however, no significant difference could be detected, and, as a result, clinical development of this compound has been discontinued.

Brequinar Sodium

Brequinar sodium is an immunosuppressive agent with a mode of action very similar to that of MMF. Rather than impairing purine metabolism, however, it impairs pyrimidine metabolism. Phase I and II clinical trials were commenced but not completed. Clinically significant thrombocytopenia has been associated with its use.

Leflunomide

Leflunomide is a promising new immunosuppressive agent. It is structurally unrelated to any of the compounds currently in use or under investigation. It appears to act by blocking T and B cell responsiveness to IL-2 and other cytokines. In small and large animal models, it has been shown to reverse acute rejection without major toxicity. Its action may be synergistic with cyclosporine. Leflunomide is not currently being developed for use in clinical transplantation.

NEW MONOCLONAL ANTIBODIES

The increasingly detailed understanding of the immune response, together with biotechnological developments, has led to the production of several potentially therapeutically valuable monoclonal antibodies targeted at different facets of the immune response. Despite several years of work on these compounds, however, OKT3 remains the only monoclonal in routine transplantation practice.

CD45 monoclonals are directed against leukocyte common class I and class II antigens on dendritic cells or passenger leukocytes. These cells are powerful inducers of the immune response. Before transplantation, cadaveric kidneys have been perfused with these monoclonals to deplete them of their dendritic cells and hence reduce their immunogenicity. Early clinical trials have reported a decreased incidence of acute rejection episodes.

Increasing appreciation of the role of adhesion molecules in the immune response (see Chap. 2) has led to the development of antibodies directed against them. **BIRR1** is a murine monoclonal antibody against **ICAM-1** (intercellular adhesion molecule-1 [CD54]). Phase 1 clinical trials suggest safety and effectiveness. The antibody against its ligand **leukocyte function–associated molecule-1** (LFA-1) has been shown to be effective in animal models.

Monoclonal antibodies directed against the alpha chain of the IL-2 receptor, so-called **anti-Tac** antibodies, prevent allograft rejection in animals and are as effective as antithymocyte globulin in early clinical trials, perhaps with fewer side effects. Promising early results have been obtained with an antibody directed against the T cell antigen-receptor complex (**T10 B9**). **IL-2 toxin** is a genetic construct chimeric toxin with antigenic determinants of both IL-2 and diphtheria toxin. The IL-2 antigen targets the lethal diphtheria toxin onto the IL-2 receptor. This immunotoxin has produced dramatic antigen-specific immunosuppression in animal models, with the only cells affected being activated T cells with high-affinity IL-2 receptors. **Anti-CD4** monoclonal antibodies may block the interaction between the T cell receptor and the polymorphic determinants of class II antigens. Both the IL-2 toxin and the anti-CD4 monoclonal have potential as tolerance-inducing agents for future clinical use.

Humanized Monoclonal Antibodies

All rodent-derived monoclonal antibodies have intrinsic disadvantages, including a propensity to elicit human anti-mouse antibodies, variable effectiveness in triggering human effector functions, and a short half-life. **"Humanized"** monoclonal antibodies exploit genetic engineering techniques to combine a rodent-derived antibody binding site with a human antibody framework. The first generation of humanized antibodies were simple chimeric antibodies in which the rodent variable domains were attached to the constant domains of human antibodies. In the second-generation antibodies, so-called **complimentary determining regions (CDR)**–grafted antibodies, antigen-binding loops of rodent monoclonal antibodies have been built into human antibodies.

Attempts have been made to humanize several of the rodent antibodies noted above. The most successful product to date is the monoclonal **humanized anti-Tac** (Zenapax) (HAT). HAT binds to the p55 subunit of the IL-2 receptor and blocks the formation of the high-affinity receptor and its subsequent activation by IL-2. Phase 1 clinical trials with this antibody suggest that it is safe for human use and effective in preventing rejections. As anticipated, HAT has a long half-life and is administered every other week. A first-dose reaction, such as is seen following administration of OKT3, has not been observed. A double-blind, randomized, placebo-controlled trial is in progress using HAT for induction immunosuppression in combination with standard immunosuppressive agents. A similar study is in progress using **CHI 621**, a chimeric humanized monoclonal antibody also targeted against the IL-2 receptor.

As a result of genetic engineering techniques, a variety of recombinant products has been produced designed to impair the function of the ligand-receptor accessory molecules (see Chap. 3). Of these, the **CTLA4Ig fusion protein** is the most promising and has been shown to be capable of inducing tolerance in animal models.

DONOR-SPECIFIC BONE MARROW AND BLOOD TRANSFUSIONS

Infusion of donor-specific bone marrow in combination with short-term nonspecific immunosuppression using polyclonal antibodies has produced long-term graft survival in the absence of immunosuppressive therapy in experimental and clinical organ allografts. The donor bone marrow provides an as yet unidentified signal for tolerance. The cellular components of the bone marrow that may be responsible for its tolerance-inducing effect are so-called **veto cells**. These cells are a small subpopulation of donor marrow cells with powerful suppressor cell functions. The tolerogenic effect of bone marrow and blood may also be due to the development of a state of microchimerism (see Chap. 2). Clinical trials are in progress to test the potential benefit of perioperative donor-specific blood transfusion in live-related transplantation.

Part III: Immunosuppressive Protocols

There are currently a limited number of immunosuppressive drugs available for use in clinical transplantation, yet there is a wide variety of permutations of these drugs that make up immunosuppressive protocols. Transplant centers tend to be loyal to their own protocols, which often have been developed in response to local needs and experience. Protocols should be regarded as guides for therapy that need not necessarily be adhered to slavishly and may require modification from patient to patient and with new knowledge and experience. In an era where short-term success rates for cadaveric transplants of greater than 85% are commonplace, it may take experience with hundreds of patients followed for prolonged periods to prove the benefit of a new or modified approach. There is still very little data on the impact of different protocols on 5- and 10-year graft survival.

Certain principles should guide all transplant protocols:
1. The risk of acute rejection is highest in the first weeks and months post-transplant and diminishes thereafter. Immunosuppression should be at its highest level in this early period and should be reduced for long-term therapy.
2. All patients are not equal with respect to the chances of rejection, and the dangers of immunosuppression and protocols should take this into account. Multiply transplanted patients and patients with high levels of preformed antibodies may require more intense therapy. Older patients may not tolerate heavy immunosuppression. Recipients of live-related transplants may require less immunosuppression.
3. The most feared side effects of immunosuppression—infection and malignancy—tend to reflect the total amount of immunosuppression given rather than the dosage of a single drug. The total quantity of immunosuppression should be monitored and considered when deciding to prolong therapy or treat refractory rejection.
4. Delayed graft function complicates early transplant management and may have an unfavorable impact on long-term function. Cyclosporine has been implicated in the prolongation and perhaps production of delayed graft function. Many centers avoid cyclosporine, reduce its dose, or add other agents for grafts with delayed function.
5. Corticosteroids are valuable adjuncts to the basic immunosuppressive protocol. There is still no consensus as to their best application. Not all patients need steroids, although it is not yet possible to clearly identify those patients who do not. Protocols that avoid or discontinue corticosteroids should be used selectively and with great care (see the section on steroid withdrawal)
6. Established chronic rejection does not respond to high-dose immunosuppression. Immunosuppression of a failing graft should be kept to a minimum, and potentially reversible causes of graft dysfunction should be ruled out (see Chap. 9).
7. The minimal mortality nowadays associated with kidney transplantation is due to a large degree to an appreciation of when to minimize or stop immunosuppression and abandon a kidney. Although each case must be considered individually, patients with deteriorating graft function despite more than two or three appropriately treated rejections are better allowed to return to dialysis and seek another transplant. As the new generation of immunosuppressive agents enters routine clinical practice, great care and judgment will be needed to avoid the temptation of excessively adding or exchanging new agents.
8. Kidney allografts have long memories! Immunosuppression is required for the functional life of the graft even if it is 20 years or more. Discontinuation of immunosuppressive drugs, even many years post-transplant, may lead to late acute rejection or accelerated chronic rejection. Discontinuation should be considered only if there is a specific, overriding indication, such as malignancy (see Chap. 9).

PROTOCOLS FOR CADAVERIC TRANSPLANTS

Cyclosporine

Cyclosporine, 10–14 mg/kg/day PO (3–4 mg/kg/day IV), is given as a single dose or twice daily starting immediately prior to transplant.

**Table 4-7. Approximate therapeutic ranges for
cyclosporine (μg/liter)**

Months post-transplant	HPLC and monoclonal RIA	Monoclonal FPIA	Polyclonal FPIA
0–2	150–350	250–500	500–900
2–6	100–250	175–350	400–700
>6	~100	~150	300–400

HPLC = high-performance liquid chromatography; RIA = radioimmunoassay;
FPIA = fluorescent polarization immunoassay.

The IV infusion is given over at least 4 hours or can be given as a constant infusion over 24 hours. Some programs prefer to omit the preoperative dose or avoid IV cyclosporine altogether. Doses are reduced to maintain levels within the ranges given in Table 4-7. It is wise to continue to monitor trough levels of cyclosporine, although the degree of reliance on these levels varies from program to program. The desired dose and target level is influenced by concomitant use of adjunctive agents and history of rejections. By 3 months post-transplant, most patients are receiving cyclosporine in a dose of 3–5 mg/kg.

There is still no clear consensus regarding the best dose or drug level for long-term cyclosporine use, and it is unfortunate that prospective randomized trials comparing cyclosporine dose ranges are not available. Fear of progressive nephrotoxicity has tempted many clinicians to permit low levels, yet such a policy may allow for the insidious development of chronic rejection. Retrospective studies have shown that continued use of cyclosporine is conducive to prolonged adequate graft function and that, within the range of the recommended doses, higher doses may be better than lower doses. Far more kidneys are lost to chronic rejection than to chronic cyclosporine toxicity.

Sandimmune/Neoral Switch

Many patients are now switching from Sandimmune to Neoral cyclosporine in anticipation of the eventual discontinuation of Sandimmune production. This switch requires care because of the different pharmacokinetics of the two formulations (see the section on cyclosporine's pharmacokinetics). Though a 1:1 dose ratio is recommended, some patients require somewhat less Neoral than Sandimmune. Even in stable patients, cyclosporine blood levels should be monitored more carefully in the month following the switch and dose adjustments made. An elevation of the creatinine level soon after a switch is more likely to be due to nephrotoxicity than rejection.

Cyclosporine Withdrawal

Several studies have shown that it may be possible to withdraw cyclosporine in some stable patients. Such a policy is discouraged, however, since it may increase the risk of late rejections and graft loss, particularly when the transplant was not well-matched. There is also little to gain from cyclosporine withdrawal, since continued use of the drug is conducive to prolonged graft function.

Corticosteroids

Methylprednisolone is given intraoperatively in a dose of up to 1 g. The dose is then reduced rapidly from 150 mg on day 1 to 20–30 mg on day 14. Some programs avoid the steroid cycle altogether, modifying it or starting at 30 mg daily or even less. There is some evidence that the use of high-dose steroids in the early post-transplant period may minimize the incidence of acute rejection. The maximal oral dose of prednisone at 1 month should be 20 mg and 15 mg at 3 months. After a year, many patients tolerate an every-other-day regimen. The low long-term maintenance doses that patients typically receive (5.0–7.5 mg daily) should be regarded with great care and respect. Rejection episodes may occasionally occur when even very small dose reductions are made.

Steroid Withdrawal

Steroid withdrawal implies the discontinuation of steroid administration post-transplant and needs to be differentiated from **steroid avoidance**, in which steroids are administered only in the event of rejection. Steroid avoidance has never been popular in the United States, although it has been applied in Europe. Many patients who avoid steroids end up receiving them for rejection anyway. Steroid withdrawal is a more tempting ploy that may be considered in selected patients, although the anxiety associated with withdrawal (for both the patients and their physicians) has understandably dampened its popularity. Steroid withdrawal should be considered only in patients who are at least several months post-transplant, have not suffered recent or recurrent rejections, have excellent graft function, and are receiving relatively high doses of cyclosporine. There is some evidence that black transplant recipients may not be good candidates for withdrawal. A clear-cut benefit of withdrawal, in terms of certain steroid-related side effects (e.g., bone disease, hyperlipidemia) has not been demonstrated. There may be long-term deterioration in graft function in steroid-withdrawn patients, who should be forewarned.

Azathioprine

The addition of azathioprine (1–2 mg/kg) to cyclosporine and prednisone in the early days post-transplant is known as **triple therapy**. This regimen has become popular, although its benefits are unproved. Theoretically, triple therapy may allow for a lower dose of cyclosporine to minimize short- and long-term nephrotoxicity. It may also serve to "protect" the patient against transient low levels of cyclosporine. In the long-term, rejection episodes may be more frequent if cyclosporine levels are very low, even in the presence of azathioprine. The introduction of mycophenolate mofetil into routine clinical practice will likely further limit the use of azathioprine.

Mycophenolate Mofetil

MMF became available for routine clinical use in mid-1995 following FDA approval of its use for the prevention of acute allograft rejection (see the section on MMF's clinical trials). Clinical experience with this drug since its release suggests that its benefit, in terms of prevention of acute rejection, may be even greater than that reported in the blinded trials. It is always used as an adjunctive agent with cyclosporine and prednisone. The standard dose for adults is 1,000 mg bid (four capsules of 250 mg), although black patients may benefit from a larger dose (1,500 mg bid). It is not necessary to measure

**Table 4-8. Potential advantages and disadvantages
of sequential and induction therapy**

Potential advantages	Potential disadvantages
1-yr cadaveric function of 90% reported	Risk of first-dose reaction with OKT3
Period of delayed graft function may be foreshortened	May prolong hospital admission stay
Onset of first rejection delayed	Greater cost
Obviates early use of cyclosporine	Higher incidence of cytomegalovirus infection
	Occasional limitation of future treatment options

blood levels of MMF, and the dose can be safely reduced or held for short periods in the event of side effects as long as cyclosporine and prednisone doses are maintained. As with any new drug, clinicians should be alert for side effects and drug interactions not encountered in the clinical trials. Combinations of MMF with other agents have not been rigorously tested and are discouraged; the "steroid sparing" effect of MMF has also not been tested. Recommendations for long-term use of MMF will need to await the results of ongoing clinical trials.

Induction and Sequential Therapy

Induction therapy refers to the use of OKT3 or a polyclonal antibody in the first 7–10 days post-transplant. Cyclosporine is either withheld, or its dose kept to a minimum until 2–3 days before the antibody course is completed. In **sequential** therapy, cyclosporine is introduced only when renal function has reached a predetermined level (e.g., a plasma creatinine of 3 mg/dl). OKT3 or the polyclonal antibody is discontinued as soon as adequate cyclosporine levels are achieved. A patient with a well-functioning graft may thus receive only a few days of antibody treatment.

Sequential and induction protocols represent the major alternative to the use of cyclosporine in the early post-transplant period. The comparative advantages and disadvantages of this approach are listed in Table 4-8. Some transplant programs employ sequential or induction therapy for all cadaveric recipients, although increasingly its use is being reserved for immunologically high-risk recipients or for patients with delayed graft function. The introduction of mycophenolate mofetil into clinical practice may further limit the necessity for induction-type protocols.

PROTOCOLS FOR LIVE TRANSPLANTS

Excellent results were achieved for 2-haplotype–matched live-related transplants immunosuppressed with azathioprine and prednisone alone before the introduction of cyclosporine into routine clinical practice. Despite this experience, many transplant programs now use cyclosporine-based protocols for these patients because of the lesser incidence of acute rejection. Two-haplotype–matched transplant recipients receiving cyclosporine may be good candidates for eventual steroid withdrawal.

For all other live donor transplants, a cyclosporine-based protocol should be employed similar to that described for cadaveric transplants. A minority of transplant programs also use induction protocols for these transplants. The technique of donor-specific transfusions was once applied widely for less than 2-haplotype–matched transplants but has largely been superseded by cyclosporine use.

MANAGEMENT OF ACUTE REJECTION

First Rejection

Pulse Steroids

High doses of pulse steroids reverse approximately 75% of first acute rejections. There are numerous ways to pulse a patient, and there is no good evidence that the higher-dose pulses (500–1000 mg methylprednisolone for 3 days) are necessarily more effective than the lower-dose pulses (120–250 mg oral prednisone or methylprednisolone for 3–5 days). Most programs still prefer to use IV methylprednisolone, which is given over 30–60 minutes into a peripheral vein. Pulse therapy is suitable for outpatient use when clinically indicated. The dose of prednisone can be continued at its previous level when the pulse is completed, although some programs elect to recycle the prednisone dose after the pulse has been completed.

OKT3

The use of OKT3 (or polyclonal antibodies) is a highly effective therapy for the management of a first acute rejection, and approximately 90% of such rejections will be reversed. Despite the greater effectiveness of OKT3, most programs still prefer to use pulse steroids as their first-line acute rejection therapy because of their convenience and lower risks. OKT3 may be a better first-line option for particularly severe or vascular rejections. There is some evidence that using OKT3 rather than steroids to treat a first acute rejection may reduce the chances of eventual development of chronic rejection (see Chap. 9), possibly because OKT3 more completely clears the inflammatory process.

Recurrent and Refractory Rejections

Repeated courses of pulse steroids may be effective in reversing acute rejections, but it is probably not wise to administer more than two courses of pulse therapy before resorting to OKT3 or polyclonal antibodies. Many programs use OKT3 for all second rejections unless the rejection is clinically mild or separated from the first by at least several weeks. OKT3 is particularly valuable for rejection episodes that are **steroid-resistant** and may succeed in reversing a high percentage of such rejections. Some programs commence OKT3 if there is not an immediate response to pulse therapy while others wait several days. If renal function is deteriorating rapidly in the face of pulse steroids, it is probably wise to start OKT3 early.

The term **refractory rejection** is not well defined. It usually refers to ongoing rejection despite treatment with pulse steroids and OKT3. The management of these patients is problematic. Second courses of OKT3 can be given in selected patients, and long-term graft function can be achieved in 40–50% of such patients. When deciding whether to give a second course of OKT3, the clinician should bear in mind the severity and potential reversibility of rejection on biopsy; the increased risk of infection and malignancy that ensues, particularly if two courses are given close together; and the possibility of generating high levels of anti-OKT3 antibodies that might limit treatment options for a future transplant.

Now that tacrolimus has been approved for use in liver transplantation, it is being employed "off label" for the management of refractory kidney rejection. Nonrandomized studies have shown that up to 75% of such rejections can be reversed. If a decision is made to change to tacrolimus, it is important that cyclosporine be discontinued and its levels be allowed to fall to less than 100 ng/ml on a specific assay before tacrolimus is introduced. It may be wise to "cover" the period between adequate cyclosporine and tacrolimus levels with high-dose steroids. It is probably unnecessary to use azathioprine with tacrolimus. Mycophenolate mofetil is a valuable alternative for the treatment of refractory rejection (see the section on MMF's clinical trials).

Late Rejections

The terms **early** and **late rejection** are not well-defined. The differentiation between early and late rejection is not just semantic; each may respond differently to therapy. For practical purposes, a late rejection is one that occurs more than 3–4 months post-transplant and may be a first, or more frequently, a recurrent rejection. Late rejections can also be divided up into those that occur in the face of apparently adequate immunosuppression and into those that occur as a result of obviously inadequate immunosuppression, typically in noncompliant patients. Late rejections are often a prelude to chronic rejection and accelerated graft loss.

The initial treatment for a late rejection is pulse steroids. The effectiveness of OKT3 for acute rejection treatment tends to diminish with time so that by 3–4 months post-transplant, only 40–50% of episodes will respond to OKT3 treatment. By 1 year post-transplant, this figure may be only approximately 20%, and at this stage it may not be worth the risks associated with therapy. There is evidence that late rejections associated with noncompliance are more likely to respond to therapy. Use of polyclonal antibodies for late steroid-resistant rejection has not been systematically studied.

Thus, there are limited therapeutic options for late steroid-resistant rejection, which often occurs in a background of chronic rejection. It may often be wiser to accept graft dysfunction or loss rather than use potent high-dose immunosuppression in an already chronically immunosuppressed patient.

SELECTED READINGS

Part I

Abramowicz D, DePauw LD, LeMoine A et al. Prevention of OKT3 nephrotoxicity after kidney transplantation. *Kidney Int* 49:539, 1996.

Batiuk TD, Feldzgeritta P, Halloran P. Calcineurin activity is only partially inhibited in leukocytes of cyclosporine-treated patients. *Transplantation* 59:1400, 1995.

Burke JF, Pirsch JD, Ramos EL et al. Long-term efficacy and safety of cyclosporine in renal transplant recipients. *N Engl J Med* 331:358, 1994.

Campana C, Regazzi MB, Buggia I et al. Clinically significant drug interactions with cyclosporine. *Clin Pharmacokinet* 30:141, 1996.

Chan GL, Sinott JT, Emmanuel PJ et al. Drug interactions with cyclosporine: Focus on antimicrobial agents. *Clin Transplantation* 6:141, 1992.

Fryer JP, Granger DK, Leventhal JR et al. Steroid-related complications in the cyclosporine era. *Clin Transplantation* 8:224, 1994.

Kahan BD, Dunn J, Fitts C et al. The Neoral formulation: Improved correlation between cyclosporine trough levels and exposure in stable renal transplant recipients. *Transplant Proc* 26:2940, 1994.

Khanna A, Li B, Sehajpal PK et al. Mechanism of action of cyclosporine: A new hypothesis implicating transforming growth factor-β. *Transplantation Rev* 9:41, 1995.

Luke RG. New issues in therapy after renal transplantation. *N Engl J Med* 331:393, 1994.

Lum CT, Umen EJ, Kasiske B et al. Clinical impact of replacing Minnesota antilymphocytic globulin with ATGAM. *Transplantation* 59:371, 1995.

Norman DJ. Rationale for OKT3 monoclonal antibody treatment in transplant patients. *Transplant Proc* 25:1, 1993.

Tornatore KM, Biocevich DM, Reed K et al. Methylprednisolone pharmacokinetics, cortisol response, and adverse effects in black and white renal transplant recipients. *Transplantation* 59:729, 1995.

Part II

Baliba P, Chavin KD, Qin L et al. CTLA4Ig prolongs allograft survival while suppressing cell-mediated immunity. *Transplantation* 58:1082, 1994.

Cosimi AB. Current and future applications of monoclonal antibodies in clinical immunosuppressive protocols. *Clin Transplantation* 9:219, 1995.

Danovitch GM. Mycophenolate mofetil: Experience from the U.S. clinical trials. *Kidney Int* 48:S93, 1995.

Gregory CR, Huang X, Pratt RE et al. Treatment with rapamycin and mycophenolic acid reduces arterial intimal thickening produced by mechanical injury and allows endothelial replacement. *Transplantation* 59:655, 1995.

Halloran PF. Aspects of allograft rejection, IV: Evaluation of new pharmacologic agents for prevention of allograft rejection. *Transplantation Rev* 9:138, 1995.

Halloran PF, Batiuk TD, Goes NB et al. Strategies to improve the immunologic management of organ transplants. *Clin Transplantation* 9:227, 1995.

Manez R, Jain A, Marino IR et al. Comparative evaluation of tacrolimus (FK506) and cyclosporine A as immunosuppressive agents. *Transplantation Rev* 9:63, 1995.

Morris RE. Mechanism of action of new immunosuppressive drugs. *Kidney Int* 49:S26, 1996.

Nickerson PW, Steurer W, Steiger J et al. In pursuit of the "Holy Grail": Allograft tolerance. *Kidney Int* 45:S40–S49, 1994.

Sollinger HW for the U.S. Renal Transplant Mycophenolate Mofetil Study Group. Mycophenolate mofetil for the prevention of acute rejection in primary cadaveric renal allograft recipients. *Transplantation* 60:225, 1995.

Part III

Delminico FL, Tolfoff-Rubin N, Aucinloss JH et al. Management of the renal allograft recipient: Immunosuppressive protocols for long-term success. *Clin Transplantation* 8:34, 1994.

Helderman JH, Van Buren DH, Amend WJ et al. Chronic immunosuppression of the renal transplant patient. *J Am Soc Nephrol* 4:S2, 1994.

Hricik DE, Seliga RM, Fleming-Brooks S. Determinants of long-term allograft function following steroid withdrawal in renal transplant recipients. *Clin Transplantation* 9.419, 1995.

Hricik DE, Almawi WY, Strom TB. Trends in the use of glucocorticoids in renal transplantation. *Transplantation* 57:979, 1994.

Montagnino G, Tarantino A, Banfi G et al. A randomized trial comparing triple-drug and double-drug therapy in renal transplantation. *Transplantation* 58:149, 1994.

Paul LC, Zaltzman JS, Cardella CJ. Prohylactic anti-lymphocytic antibody therapy in kidney transplantation: Quo vadis? *Transplantation Rev* 9:168, 1995.

Suthanthiran M, Strom TB. Renal transplantation. *N Engl J Med* 331:36, 1994.

Wilkinson AH, Rosenthal JT, Danovitch GM. Developments and dilemmas in renal transplantation. *Adv Renal Replacement Ther* 1:32, 1994.

5

Live-Related and Cadaveric Kidney Donation

J. Thomas Rosenthal and Gabriel M. Danovitch

Kidney transplantation cannot proceed without kidney donors, and although much emphasis is given to post-transplant patient management, the appropriate identification and preparation of donors contribute critically to the success of the transplant endeavor on both the individual and the national levels. Tables 5-1 and 5-2 list the potential advantages and disadvantages of live-related versus cadaveric transplantation. Living donors are used for approximately 25% of all kidney transplants performed in the United States, and most transplant centers regard them as the preferred donation modality despite the potential morbidity associated with them.

Figure 1-1 in Chapter 1 illustrates graphically the inexorably widening gap between the demand for donor kidneys and their supply. The number of cadaver donors has remained essentially stable over the last decade, while the number of potential recipients rises each year. The inevitable impact of this discrepancy is an increase in the waiting time for cadaveric kidneys, which is now often measured in months and years (see Chap. 3). Surveys suggest that although almost all Americans are aware that kidney transplants are performed and as many as 75% express willingness to donate an organ after death, only approximately 40% of all potential cadaveric organ donors actually become donors. Some possible reasons for this discrepancy are discussed below. The transplant community now finds itself critically re-examining some long-held tenets regarding the suitability of certain types of live and cadaveric donors and carefully re-evaluating the manner in which potential donors and their loved ones are approached.

LIVE KIDNEY DONATION

Who Can Be a Live Donor?

For many years, only first-degree relatives—parents, children, and siblings who were at least 1-haplotype–matched (see Chap. 3)—were deemed suitable live kidney donors. This policy was largely based on the premise that the matching of these kidneys compared with all others so improved their prognosis, or "utility," for the recipient that the risk to the donor was justified. The advent of cyclosporine and the widening gap between the supply and demand for cadaveric kidneys is changing this attitude. It is now clear that the results of zero-haplotype–matched sibling transplants and transplants from more distant relatives and biologically unrelated donors are excellent and are similar or even better than those of 6-antigen–matched cadaveric transplants (see Chap. 3). This suggests that it is not just the matching of the live donor kidney that determines its benefits for the recipient but the excellent condition of the kidney at the time of its transplantation. There is also a widespread realization that it is highly unlikely that the cadaveric organ supply will ever keep pace with the need for organs. As a result, there has been a gradual broadening of the definition of who can be a live donor.

Table 5-1. Potential advantages of live versus cadaveric kidney donation

1. Better short-term results (approximately 95% versus 85% 1-yr function)[a]
2. Better long-term results (half life of 12–20 yrs versus 7–8 yrs)[a]
3. More consistent early function and ease of management
4. Avoidance of long wait for cadaveric transplant[a]
5. Capacity to time transplant for medical and personal convenience
6. Immunosuppressive regime may be less aggressive[b]
7. Helps relieve stress on national cadaver donor supply
8. Emotional gain to donor[c]

[a]See Chap. 3.
[b]See Chap. 4.
[c]See Chap. 15.

Table 5-2. Potential disadvantages of live donation

1. Psychological stress to donor and family*
2. Inconvenience and risk of evaluation process (i.e., intravenous pyelogram and angiogram)
3. Operative mortality (approximately 1/2000)
4. Major postoperative complications (approximately 2%)
5. Minor postoperative complication (up to 50%)
6. Long-term morbidity (possibly mild hypertension and proteinuria)
7. Risk of traumatic injury to remaining kidney

*See Chaps. 15 and 16.

Many centers now routinely accept as donors zero-haplotype-matched siblings and second-degree relatives (e.g., cousins, uncles, aunts). Biologically unrelated transplant donors are most frequently spouses or individuals who have a clearly definable emotional relationship to the recipient (e.g., adopted siblings, fiancees, best friends). The term **emotionally related donor** is a good one, since it emphasizes the importance of the personal relationship between the donor and the recipient. The definition of this relationship is all the more important because financial incentives for donation are illegal in the United States and in most industrialized countries (see Chap. 16). The wisdom of this policy is borne out in part by the clearly inferior results reported from countries where financial incentives are permitted or even encouraged. Live kidney donation, biologically or emotionally related, is an extraordinary act of altruism and love by one individual for another. Transplant centers in the United States vary in the degree to which they encourage unrelated donation.

A careful family history should be a routine part of the evaluation of all potential transplant recipients, and the advantages and disadvantages of live donation should be discussed when relevant. A brief screening often rules out obviously inappropriate donors. Patients should not be pressured into approaching family members for donation when they are uncomfortable doing so, nor should potential donors be pressured into the evaluation process. It is often a good prognostic sign when the donor accompanies the recipient to his or her pretransplant evaluation appointments. The first approach to the potential donor should ideally come from the patient and not from the patient's nephrologist or transplant physician or surgeon.

Table 5-3. Suggested evaluation process for potential live donors

Donor screening
   Educate patient regarding cadaveric and live-related donation
   Take family history and screen for potential donors
   Review ABO compatibilities of potential donors
   Tissue-type and crossmatch ABO-compatible potential donors
   Choose primary potential donor with patient and family
   Educate donor regarding process of evaluation and donation
Donor evaluation
   Complete history and physical examination
   Comprehensive laboratory screening to include complete blood
      count, chemistry panel, human immunodeficiency virus, very-low-
      density lipoprotein, HBsAg, anti-hepatitis C virus,
      cytomegalovirus, glucose tolerance test (for diabetic families)
   Urinalysis, urine culture, pregnancy test
   24-hr urine collection for protein (twice)
   24-hr urine collection for creatinine (twice)
   Chest x-ray, cardiogram, exercise treadmill for patients older than
      50 yrs of age
   Intravenous pyelogram*
   Psychiatric evaluation
   Renal angiogram*
   Repeat crossmatch prior to transplant

*May be replaced by helical CT urogram in some centers (see Chap. 11).

Some patients find it difficult to approach family members, and the nephrologist and transplant team should be prepared to facilitate the discussion of donation. Written material explaining the donation process often can help to alleviate the fears and anxiety of potential donors.

Donor Evaluation

Evaluation of living donors is a stepwise process that progresses from initial screening through noninvasive to invasive evaluation and surgery. A practical schema for the process is shown in Table 5-3. Certain basic principles are consistent in the manner that all programs approach and evaluate donors, although details of policy may differ (see Kasiske and Bia, 1995). The pace of the evaluation is often made by the donors, who must appreciate that the process is not irreversible. The donor can withdraw at any time, although clearly it is wasteful to do so at the more advanced stages of evaluation. Precise definition of renal anatomy with intravenous pyelogram and angiography or with the spiral CT scan (see Chap. 11) is the final step in the process and should follow psychiatric or social worker evaluation (see Chap. 15) and completion of the recipient workup. The donor who has second thoughts about donation should be provided, if he or she wishes, with a medical alibi to justify his or her hesitation to the family.

Exclusion Criteria

Potential donors are excluded on medical grounds when it is believed that there may be a risk of unrecognized kidney disease or an

Table 5-4. Exclusion criteria for live-related donors

Age <18 yrs or >65 yrs
Hypertension (>140/90 or necessity for medication)
Diabetes (abnormal glucose tolerance test or HbA_{1c})
Proteinuria (>250 mg/24 hr)
History of kidney stones
Abnormal glomerular filtration rate (Ccreat < 80 ml/min)[a]
Microscopic hematuria
Urologic abnormalities in donor kidneys
Significant medical illness (e.g., chronic lung disease, recent
  malignancy)
Obesity (30% above ideal weight)
History of thrombosis or thromboembolism
Psychiatric contraindications[b]

[a]Measured by either creatinine clearance or a radiolabeled filtration marker.
[b]See Chap. 15.

increased risk of short- or long-term morbidity and mortality from
the operative procedure itself. Table 5-4 reviews some frequent criteria for excluding potentially compatible donors. Many of these criteria are not absolute, and when findings are borderline, it is always
wise to err on the side of donor safety, since the donor, unlike the
recipient, does not need the operation to improve his or her health.
Some centers adhere rigidly to an upper age limit, while other centers attempt to judge biological rather than chronological age. A
glomerular filtration rate (GFR) of 80 ml/minute or more has generally been believed to be adequate to permit donation, although older
donors, women with low muscle mass, and vegetarians may have a
GFR of less than 80 ml/minute with no evidence of renal disease. To
avoid conflict of interest, it is preferable for a physician other than
the one caring for the recipient to determine donor suitability. It
must be clear to all concerned that donors are not to be sacrificed for
recipients even in circumstances (particularly parents to children) in
which the donor is quite prepared to make the sacrifice.

Hereditary Kidney Disease

The issue of donation in families with hereditary kidney disease
occurs most frequently in families with polycystic kidney disease or
hereditary nephritis. In families with polycystic kidney disease, a
negative ultrasound or computed tomography (CT) scan in a potential donor older than age 30 years safely rules out the disease and
permits donation. Since the polycystic kidney gene is a dominant
one, the children of such a donor will not inherit the disease. In
hereditary nephritis, the situation may be more complex. A patient
in the third decade of life who is free of urinary abnormalities could
be deemed free of disease and hence be a donor. It is not inconceiv-
able, however, that the offspring of such a donor could suffer kidney
disease; this possibility may be a consideration in the potential
donor's decision, particularly when the family history is a strong one.

Which Donor to Choose?

If there is more than one donor in a family, it is logical to commence
workup on the relative who is best matched (i.e., a 2-haplotype match

versus a 1-haplotype match). If the donors are of the same match grade (i.e., a 1-haplotype parent and a 1-haplotype sibling), it may be advisable to choose the older donor with the thought that the younger donor would still be available for donation if the first kidney eventually fails. Women of child-bearing age are not at increased risk for obstetric problems after donation. Biologically related donors are generally preferred over emotionally related donors.

Surgical Evaluation of the Donor

Intravenous urography and renal arteriography are currently routinely performed before surgery in most centers (see Chap. 11). Digital subtraction angiography is not sensitive enough to detect small polar renal arteries (whose detection is one of the major reasons for the arteriogram) and hence does not replace a standard aortic angiogram. Spiral CT urography may be sufficiently sensitive to provide accurate anatomic information and has replaced arteriography in some centers. Usually the left kidney is selected for donation because the left renal vein is longer than the right vein and thus easier to transplant. If there are multiple arteries to the left kidney and a single artery to the right kidney, the right kidney can be used. If there are two arteries bilaterally, a kidney may still be used, employing one of several surgical techniques to handle multiple renal arteries. Occasionally, the donor has minor unilateral renal abnormalities, such as renal cysts, or even more severe problems, such as ureteral pelvic junction obstruction. In these situations, the most prudent approach, if such abnormalities are not too severe, is to transplant the abnormal kidney, leaving the donor with the normal one.

Donor Nephrectomy

The operation is similar to any simple nephrectomy performed for nontransplant purposes; in addition, transplant nephrectomy requires careful dissection and preservation of the renal artery, vein, and ureter. A flank incision above the twelfth rib with an extrapleural, extraperitoneal approach is usually performed, although some surgeons prefer an anterior transperitoneal approach, particularly if there are multiple renal arteries or if it is a right-sided nephrectomy. The transperitoneal approach has a higher operative morbidity. Excessive traction on the renal artery should be avoided to prevent vasospasm. Care must be made to avoid stripping the blood supply of the ureter. Donors should be hydrated the night before and morning of surgery to ensure a brisk diuresis. Mannitol is given intraoperatively. Papaverine or lidocaine may be dripped onto the renal artery if there is any suggestion of vasospasm. Systemic heparinization is not required. After removal, the kidney is placed in a basin of ice slushed and flushed with cold Collins' solution (see the section on Collins' solution versus University of Wisconsin solution). Heparin is added to the flush in lieu of systemic heparinization of the donor.

Postoperative Management

A chest x-ray is routinely obtained in the recovery room, and a chest tube placed or air evacuated if a pneumothorax is observed. A nasogastric tube is not routinely inserted. If a flank incision has been made, most patients are able to eat 24–48 hours after surgery. Early ambulation is encouraged, as is aggressive pulmonary toilet. The average hospital stay is 5–7 days. Most donors can return to all but the most strenuous exercise or work by 3–4 weeks. Complete recovery takes 6–8 weeks, although some donors complain of incisional pain for 2–3 months.

Postoperative Complications

Operative mortality is minimal but is not nonexistent. In a series of more than 8,000 living donors, there were five deaths due to myocardial infarction, pulmonary embolus, and hepatitis. The rate of major complications was 1.8%, which consisted of pulmonary emboli, myocardial infarctions, sepsis, pneumonia, wound infections, pancreatitis, and injuries to the spleen or the adrenal gland. There are also risks due to arteriography, such as femoral artery pseudoaneurysm or thrombosis. Careful and compulsive medical evaluation of the donor with adherence to strict donation criteria is the key to minimizing postnephrectomy complications.

Long-term morbidity has not proved to be a major problem; follow-up data for up to 45 years (following traumatic wartime uninephrectomy) suggest that having only one kidney does not have a significant health impact. There is a statistically higher risk of low-grade proteinuria. When large numbers of kidney donors have been followed, however, no increase in incidence of hypertension or deterioration of kidney function has been shown. Serum creatinine levels generally remain approximately 20% higher and clearance rates 20% lower than pre-donation values. Occasional cases of chronic renal failure have been observed postdonation, but it is unclear if the pretransplant workup of these donors was adequately compulsive or if the cases are a reflection of the incidence of de novo renal disease in the general population. Long-term mortality is not affected by kidney donation, and most life insurance companies do not penalize donors. The main risk of kidney failure in kidney donors is from trauma to the remaining kidney or unrecognized familial kidney disease.

CADAVERIC KIDNEY DONATION

The process of cadaveric transplantation—from recognition of a potential donor to the operation itself—is complex (Table 5-5). It represents the epitome of coordinated teamwork and institutional cooperation. It is best orchestrated by local regional **organ procurement organizations** (OPOs) (see Chap. 3), which provide a nationally integrated 24-hour service.

The responsibility for identifying potential donors and notifying the OPOs belongs to every health professional and hospital involved in acute patient care; it has been legally established in **"required request"** legislation (see Chap. 16). The benefits of this legislation have been less than expected, however. It has been estimated that more than 25% of the families of potential cadaveric donors are not approached, and more than half of the families that are approached decline to permit donation. The most difficult and sensitive part of the donation process—the approach to the recently bereaved family—should be handled by trained organ procurement professionals. Family members are more likely to permit donation if they are given time to accept the fact that their relative is brain-dead before organ donation is discussed. **"Uncoupling"** of the discussion of death and donation significantly increases the likelihood of family consent.

**Table 5-5. Sequence of events preceding
cadaveric donor transplantation[a]**

1. Recognition of potential donor (see Table 5-6)
2. Notification of organ procurement organization
3. Diagnosis of brain death made by attending physicians; family informed
4. Permission for organ donation obtained from family
5. Suitability of donor ascertained
6. Tissue typing and ABO blood typing of donor[b]
7. Kidneys removed and stored
8. Review local and national computer listing of all potential recipients
9. Top recipient selected by ABO blood type and United Network for Organ Sharing scoring system[b]
10. Notify top recipient patient and admit to hospital
11. Prepare "backup" recipient if recipient panel-reactive antibodies are high
12. Crossmatch between donor serum and recipient lymphocytes[b]
13. Preoperative history and physical examination
14. Preoperative chest x-ray, electrocardiogram, ABO blood typing, and routine chemistry
15. Dialyze if necessary
16. Transplant

[a]The precise sequence may vary in individual cases.
[b]See Chap. 3.

Although organ donor cards are in themselves valid legal documents, all OPOs request specific permission from families in order to maintain a high degree of public trust and acceptance. Discussion among family members of their attitudes toward organ donation should be encouraged so that the wishes of the deceased can be respected in the event of a catastrophe. Ongoing education by the transplant community of both health care professionals and the lay public is central to the maintenance of the cadaveric organ supply.

Who Is a Donor?

Currently, all solid organ donors are brain-dead cadavers, most of whom are "heart-beating" and are victims of head trauma, vascular catastrophes, cerebral anoxia, and nonmetastasizing brain tumors. It is best to regard all such patients as potential donors and then to rule out inappropriate candidates (Table 5-6). The criteria for donor acceptance are not all absolute, and many are controversial.

Donor Age

The use of organs from donors under the age of 5 or 6 is associated with an increased risk of urologic complications and impaired tolerance to episodes of graft dysfunction. Favorable results have been reported by some programs by transplanting both infant kidneys with their attachment to the great vessels—so-called **en bloc** transplantation. Organs from donors in their late 50s and 60s may be acceptable, although the long-term outcome of these kidneys may be impaired, particularly if the cause of the donor's death was vascular rather than traumatic. Older kidneys may be more sus-

Table 5-6. Contraindications to cadaveric donation

Absolute	Relative
Age >70 yrs	Age >60 yrs
Chronic renal disease	Age <6 yrs
Potentially metastasizing malignancy	Mild hypertension
Severe hypertension	Treated infection
Bacterial sepsis	Donor acute tubular necrosis
Intravenous drug abuse	Donor medical disease (diabetes, systemic lupus erythematosus)
HBsAg-positive	
Human immunodeficiency virus–positive	
Intestinal perforation	Prolonged cold ischemia
Prolonged warm ischemia	Positive for hepatitis C virus

ceptible to acute tubular necrosis, particularly if the cold ischemia time is prolonged. A biopsy of the potential allograft can be performed to assess the degree of glomerular sclerosis; some programs will not accept kidneys if more than 20% of glomeruli are sclerosed. A borderline or **"marginal"** kidney (e.g., from a 62-year-old donor with mild hypertension and a cold ischemia time of 30 hours) may be regarded as acceptable for a patient with a high percentage of panel-reactive antibodies and failing dialysis access but unacceptable for a young patient in good medical condition without antibodies. The final decision to offer a kidney to a patient is made by a transplant clinician equipped with information on the donor characteristics, the tissue match grade, and the recipient's clinical status.

Kidneys from donors who are male, non-black, of intermediate age, with immediate postoperative function, and a good tissue match may be less susceptible to chronic allograft failure than kidneys from poorly matched, female, black donors who are older than 60 years old or less than 3 years old with delayed initial function (see Chap. 9) The common factor explaining these findings may be the relative **"nephron dose"** that is transplanted (see Chap. 3). Currently, no systematic attempt is made to match the kidney size and nephron number to the size of the patient, and retrospective analysis suggests that such a policy would not necessarily be beneficial.

Contraindications to Donation

Positive serology for the human immunodeficiency virus (HIV) is a contraindication to the use of a cadaver kidney. Concern regarding transmission of HIV and the possibility of a false-negative HIV test result is such that HIV-negative donors are excluded if they are deemed to be at high risk for HIV infection because of IV drug use or because of high-risk sexual behavior. Hepatitis B surface antigen positivity is a contraindication to donation, although kidneys from donors that are hepatitis B core antibody–positive (but IgM-negative, indicating distant infection) can be safely transplanted.

The prevalence of hepatitis C virus (HCV) infection in the cadaveric donor population is approximately 2–3%, and since HCV can be transmitted by transplantation, the use of these kidneys for transplantation is controversial. In the short-term, it may be safe to transplant HCV-positive kidneys, since the progression of liver disease in the recipient is typically very slow. Some programs now routinely accept HCV-positive kidneys for their older recipients or for patients who are anti-HCV–positive. Occasional cases of fulminant HCV infection have been reported in recipients of HCV-positive kidneys.

Cancer can be transmitted by donor organs and, other than for some specific exceptions, is a contraindication to donation. Rare but well-documented cases of transplanted cancer have been described as a result of covert malignancy in the donor. Primary brain tumors are generally not regarded as a contraindication to transplantation, since, in the absence of a systemic shunt, they rarely metastasize. Confirmation of histology is mandatory to ensure that the tumors are not metastases.

Non–Heart-Beating Cadaver Donors

To reduce the shortage of kidneys for transplantation, attempts have been made to use organs from non–heart-beating donors. In the past, these organs have not been used because of the fear of irreparable ischemic damage. Protocols have been developed to minimize ischemia by rapid placement of IV cannulas to cool the organs between the time of irreversible cardiac arrest and harvesting. In reality, the practical obstacles to this process for most cases of unexpected cardiac arrest are overwhelming. Use of non–heart-beating donors has proved practical, however, in cases of brain-injured patients who are not expected to survive but in whom brain-death criteria are not met before hemodynamic deterioration. In these circumstances, consent can be obtained, and potentially well-functioning organs can be harvested before brain-death criteria are met. Protocols for non–heart-beating donors have to be carefully crafted to respect the feelings of donor families and avoid the appearance of conflicts of interest.

Diagnosis of Brain Death

Cadaveric solid organ transplantation requires that the organ or organs to be transplanted be maintained in a state of good function until the moment of harvest. Somatic death and cardiac standstill tend to follow brain death by 2–3 days, and by this time, organ function is often irreversibly impaired. Societal acceptance and the legal and medical establishment of brain-death criteria are essential components of cadaveric transplantation (see Chap. 16); countries that do not have such criteria do not have well-developed cadaveric transplant programs.

The diagnosis of brain death should be made by a physician who is independent of the transplant team and thus free of conflict of interest. Clinically, the diagnosis requires irrefutable documentation of the irreversible absence of cerebral and brain stem function (Table 5-7). Electroencephalogram and isotope and dye angiography can be used to support the diagnosis, but they are not mandatory. Once the diagnosis of brain death has been made in a potential donor, steps must be taken to maintain adequate circulatory and respiratory function until permission for donation is given. Harvesting should then be performed as expeditiously as possible.

Table 5-7. Clinical criteria for diagnosis of brain death

Irreversibility
    No sedating, paralyzing, or toxic drugs
    No gross electrolyte or endocrine disturbances
    No profound hypothermia
Absent cerebral function
    No seizures or posturing
    No response to pain in cranial nerve distribution*
Absent brain stem function
    Apnea in response to acidosis or hypercarbia
    No pupillary or corneal reflexes
    No oculocephalic or vestibular reflexes
    No tracheobronchial reflex

*Spinal reflexes may be present.

Management of the Brain-Dead Donor

Maintenance of cardiovascular stability becomes more and more difficult the longer the period of brain death. At the time of diagnosis, patients are often relatively hypovolemic because of prior therapeutic attempts to minimize brain swelling by inducing dehydration. A diabetes insipidus–like state may accompany head injuries and brain death, resulting in obligatory urine outputs of up to a liter an hour.

Blood pressure should be maintained at greater than 100 mm Hg by aggressive administration of crystalloids, colloids, or blood products. Central venous pressure should be monitored and maintained at greater than 10 mm Hg. If urine output tends to fall (to less than approximately 40 ml/hour) in a well-hydrated donor, furosemide or mannitol may be given. Insulin administration may be necessary to minimize hyperglycemia and glycosuria. If, despite good hydration, blood pressure remains low, low-dose dopamine and other inotropic agents such as dobutamine or norepinephrine are sometimes required. If a hypotonic diuresis ensues, suggesting a diagnosis of diabetes insipidus, a hypotonic infusion should be used to replace the urine output. Dextrose infusion, which may induce an additional osmotic diuresis, should be avoided; a vasopressin infusion may be required if the hypotonic urine volume is massive (more than 500 ml/hour).

Technique of Cadaveric Organ Harvesting

The principles of the harvesting operation are similar regardless of the organs to be removed. Wide surgical exposure is obtained. Each organ to be removed is dissected with its vasculature intact. There is no dissection into the renal hila in order to avoid damage to the vasculature and to prevent delayed graft function caused by vasospasm. Cannulas are placed for in situ cooling. At the time of aortic cross-clamping, flush and surface cooling is begun. The organs are removed in an orderly fashion. The kidneys are removed en bloc with the aorta and vena cava (Fig. 5-1). If multiple organs are to be removed, the preferred sequence is heart or lung first, liver and/or pancreas second, and kidneys last. The kidneys are protected against ischemia by the cold flush and surface cooling during the 10–15 minutes that it takes to remove the other organs.

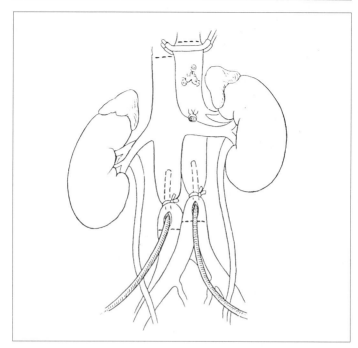

Fig. 5-1. En bloc dissection for cadaveric kidney donation with cannulas in place for in situ perfusion. Perihilar and periureteral fat are left in place.

Two variations of this approach have been described. One is a rapid infusion technique whereby cannulas are placed immediately, the aorta cross-clamped, and the dissection completed under cold infusion. The other variation is to place the donor on cardiopulmonary bypass. The donor is then cooled on bypass, and the dissection completed. Neither variation has yet found widespread use.

Kidneys Alone

Fewer than 50% of all organ donations are for kidneys only. In these circumstances, either a long midline incision from pubic notch to sternal notch can be used, splitting the sternum, or a cruciate midline incision can be made. The right colon and duodenum are mobilized, exposing the great vessels. The aortic bifurcation is isolated. The inferior mesenteric artery and vein are ligated. The aorta is controlled above the takeoff of the celiac trunk. Exposure can be achieved either by mass ligation of the porta hepatis to expose the superior mesenteric and celiac arteries or by mobilization of the left lateral segment of the liver, splitting the diaphragmatic crus, controlling the aorta, and mass-clamping the superior mesenteric and celiac arteries. The supraceliac aorta can also be controlled in the left chest behind the heart before the thoracic aorta enters the abdomen. The ureters are divided deep in the pelvis, maintaining a long segment and leaving all periureteral tissue. The aorta is cannulated at the bifurcation of the iliac arteries, and the proximal aorta is cross-clamped. An ice flush solution is begun. The kidneys are then widely mobilized, leaving Gerota's capsule intact, and removed en bloc with the abdominal aorta and vena cava. If the heart and kidneys are being donated, the procurement is similar, except that the heart team mobilizes the heart before cross-clamping the aorta, and the heart is removed first. The kidneys are separated in slush on a back table. The left renal vein is taken off the cava with a small cuff of vena cava. The remainder of the vena cava is left with the right kidney. The aorta is divided longitudinally, leaving the renal arteries attached to cuffs of aorta on each side.

Kidneys with Other Abdominal Organs

If the liver and pancreas are removed, their removal precedes kidney removal. The lower border of their dissection is the vena cava, just above the insertion of the renal veins, and the aorta, at or just below the takeoff of the superior mesenteric artery. After their removal, the abdominal landmarks are usually obscured. En bloc kidney removal as described in the section on kidneys alone is carried out by dissecting widely around the kidneys to avoid damage to the important hilar structures.

Pharmacologic Adjuncts

Most cadaver donors are given large doses of corticosteroids to deplete circulating donor lymphocytes. Mannitol in doses of up to 1 g/kg is also given to ensure diuresis and to possibly minimize ischemic injury. There is some evidence that alpha-blockers or calcium channel blockers given IV before kidney manipulation may lower the rate of delayed graft function. Phentolamine (Regitine), 10–15 mg, may be used just before cross-clamping of the aorta, since earlier use would cause significant hypotension. Systemic heparinization is carried out at the time of cannula placement with doses of 10,000–20,000 units.

Ischemia Times

Warm ischemia time refers to the period between circulatory arrest and commencement of cold storage. With modern in situ perfusion techniques, the warm ischemia time is essentially zero, although there will be warm ischemia if hemodynamic deterioration or cardiac arrest occurs before harvest. A kidney may function after up to 20 minutes of warm ischemia, but rates of delayed function and nonfunction increase markedly thereafter.

Cold ischemia time refers to the period of cold storage or machine perfusion (see the section on cold storage versus machine perfusion). **Rewarm time** is the period from removal of the kidney from cold storage or perfusion to completion of the renal arterial anastomosis. Rewarm time can be minimized by cooling the kidney during surgery (see Chap. 7).

Cadaveric Kidney Preservation

Cold Storage Versus Machine Perfusion

Harvested kidneys must be stored for a period of time before transplantation, either by cold storage on ice or by machine perfusion.

Table 5-8. Comparison of contents of flush solutions for kidney preservation

University of Wisconsin solution	Collins' solution
Modified hydroxyethyl starch	Potassium phosphate
Lactobionic acid	Potassium chloride
Potassium phosphate	Sodium bicarbonate
Magnesium sulfate	Glucose
Raffinose	Magnesium sulfate
Adenosine	
Allopurinol	
Glutathione	

For cold storage, the kidneys are flushed and separated and then placed on ice in sterile containers for transport. For machine perfusion, they are flushed and separated and then placed on specially designed perfusion machines that pump a cold colloid solution continuously through the renal artery until the time of transplant. Machine perfusion may allow a longer preservation time. Rates of delayed graft function of around 25% are obtained with simple static cold storage with cold ischemia times of up to 30 hours. After 30 hours, the rate of delayed graft function rises significantly. Most centers prefer not to use kidneys that have been in cold storage for longer than 48 hours. Delayed graft function rates of around 25% are obtainable with up to 48 hours of machine perfusion. Machine preservation is expensive and complex, and currently most transplant centers prefer simple static cold preservation, attempting to keep cold ischemia times under 30 hours.

Collins' Solution Versus University of Wisconsin Solution

For many years, kidneys have been flushed with modifications of a solution called Collins' solution during harvesting to achieve rapid cooling and blood washout. This solution is high in potassium, is hyperosmolar, and has an intracellular-like composition (Table 5-8) to stabilize cell membranes and prevent cell swelling.

The University of Wisconsin (UW) solution for flushing cadaveric organs is clearly superior to Collins' solution for liver and pancreas preservation. It may also be preferable for kidneys with prolonged preservation times. UW solution contains a number of components (see Table 5-8), and the importance of each has not been fully resolved. Glutathione may serve to facilitate the regeneration of cellular adenosine triphosphate (ATP) and maintain membrane integrity, and adenosine may provide the substrate for regeneration of ATP during reperfusion. The introduction of UW solution has had a major impact on nonrenal solid organ transplantation by allowing much longer cold ischemia times.

SELECTED READINGS

Alexander JW, Zola JC. Expanding the donor pool: Use of marginal donors for solid organ transplantation. *Clin Transplantation* 10:1, 1996.

Gaber LW, Moore LW, Alloway RR et al. Glomerulosclerosis as a determinant of posttransplant function of older donor renal allografts. *Transplantation* 60:334, 1995.

Gaston RS, Hudson S, Julian BA et al. Impact of donor/recipient size matching on outcomes in renal transplantation. *Transplantation* 61:383, 1996.

Gonwa TA, Atkins C, Zhang YA et al. Glomerular filtration rates in persons evaluated as living related donors—Are our standards too high? *Transplantation* 55:983, 1993.

Jacobbi LM, McBride VA, Etheridge EE et al. The risks, benefits, and costs of expanding donor criteria. *Transplantation* 60:1491, 1995.

Kasiske BL, Bia MJ. The evaluation and selection of living kidney donors. *Am J Kidney Dis* 26:387, 1995.

Kasiske BL, Ma JZ, Louis TA et al. Long-term effects of reduced renal mass in humans. *Kidney Int* 48:814, 1995.

Morales JM, Campistol JM, Castellano G et al. Transplantation of kidneys from donors with hepatitis C antibody into recipients with pretransplantation anti-HCV. *Kidney Int* 47:236, 1995.

Peters TG, Shaver TR, Ames JE et al. Cold ischemia and outcome in 17,937 cadaveric kidney transplants. *Transplantation* 59:191, 1995.

Portolés J, Macañes A, Prats D et al. Double renal transplant from infant donors. *Transplantation* 61:37, 1995.

Rosenthal JT. Expanded criteria for cadaver organ donation in renal transplantation. *Urol Clin North Am* 21:283, 1994.

Siminoff LA, Arnold RM, Caplan AL et al. Public policy governing organ and tissue procurement in the United States. *Ann Intern Med* 123:10, 1995.

Spital A. Do U.S. transplant centers encourage emotionally related kidney donation? *Transplantation* 61:374, 1996.

Terasaki PI, Cecka JM, Gjertson DW et al. High survival rates of kidney transplants from spousal and living unrelated donors. *N Engl J Med* 333:333, 1995.

Veller MG, Botha JR, Britz RS et al. Renal allograft preservation: A comparison of University of Wisconsin solution and of hypothermic continuous pulsatile perfusion. *Clin Transplantation* 8:97, 1994.

Winen RM, Booster MH, Stubenitsky BM et al. Outcome of transplantation of non–heart-beating donor kidneys. *Lancet* 345:1067, 1995.

Evaluation of the Transplant Recipient

Alan H. Wilkinson

The potential kidney transplant recipient must be evaluated by the transplant team to determine if he or she is a suitable candidate. The patient must also make a personal evaluation of the transplantation option, and the transplant team must see to it that this evaluation is an educated one. The excellent statistics achieved by most transplant centers for graft survival and morbidity have changed the attitude of both physicians and patients regarding the appropriateness of transplantation. Whereas transplantation was once reserved for "ideal" candidates who were either particularly brave or particularly desperate, nearly all patients with end-stage renal disease (ESRD) can now be regarded as potentially acceptable candidates for transplantation. Instead of denying the option to broad groups of patients, such as the elderly or those with diabetes mellitus, each person's candidacy should be evaluated individually. As part of the evaluation, factors that need to be corrected before the transplant takes place need to be identified.

Clinical practice guidelines for the evaluation of renal transplant candidates have been developed by the Patient Care and Education Committee of the American Society of Transplant Physicians. These guidelines provide a detailed algorithmic approach to the process of transplant evaluation (see the article by Kasiske et al. in the Selected Readings).

CONTRAINDICATIONS TO KIDNEY TRANSPLANTATION

Malignancy

There are two major reasons for excluding patients with malignant disease. The first is that immunosuppressive drugs may unfavorably influence the natural history of the malignancy. The second is that it is not reasonable for someone whose life expectancy is significantly curtailed by the presence of malignant disease to undergo transplantation. Much of the data on which transplant recommendations have been made have come from the **Cincinnati Transplant Tumor Registry**, an international registry for malignancy in solid organ transplant recipients. Most centers require at least a 2-year disease-free interval after the treatment of a malignant tumor, although a 5-year waiting period would exclude the great majority of patients who would develop recurrence. The precise waiting period, however, should be determined by the nature of the tumor; oncologic consultation may be wise. Guidelines for waiting periods for commonly encountered tumors in potential transplant recipients are shown in Table 6-1.

Chronic Infection

The presence of any chronic infection precludes transplantation and the use of immunosuppressive therapy. Osteomyelitis should be treat-

Table 6-1. Guidelines for recommending tumor-free waiting periods for common pretransplant malignancies

Site	Waiting period
Renal	
Incidental, asymptomatic	None
Large, infiltrating	At least 2 yrs
Wilms' tumor	At least 2 yrs
Bladder	
In situ	None
Invasive	At least 2 yrs
Uterus	
In situ cervical	None[a]
Invasive cervical	5 yrs
Uterine body	At least 2 yrs
Testis	At least 2 yrs
Thyroid	At least 2 yrs
Breast	At least 5 yrs[b]
Colorectum	At least 2 yrs[b]
Prostate	At least 2 yrs
Lymphoma	At least 2 yrs
Skin	
Melanoma	At least 5 yrs[b]
Squamous cell	2 yrs
Basal cell	None

[a]Routine cytologic screening required.
[b]In situ lesions may not require a waiting period.

ed, and, if necessary, the infected part should be removed surgically to prepare a patient for transplantation. Diabetic foot ulcers must be healed before transplantation. Tuberculosis requires a full course of therapy and preferably 1 year of subsequent observation for relapse. Infection with the human immunodeficiency virus (HIV) is an absolute contraindication to kidney transplantation. Recurrent urinary tract infection and peritonitis are discussed in the section on urologic evaluation and candidates on peritoneal dialysis.

Severe Extrarenal Disease

Most patients who have evidence of extrarenal disease are acceptable transplant candidates. In certain circumstances, however, extrarenal disease may preclude transplantation either because the patient is not an operative candidate or because the transplant and associated immunosuppression may accelerate disease progression. Chronic liver disease and advanced uncorrectable heart disease are contraindications to kidney transplantation alone, although these patients may benefit from combined organ transplantation. Chronic lung disease may preclude safe general anesthesia. Severe peripheral vascular disease may make arterial anastomosis technically difficult or endanger limb viability.

Noncompliance

Any patient with a history of repeated noncompliance with previous medical therapy should be considered at an extremely high risk for graft loss. It is wise to demand a period of acceptable compliance as a condition for being placed on the waiting list. Assessment of compliance is discussed in Chap. 15.

Psychiatric Illness

Organic mental syndromes, psychosis, and mental retardation of a degree that seriously impairs the patient's capacity to understand the transplant procedure and its complications are contraindications to transplantation. Any patient addicted to alcohol or any other drug should enter and successfully complete a rehabilitation program before being offered a transplant (see Chap. 15).

RECIPIENT EVALUATION

General Medical Evaluation

All patients referred to a transplant center should provide details of their medical history at the time of the initial evaluation. Particular emphasis should be placed on preexisting cardiovascular and GI diseases. The family history is very important, as it may provide information regarding the nature of the kidney disease and also allows the physician to introduce a discussion about potential living-related donors. The physical examination must be equally thorough. Care should be taken to document the presence of dental disease. A stool sample should be checked for the presence of blood. In men, the prostate must be palpated, and the prostate-specific antigon level should be routinely checked in men older than age 40 years. Many patients will be oliguric or anuric and may not be aware of prostatic hypertrophy. All women should have a Papanicolaou smear and pelvic examination, and women older than age 40 years should have a mammogram. Suggested laboratory and radiologic tests are listed in Table 6-2. Older patients and patients with multiple risk factors for coronary artery disease should undergo exercise stress testing. Cigarette smokers should be encouraged to break the habit and offered professional help to do so.

Urologic Evaluation

Ideally, the lower urinary tract should be sterile, continent, and compliant before transplantation. Urinalysis and urine culture should be performed on all urinating patients, and some programs obtain bladder washings from anuric patients. A voiding cystourethrogram should be performed in patients in whom a voiding or genitourinary abnormality is suspected.

Graft implantation into the native bladder is always preferred. Diverted urinary tracts should be undiverted where possible to make the lower urinary tract functional before transplantation. Even a very small bladder may develop normal compliance and capacity after transplantation. Transplantation is possible in patients whose urinary tracts have been diverted into ileal conduits and cannot be undiverted. The rate of urologic complications is high, but the overall patient and graft survival is not different from patients with intact urinary tracts.

Indications for pretransplant native nephrectomy are listed in Table 6-3. If nephrectomy is performed, it should be done at least 6 weeks to 3 months pretransplant.

Table 6-2. Routine and elective pretransplant evaluations

Routine	Elective
Full history and physical exam	Voiding cystourethrogram
Complete blood count and chemistry panel	Exercise treadmill
	Echocardiogram
Prothrombin time and partial thromboplastin time	Coronary angiogram
	Mammogram
Blood type	Noninvasive vascular studies
HBsAg, HBsAb, HepCAb, VDRL, HIV, HSV, and CMV titers	Right upper quadrant ultrasound
Pelvic exam and Pap smear	Upper GI and upper endoscopy
Chest x-ray	Barium enema and lower endoscopy, prostate-specific antigen test
Electrocardiogram	Immunoelectrophoresis
Tissue typing and cytotoxic antibodies	EBV, VZV, HSV, toxoplasmosis titers
	Lipid profile
	Purified protein derivative (tuberculin)

CMV = cytomegalovirus; EBV = Epstein-Barr virus; HIV = human immunodeficiency virus; HSV = herpes simplex virus; VZV = varicella-zoster virus.

Table 6-3. Indications for pretransplant native nephrectomy

Chronic renal parenchymal infection
Infected stones
Heavy proteinuria
Intractable hypertension
Polycystic kidney disease[a]
Acquired renal cystic disease[b]
Infected reflux[c]

[a]Only when the kidneys are massive, recurrently infected, or bleeding.
[b]When there is suspicion of adenocarcinoma.
[c]Uninfected reflux does not require nephrectomy.

Older men frequently have prostatic enlargement and may develop outflow tract obstruction post-transplant. In general, if patients are still passing sufficient volumes of urine, the prostate should be resected preoperatively. Otherwise, the operation should be postponed until after the transplantation has been successfully performed. These patients may require an indwelling bladder catheter until the prostate has been resected.

Patient Education

At the time of the evaluation, the physician or transplant nurse coordinator should inform the patient of the risks of the operation and of the side effects and risks associated with immunosuppression. The surgical procedure and its complications should be discussed in lay terms. The nature of rejection should be explained and mention made of the increased risk of infection and of post-transplant malignancy and the occasional mortality from these complications. Patients need to understand that immunosuppressive therapy must be continued for as long as the graft survives. The benefits of live donor transplantation and cadaveric transplantation should be compared and contrasted (see Chap. 5). Each center will have its own graft survival and morbidity statistics, and these should be shared with the patient. It is wise to emphasize the improved quality of life after transplantation rather than improved length of life, since the former has been better documented (see Chap. 1).

Patients should be warned that even successful transplants do not last forever and that they may, at some point, require a return to dialysis or repeat transplantation. The importance of compliance with dialysis and dietary prescriptions while waiting for a transplant should be emphasized. The possibility of post-transplant pregnancy should be discussed with women of child-bearing age (see Chap. 9).

Special Features Related to the Primary Kidney Disease

The impact of recurrent renal disease on the post-transplant course is discussed in Chap. 9. The following section considers the aspects of the primary kidney disease that are relevant to the pretransplant workup.

Diabetes Mellitus

Diabetic nephropathy accounts for approximately 30% of ESRD in the United States. The evaluation of diabetic patients is discussed in Chap. 13. Both coronary artery and peripheral vascular disease are frequently present in these patients and must be rigorously assessed.

Systemic Lupus Erythematosus

The reported results of kidney transplantation in patients with systemic lupus erythematosus (SLE) are variable. In some studies graft survival results cannot be distinguished from those in other "low-risk" patient groups, whereas other studies report an increased tendency to rejection episodes and graft loss. Patients who still have evidence of clinically active disease are generally not candidates for transplantation. Serologic evidence of disease may persist despite clinical inactivity and is not a contraindication to transplantation. Fortunately, nearly two-thirds of patients with SLE are clinically inactive at the commencement of dialysis, and this fraction tends to rise with time. Every attempt should be made to discontinue prednisone before transplantation; transplantation is probably not wise for patients requiring more than 10 mg daily. Patients with SLE who have a history of thrombosis should be tested for the presence of lupus anticoagulant and anticardiolipin antibodies, which may predispose them to post-transplant thrombotic episodes.

Focal Glomerulosclerosis

Focal glomerulosclerosis may recur very rapidly after transplantation, presumably as the result of an unidentified serum factor that affects the permselectivity of the glomerular basement membrane

(GBM). Approximately 25% of patients develop recurrence, usually within days or weeks of transplantation. Recurrence is more common in younger patients, in patients whose initial presentation was florid, and in patients whose initial biopsy also showed mesangial hypertrophy. Patients should be forewarned of the possibility of recurrence, the chances of which are very high in a second transplant if the first was affected. The specter of recurrence may make cadaveric transplantation the preferred donor source, particularly if the first transplant was affected.

Goodpasture's Syndrome

When the primary disease is the result of antibodies directed against the GBM, transplantation should be deferred until the patient is clinically stable and anti-GBM antibody levels are undetectable. If these guidelines are followed, this group of patients does well following transplantation, and recurrence is rare. Pretransplant native nephrectomy was once recommended for these patients but is no longer regarded as necessary.

Alport's Syndrome

Patients with Alport's syndrome have a hereditary abnormality of the GBM that lacks the Goodpasture antigen. When exposed for the first time to a normal basement membrane in the allograft, they may develop de novo anti-GBM antibody disease, with a crescentic glomerulonephritis characterized by linear immunofluorescence staining of the GBM. Aggressive treatment has been tried with protocols similar to those used for primary anti-GBM disease, including plasmapheresis. The outcome is poor. The incidence of this catastrophic complication is probably less than 10%. The great majority of patients with Alport's syndrome who do not develop this complication do well post-transplant. The presence of inherited kidney disease mandates intensive family screening before consideration of live-related donation.

Amyloidosis

Patients with amyloidosis have a higher-than-average mortality rate after transplantation. The rate may be as high as 45% at 1 year and depends on the extent to which amyloid has been deposited in the heart, liver, spleen, and GI tract. Infection is a common complication. Some patients without severe extrarenal disease may be considered acceptable candidates, particularly if the amyloidosis is due to chronic inflammation. An echocardiogram should be performed to assess the extent of myocardial infiltration. The subgroup of patients with amyloidosis complicating familial Mediterranean fever may not tolerate cyclosporine therapy as a consequence of systemic and GI symptoms. Patients with primary amyloidosis, a manifestation of a plasma cell dyscrasia, have a very poor prognosis no matter what form of therapy is used.

Paraproteinemia

In patients older than age 60 years and in patients with ESRD of uncertain etiology, the pretransplant evaluation should include a plasma immunoelectrophoresis to screen for the presence of a paraprotein. Where a benign monoclonal gammopathy is identified, serial evaluations should be performed during the next 12 months to exclude the development of myeloma or macroglobulinemia. If the patient is free of myeloma or macroglobulinemia after the 12 months, it is probably safe to progress with transplantation, although surveillance should continue. There are reports of successful transplantation in patients whose original kidney disease was due to myeloma, light chain disease, or macroglobulinemia. These patients may be at particular risk for infection in the post-transplant period and for other causes of renal impairment such as dehydration, nephrotoxicity, hypercalcemia, and hyperuricemia. Some programs regard frank paraproteinemia as a contraindication to transplantation. At the very least, patients should be apprised of their high-risk status, and they may elect to remain on dialysis.

Polycystic Kidney Disease

The transplant prognosis of patients with polycystic kidney disease is not different from other "low-risk" groups. Very rarely the polycystic kidneys are so large that a pretransplant nephrectomy must be performed to create a space for the allograft. Recurrent infection or hemorrhage may be an indication for pretransplant nephrectomy. The possibility of live-related donation in families afflicted with polycystic kidney disease is discussed in Chap. 5.

Fabry's Disease

Some programs exclude patients with Fabry's disease from transplantation, although it is best to consider patients on an individual basis. Early hopes that the underlying defect in glycosphingolipid metabolism would be reversed by transplanting the missing enzyme have not been fulfilled. Infection, poor wound healing, and progression of the disease contribute to a high mortality.

Scleroderma

There is little documented experience of transplantation outcome in patients with scleroderma. As in patients with amyloidosis and Fabry's disease, the extent of generalized systemic involvement must be assessed in each patient. Wound healing is not usually impaired, and extrarenal complications may improve following transplantation. Cyclosporine is now being investigated as a therapeutic agent for the treatment of scleroderma. Tight control of blood pressure is required, and the early use of angiotensin-converting enzyme inhibitors may be indicated.

Primary Hyperoxaluria

Primary hyperoxaluria type I is an inborn error of metabolism with an autosomal recessive inheritance. The underlying defect is a deficiency of the peroxisomal enzyme alanine glyoxylate aminotransferase, which is found primarily in the liver. Deposition of oxalate leads to end-stage renal failure, and, following transplantation, rapid deposition of oxalate in the allograft leads to graft failure. Failure of the graft usually occurs despite intensive therapy with perioperative plasma exchange, high-dose pyridoxine, and oral phosphates, which are designed to minimize oxalate deposition. A more rational approach may be to consider combined liver-kidney transplantation for the management of these patients (Table 6-4). The new liver provides the missing enzyme.

Thrombotic Thrombocytopenic Purpura

Cyclosporine toxicity may be associated with a glomerular capillary thrombotic lesion very similar to that of thrombotic thrombocytopenic purpura (TTP) or hemolytic-uremic syndrome (see Chap. 4). It is probable that cyclosporine use increases the recurrence of TTP post-transplant, but even in patients treated only with prednisone and azathioprine, this condition may recur. In cases of familial TTP, it is not clear whether there is a greater risk of relapse if the graft comes from a sibling or from a cadaveric donor.

Systemic Vasculitis and Wegener's Granulomatosis

It is unusual for the vasculitides to recur if patients receive kidney transplants only after the disease is "burned out." A recurrence of up to 70% for Wegener's granulomatosis has been described, and the addition of cyclophosphamide has been recommended for control of vasculitis. It is unclear whether the monitoring of antineutrophil cytoplasmic antibody levels will prove useful for patient management.

Sickle Cell Disease

Sickle cell anemia and sickle cell disease produce a variety of renal abnormalities and may occasionally cause end-stage renal failure. The transplantation experience with these patients has been a mixed one. There is an increased incidence of severe and potentially lethal sickling crises post-transplant, presumably related to the improving hematocrit. Exchange transfusions may be effective treatment. Some programs regard sickle cell anemia as a contraindication to kidney transplantation.

Risk Factors Related to Organ System Diseases

Cardiovascular Disease

Cardiovascular disease is one of the leading causes of death in the years after kidney transplantation. Diabetic patients frequently suffer from covert coronary artery disease and should be specifically evaluated with this in mind (see Chap. 13). Older patients and patients with multiple risk factors for coronary artery disease should undergo stress testing and, when indicated, coronary angiography. Prior angioplasty or coronary artery bypass grafting is not a contraindication to transplantation as long as the patient has a nonischemic treadmill test.

Symptoms and signs of peripheral and cerebrovascular disease should be elicited and evaluated and, if indicated, corrected before transplantation. It is prudent to obtain a vascular surgery consultation. Patients who have suffered cerebrovascular accidents are generally poor transplant candidates both in terms of their perioperative risk status and the rehabilitative potential of the transplant. Patients who have required intra-abdominal reconstructive arterial surgery represent a formidable surgical challenge, and transplantation may be contraindicated.

Some dialysis patients manifest symptomatic heart failure of nonischemic origin. The term **uremic cardiomyopathy** has been

Table 6-4. Indications for combined kidney and liver transplantation

OLT candidate with severe[a] irreversible renal dysfunction due to:
1. Polycystic kidneys with massive hepatomegaly
2. Glomerulonephritis (typically IgA nephropathy)
3. Failing kidney transplant with end-stage liver disease (typically HCV- or HBV-related)
4. Repeat OLT with cyclosporine nephrotoxicity
5. Oxalosis
6. Prolonged pre-OLT dialysis dependence[b]
7. Diabetic nephropathy

OLT = orthotopic liver transplantation; HBV = hepatitis B virus; HCV = hepatitis C virus.
[a]"Severe" indicates that the patient is or would become dialysis-dependent post-transplant.
[b]Hepatorenal syndrome may become irreversible after weeks of dialysis dependence.

applied to this condition, and cardiac function may improve markedly post-transplant. Symptomatic heart failure of nonischemic origin is not an absolute contraindication to kidney transplantation.

Gastrointestinal Disease

A number of GI diseases can lead to severe morbidity after transplantation.

Peptic Ulcer Disease.   Before the introduction of effective therapy in the form of histamine antagonists, post-transplant upper GI bleeding was a common and feared complication, and all patients underwent pretransplant upper GI evaluation. This precaution may now be reserved for patients with symptoms or a history of peptic ulcer disease. Active peptic ulcer disease is a contraindication to transplantation, and if the disease persists despite medical therapy, surgical intervention may be indicated.

Pancreatitis.   A pretransplant history of pancreatitis increases the risk of post-transplant pancreatitis. Both prednisone and azathioprine have been implicated in the etiology of pancreatitis. Hyperparathyroidism should be excluded as a possible factor.

Cholelithiasis.   Patients with active cholecystitis and diabetic patients with asymptomatic cholelithiasis should undergo cholecystectomy before transplantation. In diabetics, post-transplant cholecystitis may be difficult to diagnose, and post-transplant operative intervention may be complicated. Some transplant programs routinely perform right upper quadrant sonography to exclude cholelithiasis.

Diverticulitis.   Routine colonic screening of asymptomatic older transplant candidates is probably unnecessary. When diverticulitis has been recognized to be a cause of significant symptomatology, it may be necessary to consider pretransplant colectomy.

Liver Disease

Hepatic cirrhosis and clinically active hepatitis and chronic liver disease are contraindications to kidney transplantation; these diseases may progress to end-stage liver disease post-transplant, usually as a consequence of immunosuppression. Patients with advanced or end-stage kidney and liver disease may become candidates for combined kidney-liver transplantation (see Table 6-4). The decision to transplant patients with serologic evidence of prior hepatitis B or C infection who are clinically quiescent may be a difficult one.

Hepatitis B. Some studies have reported a high incidence of post-transplant cirrhosis and death from hepatoma and hepatic failure in hepatitis B virus (HBV)–positive patients, whereas others have described a benign course with both clinical and histologic stability. Many centers regard HBeAg positivity and evidence of active viral replication as contraindications to kidney transplantation; Asian patients who areHBV-positive appear to be at particular risk for progressive liver disease after kidney transplantation. All patients should be warned, however, of the potential for progressive liver disease. Alpha-fetoprotein levels should be monitored to screen for occult hepatocellular carcinoma. Some centers base their decision to transplant on histologic criteria of disease prognosis.

Hepatitis C. Reports of the natural history of hepatitis C virus (HCV) infection post-transplant are also conflicting. HCV-infected dialysis patients may have liver enzyme levels in the normal range despite advanced histologic lesions. For this reason, many transplant centers require all HCV-positive potential transplant recipients to undergo liver biopsy pretransplant. It is probably safe to transplant patients with chronic persistent hepatitis, which is a relatively benign lesion; however, it may be wiser for patients with chronic active hepatitis to remain on dialysis. There is limited experience on the use of interferon-alpha to slow the progression of HBV and HCV in infected dialysis patients.

Seizure Disorders

The major antiepileptic agents all increase the rate of metabolism of cyclosporine. When patients who are being treated for a seizure disorder are referred for transplantation, note should be made of the anticonvulsant regimen, and a neurologic consultation should be obtained to determine which, if any, of the anticonvulsants are mandatory. If patients need to continue anticonvulsant therapy, the immunosuppressive protocol may need to be adjusted (see Chap. 4).

Chronic Pulmonary Disease

Perioperative risks associated with severe lung disease include ventilator dependency and infection. Patients with suppurative bronchiectasis or chronic fungal disease are not candidates for kidney transplantation. Pulmonary function testing may help determine suitability for transplantation. Patients who smoke should be strongly advised to stop before transplantation; smoking cessation programs may be helpful.

Risk Factors Related to Individual Patient Characteristics

Age

Both the very young and older patients have an increased risk of graft loss and morbidity, although most centers no longer have an arbitrary upper age at which patients are no longer accepted for transplantation. Several studies have reported that patients between the ages of 55 and 65 years are not at a significantly increased risk of post-transplant morbidity as long as they do not suffer from significant vascular disease and their general medical evaluation is unremarkable; moreover, life expectancy may be better with transplantation than dialysis in this group. It is wise to rule out covert coronary artery disease with stress testing before transplantation in older patients. Experience with transplant recipients in their late 60s and 70s is limited. Each case should be examined on its merits; patients should not be arbitrarily excluded from transplantation because of their age. There is some evidence that older patients may be immunologically less aggressive and that the metabolism of cyclosporine by the P450 system in the liver (see Chap. 4) may be slowed. Transplantation in pediatric patients is discussed in Chap. 14.

Obesity and Malnutrition

Severe malnutrition is less frequent now that patients with ESRD are starting dialysis earlier. Dialysis units should ensure that patients are adequately dialyzed and nourished, as malnourished patients are at greater risk of infection and poor wound healing. Obese patients are also at greater risk in the perioperative period from wound complications and pulmonary infections. The long-term risks from cardiovascular disease secondary to hypercholesterolemia and from hypertension are compounded by obesity. Prednisone therapy may induce very rapid weight gain, and these patients must be encouraged to lose as much excess weight as possible before transplantation. The nutritional assessment of dialysis patients is discussed in Chap. 17.

Candidates on Peritoneal Dialysis

Patients frequently ask whether it is preferable to be on hemodialysis or peritoneal dialysis while they are on the transplant waiting list. In general, the form of dialysis has no bearing on suitability for transplantation. If necessary, it is usually possible to continue to use peritoneal dialysis after the transplant, unless the surgeon has entered the peritoneum during the transplantation. Peritonitis and exit site infections must be adequately treated, and about 6 weeks should elapse after an episode of peritonitis before patients are put on the active cadaveric waiting list. Occasionally, the location of the exit site of the dialysis catheter may prevent the use of that side for transplantation.

Predialysis Transplantation

Five to 10% of kidney transplants are now performed on patients with advanced chronic kidney disease who are not yet dependent on dialysis. Diabetic patients, in particular, should be considered for predialysis transplantation to obviate the development of diabetic complications (see Chap. 13). Diabetic patients should be referred to transplant centers for evaluation as soon as they have established kidney disease because their disease progression may be rapid and it may require months to prepare a live-related donor or even years to obtain a cadaveric kidney.

For other forms of chronic kidney disease in which disease progression may be slow (e.g., chronic interstitial nephritis, polycystic kidney disease), careful clinical judgment is required to time the transplant. If a living donor is available, it may be possible not to place a dialysis access and either transplant the patient when the earliest uremic symptoms develop or wait until an accurately measured glomerular filtration rate is less than 10–15 ml/minute. For potential cadaveric kidney recipients, it is wise to place a dialysis access (or plan for peritoneal dialysis) as ESRD approaches and the patient is placed on the waiting list. There are currently no defined criteria to determine when a patient can be placed on the cadaveric waiting list, although **listing criteria** are being developed. It must be emphasized to patients that preparation for transplantation and preparation for dialysis are not mutually exclusive, but can be performed in parallel. It is unwise to get into a "race against time" to find a kidney for patients who are reluctant to start dialysis.

Patients seeking predialysis transplantation should clarify their health insurance status to ensure that the cost of their evaluation and preparation of live donors is financially covered. In the United States, Medicare ESRD benefits do not currently commence before dialysis and transplantation. Patients who receive a transplant before the development of frank uremic symptoms or commencement of dialysis may not feel the improved sense of well-being typically enjoyed by dialysis patients post-transplant. They should be warned of such.

Highly Sensitized Patients

Approximately 40% of the national pool of patients awaiting cadaveric transplants have high levels of preformed cytotoxic antibodies that may prevent them from receiving a kidney or prolong their wait considerably. Cytotoxic antibodies result from failed prior transplants, multiple pregnancies, and multiple blood transfusions. Attempts have been made to reduce the antibody levels by plasma exchange with cyclophosphamide and immunoabsorption, but these techniques have not yet proved to be clinically effective and practical. Patients with high levels of antibodies should be warned of the probability of a prolonged wait for a kidney. There is reason to hope that the widespread use of erythropoietin in dialysis patients will lower the level of preformed antibodies by minimizing blood transfusion requirements.

Previously Transplanted Candidates

The fate of second and multiple transplants is dependent to a considerable extent on the rate and etiology of the prior transplant loss. Patients who lost kidneys because of surgical complications or have kidneys that functioned for more than a year have a prognosis that is not significantly different from patients with primary transplants. If the primary transplant is lost to early rejection, the prognosis for another transplant is impaired, and the patient will do best with a highly matched cadaveric transplant or a 2-haplotype–matched live-related transplant if a suitable donor is available. Patients must be made aware of their impaired prognosis.

The process of evaluating a patient for a repeat transplant is the same as for a primary transplant. In patients whose first transplant life was prolonged, special attention should be paid to the possibility of covert coronary artery disease or malignancy.

Candidates for Double Organ Transplants

Patients with end-stage liver disease (ESLD) who are candidates for orthotopic liver transplantation (OLT) frequently have impaired renal function as a result of hepatorenal syndrome, "pre-renal" dysfunction, acute tubular necrosis, or nephrotoxicity. In the great majority of cases, renal function will improve following successful OLT despite what is often a prolonged period of dialysis dependence. Concomitant renal transplantation is therefore *not* indicated when it is anticipated that native renal function will improve.

Irreversible renal dysfunction may accompany ESLD; in these cases, it is logical to consider a combined procedure (see Table 6-4). The addition of a kidney transplant adds relatively little to the considerable morbidity of an OLT, but a well-functioning kidney may facilitate post-transplant management. The immunosuppressive regimen does not need to be modified. Results of the combined procedure are similar to those of OLT alone.

Experience with combined heart and kidney transplants is more limited. The same principles regarding reversibility of renal dysfunction apply. Combined kidney and pancreas transplantation is discussed in Chap. 13.

Waiting Period for a Cadaveric Transplant

More than 31,000 patients with ESRD await cadaveric kidney transplants in the United States. The length of the waiting period is often measured in months and years and is determined by blood group, the presence of preformed antibodies, and local factors. During the waiting period, patients must remain compliant to their dialysis regime and attempt to improve their physical and emotional health and rehabilitation. Close liaison between the personnel of the dialysis unit and the transplant program is essential, and the transplant program must be kept updated regarding significant medical developments. The transplant program should maintain contact with the patients either by routine visits or by telephone. This contact ensures that the program is updated with medical and demographic data and that the patient does not feel forgotten or disheartened by a prolonged wait.

SELECTED READINGS

Boletis J, Delladetsima J, Psimenou E et al. Liver biopsy is essential in anti-HCV positive renal transplant patients irrespective of liver function tests and serology for HCV. *Transplant Proc* 27:945, 1995.

Frazier P, Davis-Ali S, Dahl K. Correlates of noncompliance among renal transplant recipients. *Clin Transplant* 8:550, 1994.

Ismail N, Hakim RM, Helderman JH. Renal replacement therapies in the elderly: Part II. Renal transplantation. *Am J Kidney Dis* 23:1, 1994.

Kasiske BL, Ramos EL, Gaston RS et al. The evaluation of renal transplant candidates: Clinical practice guidelines. *J Am Soc Nephrol* 6:1, 1995.

Katz SM, Kerman RH, Golden D et al. Preemptive transplantation—An analysis of benefits and hazards in 85 cases. *Transplantation* 51:351, 1991.

Le A, Wilson R, Douek K et al. Prospective risk stratification in renal transplant candidates for cardiac death. *Am J Kidney Dis* 24:65, 1994.

Levinson JL, Olbrisch ME. Psychosocial evaluation of organ transplant candidates. A comparative survey of process, criteria and outcomes in heart, liver and kidney transplantation. *Psychosomatics* 34:314, 1993.

Lochhead KM, Pirsch JD, D'Alessandro AM et al. Risk factors for renal allograft loss in patients with systemic lupus erythematosus. *Kidney Int* 49:512, 1996.

Parfrey PS, Harnett JD, Foley RN et al. Impact of renal transplantation on uremic cardiomyopathy. *Tranoplantation* 60:908, 1995

Penn I. The effects of transplantation on preexisting cancers. *Transplantation* 55:742, 1993.

Ramos EL, Kasiske BL, Alexander SR et al. The evaluation of candidates for renal transplantation: The current practice of U.S. transplant centres. *Transplantation* 57:490, 1994.

Ramos EL, Tisher CC. Recurrent disease in the kidney transplant. *Am J Kidney Dis* 24:152, 1994.

Schaubel D, Desmeules M, Mao Y et al. Survival experience among elderly end-stage renal disease patients. *Transplantation* 60:1389, 1995.

Shandera K, Sago A, Angstadt J et al. An assessment of the need for voiding cystourethrogram for urologic screening prior to renal transplantation. *Clin Transplant* 7:299, 1993.

The Transplant Operation and Its Surgical Complications

J. Thomas Rosenthal

Kidney transplantation is an elective or semielective surgical procedure performed on patients who have undergone careful preoperative assessment and preparation. Chronic dialysis allows patients to
be maintained in optimal condition and provides time to address
potentially complicating medical and surgical issues. Chapter 6
describes these preparations. In this respect, kidney transplantation
differs somewhat from heart or liver transplantation, where the
condition of the patient is often deteriorating rapidly in the pretransplant period.

TRANSPLANT OPERATION

Immediate Preoperative Preparations

Chapter 5 describes the process of kidney transplant donation and
provides a standard preoperative checklist (see Table 5-5). If transplant candidates have been well prepared, it is rarely necessary to
call off surgery because of last-minute findings. Occasionally,
recent events such as peritonitis, pneumonia, GI bleeding, or new
onset of chest pain or cardiographic changes require cancellation
of surgery.

The decision to dialyze a patient before transplantation depends
on the timing of the previous dialysis, clinical assessment of volume
status, and serum electrolyte levels, particularly potassium.
Because of the danger of intraoperative or postoperative hyperkalemia in oliguric patients, it is wise to dialyze patients with a
serum potassium level of more than 5.5 mEq/liter. In well-dialyzed
patients, preoperative dialysis for fluid removal is usually unnecessary. If fluid is removed, it should be done with care to maintain the
patient at, or somewhat above, his or her dry weight to facilitate
postoperative diuresis. If time constraints demand it, a brief preoperative dialysis lasting 1–2 hours may be all that is necessary to
reduce potassium levels and optimize the hemodynamic status.

Operative Technique

Because all kidney transplant recipients receive immunosuppressive
drugs and many are anemic or malnourished at the time of surgery,
wound healing is potentially compromised. Meticulous surgical technique, attention to detail, strict aseptic technique, and perfect
hemostasis are essential. Drains are best avoided, but if they are
used they should be closed systems and should be removed as quickly as possible.

Incision

An oblique incision is made from the symphysis in the midline curving in a lateral superior direction to the iliac crest (Fig. 7-1). It can
be extended into the flank or as high as the tip of the twelfth rib if
more exposure is needed. In a first transplant, the incision site may

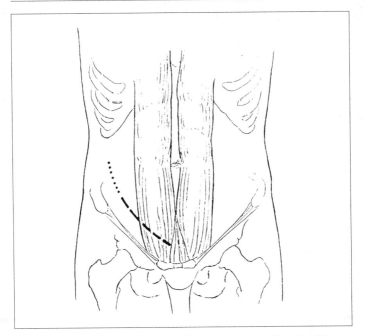

Fig. 7-1. Standard incision for adult kidney transplantation. An oblique incision is made from the symphysis in the midline curving in a lateral and superior direction to the iliac crest.

be in either lower quadrant. There are different approaches to the decision regarding which side to use. One approach has been to always use the right side, regardless of the side of origin of the donor kidney, because the accessibility of the iliac vein makes the operation easier than on the left side. Another approach is to use the side contralateral to the side of the donor kidney; that is, a right kidney is put on the left side, and vice versa. This technique was used when the hypogastric artery was routinely used for the anastomosis because the vessels lie in a convenient position and the renal pelvis is always anterior, making it accessible if ureteral repair is needed. The third approach has been to use the side ipsilateral to the donor kidney; that is, a right kidney is put on the right side, and vice versa. This choice is best when the external iliac artery is used for the arterial anastomosis. The vessels then lie without kinking when the kidney is placed in position. In repeat transplants, the side opposite the original transplant is generally used. In further transplants, the decision where to place the kidney is more complex; a transabdominal incision may be necessary, and more proximal vessels may be used. The retroperitoneal space is entered, and a pocket is made for the kidney.

Vascular Connections

Figure 7-2 shows the vascular connections for a kidney transplant.

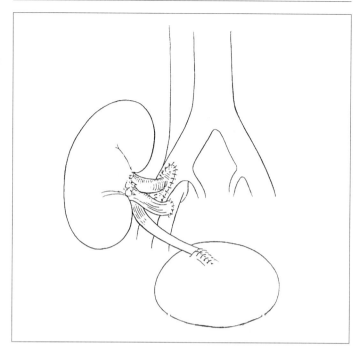

Fig. 7-2. The standard "hookup." The donor renal artery is shown anastomosed end-to-end on a Carrel aortic patch to the recipient external iliac artery. The donor renal vein is anastomosed to the recipient external iliac vein. The donor ureter is anastomosed to the recipient bladder with an antireflux technique.

Renal Artery.   The donor renal artery may be sewn to the external iliac artery in an end-to-side fashion or to the hypogastric artery in an end-to-end fashion. In a cadaveric kidney transplant, the donor renal artery or arteries are usually kept in continuity with a patch of donor aorta called a **Carrel patch**, which makes the end-to-side anastomosis much easier and safer and facilitates the anastomosis of multiple renal arteries. In a live-related transplant, a Carrel patch is not available, and the renal artery itself is sewn to the recipient artery. If an end-to-side anastomosis is chosen, a 4-mm aortic punch is useful in creating the recipient arteriotomy. A fine nonabsorbent monofilament suture, such as 5-0 or 6-0 Proline, is usually chosen. In small children and in patients undergoing repeat transplants on the same side, it may be necessary to use arteries other than the external iliac or hypogastric. The common iliac artery or even the aorta may sometimes be used.

Multiple Arteries.   A variety of techniques have been proposed for handling multiple donor renal arteries. In cadaveric transplants, it is best to keep them all on a single large Carrel patch, which minimizes the likelihood of damage to a small polar artery. In no case should polar arteries be sacrificed. Ligation of a lower pole artery may lead to ureteral necrosis. There may be visible capsular vessels that supply a tiny part of the cortical surface of the kidney. These vessels may be ligated, and tiny superficial ischemic areas on the surface of the kidney may result. If there are multiple arteries in a live transplant or if a Carrel patch is not available, the donor arteries can be anastomosed individually or anastomosed to each other before being anastomosed to the recipient vessel.

Renal Vein. The renal vein is sewn to the external iliac vein. Suture material similar to that used for the arterial anastomosis is usually chosen. If there are multiple renal veins, the largest may be used; the others can be ligated safely due to internal collateralization of the renal venous drainage.

Ureter. The ureter can be placed either into the recipient's bladder or into the ipsilateral native ureter as a ureterostomy. The native ureter may also be brought up to the allograft renal pelvis as a ureteropyelostomy. Most surgeons use the bladder whenever possible. Preferably, the recipient's bladder will have been shown to be functional before the transplant operation, although even small, contracted bladders that have not "seen" urine for prolonged periods can function well. If necessary, the ureter can be placed in a previously fashioned ileal or colonic conduit.

Establishing an antireflux mechanism is important to prevent post-transplant pyelonephritis. In one method, the bladder is opened, the ureter is brought into the bladder by a separate opening posteriorly, and laterally, a submucosal tunnel is created. The ureter is sewn into the bladder from within, and the bladder is then closed. This technique is similar to a so-called **Leadbetter-Politano reimplant**.

The other approach is to make a single, small opening into the bladder and sew the ureter in from the outside. Bladder muscle is then brought over the ureter to create the antireflux mechanism (Fig. 7-3). This technique is similar to a so-called **Liche reimplant**. Because of its simplicity, many surgeons have adopted this extravesical approach. Indwelling stents are not usually required but may be used if there is any question about the reimplant. A 4.8-mm double-J stent is useful in this setting. Foley catheter drainage of the bladder is required for 1–3 days unless there are bladder abnormalities.

Drains

Drains may be placed through a separate small incision into the perirenal space to drain blood, urine, or lymph. Some surgeons routinely place drains, whereas others do not. Closed drains such as the Jackson-Pratt are preferred over the open Penrose type drains because of a lower risk of wound infection. When drains are used, they should be removed as soon as there is no longer significant drainage, typically 24–48 hours post-transplant.

Surgical Considerations in Young Children

The procedure for children who weigh more than 20–25 kg is the same as the procedure for adults. In smaller children, comparatively large adult-sized kidneys are implanted, since kidneys from equivalently sized infant donors typically do not function well (see Chap. 5). A larger incision and more proximal blood vessels are used for implantation. The common iliac artery and vein or even the aorta and vena cava may

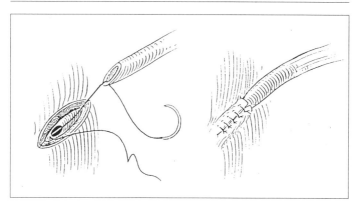

Fig. 7-3. A Liche reimplant. A single, small opening is made in the bladder, and the ureter is sewn in from the outside. Bladder muscle is used to create an antireflux mechanism.

be used. In children weighing more than 10–12 kg, an extraperitoneal approach may still be used. The right side is almost always preferable because of the easy exposure of the common iliac vein. In children weighing less than 10–12 kg, a midline transabdominal approach is necessary. The great vessels are approached by mobilizing the cecum, and the kidney is placed behind the cecum. To provide room for a large kidney in the right flank, a right native nephrectomy is sometimes necessary at the time of the transplant to create room for the allograft. Careful intraoperative fluid management is critical to prevent thrombosis of large kidneys in small children.

Intraoperative Fluid Management

Adequate perfusion of the newly transplanted kidney is critical for the establishment of an immediate postoperative diuresis and the avoidance of acute tubular necrosis (see Chap. 9). Volume contraction should be avoided and mild volume expansion maintained, conducive to the recipient's cardiac status. Central venous pressure should be maintained at approximately 10 mm Hg with the use of isotonic saline and albumin infusions, and systolic blood pressure should be kept above 120 mm Hg. If blood is required, cytomegalovirus–negative units should be used.

Immediately before the release of the vascular clamps, a large dose of methylprednisolone is usually given (up to 1 g in some programs; see Chap. 4). Mannitol (12.5 g) and furosemide (up to 200 mg) are also given, and fluid replacement is maintained accordingly. Direct injection of the calcium channel blocker verapamil in a dose of 5 mg into the renal artery reduces capillary spasm and improves renal blood flow. Postoperative management is discussed in Chap. 8.

SURGICAL COMPLICATIONS OF KIDNEY TRANSPLANTATION

The clinical presentation of surgical and nonsurgical complications of kidney transplantation may be very similar. Graft dysfunction may reflect an acute rejection or a urine leak; fever and graft tenderness may reflect wound infection or rejection. Post-transplant events have a broad differential diagnosis that must include technical complications of surgery as well as immunologic and other causes.

The fundamental algorithm in the management of post-transplant graft dysfunction requires that vascular and urologic causes of graft dysfunction be ruled out before concluding that an event is due to a medical cause such as rejection or cyclosporine toxicity. The differential diagnosis of postoperative graft dysfunction is discussed in Chap. 8, and the radiologic diagnostic tools are discussed in Chap. 11. Doppler ultrasound is invaluable in the differentiation of medical and surgical postoperative complications.

Wound Infection

In the 1960s and 1970s, wound infection rates after kidney transplantation were as high as 25%. Wound infections should not now occur in more than 1% of cases. This improvement is due to several factors: patients receiving transplants are healthier; lower steroid doses are used for both maintenance and treatment of rejection; and perioperative antibiotics are routinely used. In most cases, a first-generation cephalosporin is sufficient (see Chap. 10). Obviously, strict aseptic technique in the operating room is essential to prevent wound infection. If infections do occur, they should be treated with drainage and systemic antibiotics to avoid contamination of the vascular suture line and possible mycotic aneurysm formation. The risk of infection or other wound problems is significantly higher in obese patients.

Lymphocele

Presentation

Lymphoceles are collections of lymph caused by leakage from severed lymphatics that overlie the iliac vessels. They may develop and present 1 week to several weeks after transplantation. The incidence of lymphoceles reported in the literature ranges from less than 1% to 10%. Some lymphoceles are small and asymptomatic. Others are large and produce symptoms. Usually, the larger the lymphocele, the more likely it is to produce symptoms and require treatment, although there are some cases of very small but strategically placed lymphoceles producing ureteral obstruction. Lymphoceles may present by producing ureteral obstruction; by compressing the iliac vein, leading to deep vein thrombosis or leg swelling; or as an abdominal mass. Lymphoceles occasionally produce incontinence secondary to bladder compression, scrotal masses secondary to spontaneous drainage into the scrotum, or vena cava obstruction. Lymphoceles can be avoided by minimizing the dissection of the iliac vessels and by ligating all lymphatics. Electrocoagulation is not adequate.

Diagnosis

Lymphoceles are usually diagnosed by ultrasound (see Chap. 11). The characteristic ultrasound finding is a roundish, sonolucent, septated mass. Hydronephrosis may be present, and the ureter may be seen adjacent to and compressed by the lymphocele. More complex internal echoes may signal an infected lymphocele. Usually, the clinical situation and ultrasound appearance will distinguish a lymphocele from other types of perirenal fluid collections, such as hematoma or urine leak. Simple needle aspiration of the fluid using sterile technique will make the diagnosis. The fluid obtained will be clear and have high protein content, and the creatinine concentration will be equal to that of serum.

Treatment

No therapy is necessary for the common, small, asymptomatic lymphocele. Percutaneous aspiration should be performed if there is suspicion of a ureteral leak, obstruction, or infection. The most common indication for treatment is ureteral obstruction. If the cause of the obstruction is simple compression due to the mass effect of the lymphocele, drainage alone will resolve the problem. The ureter itself is often narrowed and may need to be reimplanted because of its involvement in the inflammatory reaction in the wall of the lymphocele. Repeated percutaneous aspirations are not advised because they seldom lead to dissolution of the lymphocele and often result in infection.

Infected or obstructing lymphoceles can be drained externally using either a closed or an open system. Closed systems are superior because they control the fluid and are less susceptible to infection. Sclerosing agents such as povidone iodine (Betadine) or tetracycline can be instilled into the cavity with good results. Lymphoceles can also be drained internally by marsupialization into the peritoneal cavity, where the fluid is resorbed. Marsupialization can be done as an open surgical procedure or laparoscopically. It is important to ensure that the opening in the lymphocele is large enough to prevent peritoneal overgrowth, which can produce recurrence or bowel entrapment and incarceration. Omentum is often interposed in the opening to prevent closure. Care must be taken to avoid injury to the ureter, which may lie in the wall of the lymphocele. On rare occasions, the actual site of lymph leak can be identified and ligated.

Bleeding

Postoperative bleeding seldom arises from the vascular anastomoses unless a mycotic aneurysm ruptures or the graft itself ruptures. These events are not likely to occur until a few days after transplantation and are associated with exsanguinating hemorrhage. Early postoperative bleeding can occur from small vessels in the renal hilum, which may not have been apparent prior to closure because of vasospasm. After surgery, when perfusion improves, these hilar vessels can then bleed. Meticulous hemostasis during the operation minimizes this risk. Close observation of vital signs and serial hematocrits is necessary for the first several postoperative hours to recognize this type of bleeding. Ultrasound can confirm the presence of perigraft hematoma. Surgical exploration may be necessary. If bleeding occurs, coagulation parameters should be studied to ensure that there is no occult coagulopathy.

Late hemorrhage can result from the rupture of a mycotic aneurysm. The bleeding may be profound. Nephrectomy and repair of the artery are usually required. Rarely, the external iliac artery may have to be ligated and blood supply to the ipsilateral leg provided by extra-anatomic bypass.

Graft Thrombosis

Arterial or venous thrombosis most often occurs within the first 2–3 days after transplant, although it may occur as long as 2 months post-transplant. The reported incidence varies widely from 0.5% to as high as 8%. The early variety is most often a reflection of surgical technique; the later is most often associated with acute rejection. Patients with high platelet counts (more than 350×10^9/liter) may be more susceptible to thrombosis. If the kidney has been functioning, thrombosis is heralded by a sudden cessation of urine output and rapid rise in serum creatinine, often with graft swelling and local pain. Platelets may be consumed, and thrombocytopenia and hyperkalemia may develop. Venous thrombosis may present with severe graft swelling, tenderness, and gross hematuria. If a patient's native kidneys were making large quantities of urine, however, the only sign of thrombosis may be the rising creatinine level; if the allograft had not been functioning, there may be no overt signs of thrombosis at all. For this reason, grafts that are not functioning are routinely examined by radionuclide scan or Doppler ultrasound to ensure ongoing blood flow to the graft. Diagnosis of thrombosis is by a Doppler ultrasound or isotope flow scan (see Chap. 11). These techniques help distinguish thrombosis from other causes of acute anuria such as rejection or obstruction. Confirmed thrombosis usually requires graft nephrectomy.

The transplanted kidney has no collateral blood supply, and its tolerance for warm ischemia is short. Unless the problem can be diagnosed quickly and repair carried out immediately, the kidney will be lost. While there are a few case reports of kidney salvage after thrombosis, most grafts sustaining either arterial or venous thrombosis are lost. Streptokinase has not been reported to be useful for arterial thrombosis. It has been successfully used in a case of renal vein thrombosis that occurred late after transplant and was associated with deep venous thrombosis of the leg that extended up to the transplant vein.

Renal Artery Stenosis

Renal artery stenosis is a late complication and occurs in 2–12% of transplant cases. Its presentation, diagnosis, and management are discussed in Chaps. 9 and 11. Two major types of stenoses are seen. One is a discrete, suture line stenosis, which is most often seen following end-to-end anastomosis. The other type is a more diffuse, postanastomotic stenosis, which can occur following any type of arterial anastomosis. Table 7-1 lists potential causes of both types of stenosis. The postulate that rejection can cause renal artery stenosis has not been conclusively proved.

When technically feasible, percutaneous transluminal angioplasty offers the safest mode of treatment with a high rate of success. In one series, more than 80% of patients were cured 2 years after treatment, although recurrence may occur in up to 20% of cases. If angioplasty is not technically feasible or fails as a primary form of therapy, surgical repair is necessary. Graft loss following surgical repair has been reported in up to 30% of cases and is a reflection of the difficulty in directly approaching the vascular anastomosis in a noncollateralized kidney.

Urine Leaks
Etiology and Diagnosis

Urine leaks may occur at the level of the bladder, ureter, or renal calyx. They typically occur within the first few days of the transplant or at the onset of post-transplant diuresis. Urine leaks may be

Table 7-1. Potential causes of renal artery stenosis

1. Rejection of the donor artery
2. Atherosclerosis of the recipient vessel
3. Clamp injury to the recipient or donor vascular endothelium
4. Perfusion pump cannulation injury of the donor vessel
5. Faulty suture technique: purse string effect, lumen encroachment by the suture, improper suture material, fibrotic inflammatory reaction to polypropylene in the setting of abnormal hemodynamics
6. End-to-end anastomosis with abnormal fluid dynamics
7. Angulation due to disproportionate length between graft artery and iliac artery
8. End-to-end anastomosis with vessel size disproportion
9. Kinking of the renal artery

technical in etiology due to a non-watertight ureteral reimplant or bladder closure. They may also be due to ureteral slough secondary to disruption of ureteral blood supply; the blood supply to the distal donor ureter is the most endangered by the harvesting procedure. Leaks may also occur as a result of a tight ureteral stenosis that leads to forniceal rupture. If the wound is drained, a urine leak may present with copious drainage. If the wound is not drained, a urine leak may present with pain, rising creatinine level due to the reabsorption of urine, and a fluid density mass on ultrasound. This clinical picture may be confused with rejection. If ultrasound shows a fluid collection, the fluid should be tapped under sterile conditions and the creatinine level of the fluid compared with the serum creatinine level. A renal scan will often identify the leak by showing radioisotope outside the urinary tract. A cystogram may show leakage of contrast outside of the bladder (see Chap. 11).

Treatment

There should be no delay in instituting therapy. A Foley catheter reduces intravesical pressure and may reduce or stop leakage altogether. Percutaneous antegrade nephrostomy may be used to definitively diagnose the leak and control the flow of urine. Some leaks can be managed definitively with external drainage and stent placement alone. It may be difficult, however, to access the collecting system percutaneously, since there is often not enough hydronephrosis present. If the leak is due to a ureteral slough, percutaneous treatment will never work and only delays definitive treatment. For these reasons, when leaks occur, early surgical exploration and repair is usually required.

The type of surgical repair depends on the level of leak and the viability of the tissues. Bladder fistulas should be closed primarily. A calyceal leak that is the result of obstruction is treated by removal of the obstruction. If a ureteral leak is a simple anastomotic leak, resection of the distal ureter and **reimplantation** is the easiest solution. If the ureter is nonviable due to inadequate length of blood supply, **ureteropyelostomy** using the ipsilateral or contralateral native ureter is a good option. **Cystopyelostomy** has also been done to replace a sloughed ureter. Here, the bladder is mobilized and brought directly to the allograft renal pelvis without an intervening ureter. The advantage of using the native ureter over direct anastomosis of the bladder to the renal pelvis is that the native ureter is antireflux-ing, which may result in lower incidence of pyelonephritis. An indwelling double-J stent is usually left in place after repair of a urine leak. Nephrostomy drainage is not essential, although if a prior per-cutaneous nephrostomy has been done, it is wise to leave it in place until several days after surgery. It should be removed only after a trial of nephrostomy occlusion to ensure continuity of distal drainage. The double-J stent can be removed cystoscopically several weeks later, fol-lowed by ultrasound to ensure that urine is not recollecting.

Ureteral Obstruction

Diagnosis

Ureteral obstruction is usually manifested by impairment of graft function. Obstruction may be painless because of the absence of innervation. Hydronephrosis may be seen on ultrasound; increasing hydronephrosis is good evidence of obstruction. Low-grade dilata-tion of the collecting system secondary to edema at the implant site is often seen on early post-transplant ultrasound examinations and should not necessarily lead to the conclusion that there is obstruc-tion present. Confirmation of the obstruction and identification of the site can be made by intravenous pyelogram, although often graft function is not adequate to allow good visualization. Obstruction can be confirmed by retrograde pyelogram, although the ureteral orifice may be difficult to catheterize. Renal scan with furosemide washout is a good screening test but does not provide clear anatom-ic detail. The most effective way to visualize the collecting system is by percutaneous antegrade pyelography.

Etiology and Treatment

Acute postoperative obstruction usually requires surgical repair. Blood clots, a technically poor reimplant, and ureteral slough are the common causes of early acute obstruction after transplantation. Ureteral fibrosis secondary to either ischemia or rejection can cause an intrinsic obstruction. Extrinsic obstruction can be caused by ureteral kinking or periureteral fibrosis from lymphoceles or graft rejection. Calculi are rare causes of transplant obstruction.

Intrinsic ureteral scars can be treated effectively by endourologic techniques in an antegrade (Fig. 7-4) or retrograde approach. If graft dysfunction is associated with significant or increasing hydronephrosis, obstruction is confirmed with a fine needle percuta-neous nephrostogram (see Chap. 11 and Fig 7-4A). If obstruction is confirmed, a guide wire is passed endoscopically through the stric-ture (see Fig. 7-4B). If the stricture is short (i.e., less than 2 cm), bal-loon dilatation allows a working element to be passed, and under direct vision the stricture is incised with a cold knife (see Fig. 7-4C). The stricture can also be approached retrograde via the bladder cys-toscopically. A stent is left indwelling (see Fig. 7-4D) and removed cystoscopically after 2–6 weeks. The nephrostomy is removed after an antegrade nephrostogram has confirmed that the urinary tract is unobstructed. Early reports suggest success rates of 70–80% with these techniques. Endourologic techniques can also be used to remove calculi, which can also be destroyed by extracorporeal shock wave lithotripsy.

Extrinsic strictures or strictures that are longer than 2 cm are less likely to be amenable to percutaneous techniques and require surgi-

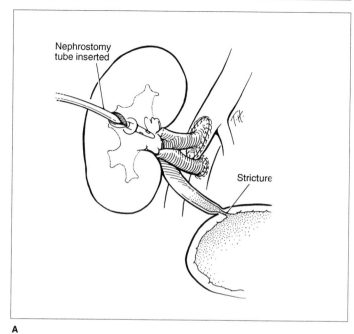

A

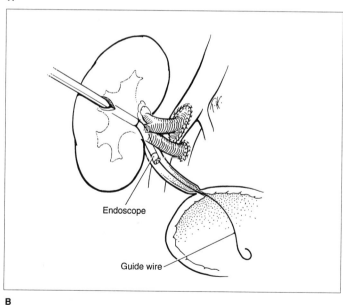

B

Fig. 7-4. Stages in the endourologic treatment of ureteral structure. See text for description of steps.

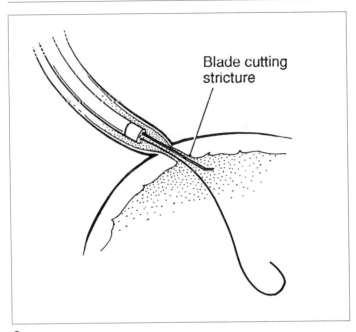

C

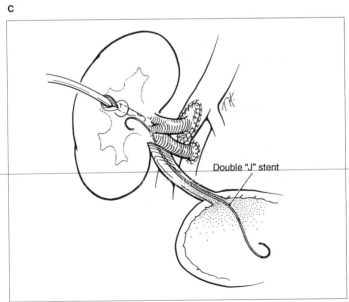

D

Fig. 7-4 *(continued).*

cal treatment as do those strictures that fail endourologic incision. The same surgical options are used as for ureteral leaks: direct reimplantation of the ureter above the stricture or anastomosis of the native ureter or bladder to the renal pelvis if the stricture is high.

ALLOGRAFT NEPHRECTOMY

Indications

Kidneys that have failed either for technical reasons or from rejection may need to be removed. Indications for allograft nephrectomy are symptoms and signs that typically occur when immunosuppression is withdrawn but may be delayed by weeks or months. These may include low-grade fever, graft tenderness and swelling, malaise, thrombocytopenia, and hematuria. It may be possible to lessen the symptoms and avoid nephrectomy by temporary reinstitution of small doses of steroids. Avoidance of nephrectomy is preferred, since the procedure may have an unfavorable impact on the prognosis of a future transplant and may cause a steep elevation in the percentage of preformed cytotoxic antibodies (see Chap. 3). If the graft loss is acute and occurs within 1 year of transplantation, nephrectomy may be necessary in up to 90% of cases. Graft loss from chronic rejection after 1 year results in nephrectomy in up to 50% of cases. The rejected graft that remains in situ typically becomes a small fibrotic mass. Acquired cystic disease may develop as described in chronically diseased native kidneys.

Procedure

The removal of a failed allograft may be technically more difficult than the transplant operation itself because of the inflammatory response and scarring due to rejection. Usually, the old incision is reopened. Care must be made to avoid the peritoneum, which may have become draped across the surface of the kidney. If the nephrectomy is performed soon after transplantation, especially if there has not been a great amount of rejection, the kidney can be removed entirely, since it is not very adherent to surrounding structures. If there has been recurrent rejection, the kidney usually adheres to surrounding structures and needs to be removed subcapsularly. The hilar vessels are friable and should be ligated and suture ligated. It is almost always safe to leave a small amount of donor vessel in the recipient so that repair of the recipient iliac vessels is not necessary.

Hemostasis should be meticulous. Some dead space is always left after nephrectomy. If this fills with blood, abscess formation is more likely. While a closed drain may be used, it may inadequately drain the blood and create the potential for infection by its presence. Electrocoagulation of the entire raw surface of the capsule should be performed, and spraying thrombin topically may improve hemostasis. Topical and parenteral antibiotics are routinely used.

Complications

Although there are few series in the literature, the reported morbidity for allograft nephrectomy is high. The potential complications include acute bleeding during surgery secondary to injury to the iliac artery or vein; injury to other surrounding structures, such as bowel; infection; and lymph leaks. Leaving small segments of the allograft renal artery or vein does not usually cause any long-term

Table 7-2. Precautions for post–kidney transplant patients undergoing surgical procedures

1. Maintain hydration.
2. Use non-nephrotoxic prophylactic antibiotics.
3. Modify intravenous cyclosporine dose.
4. Provide perioperative steroid coverage.
5. Avoid nephrotoxic antibiotics and analgesics.
6. Monitor graft function and plasma potassium, and acid-base status.
7. Consider wound healing impairment.

problems, although rupture can occur if they become secondarily infected. Likewise, leaving a small amount of allograft ureter in place can result in some gross hematuria after the allograft nephrectomy; the hematuria is almost always limited and usually does not require reoperation.

NON–TRANSPLANT-RELATED SURGERY

Immunosuppressed transplant patients may occasionally require significant surgical intervention not directly related to the transplant itself, such as coronary artery bypass, cholecystectomy, or hip replacement. Nephrologists or members of the transplant team will often be requested to aid in the perioperative management of such patients, and certain precautions are required (Table 7-2).

The renal function of many transplant patients is impaired to varying degrees, and the capacity to concentrate urine and lower urinary sodium concentration may be limited. Maintenance of hydration is, therefore, particularly important perioperatively to avoid further reduction in renal function. If a patient will be unable to take immunosuppressive medications orally for more than 24 hours, cyclosporine should be given IV in a dose that is approximately one-third of the total daily oral dose (see Chap. 4) given over 4–8 hours. Although functional adrenal suppression in patients on 10 mg of prednisone per day or less is uncommon, 100 mg of hydrocortisone is typically given every 6 hours postoperatively until the patient can return to the preoperative oral prednisone dose. For patients receiving triple therapy (see Chap. 4), azathioprine can be safely withheld for 2–3 days, as can mycophenolate mofetil. Non-nephrotoxic antibiotics should be given prophylactically, and if IV contrast is required for radiologic studies, a saline diuresis should be maintained. In patients with markedly impaired graft function, careful monitoring of postoperative plasma potassium levels and acid-base status is mandatory.

SELECTED READINGS

Aboaljoud MS, Deierhoi MH, Hudson SL et al. Risk factors affecting second renal transplant outcome with special reference to primary allograft nephrectomy. *Transplantation* 60:138, 1995.

Churchill BM, Steckler RE, McKenna PH et al. Renal transplantation and the abnormal urinary tract. *Transplant Rev* 7:21, 1993.

Davidson I, Ar'Rajab A, Dickerman B et al. Perioperative albumin and verapamil improve early outcome after cadaver renal transplantation. *Transplant Proc* 26:3100, 1994.

Gruessner RW, Fasola C, Benedetti E et al. Laparoscopic drainage of lymphocele after kidney transplantation, indications and limitations. *Surgery* 117:288, 1995.

Merkus JWS, Huysmans FTM, Hoitsma AJ et al. Treatment of renal allograft artery stenosis. *Transplant Int* 6:111, 1993.

Nargund VH, Cranston D. Urologic complications after renal transplantation. *Transplant Rev* 10:24, 1996.

Pleass HC, Clark KR, Rigg KM et al. Urologic complications after renal transplantation: A prospective randomized trial comparing different techniques of ureteric anastomosis and the use of prophylactic ureteric stents. *Transplant Proc* 27:1091, 1995.

Rosenthal JT. Complications of Renal Transplantation and Autotransplantation. In RB Smith, RM Ehrlich (eds), *Complications of Urologic Surgery*. Philadelphia: Saunders, 1990. Pp 231–256.

Wong W, Fynn SP, Higgins RM et al. Transplant renal artery stenosis in 77 patients—does it have an immunologic cause? *Transplantation* 61:215, 1996.

The First Two Post-Transplant Months

William J. C. Amend Jr., Flavio Vincenti, and Stephen J. Tomlanovich

The "early" period following renal transplantation usually refers to the first two post-transplant months. It is useful to further divide this period to allow consideration of the different diagnostic and therapeutic issues that have an impact on both routine and complicated transplant management and that tend to change with time. It is a fair generalization to say that surgical issues predominate in the first post-transplant days and medical and immunologic issues tend to predominate thereafter. During this entire period, patients should ideally be followed by a combined surgical and medical team. In this chapter, patient management on the first post-transplant day, the first 2–8 days, and the first 9–60 days are considered separately. Clearly, this breakdown is somewhat arbitrary. Patients who successfully navigate their way through these first 2 months can usually look forward to prolonged graft function. Immunosuppressive therapy during this period is discussed in Chap. 4.

FIRST POSTOPERATIVE DAY

Recovery Room Assessment

Patients should be reevaluated by the transplant team immediately on arrival from the operating room. This initial assessment should first address routine postsurgical issues such as hemodynamic and respiratory stability. Most patients will be extubated and awake. The operative record should be reviewed to assess fluid and blood loss and replacement and to ensure that intraoperative immunosuppressive protocols have been adhered to (e.g., use of corticosteroids, OKT3; see Chap. 4). The surgeon should report any untoward intraoperative events and the appearance of the transplanted organ after completion of the anastomosis and release of vascular clamps. It is often possible to anticipate early graft function based on the intraoperative perfusion characteristics of the kidney, the firmness or turgidity of the allograft, and the intraoperative urine volume. Special situations, such as the use of pediatric en bloc kidneys (see Chap. 5), transplantation into a difficult vascular bed, or the use of ureteral stents should be clearly noted.

Routine postoperative orders are reviewed in Table 8-1. The length of time a patient remains in recovery will depend on both medical and logistical factors. The postoperative nursing environment must allow for close hemodynamic and fluid management. This environment can be in an intensive care unit or a surgical "step-down" unit, depending on the facilities available in a given institution. Special considerations for the postoperative management of diabetic patients are discussed in Chap. 13.

Hemodynamic Evaluation

Postoperative hemodynamic evaluation is critical for several reasons: for routine postsurgical management, to optimize graft func-

Table 8-1. Suggested postoperative orders on transfer of kidney transplant recipient from the recovery room

Postoperative nursing orders
1. Vital signs q1h for 24 hr, then q4h when patient is stable
2. Intake and output q1h for 24 hr, then q4h
3. IV fluids per physician
4. Daily weight
5. Turn, cough, deep breathe q1h; encourage incentive spirometry q1h while awake
6. Out of bed first postoperative; ambulate daily thereafter
7. Head of bed at 30 degrees
8. Dressing changes q4h for 24 hr, then q8h and prn
9. Check dialysis access for function q4h
10. No blood pressure; venipuncture in extremity with fistula/shunt
11. Foley catheter to bedside drainage, irrigate gently with 30 ml normal saline prn for clots
12. Catheter care q8h
13. Notify physician if urine output drops to less than 50 ml/hr or if greater than 200 ml/hr
14. Notify physician if temperature is >38°C, or if systolic blood pressure is >180 mm Hg or <110 mm Hg
15. NPO until changed by surgical team
16. Chest x-ray in the morning
17. Electrocardiogram in the morning

Postoperative laboratory orders
1. Complete blood count with platelets, electrolytes, creatinine, glucose, and blood urea nitrogen q6h for 24 hrs, then every morning
2. Cyclosporine level every morning
3. Chemistry panel, urine culture and sensitivity twice a week

tion, to fully assess the significance of the urine output (or lack thereof), and to undertake therapeutic intervention.

Hemodynamic evaluation may be somewhat difficult in patients with chronic renal failure with hemodialysis fistulae or shunts. Vascular sclerosis is frequent in uremic patients, especially in elderly and diabetic patients, such that systolic hypertension is frequent. The clinician should be familiar with the patient's pretransplant blood pressure and antihypertensive medications. A review of the operative course with the transplant surgeon may be useful for blood pressure management decisions, since there is impaired intrinsic renal autoregulation and the initial blood flow to the allograft is primarily dependent on mean systemic arterial blood pressure. The surgeon can report on the intraoperative level of mean arterial blood pressure that provided the best observed allograft turgor and urine output. Excessive postoperative arterial hypertension may increase the risk of anastomotic leak and cerebrovascular catastrophes. Reduced mean arterial pressures, on the other hand, increase both the risk of postoperative acute tubular necrosis (ATN) and of irreversible vascular thrombosis at the fresh anastomotic sites. Sublingual nifedipine is effective and convenient for management of postoperative systolic hypertension. Intravenous labetalol, hydralazine, esmolol, or nitroprusside can be used in resistant cases where the systolic blood pressure is consistently over 180 mm Hg.

Many kidney transplant units use central venous pressure or pulmonary artery and pulmonary wedge pressure measurements in the first 24–48 hours post-transplant. These measurements can be useful especially when the clinical team is not sure of the need for and amount of fluid resuscitation. Since kidney transplant recipients may have varying degrees of heart failure (from uremic cardiomyopathy, hypertensive cardiomyopathy, or coronary artery disease), the more sophisticated preload monitoring techniques may be invaluable. Such patients will, ideally, have been identified in the pretransplant stage, and the results of the pretransplant cardiac evaluation (see Chap. 6) should be available to aid in their postoperative assessment. Clinical judgment, however, should supersede slavish commitment to central venous pressure parameters. Thus, a normotensive patient with a good urine output may have a low recorded central venous pressure and yet not need fluid resuscitation.

Intravenous Fluid Replacement

Several factors need to be assessed to determine the rate and form of post-transplant fluid replacement. In general, the patient should be kept euvolemic or mildly hypervolemic, and repeated hemodynamic assessment is required. Insensible fluid losses are typically 30–60 ml/hour. Vascular volume deficits can continue due to "third-spacing" over the first 12–24 postoperative hours and need to be replaced. Volume losses at the operative site must be considered, especially if there are concomitant changes in urine volume and hemodynamic status. Urine volume must be monitored hourly and replaced accordingly (see the section on urine output).

Which Intravenous Fluid?

Insensible fluid loss is essentially water loss and is replaced by a 5% dextrose solution at approximately 30 ml/hour. If the patient is deemed to be hypervolemic, it may be wise not to replace this fluid and allow the patient to gradually reach the postoperative dry weight over the ensuing days. Hourly urine output is replaced with half-normal saline on a "milliliter-for-milliliter" basis. Half-normal saline is used for urine replacement, since the sodium concentration of the urine of a newly transplanted diuresing kidney is typically 60–80 mEq/liter. If there are large nasogastric losses, these are replaced with normal saline. If the patient is deemed to be hypovolemic or if an attempt is being made to increase urine volume (see the section on urine output), isotonic saline boluses are given after bedside clinical and hemodynamic evaluation. Malnourished, hypoalbuminemic patients may benefit from albumin infusion for volume restoration.

Potassium replacement is usually not required unless urine volumes are very high and should be given with great care in oliguric patients. Lactated Ringer's solution and other premixed IV fluids are unnecessary. Their potassium and bicarbonate content is inadequate if replacement is indeed required, and it is better to supplement saline infusions with potassium, bicarbonate, and calcium on an as-needed basis. The necessity for blood transfusion is discussed in the section on early postoperative bleeding.

Urine Output

The initial urine volume can range from anuria to oliguria, "nonoliguria," or polyuria and may shift from one to the other based on parenchymal, urologic, or perfusion factors. A background knowledge of the patient's native urine output is critical to assess the origin of the early post-transplant urine output. Information about the donor kidney itself is critical. When the transplant is from a live donor, postoperative oliguria is rare because of the short ischemia time (see Chap. 5) and if it occurs must raise immediate concern regarding the vascularization of the graft. On the other hand, when a patient receives a cadaveric kidney with a prolonged ischemia time or preprocurement ATN, postoperative oliguria can be anticipated. The mate kidney from a cadaveric donor will often "perform" in a similar manner (i.e., exhibit ATN or not) in both recipients, and it can be informative to call the transplant center receiving the other kidney to inquire about its performance.

Various techniques and protocol modifications have been made to encourage postoperative diuresis (see Chap. 4). Some protocols do not permit the use of IV cyclosporine in the early postoperative period. Dopamine infusions at "renal dose" levels of 1–5 μg/kg/min are used routinely at some centers to promote renal blood flow and counteract cyclosporine-induced renal vasoconstriction. Perioperative calcium channel blockers are also sometimes used.

The Anuric and Oliguric Patient

Anuria is easy to define. Oliguria is relative and in the post-transplant situation usually refers to urine outputs of less than approximately 50 ml/hour. Before addressing the low urine output therapeutically and diagnostically, the patient's volume status and fluid balance must be assessed, and the Foley catheter must be irrigated to ensure patency. If there are clots and an associated ball-valve effect at the catheter's internal ostium, the catheter should be removed while applying gentle suction in an attempt to capture the offending clot. Thereafter, a larger-sized catheter may be required. If the Foley catheter is patent and the patient is clearly hypervolemic (i.e., edematous, with congested pulmonary vasculature on chest x-ray, or with elevated venous or wedge pressures), up to 200 mg of furosemide should be given IV. If the patient is judged to be hypovolemic, isotonic saline should be given in boluses of 250–500 ml, the response assessed, and the IV infusion repeated if necessary. If the patient is judged to be euvolemic or a confident clinical assessment cannot be made, a judicious isotonic saline challenge should be given, followed by a high dose of furosemide.

If a diuresis follows these maneuvers, urine output is again replaced milliliter-for-milliliter with half-normal saline. The volume challenge and furosemide dose may be repeated if urine volume falls off, but only after careful hemodynamic assessment. A constant infusion of furosemide in a dose of 5–10 mg/hour is employed in some centers. An algorithmic approach to the management of postoperative oliguria is suggested in Fig. 8-1.

Diagnostic Studies in Persistent Oliguria or Anuria

If the volume challenge, furosemide use, and volume replacement have no significant impact on the post-transplant urinary output, diagnostic studies should be carried out to determine the cause of the early post-transplant oliguric state (see Chap. 11). The urgency of this workup depends somewhat on the clinical circumstances. If diuresis is anticipated, such as after a live donor kidney transplant,

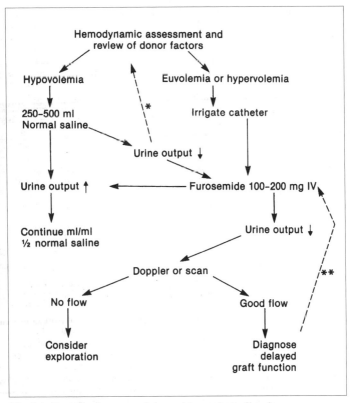

Fig. 8-1. Algorithmic approach to post-transplant oliguria.
*The volume challenge can be repeated, but only after careful reassessment of the volume status and fluid balance.
**Repeated doses of IV furosemide or furosemide "drips" may be valuable in patients whose urine output fluctuates. Persistent oliguria will usually not respond to a repeat dose.

diagnostic studies should be performed immediately—in the recovery room if necessary. If oliguria is anticipated, studies can usually be safely delayed by several hours.

The purpose of diagnostic studies is to confirm the presence of blood flow to the graft and the absence of a urine leak or obstruction. Blood flow studies are performed scintigraphically or by Doppler ultrasound. If the flow study reveals no demonstrable blood flow, a prompt surgical re-exploration is necessary to attempt to repair any vascular technical problem and diagnose hyperacute rejection. These kidneys are usually lost, however, and are removed during the second surgery.

If adequate blood flow is visible with the scintiscan or Doppler studies, the possibility of ureteral obstruction or urinary leak needs to be considered and can be evaluated by the same imaging studies. In the first 24 hours post-transplant, as long as the Foley catheter has been providing good bladder drainage, the obstruction or leak is almost always at the ureterovesical junction and represents a technical problem that needs surgical correction. To avoid this complication, some surgeons place a ureteral stent at the time of transplantation. This can be attached to the Foley catheter and subsequently removed with the catheter, or it can be removed cystoscopically several weeks post-transplant (see Chap. 7).

The Polyuric Patient

Occasionally, patients, usually recipients of live-donor transplants, pass massive amounts of urine (>500 ml/hour) in the early post-transplant period. Generally, these patients are hypervolemic, and it is safe for urine replacement to be reduced stepwise to a less than milliliter-for-milliliter replacement. If a negative fluid balance is permitted, the volume status must be reassessed at frequent intervals and the fluid replacement returned to milliliter-for-milliliter when the urine volume becomes more manageable or if the patient becomes relatively hypotensive. Potassium and calcium may need to be replaced in the polyuric patient.

Early Postoperative Bleeding

The possibility of surgical postoperative bleeding must be considered in any patient with a rapidly falling hematocrit and saline-resistant hypotension. If a drain is present, it may repeatedly fill with blood, or there may be a palpable or visible perinephric hematoma. Most hematomas will spontaneously tamponade and do not require reoperation as long as the patient can be maintained hemodynamically stable with crystalloid and colloid solutions and/or blood. The threshold for postoperative blood transfusion will depend on the clinical circumstances. Older or diabetic patients who may have covert coronary artery disease should be transfused earlier rather than later. If possible, blood from cytomegalovirus (CMV)-negative donors should be given. At reoperation, an identifiable bleeding site is not uniformly discovered (see Chap. 7), and the bleeding may represent tissue oozing exaggerated by a uremic bleeding diathesis. In such cases, administration of IV desmopressin acetate (DDAVP) at 0.3–0.6 μg/kg can be useful.

Postoperative Hemodialysis

If the patient is well-dialyzed preoperatively and enters the operation normokalemic, early postoperative dialysis is usually not required. Oliguric patients, especially those with bleeding complications, may develop dangerous hyperkalemia and may require urgent therapy with IV calcium, bicarbonate, or insulin and glucose combinations. Sodium polystyrene sulfonate (Kayexalate) enemas should be avoided in the early postoperative period, as they may cause colonic injury. Patients with persistent hyperkalemia should be dialyzed. A no-heparin protocol should be used, a bicarbonate bath is preferred, and ultrafiltration should be avoided to prevent hypotension. A 2- or 3-hour dialysis is usually adequate.

If the patient was on chronic ambulatory peritoneal dialysis before transplant and the Tenckhoff catheter is in place, it may be possible to adequately peritoneally dialyze the patient postoperatively. Generally, hemodialysis is preferred because of the possibility of a peritoneal leak or infection; a temporary hemodialysis catheter may be required for access in these circumstances.

FIRST POSTOPERATIVE WEEK

The first postoperative week is generally characterized by progressive improvement in the patient's overall condition in conjunction with steady improvement in kidney function. Most patients can leave the intensive care setting after 24–48 hours. Continued close observation of urine output is still indicated; however, fluid replacement need not be adjusted on an hourly basis and can be ordered on a 4- to 8-hour record of urine output. The urine volume is a useful indicator of kidney allograft function but may be misleading in patients who had appreciable urine output from their native kidneys. Mild fluctuations in urine volumes are acceptable, but a persistent drop in urine volume of more than 50% or the sudden onset of oliguria or anuria must be promptly investigated (see the section on patients with delayed graft function). The Foley catheter usually can be removed after 2–4 days. Patients should void frequently after catheter removal to avoid overdistention of the bladder.

Patients should be ambulated within 24 hours of surgery. They are usually started within 72 hours on a liquid diet and progress thereafter as tolerated. Abdominal distention and pain and the prolonged absence of bowel sounds require investigation by abdominal x-rays and consideration of the occasional occurrence of intra-abdominal catastrophes. Incisional pain may persist throughout the first postoperative week but is usually mild. Severe pain or a change in the pain pattern should be thoroughly investigated to rule out rejection, perinephric hematoma, and urine leaks. Fever is not uncommon in the first week and is most commonly due to postoperative atelectasis. Opportunistic infections do not occur at this time, and extensive workup of fever is usually not indicated. Persistent fever with no obvious infectious source may be a manifestation of unrecognized rejection.

The management of the transplant patient in the first week is largely determined by the quality of function of the allograft. Patients typically exhibit one of three patterns of function: excellent graft function, moderate graft dysfunction, or delayed graft function.

Patients with Excellent Graft Function

In ideal circumstances, graft function and diuresis are excellent postoperatively, dialysis is not required, and the serum creatinine level declines rapidly so that patients achieve stable kidney function within the first post-transplant week (the serum creatinine level may reach <2.5 mg/dl). Almost all the recipients of kidneys from live donors as well as 30–50% of cadaveric kidney recipients enjoy such a favorable postoperative course. In patients with excellent early function, both the urine volume and serum creatinine levels are useful markers to monitor for the occurrence of early rejection, cyclosporine toxicity, and other underlying pathologic events in the allograft.

If the course of these patients remains uneventful, it is not mandatory to routinely perform imaging studies. Some transplant centers elect to perform renal ultrasound and scintiscans to provide baseline data.

Patients with Moderate Graft Dysfunction

Patients with moderate graft dysfunction are nonoliguric and exhibit modest daily declines in serum creatinine levels. These patients do

Table 8-2. Causes of delayed graft function

Donor factors
    Donor age >55 yrs
    Donor acute tubular necrosis
    Prolonged cold or warm ischemia time
Intraoperative factors
    Prolonged rewarm time
    Intraoperative hypotension
    Negative intraoperative fluid balance
Recipient factors
    Prior failed transplants
    Postoperative hypotension or hypovolemia
    Early high-dose cyclosporine
    Early OKT3 use

not usually require dialysis but will not normalize their kidney function within the first postoperative week. In these patients, the urine volume and the daily serum creatinine concentration are useful markers to monitor the development of complications. Depending on the rate of decline in the serum creatinine concentration, it may be wise to obtain imaging studies to rule out the possibility that urine leak or partial obstruction is accounting for the slow improvement of function. Studies should certainly be performed if the serum creatinine concentration plateaus at a high level or begins to rise. The pathophysiology of the slow improvement in function in these patients is usually ATN, which may be exaggerated by cyclosporine toxicity (see Chap. 4).

Patients with Delayed Graft Function

A varying percentage of cadaveric transplant recipients remain anuric or oliguric and dependent on dialysis in the early post-transplant period. The frequency of delayed graft function may be as low as 10% and as high as 50% in some programs. In recipients of transplants from live donors, this occurrence is exceptional and almost always portends a serious complication. In patients who have had previously failed transplants, delayed graft function is more common, an observation that suggests an immunologic etiology. Potential causes of delayed graft function are listed in Table 8-2.

The terms **delayed graft function** and **ATN** are often used interchangeably; however, it is wise to differentiate them. Not all delayed graft function is due to ATN, and covert accelerated acute rejection and technical complications such as vascular thrombosis will account for some of the cases and cause permanent or so-called **primary nonfunction**. When differentiated from other causes of delayed graft function, ATN appears to be a relatively benign condition that resolves spontaneously over days and sometimes weeks. Recovery is usually first recognized by the patient and is heralded by a steady increase in urine output, diminution in intradialytic rise in creatinine concentration, and eventual steady improvement in kidney function.

Prognostic Implication

The reported impact of delayed graft function on long-term graft survival and function has been the subject of much controversy.

Some studies report little or no impact, while others report a greater than 20% reduction in one-year graft survival when early graft function is impaired. Much of the discrepancy can probably be accounted for by failure to differentiate between ATN and other causes of delayed function. Highly matched kidneys may be less susceptible to the harmful affects of delayed graft function and it has been suggested that ATN exposes the mismatched kidney to a more aggressive immune attack. Marginal kidneys (see Chap. 5) may be more susceptible to the harmful effects of delayed graft function. Even if the ultimate impact of delayed graft function is not great, it certainly complicates patient management, and every attempt should be made to minimize its frequency and severity.

Management

Delayed graft function complicates management because it masks clinical detection of post-transplant events. Graft thrombosis and acute rejection are difficult to detect in an anuric or oliguric patient, and a urine leak will not manifest itself if the kidney does not make urine! Thus, in this situation, there must be greater reliance on noninvasive imaging studies to assess the status of the allograft. Doppler ultrasound or scintiscans should be performed at regular intervals to ensure maintenance of blood flow and to rule out urine leaks and obstruction (see Chap. 11). Fine-needle aspiration biopsy is particularly useful in this setting (see Chap. 12) because it allows repeated, minimally invasive monitoring of intragraft events. Core biopsy is performed at intervals in some centers to ensure that the diagnosis is indeed ATN and not covert rejection.

Some transplant programs modify their immunosuppressive protocols in the presence of ATN, usually on the premise that cyclosporine or tacrolimus administration should be avoided or minimized in this situation (see Chap. 4). Avoidance of cyclosporine and tacrolimus may reduce the length of the oliguric period, but the incidence of delayed graft function is not clearly lower with alternative protocols. Criteria for dialysis and dietary management during this period are the same as for any postoperative end-stage renal failure patient.

Rejection in the First Week Following Transplantation

Accelerated Acute Rejection

Accelerated rejection is due to presensitization and is mediated by antibodies to donor human leukocyte antigens (HLAs). The rejection occurs after an anamnestic response and a critical level of antibodies is produced that results in an irreversible vascular rejection. Accelerated rejection can occur immediately post-transplant (**hyperacute rejection**), or it may be delayed by several days (**delayed hyperacute rejection**). Patients are usually anuric or oliguric and often have fever and graft tenderness. The renal scan shows little or no uptake, and there may be evidence of intravascular coagulation. The differential diagnosis in this setting includes both arterial and venous thrombosis; however, patients with these vascular complications are frequently asymptomatic. Prompt surgical exploration of the allograft is indicated; when in doubt, an intraoperative biopsy is performed to determine its viability. Most allografts need to be removed.

The pathology of accelerated acute rejection is discussed in Chap. 12. Because of assiduous attention to the pretransplant crossmatch (see Chap. 3), it occurs rarely. A form of anti-HLA class I–mediated rejection has been described where the pretransplant crossmatch is negative yet becomes positive post-transplant. These patients are oliguric but have persistent blood flow. Histologic studies show absence of typical cell-mediated rejection but evidence of glomerular endothelial injury.

Early Cell-Mediated Rejection

Classic cell-mediated rejection can be detected in the latter part of the first transplant week, although it typically occurs somewhat later. Patients who have had recent blood transfusions, especially patients who have donor-specific blood transfusions, may develop a typical, reversible, cell-mediated rejection very early in the first post-transplant week. These cell-mediated rejections can be differentiated from accelerated humoral rejection by a renal scan, which shows decreased but persistent perfusion. If in doubt, a kidney biopsy may be indicated. Treatment of acute rejection is discussed in Chap. 4, and pathology is discussed in Chap. 12.

Nonimmunologic Causes of Graft Dysfunction in the First Week

There are a variety of nonimmunologic causes of graft dysfunction in the first post-transplant week. Technical vascular complications such as renal artery or renal vein thrombosis may result in abrupt loss of function. Urologic complications, such as obstruction, urine leaks from the ureteroneocystostomy, and necrosis of the ureter, can present with deterioration in kidney function, increased pain over the allograft, or drainage of fluid through the wound. The combination of Doppler ultrasound and scintiscan can be extremely useful in determining the diagnosis. In cases of obstruction, an antegrade pyelogram provides the most accurate localization of the obstruction (see Chap. 11). In patients with a suspected urine leak associated with wound drainage, a prompt diagnosis can be made if the creatinine concentration of the fluid is greater than the simultaneously measured plasma level. Any excessive drainage from the incision or a surgical drain should be sent for creatinine estimation.

The use of cyclosporine or tacrolimus during the first week after transplantation may result in abnormalities in graft function (see Chap. 4). The recovery from ATN may be delayed, and even in patients with excellent graft function, cyclosporine can, on occasion, cause an abrupt deterioration in function that needs to be differentiated from early rejection and graft thrombosis. This response is most likely due to renal vasoconstriction and can be reversed by decreasing the cyclosporine or tacrolimus dose.

Use of both cyclosporine and tacrolimus may be associated with a drug-induced hemolytic-uremic syndrome (HUS) (see Chap. 4). HUS may be evident clinically by virtue of the typical laboratory findings of intravascular coagulation (e.g., thrombocytopenia, distorted erythrocytes, elevated lactic dehydrogenase levels) accompanied by an arteriolopathy and intravascular thrombi on transplant biopsy (see Chap. 12). Development of HUS may be covert, however, and the laboratory findings may be inconsistent. The initial transplant biopsy may also be misleading, so a high level of clinical suspicion is required. It is critical to make the diagnosis, since improvement in transplant function may follow discontinuation or reduction of cyclosporine and institution of plasmapheresis.

Medical Management in the First Week

Cardiovascular and hemodynamic stability remain extremely important during the first week following transplantation to ensure adequate perfusion of the allograft. Drugs that can alter intrarenal hemodynamics, such as angiotensin-converting enzyme (ACE) inhibitors or nonsteroidal anti-inflammatory agents, should be avoided. While control of hypertension during the first week following transplantation is important, tight control should be avoided to prevent episodes of hypotension. Calcium channel blockers are effective and well-tolerated antihypertensive agents, and they have some theoretical and practical advantages over other agents (see Chaps. 4 and 9).

Changes in immunosuppressive strategy during the first week following transplantation should be based as much as possible on the results of diagnostic studies. Combined therapeutic and diagnostic maneuvers can be useful on a short-term basis—for example, a decrease in graft function after introduction of cyclosporine or tacrolimus may be managed by withholding or reducing the dose for a day or two; a rise in the serum creatinine concentration within days of transplantation in recipients of live-related transplants pretreated with donor specific transfusions can be assumed to be due to early cell-mediated rejection and treated with a steroid pulse. In both examples, other causes of kidney dysfunction must be ruled out first by noninvasive studies.

More aggressive pursuit of a definitive diagnosis with core kidney biopsy or angiogram should be considered in patients with significant risk factors, including highly sensitized individuals; patients who have had a previous, rapidly rejected kidney transplant; and patients who have native kidney diseases with a high risk of early recurrence. Generally speaking, core kidney biopsies should be avoided in the first week because there may be a greater incidence of bleeding. Finally, particular attention should be paid to the nutritional support of these highly catabolic patients (see Chap. 17), and ambulation should be encouraged in anticipation of discharge.

The Surgical Incision

With modern surgical techniques and prophylactic perioperative antibiotics, significant wound infections and problems have become infrequent following transplantation. Obese patients are more susceptible to wound dehiscence and infection. A serosanguineous incisional ooze is not uncommon post-transplant; however, if it is profuse enough that it can be collected into a syringe, its creatinine concentration should be measured to ensure that it is not a urine leak. Staples and sutures are usually removed at 12–14 days.

THE FIRST TWO POSTOPERATIVE MONTHS

The next 2-month period is characterized by the transition from inpatient to outpatient management. Most stable patients are discharged 5–14 days postoperatively. Transplant centers vary with respect to their enthusiasm for early discharge; logistical issues such as travel distance to the transplant center, the availability of a help-mate, and the frequency of outpatient clinics need to be considered. Before discharge, it is critical to counsel the patient about his or her medications. The patient should be familiar with their names, doses, and purpose as well as their side effects and possible drug interactions, especially with cyclosporine and tacrolimus. Diet, exercise, and wound care are discussed. The patient can be encouraged to ambulate and to begin light aerobic exercise by walking or exercise-biking. Premenopausal, sexually active female patients must receive contraceptive counseling because many women presume, often mistakenly, that they are still infertile. Patients must be taught to recognize the symptoms and signs of infection and rejection. It is wise to instruct patients to maintain a diary of their vital signs, urine output, and medications. Patients should be warned and prepared for the possibility of readmission to the hospital.

Discharge from the hospital often engenders anxious anticipation in both the patient and family members; empathic counseling should be available on an informal and formal level.

Clinical Course

By the second post-transplant week, the graft function of most patients with delayed graft function due to ATN begins to improve. Some patients remain oliguric for several weeks, and constant surveillance for covert rejection and urologic complications is required (see the section on patients with delayed graft function). Patients who still require dialysis can receive it on an outpatient basis.

Because many of the patients are at home during this period, close attention to the development of allograft pain, fever, weight gain, or decreased urine output is important. If any of these signs or symptoms occur, patients are instructed to contact the transplant team, whose representatives must be available on a 24-hour basis. Patients without complications generally should be seen as outpatients at least twice weekly for the first month and weekly for the following month. During each outpatient visit, a routine physical examination is required to assess the urine volume status; adjust blood pressure medications; and examine the allograft to detect enlargement, tenderness, or the presence of a new bruit. Routine laboratory work should include a urinalysis, complete blood count, plasma creatinine and blood urea nitrogen levels, and an electrolyte panel that includes phosphate and calcium levels. Hepatic enzyme levels should be checked regularly.

At each clinic visit, the medications should be carefully reviewed with the patient, and changes, particularly of critical immunosuppressive medications, should be explained with great care. At this stage, the patient is often taking a multitude of medications: immunosuppressives, antihypertensives, and infection prophylactic agents. Every attempt should be made to simplify the therapeutic regimen and re-emphasize the importance of adherence. Meticulous attention to detail is crucial in this post-transplant period, and early intervention is necessary to minimize morbidity and mortality.

Well patients should gradually return to normal activity; some patients will wish to return to work after 4–6 weeks. A 3-month leave of absence from work is legitimate. Regular, graduated aerobic exercise should be encouraged, and normal social and family life should resume.

Differentiation of Infection, Rejection, and Cyclosporine Toxicity

The accurate recognition and treatment of infection, rejection, and cyclosporine toxicity and their differentiation from surgical post-transplant complications are constant concerns in the early post-transplant period. The treatment of common post-transplant infections is discussed in Chap. 10 and the treatment of rejection in Chap. 4.

Fever

Fever may indicate either rejection or infection. Infection during the first month is rarely due to opportunistic organisms and usually results from bacterial pathogens in the wound, urinary tract, or respiratory tract. CMV infection may mimic acute rejection. It occurs in approximately 20–30% of patients 1–6 months post-transplantation (see Chap. 10), and its possible presence needs to be constantly considered, particularly in recipients of kidneys from CMV-positive donors.

Post-transplant fever must always be taken seriously. Acute rejection will often be present with seemingly innocuous flu-like symptoms or upper respiratory tract infection. The fever and the symptoms consistently and rapidly resolve when the rejecting patient receives pulse steroids (see Chap. 4). Rejection is often not associated with fever, particularly in patients receiving cyclosporine. Febrile patients should have a chest x-ray and be fully cultured. They usually require readmission to the hospital or very close outpatient follow-up.

Elevated Creatinine Level

Measurement of the serum creatinine level is a simple, inexpensive diagnostic test that lies at the core of early post-transplant management. Its significance is not lost on patients, who often wait in trepidation at each clinic visit for their creatinine "verdict." Large elevations in plasma creatinine concentration (i.e., greater than 25% from baseline) almost always indicate a significant, potentially graft-endangering event. Smaller elevations may represent laboratory variability; recognition of their significance is sometimes more of an art form than a science! If there is any question regarding a small asymptomatic rise in the plasma creatinine concentration, the test should be repeated within 48 hours; the directional change will usually facilitate its clinical evaluation.

Anatomic or surgical problems must be ruled out before "medical" diagnoses are made to explain deteriorating graft function. Doppler ultrasound is invaluable (see Chap. 11); it should be performed before any major therapeutic intervention. Scintiscans are nonspecific in the settings of ATN, rejection, and drug toxicity and are of limited diagnostic value at this stage.

The gold standard diagnostic tool is either the kidney biopsy or fine-needle aspiration biopsy (see Chap. 12). The timing and frequency of kidney biopsies vary between centers. One clinical approach to graft dysfunction is to make a therapeutic intervention empirically based on the clinical presentation and laboratory values. A favorable response confirms the diagnosis, but a lack of a response will likely require a tissue diagnosis. Some programs insist on a tissue diagnosis of rejection before embarking on a course of OKT3 or polyclonal antibodies. This policy is wise because occasionally CMV infection may present as fever and graft dysfunction, in which case potent immunosuppressive therapy could be catastrophic.

Another, more aggressive approach to graft dysfunction is to perform a kidney biopsy whenever the serum creatinine rises 25% above the baseline value. Therapy is then based on the histologic findings. This approach should be considered in patients deemed to be at particular immunologic risk because of high levels of panel reactive antibodies, retransplant, or kidney diseases associated with early recurrence. The core biopsy is, however, an invasive procedure that is limited by the frequency with which it can be used. The aspiration biopsy overcomes these limitations. Aspiration biopsy can be repeatedly used with little or no risk to the allograft. It can be done in the outpatient clinic, and results obtained within hours. It does require an experienced cytologist for a reliable interpretation, and it has significant diagnostic limitations. In each transplant center, a protocol should be developed that logically incorporates both noninvasive and invasive techniques to evaluate allograft dysfunction during this time period.

Cyclosporine Levels

Despite nearly a decade of experience with cyclosporine, there remains a lack of uniformity regarding the use of trough blood levels in routine patient management. Guidelines are provided in Chap. 4. It is clear that high blood levels of cyclosporine do not preclude a diagnosis of rejection and that nephrotoxicity may occur at apparently low levels. Nephrotoxicity and rejection may coexist. With these provisos, however, it is fair to initially presume that a patient with deteriorating graft function and a very high cyclosporine level is probably suffering from nephrotoxicity and that a patient with deteriorating graft function and very low levels is probably undergoing acute rejection. If the appropriate clinical therapeutic response does not have a salutary effect on graft function, the clinical premise needs to be reconsidered. Cyclosporine toxicity usually resolves within 24–48 hours of a dose reduction. Progressive elevation of the plasma creatinine level even in the face of persistently high cyclosporine levels is highly suggestive of rejection.

Acute rejection may present as dramatic deterioration of graft function, whereas it is unusual for cyclosporine toxicity to produce a greater than 50% elevation of the plasma creatinine level. The degree of renal impairment associated with HUS is variable, as are the levels of cyclosporine (see the section on patients with delayed graft function).

Experience with tacrolimus use in the early post-transplant period is limited. The same principles used to differentiate between cyclosporine nephrotoxicity and rejection would seem to apply to the differentiation of tacrolimus nephrotoxicity and rejection.

Graft Tenderness

Graft tenderness on palpation in the first few days post-transplant is usually an innocuous finding related to recent surgery. In a stable patient, it is important to regularly palpate the graft to determine a clinical baseline for future changes. The development of graft tenderness in a previously pain-free, stable patient is a significant symptom that needs to be evaluated. A tender, swollen graft in a patient with a rising creatinine concentration and fever usually indicates rejection, although the possibility of acute pyelonephritis must be considered. Cyclosporine and tacrolimus toxicity and CMV infection do not produce graft tenderness. Excruciating localized perinephric pain is usually due to a urine leak.

Fluid Retention and Oliguria

Both rejection and cyclosporine toxicity may produce weight gain and edema due to impaired glomerular filtration rate and avid tubular sodium reabsorption. Mild peripheral edema is common in stable patients receiving cyclosporine and usually responds to oral furosemide. Both acute rejection and cyclosporine or tacrolimus toxicity can produce graft dysfunction in the absence of oliguria. Oliguria is common in acute rejection but makes a diagnosis of drug toxicity unlikely.

Common Laboratory Abnormalities in the Early Post-Transplant Period

Urinalysis

Examination of the urine for the presence of red and white blood cells, bacteria, and protein should be part of the routine outpatient visit. Pyuria can indicate either rejection or infection, and the urine should be cultured. The presence of proteinuria may herald the early recurrence of the primary kidney disease or chronic rejection. In the case of patients at risk for recurrent focal sclerosis, the finding of proteinuria is an indication for graft biopsy, since plasmapheresis may be indicated (see Chap. 9). Trace or "one plus" proteinuria amounting to less than 500 mg daily is usually not a morbid finding. Transient microscopic hematuria is common posttransplant but requires urologic evaluation if it is persistent.

Hyperkalemia

Elevated serum potassium levels are not uncommon in the first few post-transplant months in patients receiving cyclosporine or tacrolimus. The mechanism of the hyperkalemia is discussed in Chap. 4. As long as the patient is not oliguric and kidney function is good, this hyperkalemia is rarely dangerous and can usually be managed safely with dietary potassium restriction and diuretics. Care should be taken to avoid concomitant use of drugs that may further exaggerate hyperkalemia, such as ACE inhibitors, beta blockers, and oral phosphate supplements.

Hypophosphatemia, Hypercalcemia, and Hypomagnesemia

The mechanisms of post-transplant hyperphosphatemia and abnormalities of divalent ion metabolism are discussed in Chap. 9. Profound hypophosphatemia may develop in the first few weeks post-transplant, particularly in patients with excellent graft function. Phosphate supplements in a dose of 250–500 mg tid should be given if the serum phosphate levels fall below 2 mg/dl (see Chap. 17). Phosphate supplementation is usually adequate to control mild post-transplant hypercalcemia. Magnesium supplements should probably be given for cyclosporine or tacrolimus-induced hypomagnesemia if the serum magnesium level falls below 1.5 mg/dl, although they are often ineffective.

Hyperchloremic Metabolic Acidosis

Proximal, distal, and type IV renal tubular acidosis have been described to occur post-transplant, and mild hyperchloremia and hypobicarbonatemia are common. Renal tubular acidosis may be a manifestation of immune-mediated impairment of hydrogen ion secretion, of acute or chronic interstitial renal disease impairing tubular ammonia secretion, of parathyroid hormone-induced reduction in proximal tubular bicarbonate reabsorption, or of cyclosporine-induced impairment in tubular aldosterone responsiveness. The ensuing metabolic acidosis is usually not severe enough that it requires therapeutic intervention, and the finding is too non-specific to be of much diagnostic value.

Anemia

Profound anemia at the time of transplantation is much less common in the present erythropoietin era. Erythropoietin is usually discontinued at the time of transplantation, and the hematocrit level may fall post-transplant and then rise toward normal over weeks and months. Post-transplant polycythemia is discussed in Chap. 9. Resistant anemia needs to be evaluated, with the possibility of GI bleeding high on the differential diagnosis. Patients receiving azathioprine often develop macrocytosis (see Chap. 4).

SELECTED READINGS

Carmellini M, Romagnoli PC, Giulianotti A et al. Dopamine lowers the incidence of delayed graft function in transplanted kidney patients treated with cyclosporine A. *Transplant Proc* 26:2626, 1994.

Danovitch GM, Nast CC, Wilkinson A et al. Evaluation of fine needle aspiration biopsy in the diagnosis of renal transplant dysfunction. *Am J Kidney Dis* 17: 206, 1991.

Halloran PF, Wadgymar A, Ritchie S et al. The significance of the anti-class 1–mediated response: Clinical and pathological features of anti-class 1–mediated rejection. *Transplantation* 49:85, 1990.

Howard RJ, Pfaff WW, Brunson ME et al. Increased incidence of rejection in patients with delayed graft function. *Clin Transplantation* 8:527, 1994.

Katznelson S, Wilkinson AW, Rosenthal TR et al. Cyclosporine-induced hemolytic-uremic syndrome: Factors that obscure its diagnosis. *Transplant Proc* 26:2608, 1994.

Olsen S, Burdick JF, Keown PA et al. Primary acute renal failure ("acute tubular necrosis") in the transplanted kidney: Morphology and pathogenesis. *Medicine* 68:173, 1989.

Shoskes D, Hodge E, Goormontie M et al. Six-antigen matched kidneys may be less susceptible to the harmful effects of delayed graft function. *Transplant Proc* 27:1068, 1995.

Toogood GJ, Roake JA, Morris PJ. The relationship between fever and acute rejection or infection following renal transplantation in the cyclosporine era. *Clin Transplantation* 8:373, 1994.

Troppman C, Gillingham KJ, Benedetti E et al. Delayed graft function, acute rejection and outcome after cadaver renal transplantation. *Transplantation* 59:962, 1996.

9

Long-Term Post-Transplant Management and Complications

Mary M. Meyer, Douglas J. Norman, and Gabriel M. Danovitch

Among both physicians and patients, there has been an understandable yet perhaps naive tendency to emphasize the early results and impact of kidney transplantation. Success has typically been measured in terms of 1- and 2-year graft and patient survival. While such short-term success is obviously important, it is clearly not the ultimate purpose of the transplantation enterprise. Success is better measured in terms of long-term graft function; freedom from morbidity; and personal, social, and vocational rehabilitation.

Kidney transplants do not last forever; although they have the capacity to function for decades, their life is often foreshortened. Whereas 1-year graft survival rates have improved by as much as 30% since the introduction of cyclosporine in the early 1980s, this dramatic change has had little or no impact on the subsequent annual rate of graft loss. The mean half-life of a cadaveric transplant is currently approximately 8 years. When patient populations are matched, the mortality rate after cadaveric transplantation for nondiabetic patients is not markedly different from that after the commencement of chronic hemodialysis. The sense of well-being and potential for rehabilitation that frequently accompanies a functional transplant may be clouded by long-term complications, although many patients will enjoy years of post-transplant life without these complications having a significant impact on the quality of their lives. As more and more patients choose the transplantation option for end-stage renal disease and as improved immunosuppression provides better early transplant results, an enlarging population of transplant recipients has become susceptible to long-term complications.

This chapter considers the impact of time on kidney transplants and their recipients. Part I considers the causes of graft loss after the first few post-transplant months. Part II considers long-term post-transplant organ system function and dysfunction and the rehabilitative potential of successful transplants. The statistical aspects of graft and patient longevity are described in Chaps. 1 and 3.

Part I: Late Causes of Graft Loss

Table 9-1 lists the causes of graft loss after the first post-transplant year. The wide range in reported etiologic frequency reflects different patient populations and diagnostic overlap. Chronic rejection, death, and noncompliance are the most common causes in the majority of reported series.

Table 9-1. Causes of renal allograft loss after 1 year

Cause	Percentage of patients (%)
Chronic rejection[a]	24–67
Patient death[b]	22–48
Noncompliance	4–28
Recurrent disease	2–9
Other[c]	2–13

[a]Percentage of graft loss ascribed to chronic rejection is highest when patient death is excluded from analysis.
[b]Death usually due to infection or a cardiovascular event.
[c]Other includes renal artery stenosis, technical failures, obstruction.
Source: Modified from MJ Bia. Nonimmunologic causes of late renal graft loss. *Kidney Int* 47:1470, 1995.

CHRONIC REJECTION (CHRONIC ALLOGRAFT NEPHROPATHY)

Chronic rejection is a widely used term that is being replaced by the less specific but more accurate term **chronic allograft nephropathy.** This change in nomenclature is not just semantic; it reflects the growing appreciation of the fact that many of the factors leading to late graft failure are not solely immune in nature but are similar to the factors that cause inexorable loss of function in diseased native kidneys. The causes of chronic allograft nephropathy can be divided into immunologic, or **alloantigen-dependent**, causes and nonimmunologic, or **alloantigen-independent**, causes (Table 9-2). Figure 9-1 illustrates how these factors may interact to produce the pathologic changes of chronic allograft nephropathy (see Chap. 12).

Alloantigen-Dependent Factors

Acute Rejection Episodes

Numerous studies have shown that the most significant predictive factor for the development of chronic allograft nephropathy is the incidence of acute rejection episodes within the first post-transplant year. In some studies, even a single, early (<2 months) episode has a predictive impact, although multiple episodes and late episodes are more powerful predictors. It has been estimated that the half-life of allografts with no rejection episodes is 13 years, compared with 6 years for allografts with more than one episode.

Histologic follow-up of apparently successfully treated acute rejection episodes frequently reveals persistent evidence of inflammation. Common features of all organ allografts undergoing so-called chronic rejection are persistent perivascular inflammation and arteriosclerosis that affects intramural arteries; acute and chronic changes are often admixed. It may well be that low-grade repetitive epithelial damage induces secretion of fibrogenic cytokines, adhesion molecules, and inflammatory mediators that are responsible for smooth-muscle cell replication and eventually lead to obliterative vasculopathy, fibrosis, and glomerulosclerosis. Intragraft expression of transforming growth factor-beta mRNA has been found to be correlated to the degree of renal allograft interstitial fibrosis (Fig. 9-2).

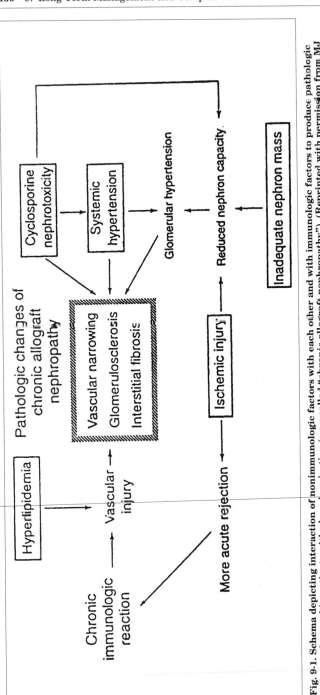

Fig. 9-1. Schema depicting interaction of nonimmunologic factors with each other and with immunologic factors to produce pathologic changes observed in patients with chronic rejection (now called "chronic allograft nephropathy"). (Reprinted with permission from MJ Bia. Nonimmunologic causes of late renal graft loss. *Kidney Int* 47:1470, 1995. Reprinted by permission of Blackwell Science, Inc.)

Table 9-2. Causes of chronic allograft nephropathy

Alloantigen-dependent	Alloantigen-independent
Acute rejection	Delayed graft function
Poor HLA match	Nephron "dose"
Prior sensitization	Hypertension
Suboptimal immunosuppression	Hyperlipidemia
Noncompliance	Late cytomegalovirus infection
	Cyclosporine toxicity

HLA = human leukocyte antigen.

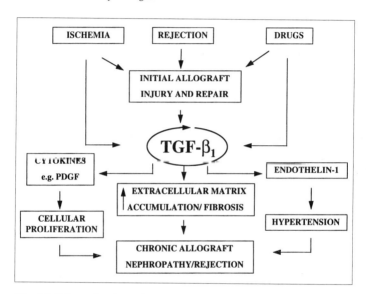

Fig. 9-2. Schema for the pathogenesis of chronic allograft nephropathy/rejection. In this fibrogenic cytokine hypothesis, intrarenal expression of transforming growth factor-beta$_1$ (TGF-β_1) represents a significant pathogenetic molecular event for the expression of chronic allograft nephropathy/rejection. The ability of TGF-β_1 to promote its production (positive feedback loop), and its additional properties (e.g., regulation of platelet-derived growth factor [PDGF] activity, stimulation of endothelin-1 production) are also incorporated into this framework. That two of the most commonly used drugs in transplantation, cyclosporine and steroids, stimulate TGF-β_1 expression is also considered in this formulation regarding the cascade of events involved in chronic allograft nephropathy/rejection. (From Sharma VK, Bologa RM, Xu GP et al. Intragraft TGF-β, mRNA: A correlate of interstitial fibrosis and chronic allograft nephropathy. *Kidney Int* 49:1297, 1996. Reprinted by permission of Blackwell Science, Inc.)

Histocompatibility

For many years, the improved long-term prognosis of living-related donor transplants compared with cadaveric donor transplants was presumed to be due to better histocompatibility matching. Although matching is, no doubt, important, the excellent short- and long-term results of spousal and living-unrelated transplants (see Chap. 3) suggest that the condition of the kidney at the time of the transplant operation is a critical, alloantigen-independent factor. The importance of matching is particularly evident for cadaveric transplants; zero-mismatched cadaveric transplants have a 5-year survival and half-life approaching 80% and 13 years, respectively, compared with approximately 50% and 8 years for completely mismatched transplants.

Suboptimal Immunosuppression

The importance of alloantigen-dependent factors is clearly illustrated by the ongoing necessity to maintain adequate immunosuppression for the life span of the graft. Noncompliance is a potent cause of late graft loss, and although occasional long-term stable patients may "get away" with discontinuation of all immunosuppression, such a policy is fraught with danger and should be discouraged unless there is a specific overriding indication (see the section on post-transplant malignancy). Acute rejection episodes have been described after 20 years of graft function. Despite the potential for cyclosporine nephrotoxicity, available evidence suggests that patients with somewhat higher cyclosporine doses and blood levels may do better in the long-term than patients with lower doses and levels (see Chap. 4). Similarly, steroid withdrawal may also have an unfavorable long-term impact.

Alloantigen-Independent Factors

Nephron Dose and Hyperfiltration

The concept of nephron "dose" is discussed in Chaps. 3 and 5. In essence, it states that circumstances associated with an unfavorable ratio between the supply of functioning nephrons transplanted and the demands of the recipient make the allograft more susceptible to chronic loss of function. The supply of functioning nephrons may be an absolute feature of the allograft (young or old age, female sex, black race, all of which are associated with a reduced nephron supply) or a feature of perioperative events such as prolonged ischemia times and acute tubular necrosis.

The relevance of the nephron dose hypothesis to human renal transplantation remains controversial. In a rat model of chronic rejection, the transplanted kidney appeared to be protected from progressive damage by the presence of a retained, functioning recipient native kidney. This finding supports the hypothesis that hyperfiltration in the remaining nephrons makes them susceptible to chronic damage in a manner similar to that proposed to explain the inexorable loss of function of the diseased nephrons of patients with chronic renal failure. Perioperative damage to the allograft may contribute to nonspecific tissue injury, cytokine release, upregulation of cell-surface markers and adhesion molecules, and chemoattraction of neutrophils with further cycles of injury and repair.

Other Factors

Systemic hypertension may exaggerate and perpetuate the vascular injury associated with allograft nephropathy, which has pathologic features in common with hypertensive nephrosclerosis. **Hyperlipidemia** has been associated with allograft nephropathy.

In animal models, the vascular lesions can be exacerbated by high lipid intake. Evidence of **cyclosporine toxicity** may also be found in chronically rejecting grafts. Late **cytomegalovirus (CMV) infection** has also been implicated.

Clinical Features

The hallmark of chronic rejection is an occlusive vascular change associated with typical interstitial and glomerular lesions. Chronic transplant glomerulopathy and de novo membranous glomeru-lonephritis are also manifestations of chronic rejection. The patho-logic features and differentiation of chronic rejection from the lesions of chronic cyclosporine toxicity and hypertension are described in Chap. 12. The severity of the histologic features of chronic rejection correlate with the duration of subsequent allograft survival.

Chronic rejection typically occurs in patients who have suffered episodes of acute rejection, particularly when these episodes are mul-tiple or late, or where recovery of graft function, as judged by the return of the serum creatinine level to baseline, is incomplete. It pre-sents clinically as deterioration of graft function, typically with pro-teinuria of varying degrees and hypertension. It rarely occurs within the first 6 months of transplantation. The time course to allograft failure is extremely variable, ranging from months to years. In most cases, the loss of graft function is inexorable, although spontaneous reduction and arrest of the rate of decline may occur. Proteinuria is usually moderate (1–3 g daily), but nephrotic-range proteinuria may occur. Chronic rejection is the most common cause of transplant nephrotic syndrome.

Renal function in chronic rejection is typically monitored by fol-lowing the rise of the serum creatinine level. The creatinine clear-ance, however, may overestimate the true glomerular filtration rate (GFR) in the presence of chronic renal failure and proteinuria. As a result, the early stages of graft dysfunction may be associated with apparently minor rises in the creatinine level, whereas small changes in the GFR produce big changes in creatinine levels as the graft approaches end-stage failure.

Differential Diagnosis

Chronic rejection needs to be differentiated from other causes of late graft dysfunction. The absence of a history of rejection, hyperten-sion, and proteinuria should arouse diagnostic skepticism. A renal ultrasound should be performed at least once to rule out obstructive causes of graft dysfunction, and the possibility of renal artery steno-sis should be considered, particularly if hypertension is severe or the hematocrit is high (see the section on hypertension below and Chap. 7). Kidney biopsy will provide a definitive diagnosis and may allow an estimate of the severity of the lesion and show the presence of coex-isting acute rejection or de novo or recurrent glomerular lesions.

Treatment

There is currently no specific treatment for chronic allograft nephropathy; the therapeutic questions and options are similar to those faced in the management of chronic renal failure in native kid-neys. A faster progression has been reported for patients with a diastolic blood pressure of greater than 90 mm Hg, so good control of blood pressure is mandatory. There may be some theoretical benefit to using angiotension-converting enzyme (ACE) inhibitors, low-protein diets, and hypolipidemic agents. ACE inhibitors should be used with care because of their potential to cause anemia, hyperkalemia, and renal dysfunction. A proposed benefit for dietary fish oil supplements could not be upheld in controlled trials.

The optimal management of immunosuppression for the chronic failing allograft has yet to be defined (see Chap. 4). If there is suspicion of an element of acute rejection, a steroid pulse should be given, but this therapy should not be repeated if it is ineffective. Monoclonal and polyclonal antibodies should not be given in the presence of chronic rejection. Intensified cyclosporine administration will often merely exaggerate nephrotoxicity. It is yet to be seen if mycophenolate mofetil will reverse or stabilize the vascular lesions of established chronic rejection, although there are theoretical reasons to hope that it might do so. This agent may serve to prevent chronic rejection by reducing the frequency of early acute rejection episodes. There are formidable obstacles to the design of clinical trials to test therapeutic interventions for chronic rejection.

End-Stage Transplant Failure

As chronic rejection inexorably progresses, there comes a time when future options must be considered in a manner similar to non–rejection-related causes of chronic renal disease. The indications for access placement and commencement of dialysis do not differ in patients with rejecting grafts. Some patients will elect to go back on a cadaveric transplant list or be fortunate enough to have a live-related transplant before recommencing dialysis. At this stage, immunosuppression should be minimized, although it should not be stopped altogether until dialysis access is available. Management of the rejecting graft in a dialysis patient is discussed in Chap. 7.

LATE ACUTE REJECTION AND NONCOMPLIANCE

Whereas episodes of acute rejection are a common and anticipated accompaniment of the first few post-transplant months, late episodes of rejection are relatively unusual. It has been estimated that acute rejection accounts for up to 10% of late graft loss, although clinically unrecognized acute rejection is probably considerably more common. The development of an acute rejection episode in a previously stable patient must arouse suspicion of noncompliance or inadequacy of the immunosuppressive regimen. In some series, varying degrees of noncompliance have been documented in up to 30% of graft losses; in adolescent patients, noncompliance is the most common cause of late graft loss. The varied demographic, behavioral, and situational factors associated with noncompliance and their recognition and management of noncompliance are discussed in Chaps. 14 and 15.

RECURRENT DISEASE

The true incidence of recurrence of the original kidney disease in the allograft is unknown. Patients often present with end-stage renal disease of uncertain etiology and may be labeled with "chronic glomerulonephritis" without biopsy documentation, making a diagnosis of recurrent disease difficult to prove. When allograft function deteriorates slowly over time, the diagnosis of chronic rejection is

Table 9-3. Recurrence rates of glomerulonephritides

Type	Reported frequency of recurrence (%)	Reported graft loss rate from recurrence (%)
Focal segmental glomerulosclerosis	23–43	11–50
Membranoproliferative type I	20–30	33
Membranoproliferative type II	88–100	50
Membranous[a,b]	10	Rare
IgA nephropathy[a]	38–50	1
Henoch-Schönlein[a] purpura	75–88	20–40
Anti-GBM nephritis	12	Rare
Hemolytic-uremic syndrome	13–25	40–50
Lupus nephritis	<1	None

GBM = glomerular basement membrane.
[a]Histologic recurrence may be more frequent in recipients of live-related transplants.
[b]Membranous nephropathy may also occur de novo after transplantation with reported incidence of 4–9% and a relatively benign course (see Chap. 12).

often assumed, no biopsy is obtained, and possible recurrent disease is missed. Recurrence of the original disease does not always portend immediate or ultimate graft failure and may be silent, only to be serendipitously discovered when a biopsy is performed. Recurrent disease has been estimated to be responsible for approximately 2% of graft losses. Individual disorders are discussed in greater depth in Chaps. 6 and 13.

Genetic and Metabolic Diseases

A variety of genetic and metabolic diseases may have an impact on long-term transplant function. Pathologic changes of **diabetic nephropathy** with impairment of graft function may develop in diabetic recipients of a kidney transplant; a simultaneous pancreas transplant may be protective. Graft loss from recurrent diabetic nephropathy is rare. Patients with **Alport's syndrome** may occasionally develop an acute anti-glomerular basement membrane–mediated glomerulonephritis. Patients with **Fabry's disease** may succumb to the vascular complications of the disease, which are not ameliorated by transplantation. Patients with **oxalosis** may lose their grafts to massive hyperoxaluria and may benefit from combined kidney and liver transplantation. Patients with **sickle cell anemia** may suffer severe sickle cell crises posttransplant and have a high incidence of early graft loss and death. Patients with **amyloidosis** tend to tolerate immunosuppression poorly. Amyloidosis may recur in the graft, but in patients with familial Mediterranean fever, this may be prevented by the continued use of colchicine.

Glomerulonephritis

Recurrent glomerulonephritis has been reported to occur in up to 10% of transplant patients but causes graft failure much less frequently. The incidence of recurrence and the propensity for causing allograft dysfunction varies with disease category (Table 9-3). Onset of recurrent disease is usually heralded by the development of proteinuria and microscopic hematuria and may be clinically difficult to separate from chronic rejection. The approach to potential transplant recipients with glomerulonephritis is discussed in Chap. 6.

Focal segmental glomerulosclerosis (FSGS) may recur in a florid fashion in the early postoperative period possibly because of a circulating plasma factor that increases glomerular permeability. Management is discussed in Chap. 14. Recurrence of other forms of primary glomerulonephritis is usually subclinical. It is well-documented as occurring in types I and II **membranoproliferative** and **membranous glomerulonephritis**, and it may occasionally produce graft failure. Clinically significant recurrence of **IgA nephropathy** is very rare given the frequency of this lesion in the dialysis population. The glomerulonephritis of the collagen vascular diseases and the vasculitides occasionally recur in the transplant; patients may benefit from the inclusion of cyclophosphamide in their immunosuppressive regimen. Recurrence of **lupus nephritis** has been reported but is rare. For reasons that are not well understood, patients with lupus who receive cadaveric transplants tend to have a worse long-term prognosis for graft function than patients without lupus (see Chap. 6).

DEATH

Graft loss because of the death of the recipient has been reported in a varying percentage of transplant recipients. This percentage will clearly vary depending on the age of the recipients and their medical condition at the time of transplantation. The incidence of myocardial infarction and cerebrovascular accidents may be 25-fold that of the nontransplant population, and atherosclerotic deaths account for up to 55% of all late transplant deaths in some series. Infectious deaths and death due to malignancy account for approximately 30–40% of late deaths and may be a reflection of excessive long-term immunosuppression. Chronic liver disease is becoming increasingly recognized as a cause of death in transplant patients. Each of these individual morbid conditions is discussed in the section on organ system dysfunction below. The incidence of suicide has been reported to be as high as 1%, which is 50-fold greater than age-matched controls.

Part II: Organ System Function and Dysfunction

HYPERTENSION

Hypertension is the most common post-transplantation complication excluding allograft rejection and is an important risk factor for the development of atherosclerotic cardiovascular disease. The prevalence is reported to be as high as 80% in the early period after transplantation, although it may drop during long-term follow-up. Much can be learned about the etiology of post-transplant hypertension by observing its prevalence in different transplant populations. Recipients of live-related transplants who have undergone bilateral native nephrectomy, who are not receiving cyclosporine, and who have excellent graft function have a prevalence of hypertension that is not different from the general population. Patients on cyclosporine who have their native kidneys in situ and who suffer from chronic allograft nephropathy are almost uniformly hypertensive. Hypertension may be the cause or the result of declining allograft function; its severity in black patients may partially explain the differences in long-term allograft survival between black and white patients.

Native Kidney–Mediated Hypertension

Hypertension is less prevalent among transplant patients who are anephric. Removal of native kidneys even several years after transplantation can return elevated blood pressures to normal. The native kidneys continue to produce renin, which causes increased intrarenal vascular resistance, reduced renal plasma flow, and systemic hypertension. Several reports have indicated that excision of native kidneys is followed by a consistent fall in blood pressure and reduction in the vascular resistance of the allograft. Although increased concentrations of renin have been measured in the renal veins of native kidneys as compared with transplanted kidneys, the renal vein renin levels of native kidneys do not appear to be a reliable indicator of the need for bilateral native nephrectomy for the treatment of recalcitrant hypertension. Before consideration is given to post-transplant native nephrectomy, other, potentially reversible, causes of hypertension need to be ruled out. Ablation of native kidneys by radiologic embolization may be an effective alternative to surgical nephrectomy, but no large series has been reported to adequately evaluate the effectiveness of this technique.

Donor Kidney–Mediated Hypertension

There is some provocative evidence that suggests that hypertension can be induced by the donor kidney itself. Cross-transplantation studies in normotensive and spontaneously hypertensive strains of rats have shown that hypertension can be cured or induced by the donor kidney. Human studies in patients with essential hypertension leading to nephrosclerosis and end-stage renal disease have shown cure of hypertension and reversal of hypertensive damage to the heart and retinal vessels after transplantation of kidneys from normotensive donors. Hypertension in the parents of cadaveric kidney donors may correlate with elevated blood pressure in the recipient, and receipt of a kidney from a donor who died of subarachnoid hemorrhage (and is thus more likely to have been hypertensive) may predispose the recipient to hypertension.

Rejection

Elevated blood pressure often accompanies acute rejection. Hypertension is especially prevalent with hyperacute and acute vascular rejection. Chronic allograft nephropathy is associated with progressive ischemia and fibrosis with secondary renin production and is the leading cause of post-transplant hypertension. Hypertension related to rejection may respond to ACE inhibition, which suggests a renin-dependent mechanism.

Renal Artery Stenosis

The prevalence of renal artery stenosis in the transplant population is difficult to assess. Functionally significant stenoses, which may require renal artery narrowing of more than 70–80%, have been observed to occur in up to 12% of patients. Stenoses may occur in the recipient artery, at the suture line, and in the donor artery. Stenoses can occur up to 2 years after transplantation but occur most commonly within the first 6 months. Stenoses along the course of the recipient artery may be due to endothelial injury induced by rejection and trauma at the time of harvesting. The surgical issues relating to renal artery stenosis are discussed in Chap. 7.

Renal artery stenosis should be suspected when persistent hypertension is difficult to control medically. It may be accompanied by the onset of diuretic-resistant edema in the absence of heavy proteinuria. Graft function is usually impaired and may vary with volume status or without obvious explanation. In the setting of a functionally solitary kidney with renal artery stenoses, ACE inhibition may result in loss of renal autoregulation of the hypoperfused kidney and an abrupt decline in GFR, particularly if there is concomitant volume contraction. The sensitivity and specificity of using ACE inhibition as a provocative test for renal artery stenosis has not yet been determined. Polycythemia in the presence of impaired graft function and hypertension suggests renal artery stenosis. The presence of a soft systolic bruit is not specific, although loud bruits, new bruits, and bruits with a diastolic component warrant suspicion.

The diagnostic reliability of Doppler studies of the renal artery for the diagnosis of renal artery stenosis is controversial. Colorflow Doppler in experienced hands may be an adequate screening test. Some clinicians, however, are distrustful of ultrasound testing in this situation and seek a definitive diagnosis with renal angiography or digital subtraction angiography in suspicious cases. Radionuclide scanning is not useful for diagnosis of renal artery stenosis in the transplant kidney, since there is not a paired kidney for comparison (see Chap. 11).

Percutaneous transluminal angioplasty of the stenotic artery is the therapeutic procedure of choice (see Chaps. 7 and 11). The initial success rate, as judged by reduction of blood pressure and the need for antihypertensive medications, has been reported to be 60–85%, although up to 30% of cases may restenose. The possibility of restenosis should be kept in mind in the follow-up of patients who have undergone angioplasty. Surgical repair of stenotic lesions is difficult, and graft loss is not uncommon (see Chap. 7).

Corticosteroids and Cyclosporine

Although "pulses" and high doses of corticosteroids may be associated with hypertension (and should not be given in the presence of uncontrolled hypertension), the low maintenance doses of prednisone given to transplant patients probably do not produce or exaggerate hypertension. There is good evidence, however, that cyclosporine is a significant contributor to post-transplant hypertension. Cyclosporine produces hypertension when administered in both transplantation and nontransplantation situations and in the presence and absence of kidney dysfunction.

Cyclosporine hypertension is produced by vasoconstriction and increased sympathetic nerve activity (see Chap. 4). Patients who have been switched from cyclosporine to azathioprine have been documented to have improved renal blood flow, decreased blood pressure, and decreased vascular resistance. In addition, cyclosporine causes sodium retention, volume expansion, and renin suppression. No significant correlation has been shown between any of these phenomena and cyclosporine dose and blood levels.

Management of Post-Transplant Hypertension

There is no clear-cut consensus regarding the therapy of post-transplant hypertension. Many patients will require two or more antihypertensive agents. In patients who are edematous, diuretics should be used with care to approach dry weight while observing graft function. Calcium channel blockers are usually well-tolerated and may serve to ameliorate cyclosporine-mediated vasoconstriction. Long-acting nifedipine, isradipine, and amlodipine are probably the most effective of these agents and do not elevate cyclosporine levels as do diltiazem and verapamil (see Chap. 4). Nifedipine may cause pedal edema and exaggerate gingival hyperplasia.

ACE inhibitors can be used and may be beneficial if there is an element of renin mediation from either the graft or native kidneys. Deteriorating graft function after therapy with ACE inhibitors must alert suspicion of renal artery stenosis but may occasionally occur even with a widely patent renal artery, particularly if patients are simultaneously volume-contracted. ACE inhibitors may increase the incidence of hyperkalemic episodes, particularly in diabetic patients, and may be a cause of post-transplant anemia.

ATHEROSCLEROSIS AND HEART DISEASE

Cardiovascular complications, including myocardial infarction, congestive heart failure, and cerebrovascular accidents, are the second leading cause of death in kidney transplant patients, exceeded only by death from infection. They are the most common cause of death after the first post-transplant year. Cardiovascular disease is very common in patients with end-stage renal disease (50% of deaths being due to cardiovascular causes for both peritoneal dialysis and hemodialysis patients), and the same risk factors present in uremia persist after transplantation: arterial hypertension, diabetes or glucose intolerance, secondary hyperparathyroidism, and hyperlipidemia. Multivariate analysis has shown that, after taking pretransplant and post-transplant vascular disease into account, age, sex, diabetes, cigarette smoking, hypertension, serum cholesterol, and the number of acute rejection episodes treated with high-dose steroids are independently linked to the risk of vascular disease after transplantation.

The risk of developing ischemic heart disease in transplant patients previously free of clinically recognized disease has been estimated to be three- to fourfold greater than for age-matched controls. Overall, the factors that represent the greatest relative risk for ischemic heart disease after transplantation are pretransplant heart disease and diabetes.

Hyperlipidemia

Patients with end-stage renal disease tend to develop hyperlipidemia with predominant hypertriglyceridemia. Following transplantation, this pattern changes; by 3 months post-transplant, approximately 50% of transplant recipients treated with cyclosporine are hypercholesterolemic. Kidney transplant patients generally exhibit hyperlipidemia of type IIa (pure hypercholesterolemia) or type IIb (combined hypercholesterolemia and hypertriglyceridemia) Hypertriglyceridemia may decline somewhat after transplantation, but hypercholesterolemia develops and persists. High-density lipoprotein (HDL) may not be protective because the HDL in transplant patients is abnormally enriched in triglyceride and cholesterol, and the HDL cholesterol-to-apoprotein A ratio is elevated. Levels of low-density lipoprotein (LDL) and very-low-density lipoprotein (VLDL) are also elevated in transplant patients.

Increasing age, diabetes mellitus, heavy proteinuria, renal dysfunction, excessive weight gain, use of beta blockers, and use of diuretics may all contribute to hyperlipidemia. A correlation has been observed between the level of both serum cholesterol and triglycerides and the cumulative corticosteroid dose. Steroids may contribute to peripheral insulin resistance by stimulating acetyl coenzyme A (CoA) carboxylase and free fatty acid synthetase, thereby enhancing lipogenesis.

Cyclosporine is associated with a Fredrickson's type IIa and IIb lipid profile and with elevated lipoprotein (a) levels, which are themselves independent risk factors for the development of coronary artery disease. Cyclosporine is lipophilic and binds to the LDL receptor and may alter feedback signals governing cholesterol synthesis. It also impairs bile acid synthesis by interfering with cholesterol conversion to bile acids and may predispose to glucose intolerance (see the section on carbohydrate intolerance).

Prevention of Atherosclerosis and Treatment of Hyperlipidemia

Diet and Weight Control

Prevention is better than cure; obese patients should be strongly counseled to lose weight before transplantation. The incidence of post-transplant atherosclerotic complications is related to the presence of pretransplant vascular disease. Risk factors should be addressed before transplant and should be constantly assessed during the post-transplant period. Undesirable weight gain is a serious and all-to-frequent post-transplant problem. Risk factors and dietary recommendations for carbohydrate and fat intake and techniques of weight reduction are important and are described in Chap. 17. Dietary compliance tends to wane with time, and diet alone is unlikely to adequately control multifactorial hyperlipidemia in transplant patients.

Corticosteroid Dose

Weight loss may be very difficult for transplant patients on steroids. Whenever possible, the steroid dose should be minimized and kept at 10 mg daily or less for long-term use. There are suggestive but not conclusive data for the beneficial impact of alternate-day steroids on the lipid profile and for the benefit of steroid discontinuation (see Chap. 4).

Treatment of Hypertension

Effective treatment of hypertension is a cornerstone in the prevention of cardiovascular disease and is discussed in the section on hypertension above.

Pharmacologic Therapy

The relationship between the reduction of lipid levels and reduced incidence of coronary artery disease that has been illustrated in the general population has yet to be proven to be applicable to the transplant population. Despite this lack of proof, it would appear wise to treat post-transplant hyperlipidemia aggressively using pharmacologic treatment when more conservative therapy fails.

Lovastatin, pravastatin, and simvastatin are hydroxymethylglutaryl (HMG)-CoA reductase inhibitors that have been shown to be effective in reducing both total and LDL cholesterol levels in kidney transplant patients. These drugs may have additional immune modulating benefits (see Chap. 4). At dosages of more than 40 mg daily, lovastatin given to patients receiving cyclosporine has been associated with rhabdomyolysis and acute renal failure. Daily doses of 20 mg or less have not been associated with rhabdomyolysis and can be used safely with supervision. This complication has not been observed with pravastatin and simvastatin. Hepatotoxicity can occur with these agents; they should be used with caution in patients receiving other potentially hepatotoxic drugs. Levels of serum creatine phosphokinase (CPK) and liver enzymes levels should be routinely followed.

There are inadequate data on the safety and effectiveness of other lipid-lowering agents. Bile-acid sequestrants such as cholestyramine and colestipol should not be used with cyclosporine or tacrolimus, which may be bound and eliminated in the stool. Nicotinic acid is poorly tolerated because of gastric upset and hepatotoxicity. The fibric acid derivatives gemfibrozil and clofibrate are generally well-tolerated but may cause myositis.

Exercise

Regular aerobic exercise has been recommended for the prevention and treatment of cardiovascular disease. Patients with end-stage renal disease are often physically deconditioned, and preliminary studies suggest that supervised exercise training after kidney transplantation is feasible and worthwhile. It has yet to be shown, however, that exercise or any of the techniques listed previously will prevent the development of vascular complications in long-term transplant recipients.

HEPATOBILIARY DISEASE

Chronic Liver Disease

Hepatic dysfunction is common after kidney transplantation, and chronic liver disease is one of the leading causes of late morbidity and mortality among recipients of long-surviving kidney allografts. In the majority of these cases, it is possible to detect either serologic or enzymatic evidence of liver disease pretransplant, and vaccination programs and careful pretransplant screening are now regarded as mandatory. Pretransplant liver biopsy is often advisable (see Chap. 6). The controversy regarding the use of cadaveric donors with evidence of prior hepatitis B and C infection is discussed in Chap. 5.

Hepatitis B

In the general population, up to 6% of HBsAg-positive carriers who develop chronic hepatitis progress to cirrhosis. In the transplant population, immunosuppressive therapy appears to potentiate hepatitis B viral replication and stimulate progression from benign to aggressive liver disease. The hepatitis B virus (HBV) appears to have a steroid-responsive enhancer sequence that may function to increase the transcription and replication of the virus in hepato-cytes. The frequency of progression of HBsAg-positive patients to chronic active hepatitis or cirrhosis varies from very low to 80% in some studies. Progression may be particularly aggressive in Asian patients. Serum transaminases may be poor predictors of disease activity on liver biopsy and may underestimate the prevalence of liver disease. The presence of HBeAg, HBV DNA, or HBV DNA poly-merase in the serum correlates with active viral replication and pro-gression of liver disease and is a better marker of disease activity. Progression of chronic hepatitis is often silent until end-stage dis-ease is approached. Serial liver biopsies may be required after trans-plantation to determine disease severity.

Management of progressive HBV disease is problematic. Immunosuppression, particularly with corticosteroids, should be minimized. Recombinant alpha-interferon has demonstrated effica-cy in the treatment of chronic HBV in immunocompetent hosts, but its immunomodulating effect may enhance graft rejection.

Hepatitis C

Since the introduction of the HBV vaccine, hepatitis C virus (HCV) has become the most common cause of acute hepatitis in the patients and staff of hemodialysis units. Seventy percent of cases of chronic liver disease in kidney transplant recipients have been attributed to HCV. After a follow-up of nearly 6 years, approximate-ly one-third of the patients with early HCV chronic hepatitis and nearly two-thirds with advanced chronic hepatitis have been report-ed to experience clinical deterioration with the development of cir-rhosis and, in some cases, have died due to liver disease. The disease typically progresses silently over many years, with mild constitu-tional symptoms and normal or fluctuating transaminase levels. HCV infection can manifest as de novo or recurrent membranopro-liferative glomerulonephritis in the transplant patient or rarely as mixed cryoglobulinemia.

Immunosuppression may have less of an impact on the progres-sion of HCV infection than on HBV infection; some studies suggest that the course of HCV infection does not differ between transplant recipients and chronic dialysis patients. Concomitant alcohol abuse and infection with a particularly pathogenic HCV strain can con-tribute to the severity of the disease process. Although alpha-inter-feron may transiently control disease activity, its side effect profile makes it unsuitable for routine use. Newer antiviral agents are being tested in clinical trials.

Cyclosporine Hepatotoxicity

Transient liver function abnormalities are commonly observed in transplant patients. Cyclosporine-induced hepatotoxicity is mani-fested by hyperbilirubinemia and mildly elevated serum transami-nase levels. Cyclosporine dose reduction usually results in a prompt decline in bilirubin and transaminase levels. Cyclosporine does not produce chronic liver disease, although occasional patients may experience recurrent or persistent liver function abnormalities and

Table 9-4. Beneficial effects of kidney transplantation on bone and mineral metabolism

1. Improvement or cure of bone pain and subperiosteal bone resorption
2. Reduction in serum alkaline phosphatase
3. Normalization of serum calcitriol
4. Reduction in serum phosphorus
5. Normalization or reduction of parathyroid hormone levels
6. Mobilization of soft-tissue calcium levels
7. Resolution of aluminum bone disease
8. Prevention of dialysis amyloid osteoarthropathy

are predisposed to develop biliary calculus disease. The etiology of the cyclosporine-induced hepatic dysfunction is unknown, but cyclosporine has been observed to reduce bile flow and bile acid secretion in rats.

Azathioprine Hepatotoxicity

A variety of hepatic lesions have been attributed to azathioprine, including veno-occlusive disease, peliosis hepatis, and cholestatic and hepatocellular liver injury. The reaction to azathioprine may be idiosyncratic or may require an associated condition, such as an underlying autoimmune disorder or viral hepatitis. In the presence of impaired liver function, azathioprine should be reduced or discontinued. The cyclosporine dose should be minimized and parent compound assays used for monitoring (see Chap. 4).

Pancreatitis and Cholecystitis

Acute pancreatitis is a rare but potentially lethal post-transplant complication with a reported mortality rate of more than 50% within the first 3 months post-transplant. Post-transplant hyperparathyroidism, hyperlipidemia, CMV infection, and the use of steroids and cyclosporine have been implicated in its induction.

Cholelithiasis and its complications are increased in frequency in patients receiving cyclosporine. The precise mechanism is unclear but may be related to the effect of cyclosporine on bile composition. Cholecystectomy is often recommended in the pretransplant period for patients with asymptomatic gallstones, particularly if they are diabetic (see Chap. 7).

BONE AND MINERAL METABOLISM

Kidney transplantation has both beneficial and detrimental effects on bone and mineral metabolism. In the majority of patients, the effects of transplantation on bone metabolism are salutary, with healing of osteodystrophy and aluminum bone disease and eventual resolution of hyperparathyroidism (Table 9-4). Post-transplant abnormalities of bone and mineral metabolism are discussed below.

Hypophosphatemia

Hypophosphatemia is the most common of the post-transplant divalent ion abnormalities. It is produced by a persistent phosphaturia that may be particularly marked in well-functioning grafts. The phosphaturia is multifactorial. Parathyroid hormone (PTH) levels may remain elevated for a year or more post-transplant, there may be a PTH-independent renal phosphate "leak," and corticosteroids may impair proximal tubule phosphate reabsorption.

Clinically significant hypophosphatemia with plasma phosphate levels of less than 2 mg/dl is most common in the early post-transplant period. If untreated, it can cause muscle weakness and osteomalacia. Dietary supplementation with phosphate in a dose of 250–500 mg tid is usually adequate, and phosphate levels should be kept above 2 mg/dl (see Chap. 17).

Calcium, Magnesium, and Aluminum

Approximately 10% of transplant recipients develop varying degrees of **hypercalcemia**. Hypercalcemia is due largely to persistent hyperparathyroidism (see below) and is less frequent now that hyperparathyroidism is better controlled in the dialysis population. Post-transplant elevations of serum albumin levels and resorption of extraskeletal calcification may also contribute to hypercalcemia.

Patients who have undergone pretransplant parathyroidectomy may develop severe post-transplant **hypocalcemia**. This has been ascribed to urinary calcium loss by the newly functioning kidney exaggerated by steroid-induced reduction in intestinal calcium reabsorption. The hypocalcemia may require intravenous calcium for its correction in addition to oral supplements and vitamin D.

Cyclosporine use is associated with **hypomagnesemia** secondary to a renal tubular magnesium leak (see Chap. 4). Hypomagnesemia may be associated with cyclosporine-induced hypertension and neurotoxicity. Magnesium supplements are usually prescribed when plasma magnesium levels fall below 1.5 mg/dl, although the effectiveness of these supplements has not been well-studied.

A well-functioning allograft excretes aluminum effectively and is the best treatment for aluminum bone disease. Successful transplantation is superior to deferoxamine therapy in lowering stainable bone aluminum and in improving bone histology.

Hyperparathyroidism

Post-transplantation hyperparathyroidism is the sequela of the secondary hyperparathyroidism of kidney failure with the induction of parathyroid gland hyperplasia. After transplantation, the glands appear to involute, and an increased number of cells become quiescent. The time course for involution is unknown but is generally believed to be quite slow due to the low rate of parathyroid cell turnover and lack of mechanism for cell deletion. The hyperfunctioning glands have been found to be responsive to changes in ionized calcium, but, for any given level of calcium, the PTH level is above normal. The elevated PTH level suggests that there is an increased parathyroid gland mass with an obligatory basal rate of cellular secretion of PTH. The well-functioning transplant tends to normalize vitamin D metabolism, and the combination of high levels of PTH and calcitriol leads to hypercalcemia and hypophosphatemia.

Severe post-transplant hypercalcemia is rare now that secondary hyperparathyroidism is better controlled in dialysis patients. Transient hypercalcemia with plasma levels ranging between 10.5 and 12.5 mg/dl usually resolves within a year post-transplant but will persist in some patients. Normocalcemic hyperparathyroidism with low levels of 1:25 vitamin D has also been described.

In most cases, the paucity of complications and the high rate of spontaneous resolution of hypercalcemia and hypophosphatemia encourage a conservative therapeutic approach to the treatment of hyperparathyroidism. Phosphate supplementation is usually all that is required to keep plasma calcium and phosphate at acceptable levels. The addition of oral 1:25 vitamin D (Rocaltrol) may also be beneficial. Persistent hypercalcemia or failure to keep levels below 12.5 mg/dl may be an indication for parathyroidectomy, particularly if there is evidence of bone demineralization, bone pain, or calcium-related graft dysfunction.

Osteopenia

Bone mineral density (BMD) is typically low in patients with end-stage renal disease and falls further in the first 2 years post-transplant. Not surprisingly, postmenopausal females are at particular risk, and their vertebral bone densities may be below the fracture threshold. Most studies suggest that the cumulative steroid dose is the preeminent factor accounting for loss of BMD; persistent post-transplant hyperparathyroidism is also important.

Corticosteroids inhibit intestinal calcium absorption and may interfere with the normal production of bone collagen by osteoblasts. In animal models, cyclosporine has been shown to have an independent catabolic effect on bone, but this has not been clearly demonstrated in humans. Progressive osteopenia has been identified in pediatric and adult transplant recipients; in adults, a progressive loss in vertebral bone has been recognized due to an inadequate amount of bone replacement during the remodeling cycle. Vitamin D supplements may be beneficial in children; calcium supplementation should be prescribed for adult women who are at high risk for osteoporosis (diphosphonates may be particularly effective for this group) (see Chap. 17). The corticosteroid dose should be kept at a safe minimum (see Chap. 4). The possibility of covert hyperparathyroidism as a cause of osteopenia should also be considered.

Osteonecrosis

Osteonecrosis, most frequently affecting the femoral head but also affecting other weight-bearing bones, is one of the most feared post-transplant complications. It may have a major impact on the rehabilitation and quality of life of the transplant recipient. The incidence varies widely, although approximately 15% of patients are afflicted in the first 3 years post-transplant. The incidence appears to be decreasing in association with better preoperative control of phosphorus and calcium levels on dialysis and with the use of cyclosporine, possibly as a result of fewer episodes of rejection requiring steroid therapy.

The pathogenesis of osteonecrosis is still not well-understood. Because it is not observed during chronic renal failure despite hyperparathyroidism and renal osteodystrophy but may occur after corticosteroid treatment for systemic lupus erythematosus or after kidney transplantation, steroid therapy is implicated as a major contributing factor. Some studies, however, have found no difference in cumulative steroid dosage or number of methylprednisolone pulses between patients with osteonecrosis of the femoral head after transplantation and those without.

Osteonecrosis of the femoral head usually presents as hip pain and limitation of movement that is exacerbated by weight-bearing. The onset may be insidious; most cases are recognized between 6 months and 5 years post-transplant. Pain may be referred to the knees, and osteonecrosis may independently affect the knees and shoulders. Symptoms may predate the earliest radiographic changes by several months. Magnetic resonance imaging is the most sensitive technique for early detection, radionuclide bone scanning may be helpful but has a high false-negative rate.

Discussion of the orthopedic evaluation and management of osteonecrosis is beyond the scope of this text. Core decompression before femoral head collapse may relieve pain but may not influence the progression of the lesion. Total hip arthroplasty is required where there is significant destruction of the acetabular cartilage and femoral head collapse.

Bone and Joint Pain

Patients receiving high doses of steroids that are then rapidly tapered may develop arthralgias, myalgias, and even joint effusions. The syndrome is transient and typically resolves when the baseline steroid dose has been attained. Episodic bone pain of unknown cause, usually affecting the knees or ankles, has also been described in patients receiving cyclosporine. This pain often responds to treatment with calcium channel blockers. Proximal myopathy, usually ascribed to steroid use, may respond to physical training and reduction of the steroid dose.

CARBOHYDRATE INTOLERANCE

Approximately 20% of post-transplant patients develop hyperglycemia, and 5–10% require therapy with oral hypoglycemic agents or insulin. Transient tubular glycosuria is also common.

Corticosteroid therapy is the most frequent cause of post-transplantation hyperglycemia. Steroids may increase production of glucose from gluconeogenesis, impair peripheral use of glucose, and cause elevation of glucogen levels by a direct anti-insulin effect at the cellular level. An undetermined threshold dose of corticosteroid may be required to provoke diabetes in susceptible individuals. Some studies have shown post-transplant diabetes to be related to steroid dose, increased patient age, black race, a positive family history of diabetes, increased body weight, and human leukocyte antigen (HLA) A28. These findings have not been consistent.

Typically, the onset of steroid diabetes is mild, without associated ketoacidosis; it may resolve on withdrawal or reduction of the steroid dose. Both cyclosporine and tacrolimus contribute to glucose intolerance by inhibiting insulin secretion by pancreatic beta cells and by inducing peripheral insulin resistance (see Chap. 4). Animal studies have revealed a decrease in islet cell insulin content as well as a severe degranulation and hydropic degeneration of islet cells after treatment with cyclosporine. Human studies have shown both improved glucose tolerance curves and insulin output after conversion from cyclosporine to azathioprine and prednisone. Cyclosporine dose reduction may improve glucose intolerance.

REPRODUCTIVE FUNCTION

Male

Following successful transplantation, approximately two-thirds of male patients observe improved libido and increased sexual activity to predialysis levels. In some patients, there is no improvement, and occasionally sexual function deteriorates. Fertility, as assessed by sperm counts, improves in 50% of patients. The sex hormone profile tends to normalize; plasma testosterone and follicle-stimulating hormone levels increase; and luteinizing hormone levels, which may be high in dialysis patients, fall to normal or low levels. Cyclosporine may impair testosterone biosynthesis through direct damage to Leydig cells and germinal cells, and a direct impairment of the hypothalamic pituitary gonadal axis has been suggested. There is no increased incidence of neonatal malformations in pregnancies fathered by transplant recipients.

Additional factors may account for failure of male sexual function to improve post-transplant. Antihypertensive medications may be responsible in some patients, autonomic neuropathy may impair erectile function, and interruption of both hypogastric arteries may occasionally impair vascular supply. Male patients should be asked about their sexual function and referred for urologic evaluation when necessary.

Female

Women with chronic renal failure demonstrate loss of libido, anovulatory vaginal bleeding or amenorrhea, and high prolactin levels. Maintenance dialysis therapy results in improvement in sexual function in only a small percentage of women, and pregnancy is rare. Within a year of successful transplantation, menstrual function and ovulation typically return, and prolactin levels fall to normal.

Family Planning

All women of childbearing age should be counseled concerning the possibility and risks of pregnancy after kidney transplantation. Psychosocial issues should be discussed, genetic counseling should be provided for those with hereditary kidney disease, and consideration should be given to the long-term prognosis of the patient and the graft. Patients can be assured that birth defects are not increased with the use of azathioprine and cyclosporine during pregnancy, although intrauterine growth retardation and prematurity are common. Data regarding the stability of graft function during and after pregnancy should be discussed. All pregnancies should be planned and prepared for. Conception should be delayed 18–24 months after kidney transplantation and contraception practiced until then. Contraceptive counseling should begin immediately post-transplant, since ovulatory cycles may begin within 1–2 months of transplant in women with well-functioning grafts.

Oral Contraceptives. Low-dose estrogen-progesterone preparations are advised. They should be used with caution because they may cause or aggravate hypertension or precipitate thromboembolism, especially in the context of cyclosporine immunosuppression. Cyclosporine levels should also be monitored soon after they are commenced.

Table 9-5. Criteria for reduction of post-transplant pregnancy risk

1. Patient should be 1½–2 years post-transplant
2. Good allograft function*
3. No recent episodes of acute rejection
4. Normotensive or minimal antihypertensive regimen
5. Minimal or no proteinuria
6. Normal allograft ultrasound
7. Prednisone less than 15 mg/day; azathioprine < 2 mg/kg/day. Cyclosporine at therapeutic levels.

*Serum creatinine level <2.0 mg/dl, preferably <1.5 mg/dl.

Intrauterine Device. The risk of infection may be increased in immunocompromised patients, and the efficacy of the intrauterine device may be compromised by the anti-inflammatory properties of the immunosuppressive agents. There is an increased incidence of ectopic pregnancy above the 0.5% incidence of ectopic pregnancy observed in patients with a kidney allograft. This form of contraception is not recommended.

Barrier Contraceptive Devices. Barrier contraception is the safest modality but depends on user compliance for efficacy.

Long-Acting Contraceptives. The long-acting, subcutaneously placed hormone preparations are highly effective and well-tolerated. They have not yet been formally tried in the transplant situation and should be used only under careful supervision.

Pregnancy

Women with end-stage renal disease sometimes seek transplantation with the knowledge that a well-functioning graft will give them the only real chance for natural motherhood. It has been estimated that 2% of women of childbearing age conceive after transplantation. The incidence of spontaneous abortion has been reported to be 13% and ectopic pregnancy 0.5%. These frequencies are not different from the normal population. Approximately one-third of pregnant transplant patients seek therapeutic abortion, a number that likely reflects inadequate family planning in women who have not previously considered themselves to be fertile. More than 90% of conceptions that continue beyond the first trimester end successfully.

Table 9-5 lists the criteria that should ideally be met before conception. A 90% incidence of successful pregnancies has been reported for women with a baseline creatinine of 1.5 mg/dl or less. Failure to meet all the listed criteria places the patient in a higher risk category but is not necessarily a contraindication to pregnancy. The U.S. National Transplantation Pregnancy Registry has been developed to provide current information concerning transplant pregnancy for the benefit of patients and their physicians.

Antenatal Care

Pregnancy in a patient with a kidney transplant should be considered a high-risk condition and should be monitored in a tertiary care center with consultation by a transplant nephrologist, obstetrician,

Table 9-6. Antepartum management of kidney transplant patients

1. Baseline data: Complete blood count, chemistry panel, CMV, HSV, HBV, HCV, and rubella serology; Rh status and antibody screen if Rh-negative; 24-hr urine for total protein and creatinine clearance; urinalysis and urine culture
2. Office visits every 2 wks until 28 weeks' gestation, followed by weekly visits until delivery. CBC, chemistry panel, urinalysis, and urine culture at each visit. Close attention to blood pressure control and cyclosporine levels.
3. CMV, HSV, HBV serology; 24-hr urine for protein and creatinine clearance every trimester
4. Pap smear and cervical culture for HSV at 30 weeks
5. Serial ultrasounds for gestational dating and evaluation for intrauterine growth retardation and congenital anomalies
6. Nonstress or contraction stress tests; fetal movement charting

CMV = cytomegalovirus; HBV = hepatitis B virus; HCV = hepatitis C virus; HSV = herpes simplex virus.

and pediatrician. The pregnancy should be diagnosed as early as possible and accurate dating obtained by fetal ultrasound. A recommended schedule for prenatal evaluation is listed in Table 9-6.

Allograft Function

In patients with good allograft function before conception, the GFR remains stable or increases as it does during a normal pregnancy. The GFR may decline to prepregnancy values during the third trimester. Most, but not all, studies suggest that pregnancy itself does not have an unfavorable impact on long-term graft function as long as baseline function is good. Proteinuria may increase to abnormal levels in the third trimester but usually resolves postpartum and is of no prognostic significance unless it is associated with hypertension.

Hypertension

Approximately 30% of pregnant patients with kidney transplants develop pregnancy-induced hypertension, a figure that is fourfold greater than in uncomplicated pregnancies. The use of cyclosporine in pregnancy tends to increase the incidence of hypertension, which has an unfavorable impact on birth weight. The diagnosis of preeclampsia is difficult to make in patients with preexisting hypertension or chronic rejection in the third trimester. Biopsy studies in women with renal parenchymal disease have shown that the clinical diagnosis of superimposed preeclampsia can be wrong more than half the time. Plasma uric acid levels and urinary protein excretion are not useful as markers for preeclampsia, since they are often elevated at any stage of gestation in pregnant transplant recipients. Allograft biopsy may occasionally be required if a precise diagnosis of preeclampsia is deemed essential.

Infection

Urinary tract infections are the most common bacterial infections and occur in up to 40% of pregnant transplant patients. Pyelonephritis may develop despite adequate antibiotic treatment. Urinary tract infections are particularly common in patients who develop end-stage renal disease due to pyelonephritis.

Viral infections are of special concern, since viruses are capable of crossing the placenta and infecting the fetus. An infant born to a HBsAg-positive mother should be given hepatitis B immunoglobulin (0.5 ml IM) within 12 hours of birth and HBV vaccine at another site within 48 hours (followed by a booster injection at 1–6 months). The combination of immunoglobulin and vaccine offers protection for more than 90% of infants. CMV surveillance buffy coat cultures and serology should be obtained routinely because virus reactivation is possible even with substantial existing antibody titers. If viral reactivation occurs, the pediatrician should be alerted to the necessity of screening the neonate for congenital CMV infection. Herpes simplex virus (HSV) infection before 20 weeks' gestation is associated with an increased rate of abortion. HSV is not thought to be a cause of intrauterine infection as long as the membranes are intact. A positive HSV cervical culture at term is an indication for cesarean section.

Immunosuppression in Pregnancy

Acute rejection episodes may occur occasionally during pregnancy and may be difficult to distinguish from acute pyelonephritis or severe preeclampsia. Ultrasound-guided kidney biopsy can be undertaken to make a definitive diagnosis. High-dose steroid therapy can be used to treat allograft rejection.

Prednisone. Prednisone crosses the placenta, but a large proportion is converted to prednisolone, which allegedly does not suppress fetal corticotropin. Adrenal insufficiency in the neonate has been reported with maternal prednisone ingestion. Very large doses of corticosteroids administered to animals have resulted in congenital anomalies (cleft lip and palate), but no consistent abnormalities have been noted in the offspring of women treated with corticosteroids during pregnancy for rheumatologic disease or kidney transplantation. Overall, prednisone is considered to be relatively safe for use in pregnancy.

Azathioprine. At doses of 2 mg/kg or less, no anomalies attributable to azathioprine have been noted in human offspring. There are minimal data, however, on the long-term effects of azathioprine on first- or second-generation offspring. Azathioprine can cause transient gaps or breaks in lymphocyte chromosomes. Germ cells and other tissues have not been studied. It is not known whether the eventual sequelae could be the development of malignancies in affected offspring or other abnormalities in the next generation.

Cyclosporine. There are no animal or human data showing teratogenicity or mutagenicity of cyclosporine, which appears to be safe to be used during pregnancy. Intrauterine growth retardation and small size for gestational age have been reported with cyclosporine use and may reflect chronic vasoconstriction. Cyclosporine is present in the fetal circulation at the same concentration found in the mother. The increased volume of distribution may produce low maternal blood levels, and dose elevations may be required.

Other Immunosuppressants. There are currently very little data concerning the safety of pregnancy for patients receiving the new generation of immunosuppressive agents (see Chap. 4); for the present, they should be avoided during pregnancy. Mycophenolate mofetil should be discontinued 6 weeks before conception is attempted.

Breast-Feeding. Steroids are secreted in breast milk but not in sufficient quantity to affect the infant at the usual therapeutic doses. A small percentage of the maternal dose of cyclosporine is excreted in breast milk; concentrations of azathioprine and its metabolites in breast milk are minimal. At the present time, there is insufficient information about the biologic effect of even small amounts of these agents on the neonate, and breast-feeding should be discouraged.

Labor and Delivery

Vaginal delivery is recommended, since the transplanted kidney is placed in the false pelvis and there is little risk of obstruction of the birth canal or of mechanical injury to the allograft. Cesarean section is usually performed only for standard obstetric reasons. Patients with bone pathology related to previous renal osteodystrophy or steroid therapy should be identified antenatally; x-ray pelvimetry should be done and cesarean section performed if necessary. Preterm delivery occurs in approximately half of transplant pregnancies because of the frequent occurrence of declining kidney function, pregnancy-induced hypertension, fetal distress, premature rupture of membranes, and premature labor. The incidence of small-for-gestational age babies is 20%. There is no increase in fetal abnormalities.

In the perinatal period, the steroid dose should be augmented to cover the stress of labor and to prevent postpartum rejection. Hydrocortisone, 100 mg q6h, should be given during labor and delivery. Maternal hypertension and fluid balance should be monitored carefully. Graft function and the immunosuppressive regimen should be monitored with particular care in the first 3 months postpartum. Occasional cases of postpartum acute renal failure resembling hemolytic-uremic syndrome have been described.

HEMATOPOIETIC ABNORMALITIES

Successful kidney transplantation corrects the anemia of chronic renal failure. Serum erythropoietin (EPO) levels before transplantation are similar to or higher than normal but are inappropriately low for the level of hematocrit. After transplantation, there is an immediate peak increase in serum EPO levels, which fall to baseline within the first postoperative week. A sustained rise in EPO levels is observed a week to a month after recovery of graft function, followed a few days later by reticulocytosis and a rise in hematocrit. EPO levels tend to decline to normal as the hematocrit rises above 32%. Many patients develop iron deficiency anemia and persistent elevation of EPO as a result of rapid mobilization of iron and depletion of ferritin. A serum ferritin level of less than 250 μg/liter before transplantation is predictive of iron deficiency posttransplantation. EPO production and reticulocytosis are suppressed during rejection and do not increase until rejection is successfully reversed. Good allograft function is a prerequisite for correction of anemia.

Persistent anemia in the presence of good graft function requires evaluation. A hypochromic anemia may suggest iron deficiency and occult bleeding. Azathioprine may produce a macrocytosis; its hematologic complications are described in Chap. 4.

Post-Transplant Erythrocytosis

Post-transplant erythrocythemia of varying degrees has been observed in up to 20% of transplant patients. It occurs most commonly within 2 years of transplantation in hypertensive males with good graft function and their native kidneys intact. Its etiology is multifactorial but most probably relates to deficient feedback regulation of EPO metabolism with a reset threshold for red cell production. EPO levels are not consistently elevated. Occasional cases of erythrocythemia are associated with renal artery stenosis and hydronephrosis, and there are reports of resolution after native kidney nephrectomy when the native renal vein EPO levels have been higher than peripheral blood levels.

Post-transplant erythrocythemia can be associated with significant morbidity from thromboembolic complications, headaches, hypertension, and reduced cerebral blood flow. Evaluation and treatment are indicated when the hematocrit is greater than the low 50s.

Treatment

Before starting treatment, causes of secondary polycythemia should be excluded. Some patients have transient erythrocythemia associated with low red blood cell mass and respond to increased salt and water intake or discontinuation of diuretics. For most patients, the most convenient and reliable form of treatment is with relatively low doses of ACE inhibitors (e.g., 2.5–5.0 mg daily of enalapril), although higher doses are sometimes required. The mechanism of action of these drugs, which can cause anemia in renal transplant recipients, has not been clearly elucidated. Their benefit is not consistently related to the measured EPO levels.

Most patients tolerate ACE inhibitors well. Some patients develop a troublesome cough, and patients with low ambient blood pressures may not tolerate their antihypertensive effect. Therapy with theophylline (200 mg bid) may be beneficial. Adenosine is an important regulator of EPO metabolism, and its action is antagonized by theophylline. Theophylline, however, may not be well tolerated. Some patients require repeated therapeutic phlebotomy.

Deep Venous Thrombosis

Using noninvasive techniques, the incidence of deep vein thrombosis (DVT) after kidney transplantation has been estimated to be 14% and increases to 24% if diabetic patients are included. Clinically overt DVTs are less common. There are two peak time periods during which DVTs are most likely to occur. The first peak occurs within the first month of transplantation and may be related to the use of cyclosporine. The second occurs at approximately 4 months posttransplant and may be related to normalization of the hematocrit and correction of uremic platelet dysfunction. There is not an increased incidence of DVT in the side of the allograft; the incidence of postoperative DVT is low.

Swelling of the leg ipsilateral to the allograft is common and usually transient after kidney transplantation. The swelling occurs as a result of partial disruption of the lymphatic drainage from the leg. Pronounced and persistent swelling should be evaluated. Compression of the iliac vein and subsequent formation of a DVT is a known complication of lymphoceles. Such patients should be evaluated with an allograft ultrasound and venography. Confirmation of the presence of a DVT mandates immediate treatment with heparin and prolonged warfarin (Coumadin) administration.

POST-TRANSPLANT SKIN DISEASE

Post-transplant dermatologic malignancies are discussed in the section on skin cancer. In addition, kidney transplant patients are subject to a variety of troublesome skin ailments.

Viral Warts

More than 50% of kidney transplant patients have viral warts that usually appear on sun-exposed areas such as the back of the hands. The prevalence of viral warts is influenced by graft survival time and length of exposure to immunosuppressive agents. The causal agent of human warts is the **human papillomavirus (HPV)**, of which 18 subtypes are recognized thus far. Subtypes 2 and 4 have been associated with viral warts and do not have malignant potential. Type 5 may be predisposed to squamous cell carcinoma. The frequency of common warts may obscure infection by a subtype that could predispose these patients to dysplastic skin lesions. Warts and skin cancers often appear in the same patient, possibly because they share common risk factors: pale skin and excessive sun exposure.

Genital Warts

Genital warts (condylomata acuminata) are verrucous growths that result from sexual transmission of an HPV and exhibit an incubation period of 3–4 months. HPV type 6 has been found in more than 90% of cases of genital warts but is not found in tissue from cervical, vulvar, or penile carcinoma. The incidence of condylomata among kidney transplant recipients is reported to be up to 4%. Preexisting lesions may become severe and difficult to treat after transplantation. New onset of condylomata usually occurs a year after transplantation. The lesions can rapidly become numerous, unsightly, uncomfortable, and a problem for personal hygiene and personal interactions. The lesions are often resistant to therapy with topical preparations. Because of continued immunosuppression, lesions may recur even after treatment by surgical removal, fulguration, cryotherapy, or laser therapy.

Both condylomata and cervical neoplasias occur with an increased incidence in kidney transplant recipients and often appear together. Some investigators have suggested that condylomata may represent a precursor lesion of cervical cancer. Condylomata should be treated aggressively, and increased surveillance for malignancy should be maintained with biannual pelvic examinations and Papanicolaou (Pap) smears.

Dermatologic Fungal Infections

Patients who tan easily are more likely to have fungal skin infections than patients who burn on skin exposure. The most common infections are tinea rubrum, molluscum contagiosum, Malassezia furfur, and *Candida*. Topical treatment is usually adequate, and systemic spread is extremely rare.

Cyclosporine Effects on Skin

The skin is one of the principal sites of accumulation of cyclosporine. The drug is highly lipophilic, and skin acts as a storage depot for the unmodified drug. Cyclosporine seems to stimulate proliferation of squamous epithelium and skin appendages, as manifested by skin thickening, hypertrichosis, and gingival hyperplasia. Cyclosporine may also cause epidermal cysts, pilar keratosis, acne, sebaceous hyperplasia, and folliculitis.

TRANSPLANT-ASSOCIATED MALIGNANCY

Fear of malignancy, lymphoma in particular, is a constant accompaniment of immunosuppression. Much can be learned from the history of this association. The first wave of lymphomas was noted in the late 1960s with the introduction of polyclonal antibody preparations. The second wave accompanied the use of high-dose cyclosporine in the early 1980s. In the late 1980s, the use of multiple immunosuppressive agents in an attempt to further improve graft survival spawned a new wave of lymphomas, sometimes of a particularly fulminant character. Post-transplant lymphoma is more frequent in heavily immunosuppressed heart and heart-lung transplant recipients than kidney recipients and is more common in the United States compared with Europe, where antilymphocytic induction protocols are not generally used. Patients who receive antilymphocytic agents, particularly two courses, are at greater risk of lymphoma than those who do not. High rates of malignancy, therefore, appear to be a reflection of the overall potency of immunosuppressive regimens rather than the responsibility of individual agents. It has been estimated that some form of cancer will develop in up to two-thirds of patients with transplants for more than 20 years. Most of these tumors are skin cancers. The overall incidence of lymphoma in kidney transplant recipients is 1–2%.

Much of our knowledge of the malignancy-transplantation association has come from the **Cincinnati Transplant Tumor Registry**, which collects data on neoplasia in organ transplant recipients from participating centers around the world. The mean incidence of malignancies of all types is approximately 6%, with a range of 1–18%. Differences in incidence arise from different intensities of immunosuppressive regimens and variability in the completeness of reporting. Skin cancers are particularly common in Australia. The use of cyclosporine in routine dosage has not increased the incidence of malignancy above that found with azathioprine, although the distribution of malignancy is somewhat different, with more lymphomas and less central nervous system malignancies with cyclosporine.

Carcinomas of the lung, prostate, colon, rectum, and breast, which occur frequently in the general population, are not increased in incidence in kidney transplant recipients. The neoplasms that do appear in increased incidence are discussed below.

Post-Transplant Lymphoproliferative Disease

Post-transplant lymphomas have several unusual features that distinguish them from those found in the general population:

1. The majority (96%) are non-Hodgkin's lymphomas (Hodgkin's disease is the most common lymphoma in age-matched controls) and are B cell in origin.
2. Extranodal involvement (central nervous system, liver, lungs, kidneys, intestines) is most common, and multiple sites are often involved. In azathioprine-treated patients, the brain is the most common site of extranodal involvement.
3. There is a high rate of association with Epstein-Barr virus (EBV) infection. Seronegative recipients of an organ from a seropositive donor are at highest risk of development of post-transplant lymphoproliferative disease (PTLD).
4. The mortality rate is nearly 50-fold greater for PTLD than for lymphomas in the general population. The course may be extremely fulminant, with progression to death within a few months of transplantation.
5. PTLD often presents as dysfunction of the transplanted organ itself and may be confused histologically with severe rejection.
6. PTLD may respond to withdrawal or drastic reduction of immunosuppressive therapy and to antiviral chemotherapy. Standard chemotherapy and irradiation are not generally helpful and may exaggerate the degree of immune compromise.
7. Prophylactic antiviral therapy, usually targeted against CMV infection (see Chap. 10), may serendipitously reduce EBV replication and the incidence of PTLD.

Role of Epstein-Barr Virus

EBV is a human DNA–transforming herpesvirus that primarily targets B lymphocytes. It is associated with an array of disorders ranging from infectious mononucleosis to nasopharyngeal carcinoma, Burkitt's lymphoma, and B cell lymphomas in immunocompromised patients.

EBV binds to epithelial oropharyngeal cells via the CD21 receptor and replicates within. It has the innate capability of transforming and immortalizing host B lymphocytes by latent infection, producing so-called **lymphoblastoid cells**. An extrachromosomal particle of EBV genome can be found within the B cell nucleus. In an immunocompetent host, a latent carrier state is established when the proliferation of the transformed B cells is contained by a normal immune response with intact cell-mediated immunity. Approximately 95% of the adult population have serologic evidence of previous EBV infection. The presence of reactive T lymphocytes inhibits infected cell proliferation in a process termed **regression.** The addition of cyclosporine or OKT3 in vitro prevents regression, and EBV-transformed cells may proliferate uncontrollably.

EBV-associated PTLD seems to progress through stages of transformation to a malignant state. The first stage resembles an infectious mononucleosis syndrome, with the development of polymorphic diffuse B cell hyperplasias without cytogenic abnormalities or gene rearrangements. The second stage produces a subpopulation of cells with cellular and nuclear atypia and cytogenic abnormalities. In the third stage, a malignant monoclonal B cell lymphoma develops composed of cells with clonal cytogenic abnormalities and immunoglobulin gene rearrangements. All stages may be present in a single lesion, and several lesions of differing monoclonality may be present within the same host in a multifocal manner consistent with an infectious etiology.

A form of fulminant EBV-associated post-transplant lymphoma has been described, often following multiple courses of OKT3. The disease may initially resemble a severe infectious mononucleosis-like illness but may progress rapidly, with death within a few months of transplantation. At a later stage, the patient may present with localized lymphoproliferative tumor masses in the brain, lung, or gastrointestinal tract.

Clonality

The issue of the clonality of post-transplant lymphomas has been a source of dispute. It has been suggested that **polyclonal B** cell lesions are more likely to be benign and to respond to withdrawal of immunosuppression and acyclovir, whereas **monoclonal** lesions are believed to be frankly malignant. In fact, polyclonal lymphoproliferative disorders may represent an early stage in a spectrum that progresses from polyclonal activation of B cells by EBV to latently infected, malignantly transformed, monoclonal B cell lymphomas.

Treatment

Restoration of host immunity is probably the most important therapy for the control of lymphoid proliferation. Patients with evidence of polyclonality or EBV infection are most likely to respond to treatment with acyclovir, which acts by inhibiting the EBV-associated DNA polymerase but does not affect episomal EBV in nonproductive, transformed lymphocytes. In patients with monoclonal tumors with or without evidence of active or episomal EBV, immunosuppression should be drastically reduced or discontinued altogether. Acyclovir is less likely to be effective in monoclonal disorders, but conventional cytotoxic therapy and radiotherapy have also had disappointing responses, with mortality remaining at greater than 80%. Most patients in whom immunosuppression is stopped will lose their grafts to inexorable rejection. Occasionally, tumors will regress, and the patients and their grafts can be maintained on very low dose immunosuppression.

Skin Cancer

Skin malignancies in kidney transplant recipients are a major problem, particularly in geographic areas and countries, such as Australia, which are exposed to intense sunlight. Aggressive skin cancer occurs, on average, 20–30 years earlier in immunosuppressed patients than in the general population. When kidney transplant patients are compared with immunocompetent patients, it has been estimated that the incidence of skin cancer is 20 times higher on sun-exposed surfaces and up to seven times higher on generally unexposed areas. The incidence tends to increase with time after transplantation. Male gender, donor-recipient mismatching at the HLA-B locus, and recipient homozygosity for HLA-DR (see Chap. 3) have been associated with an increased risk of squamous cell carcinoma.

There are several characteristics of cutaneous malignancies in kidney transplant recipients that differ from cutaneous malignancies in the general population:

1. The incidence of squamous cell carcinoma outnumbers basal cell carcinomas with a ratio of 2.3:1.0 (Canada) to 16:1 (Australia). In the general population, this ratio is 0.2:1.0.

2. Multiple skin cancers may appear at initial diagnosis. Squamous cell carcinoma may appear concomitantly with basal cell carcinoma.
3. Squamous cell carcinoma is more aggressive in behavior and metastasizes more frequently than in the general population. In Australian transplant recipients, there is a tenfold increase in mortality from squamous cell carcinoma of the skin.
4. Malignant melanomas account for approximately 5% of skin cancers in transplant recipients compared to 2.7% of the general population.
5. Dysplastic and malignant lip lesions are much more common in transplant recipients. The lesion may appear innocent. They are more common in sun-exposed males who smoke. Lipstick may be protective!

Human Papillomavirus

Many transplant patients have viral warts that are caused by numerous subtypes of HPV. HPV type 5 has been found in a high percentage of squamous cell skin cancers, although it is unlikely that HPV type 5 alone is responsible for cutaneous neoplasms among organ transplant recipients. Warts, keratoses, and neoplasms tend to occur in sun-exposed areas of the skin, which implies that ultraviolet (UV) light may be a cofactor in oncogenesis. UV light may act as a tumor promoter, with HPV 5 as the initiating agent. In animal models, immunosuppressive drugs inhibit normal repair of UV irradiation-induced DNA lesions in epidermal keratinocytes.

Kaposi's Sarcoma

The acquired immune deficiency syndrome (AIDS) epidemic has familiarized medical practitioners with Kaposi's sarcoma, a previously rare tumor. It was recognized in kidney transplant patients, however, well before the AIDS epidemic began. In some series, up to 10% of all post-transplant malignancies are Kaposi's; the most common sites of involvement are the skin, oropharyngeal membranes, and the conjunctiva. Kaposi's sarcoma presents as reddish-blue macules and plaques, and the lesions may behave aggressively and involve lymph nodes and viscera. The patient's human immunodeficiency virus (HIV) status should be determined Kaposi's sarcoma in a transplant patient is a reflection of excessive immunosuppression and may respond to its withdrawal as well as to chemotherapy and radiotherapy.

Prevention and Treatment

1. Dermatologic surveillance is an intrinsic part of long-term post-transplant follow-up. Patients who develop viral warts, actinic keratoses, genital warts, and other undiagnosed skin lesions should be followed regularly by a dermatologist.
2. Keratoacanthomas, which may be difficult to distinguish from squamous cell carcinomas, should be excised.
3. Excessive sun exposure should be avoided and protective clothing worn. Topical sunscreens with high levels of protection should be used.
4. Low-dose systemic retinoids (isotretinoin 0.2–0.5 mg/kg/day) combined with topical tretinoin may be effective in allograft

recipients with recurrent skin tumors. They can be used safely with routine immunosuppressive medications.
5. Surgical excision of suspicious lesions is the treatment of choice. Topical applications of 5-fluorouracil have been useful for multiple superficial carcinomas. Cryosurgery and radiotherapy may also be used.
6. The development of aggressive or multifocal squamous cell carcinomas is an indication to minimize the immunosuppressive regimen. The risk of metastases or uncontrollable local growth may justify discontinuing immunosuppression altogether.

Genital Neoplasia

In female transplant recipients, there is a nearly 40-fold increase in the frequency of vulvar and vaginal carcinomas and an approximately 15-fold increased incidence of frank cervical neoplasia and intraepithelial lesions. HPV and herpes simplex type II have both been linked epidemiologically to genital cancer and may interact in a way that leads to overt malignancy, especially in the immunocompromised host who either lacks the ability to mount a cytotoxic T lymphocyte response or may have an increased susceptibility to infection with oncogenic viruses. In both immunocompetent and immunocompromised subjects, however, the critical risk factor in developing genital neoplasia is the number of sexual partners, indicating that exposure to a sexually transmitted agent is a key factor.

All women with kidney transplants should undergo annual pelvic exams and Pap smears. Patients with a prior history of condylomata or anogenital neoplasms may require more frequent monitoring.

SOCIOECONOMIC FACTORS IN LONG-TERM FOLLOW-UP

Transplantation has the potential to return end-stage renal disease patients to full-time employment and reestablish them as productive members of society. Nearly 80% of transplant recipients are able to function at nearly normal levels as compared with approximately 50% of dialysis patients. Subjectively, kidney transplant recipients have a similar pattern of life satisfaction, well-being, and psychological adjustment as the general population, and these subjective evaluations are generally much superior to those on dialysis. All studies of socioeconomic impact of transplantation consistently report that the quality of life is far better after transplantation than while on dialysis, although it should be noted that most of these studies were performed before the widespread availability of EPO. Noncompliance with medication remains a major obstacle to long-term allograft success. In some areas of the country, noncompliance and inability to pay for immunosuppressive medication are major causes of allograft failure.

Through Medicare, the United States federal government pays for inpatient hospital services and preparation for transplant surgery, including the full cost for a living donor or cadaveric kidney. In addition, the U.S. Congress has directed that the first 3-year costs of immunosuppressive drug therapy also be paid for by the government. Medicare will not pay for other medications such as antihypertensive agents. After this period, however, the patient must find other sources of funding for immunosuppressive drugs, which can amount to more than $10,000 annually. At the end of the third year after transplantation, Medicare no longer acts as payer for end-stage renal disease care unless the patient is older than 65 years of age. If the individual is unable to return to work due to complications of transplantation, an application for Social Security Disability insurance can be made.

Data regarding the functional ability of patients after transplantation are discouraging. Studies have shown that less than 70% of nondiabetic patients are deemed able to work, and less than half of them are actually working. For diabetic patients, the statistics are even worse; less than 40% are deemed able to work, and half of these are working. For the most part, it appears as if pretransplant employment status is the most important predictor of post-transplant employment status. Some patients find it difficult to find or maintain employment because employers do not want the financial liability of a transplant patient for whom health insurance costs are high, and time taken from work for clinic visits, laboratory visits, and hospitalizations for transplant complications are inconvenient and costly. Other patients are financially unable to afford the transplant if they lose their Medicaid or Medicare benefits by returning to employed status.

Quality-of-life issues also have a major impact on the functional status of kidney transplant patients and remain to be explored. Although medical expertise is improving, the capacity to fully rehabilitate kidney transplant patients remains limited by factors that are beyond immediate control.

SELECTED READINGS

Part I

Bia MJ. Nonimmunologic causes of late renal graft loss. *Kidney Int* 47:1470, 1995.

De Geest S, Borgemans L, Gemoets H et al. Incidence, determinants, and consequences of subclinical noncompliance with immunosuppressive therapy in renal transplant recipients. *Transplantation* 59:340, 1995.

Hayry P. Aspects of allograft rejection, I: Molecular pathology of acute and chronic rejection. *Transplant Rev* 9:113, 1995.

Kasiske BL, Massy ZA, Guijarro C et al. Chronic renal allograft rejection and clinical trial design. *Kidney Int* 48:S116, 1995.

Massy ZA, Guijarro C, Wiederkehr MR et al. Chronic renal allograft rejection: immunologic and nonimmunologic risk factors. *Kidney Int* 49:518, 1996.

Matas A. Chronic rejection in renal transplant recipients—Risk factors and correlates. *Clin Transplantation* 8:332, 1994.

Ramos EL, Tisher CC. Recurrent diseases in the kidney transplant. *Am J Kidney Dis* 24:142, 1994.

Sharma VK, Bologa RM, Xu GP et al. Intragraft TGF-β, mRNA: A correlate of interstitial fibrosis and chronic allograft nephropathy. *Kidney Int* 1996 [in press].

Terasaki PI, Koyama H, Cecka JM. The hyperfiltration hypothesis in human renal transplantation. *Transplantation* 57:1450, 1994.

Tullius S, Tilney N. Both alloantigen-dependent and independent factors influence chronic allograft rejection. *Transplantation* 59:313, 1995.

Van Saase JL, van der Woude FJ, Thorogood J et al. The relation between acute vascular and interstitial renal allograft rejection and subsequent chronic rejection. *Transplantation* 59:1280, 1995.

Windholm A, Albrechtsen D, Frödinil et al. Ischemic heart disease—major cause of death and graft loss after renal transplantation in Scandinavia. *Transplantation* 60:451, 1995.

Part II

Cosio FG, Dillon JJ, Falkenhain ME. Racial differences in renal allograft survival: The role of systemic hypertension. *Kidney Int* 47:1136, 1995.

Danovitch GM, Jamgotchian NJ, Eggena PH et al. Angiotensin-converting enzyme inhibition in the treatment of renal transplant erythrocytosis: Clinical experience and observation of mechanism. *Transplantation* 60:132, 1995.

First MR, Neylan JF, Rocher LL et al. Hypertension after renal transplantation. *J Am Soc Nephrol* 4(Suppl):S30, 1994.

Grotz WH, Mundinger FA, Gugel B. Bone mineral density after kidney transplantation. *Transplantation* 59:982, 1995.

Hilbrands LB, Hoitsma AJ, Koene RAP. The effect of immunosuppressive drugs on quality of life after renal transplantation. *Transplantation* 59:1263, 1995.

Julian BA, Quarles D, Niemann KM. Musculoskeletal complications after renal transplantation: Pathogenesis and treatment. *Am J Kidney Dis* 19:99, 1992.

Kasiske BL, Guijarro C, Massy ZA et al. Cardiovascular disease after renal transplantation. *J Am Soc Nephrol* 7:158, 1996.

King GN, Healy CM, Glover MT et al. Increased prevalence of dysplastic and malignant lip lesion in renal transplant recipients. *N Engl J Med* 332:1052, 1995.

Kuo PC, Dafoe DC, Alfrey EJ et al. Post-transplant lymphoproliferative disorders and Epstein-Barr virus prophylaxis. *Transplantation* 59:135, 1995.

London NJ, Farmery SM, Will EJ et al. Risk of neoplasia in renal transplant patients. *Lancet* 346:403, 1995.

Markell MS, Armenti V, Danovitch GM et al. Hyperlipidemia and glucose intolerance in the post-renal transplant patient. *J Am Soc Nephrol* 4(Suppl):S37, 1994.

Rook AH, Jaworsky C, Nguyen T et al. Beneficial effect of low-dose systemic retinoid in combination with topical tretinoin for the treatment and prophylaxis of premalignant and malignant skin lesions in renal transplant recipients. *Transplantation* 59:714, 1995.

Rosen HR, Friedman LS, Martin P. Hepatitis C and the renal transplant patient. *Semin Dialysis* 9:39, 1996.

Sturgiss SN, Davison JM. Effect of pregnancy on the longterm function of renal allografts: An update. *Am J Kidney Dis* 26:54, 1995.

10

Infectious Complications of Kidney Transplantation and Their Management

Bernard M. Kubak and Curtis D. Holt

Of the solid organ transplants, kidney transplantation is associated with the lowest rates of infections. In contrast to liver, heart, or lung allograft recipients, whose clinical status often deteriorates before transplant, the elective or semielective nature of kidney transplantation along with anatomic considerations considerably lowers the risk of infection. Despite these considerations, infections in the renal transplant patient can cause significant morbidity, leading to graft dysfunction or systemic complications. Moreover, the clinical presentation of post-transplant infections can be confused with acute rejection, which may occur simultaneously. In this regard, certain viruses, such as cytomegalovirus (CMV), Epstein-Barr virus (EBV), and hepatitis B and C viruses (HBV and HCV, respectively), can display an **immunomodulating effect**. This immunomodulation may contribute to allograft rejection, obliterative transplant arteriopathy, enhancement of other opportunistic infections, and development of post-transplant lymphoproliferative disease (PTLD).

Due to the overall state of immunosuppression (see below), infections can also occur in organ systems unrelated to the transplanted kidney. Examples include invasive pulmonary aspergillosis; CMV or cryptococcal pneumonia; reactivation or newly acquired mycobacterial and mycotic diseases (e.g., histoplasmosis, coccidioidomycosis, hyalohyphomycosis); or viral diseases such as HBV and HCV infection, herpesimplex virus (HSV) infection of the skin or GI tract, and varicella-zoster virus (VZV) infection of the skin or CNS.

This chapter emphasizes the infectious disease aspects of the pretransplant donor and recipient evaluation; the post-transplant recognition, treatment, and prophylaxis of infectious agents with appropriate agents and dosages to minimize allograft toxicity; and the implications of newer antibiotics and immunosuppressive drugs on post-transplant infections.

GENERAL GUIDELINES
FOR INFECTION RECOGNITION

Recognition of the following factors may assist in the identification of the causative pathogen(s) and the initiation of appropriate therapy prior to laboratory confirmation. These include the following:

1. Preoperative recipient infectious history or exposures (e.g., to tuberculosis, hepatitis viruses, human immunodeficiency virus [HIV], VZV, CMV, EBV), immunizations, immune-altering conditions (e.g., surgical or functional asplenia, pretransplant medical conditions requiring immunosuppressive agents), substance or IV drug abuse, liver dysfunction, malnutrition, geographic/epidemiologic exposures (e.g., endemic mycoses, Toxoplasma, Strongyloides, enteric parasites)

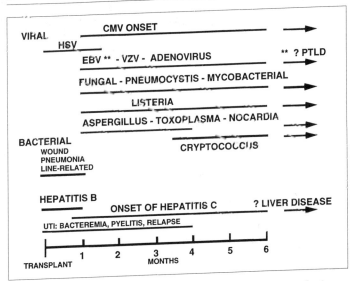

Fig. 10-1. Timetable for occurrence of infection following transplantation. CMV = cytomegalovirus; HSV = herpes simplex virus; EBV = Epstein-Barr virus; VZV = varicella zoster virus; PTLD = post-transplant lymphoproliferative disease, ** indicate possible relationship of EBV to PTLD; UTI = urinary tract infection. Arrows indicate infections or other manifestations that may present >6 months to 2 years that may present 6 months to 2 years? may present more than 2 years? post-transplantation. (Modified from RH Rubin. Infection in the Organ Transplant Patient. In RH Rubin, LS Young [eds], *Clinical Approach to Infection in the Compromised Host*. New York: Plenum, 1994.)

2. The infectious history of the donor, specifically, any infectious agent(s) that can be directly transmitted with the donor graft
3. The temporal occurrence of a presumed infectious episode relative to the date of transplantation (Fig. 10-1)
4. The **net state of immunosuppression**, a complex function that reflects the interaction of the following factors:
   a. The prophylactic immunosuppressive protocol employed
   b. Intensification of immunosuppression during episodes of rejection
   c. The presence of neutropenia
   d. Open wounds and foreign bodies (e.g., catheters)
   e. Metabolic abnormalities (e.g., malnutrition, uremia, hyperglycemia)
   f. Infection with immunomodulatory viruses

Pretransplant Screening: Recipient and Donor

Pretransplant latent infections or infectious exposures can lead to a reappraisal of transplant candidacy or, subsequently, alterations in standard post-transplant management. Preexisting infectious conditions in the donor or recipient may appear in the immediate postoperative period during induction immunosuppression, in the initial weeks post-transplant during treatment of rejection episodes, or in the later months post-transplant, depending on the overall net state

Table 10-1. Pretransplant screening

Medical conditions
    Antibiotic allergies
    Chest radiograph
    Dental assessment
    Immunizations
    Valvular repairs or replacements
    Preoperative urine culture
    PPD skin test controls
    History of sexually transmitted diseases
Serologies
    Human immunodeficiency virus
    Cytomegalovirus
    Epstein-Barr virus
    Varicella-zoster virus
    Hepatitis B virus and hepatitis C virus
    Toxoplasmosis
    Coccidioidomycosis
    Histoplasmosis

PPD = purified protein derivative (tuberculin).

of immunosuppressives. Incomplete immunizations in the recipient should be corrected prior to transplantation.

General Screening

Pretransplant evaluation is discussed in detail in Chap. 6. From the perspective of infectious diseases and their consequences, evaluation should include eliciting a history of antibiotic allergies, valvular repairs or replacements, a dental assessment, a preoperative urine culture, and a chest radiograph to exclude active pneumonic processes and identify evidence of prior granulomatous or infectious disorders (Table 10-1). A purified protein derivative (tuberculin) skin test with appropriate controls should be applied; however, suboptimal reactivity of skin testing in renal failure patients may lead to false-negative results. Isoniazid (INH) prophylaxis may be indicated with an abnormal chest x-ray result representing old tuberculosis despite a negative skin test. Precise recommendations for dosage and duration of therapy should adhere to the Centers for Disease Control guidelines on INH prophylaxis. Additional preoperative assessment should include a history of sexually transmitted diseases such as syphilis, HSV infection, viral hepatitis, and HIV infection.

Immunizations

Pretransplant candidates lacking standard pediatric or adult immunizations, splenectomized patients, and renal failure patients may benefit from pretransplant vaccinations with influenza, pneumococcal, and hepatitis B, diphtheria-pertussis-tetanus, inactivated polio, and measles-mumps-rubella (MMR) vaccines (American College of Physicians: *Guide for Adult Immunization*, 1994). Suboptimal efficacy of vaccinations in patients with renal failure must be recognized due to the effects of uremia on the immune system, however. Live vaccines should be avoided in immunocompromised patients (e.g., a renal transplant candidate with an underlying condition requiring immunosuppressive medications) and in patients who have undergone solid organ transplantation. Of particular pretransplant concern are pediatric renal failure patients with incomplete primary immunizations of live viral vaccines such as MMR. The general recommendation of avoiding live, attenuated viral vaccines in allograft recipients precludes the completion of the immunization series, thereby exposing the child to the risk of measles. Consequently, pretransplant immunization offers the opportunity to prevent the post-transplantation risks of live, attenuated viral vaccines. In this respect, measles, MMR, and varicella vaccines should, ideally, be administered several months before transplantation. Pretransplant vaccination with a live, attenuated CMV vaccine (Towne) has been reported to result in a reduction in the severity of CMV disease and improved graft survival in seronegative recipients of a CMV-positive allograft, the group considered to be at highest risk for CMV disease. Administration of this vaccine, however, has not been implemented.

Pretransplant Serologic Testing

Preoperative serologic testing can assist in the identification of at-risk candidates and should include testing for HIV (by enzyme immunoassay with Western Blot confirmation), EBV, HBV (hepatitis B surface antibody and surface antigen), HCV (by antibody screening with a confirmatory later-generation recombinant immunoblot assay or by viral-specific nucleic acid detection when warranted), VZV, CMV, and endemic mycotic antibody tests (e.g., anticoccidioidal antibody detection in any patient with endemic exposure no matter the duration).

Human Immunodeficiency Virus.   All potential transplant recipients should be tested for HIV regardless of the recognition of risk factors. HIV positivity is a contraindication to kidney transplantation because of the enhanced progression of the disease with immunosuppression and the relatively improved survival with hemodialysis. All potential transplant donors, both live and cadaveric, should be tested for HIV regardless of risk factors. Many centers will turn down kidneys from high-risk donors for fear of failure to detect antibody during the "window" after infection (see Chap. 5). Transmission of HIV by infected organs has been described, the precautions currently routinely employed have virtually eliminated the risk.

Epstein-Barr Virus.   EBV-seronegative recipients of grafts from EBV-seropositive donors may be at an increased risk for the development of PTLD (see Chap. 9), particularly if they receive prolonged or repeated courses of antilymphocytic therapy. The EBV status should be reviewed when considering heavy immunosuppression, and careful surveillance and use of prophylactic ganciclovir may be indicated.

Hepatitis B and C.   The finding of positive pretransplant HBV and HCV seroreactivity in both transplant donors and recipients has become more frequent with the availability of improved laboratory methods to detect viral-specific antibody, antigen, and nucleic acid. The impact of these test results on transplant candidacy are discussed in Chap. 6, on the use of donor kidneys in Chap. 5, and on the development of post-transplant liver disease in Chap. 9.

Cytomegalovirus. CMV infection is the most common viral infection that occurs after kidney transplantation and may vary in severity from asymptomatic infection to multiorgan involvement and death. The incidence of CMV positivity increases with age, and the majority of dialysis patients have detectable IgG antibody to CMV. The significance of the CMV antibody status of the donor and recipient is discussed in the section on specific pathogens and treatment and in Table 10-2.

Coccidioidomycosis and Histoplasmosis. The pretransplant detection of reactive *Coccidioides* complement fixation and immunodiffusion serologies or reactive *Histoplasma* serologies should alert the clinician to the possibility of reactivation post-transplant (see the section on fungal infections). In geographically high-risk areas, these tests should be performed routinely pretransplant and consideration given to the use of prophylactic antifungal agents.

Donor- and Graft-Transmitted Infections

It may be difficult to differentiate between a true donor allograft source of infection, exogenous infection, or reactivation of latent disease. The following agents have been implicated with reasonable certainty as being transmissible with the donor allograft: HIV; CMV; HBV; HCV; tuberculosis; and certain fungi, including *Histoplasma capsulatum*, *Coccidioides immitis*, *Cryptococcus neoformans*, *Candida albicans*, and *Monisporium apiospermum*. Probable transmission has been reported with HSV, aerobic grampositive and gram-negative bacteria, anaerobes, *Candida* species, *Toxoplasma*, *Strongyloides*, atypical mycobacteria, and EBV. The incidence of true donor-transmitted infection can be reduced by scrupulous donor screening and epidemiologic evaluation (see Chap. 5).

APPROACH TO INFECTION IN KIDNEY ALLOGRAFT RECIPIENTS

Several host factors, epidemiologic factors, and iatrogenic factors predispose renal allograft recipients to infection (Table 10-3). Obviously, the overall state of health and urgency of the transplant may affect the type and severity of postoperative infections. Previous medical conditions other than those pertaining to renal disease may confer increased susceptibility to infections. Furthermore, exposure of patients to broad-spectrum antibiotics or to the hospital environment immediately before transplant can result in colonization with resistant bacteria or fungi. Preexisting latent infections such as herpes viruses, CMV infection, tuberculosis, or toxoplasmosis may reactivate and cause morbidity. Potential environmental pathogens include *Pseudomonas* and *Legionella* species, which may be present in water supplies; *Listeria*, which has been associated with food-related epidemics; *Aspergillus* residing in hospital ventilation systems; and endemic mycoses such as *Coccidioides immitis* or *Histoplasma capsulatum*. Equally important are factors pertaining to the surgical procedure, such as the incidence of urine

Table 10-2. Relationship of incidence of cytomegalovirus infection and disease to seropositivity of donor/recipient

Cytomegalovirus status		Terminology	Infection incidence (%)	Disease incidence (%)	Pneumonitis incidence (%)
Donor	Recipient				
Positive	Negative	Primary infection	70–88	56–80	30
Negative	Positive	Reactivation	0–20	0–27	Rare
Positive	Positive	Reinfection	70	27–39	3–14
		Reactivation	15–30		

Source: CL Davis. The prevention of cytomegalovirus disease in renal transplantation. *Am J Kidney Dis* 16:175, 1990.

Table 10-3. General risk factors for infection in renal transplantation

1. Technical aspects of the transplant surgery
2. The duration of the surgery
3. The amount of blood products received
4. The donor graft status
5. Preexisting or latent infection in the recipient
6. Dose and duration of immunosuppressive therapy
7. The frequency of rejection episodes
8. The time period following renal transplant

leaks, wound hematomas and lymphoceles, and the type of immuno-suppression (dose, duration, and temporal relationship). Various catheters and instrumentations disrupt physical barriers and produce portals of entry for endogenous and nosocomial flora. The transplanted organ may also be or become a focus of infection as a result of an infected donor at the time of transplantation, vascular-related ischemia, and damage caused by rejection following transplantation. Transfusion-associated infections (CMV, hepatitis viruses, HIV infections) may also develop in patients receiving large numbers of blood products.

Incidence and Types of Infections

Approximately 80% of all infections in kidney transplant recipients are bacterial (Table 10-4). They generally occur within the first month post-transplant and may be associated with pretransplant conditions or postoperative complications. Historically, urinary tract infections (UTIs) were the most common infectious complication in renal allograft recipients, occurring in 35–79% of cases. Fortunately, antimicrobial prophylaxis with trimethoprim-sulfamethoxazole (TMP-SMX) or ciprofloxacin decreases the frequency of UTIs to less than 10% and essentially eliminates urosepsis unless urine flow is obstructed. TMP-SMX can also reduce the incidence of *Nocardia asteroides* infection and sepsis related to *Listeria* monocytogenes. Wound infection is encountered following renal transplantation with a reported incidence varying from 1.8–56.0%. Wound infections can involve the perinephric space or cause mycotic aneurysms at the site of vascular anastomosis, necessitating nephrectomy of the transplanted kidney. Less frequent sources of bacterial infection include the respiratory tract, GI or hepatobiliary systems, vascular access sites, and sequestered sites (paranasal sinuses, middle ear, meninges, perirectal area, and prostate).

Diagnosis

Bacterial infections in the renal transplant population can be difficult to diagnose. Signs and symptoms such as fever and leukocytosis may be masked or absent in patients receiving high-dose corticosteroids, and infection may be difficult to differentiate from other causes of graft dysfunction. Diagnosis of wound infections should include aspiration of pus or a swab specimen from the wound site. For UTIs, a clean-catch midstream urine specimen should be submitted for quantitative culture; in renal transplant recipients, lower levels of bacteriuria may be a significant risk factor for systemic infection. For detection of bacteremia, blood cul-

Table 10-4. Common bacterial pathogens listed by site of infection

Intra-abdominal	Septicemia	Urinary tract	Pneumonia	Wound
Enterobacteriaceae	*Enterobacteriaceae*	*Enterobacteriaceae*	*Enterobacteriaceae*	Mixed infection
Enterococcus species	*Pseudomonas aeruginosa*	*P. aeruginosa*	*P. aeruginosa*	*Enterobacteriaceae*
Anaerobes (*Bacteroides*)	*Staphylococcus aureus*	*Enterococcus*	*S. aureus*	*Pseudomonas* species
S. aureus	*Enterococcus*		*Streptococcus pneumoniae*	*Enterococcus* species
Mixed infection	Anaerobes (*Bacteroides*)		*Nocardiosis*	*S. aureus*
			Legionella species	Anaerobes (*Bacteroides*)

tures should be drawn before initiation of antimicrobial therapy. Specimens for post-transplant pneumonia include blood, sputum, tracheal suction in ventilated patients, bronchoalveolar lavage (BAL) fluid, transthoracic fine-needle aspirate, and, occasionally, lung biopsy. Blood cultures are not always useful in the diagnosis of pneumonia, since only 10–15% of patients with pneumonia are bacteremic. *Nocardia* species can be presumptively diagnosed if staining reveals delicately branching, gram-positive, beaded filaments. *Legionella* species can be cultured from respiratory specimens, but immunofluorescent or nucleic acid detection of specific antigens in respiratory specimens and urinary antigen detection may prove useful. The diagnosis of *Pneumocystis carinii* pneumonia can be made by indirect and direct fluorescent antibody stains from BAL and transbronchial biopsy specimens.

Approach to the Kidney Transplant Patient with Fever

The differential diagnosis of fever for nonimmunosuppressed patients needs to be broadened for kidney transplant patients to include the possibility of opportunistic infection, rejection, drug reaction, or a systemic inflammatory response. Fever may be the sole manifestation of acute rejection, which may also coexist with infection. In addition to a thorough history and physical examination, febrile patients should have urinalysis and urine and blood cultures to include fungal cultures and CMV cultures. It is often wise to obtain a chest radiograph even in the absence of pulmonary symptoms. In appropriate settings, CMV studies should include a polymerase chain reaction (PCR) or early antigen detection in blood or body fluids and serologic analysis.

SPECIFIC PATHOGENS AND TREATMENT

Bacterial Infections

The types of bacterial pathogens encountered in renal transplantation vary from center to center. Common pathogens encountered in renal allograft recipients include aerobic gram-negative bacilli (Enterobacteriaceae, *Escherichia coli*, *Pseudomonas* species), followed by aerobic gram-positive cocci (*Enterococcus*) (Table 10-5). These pathogens, among others, can occur alone or as part of a mixed infection involving multiple sites. When implementing antibacterial therapy, the following approaches will determine the agent used: (1) surgical prophylaxis (antimicrobial agents used to prevent a commonly encountered infection in the immediate postoperative setting), (2) empiric therapy (antimicrobials initiated without identification of the infecting pathogen), and (3) specific therapy (antimicrobials administered to treat a diagnosed pathogen).

Surgical Prophylaxis

Perioperative prophylaxis reduces the frequency of wound infection in the immediate postoperative setting. At some institutions, however, the incidence of infection without prophylaxis has been reported to be less than 0.5%. Generally, if prophylaxis is administered, the antibiotics should be directed against skin pathogens (e.g., staphylococci, streptococci) and urinary tract pathogens (*E. coli*, *Klebsiella* species, and *Proteus* species). Cefazolin is useful perioperatively and

Table 10-5. Pathogens, sites of infection, and antimicrobial treatment

Organisms	Common site	Antibiotic of choice	Alternative regimen
Aerobic gram-negative rods			
Escherichia coli, Proteus mirablis	Blood, intra-abdominal, wound	TG, ampicillin (if sensitive)	Aminoglycoside, TMP-SMX,
	Urinary tract infection	Ampicillin, TMP-SMX,	fluoroquinolon, FGC, SGC
		cephalosporin, antipseudo-	Fluoroquinolone, aztreonam
		monal penicillin	
Klebsiella pneumoniae, K. oxytoca	Blood, intra-abdominal, lung,	TGC	TMP-SMX, fluoroquinolone,
	urinary tract infection	TMP-SMX, cephalosporins	aminoglycoside, antipseudo-
			monal penicillin, beta-lacta-
			mase inhibitor
			Aminoglycoside, beta-lacta-
			mase inhibitor, fluoro-
			quinolone
Enterobacter aerogenes, E. cloacae	Urinary tract, lung, blood,	Aminoglycoside, TMP-SMX,	Imipenem, antipseudomonal
	gastrointestinal tract, abdomen	fluoroquinolone	penicillin
Serratia marcesens	Urinary tract, blood, lung	TGC	TMP-SMX, antipseudomonal
			penicillin ± aminoglycoside,
			fluoroquinolone, imipenem
Citrobacter freundii	Blood, wound, lung	Aminoglycoside, TMP-SMX,	Imipenem, antipseudomonal
		fluoroquinolone	penicillin. TGC
Pseudomonas aeruginosa	Intra-abdominal, lung, blood	Aminoglycoside + ceftazidime	Imipenem ± aminoglycoside,
		or antipseudomonal	fluoroquinolone, aztreonam ±
		penicillin	aminoglycoside
Acinetobacter anirctus	Blood, lung	Imipenem, aminoglycoside +	Fluoroquinolone, TGC,
		ceftazidime or antipseudo-	ampicillin/sulbactam
		monal penicillin	

Organism	Site	Treatment	Alternatives
Haemophilus influenzae	Paranasal, sinuses, blood, lung	Ampicillin, amoxicillin ± clavulanate, TMP-SMX, SGC, TGC, TMP-SMX	Erythromycin, fluoroquinolone; Beta-lactamase inhibitor
Legionella species	Lung, blood	Erythromycin (± rifampin)	Clarithromycin, TMP-SMX, fluoroquinolone
Anaerobic gram-negative rods *Bacteroides fragilis, Fusobacterium* species	Abdomen, liver abscess, blood	Metronidazole, clindamycin, cefoxitin	Antipseudomonal penicillin, beta-lactamase inhibitor, imipenem
Anaerobic gram-positive rods *Clostridium perfringens*	Skin, wound, abdomen, blood	Penicillin	Clindamycin, metronidazole, antipseudomonal penicillin, imipenem
C. difficile	Gastrointestinal tract	Vancomycin (oral), metronidazole (oral)	Bacitracin (oral), cholestyramine, lactobacilli
Anaerobic gram-positive cocci *Peptococcus, Peptostreptococcus*	Abdomen, skin, wound, blood	Penicillin, ampicillin, amoxicillin	Clindamycin, metronidazole, cephalosprins, erythromycin, vancomycin, imipenem
Aerobic gram-positive cocci *S. aureus* (MS)	Blood, lung, wound, line site	Penicillinase-resistant penicillins, FGC, SGC	Beta-lactamase inhibitor, vancomycin, imipenem, clindamycin, erythromycin, TMP-SMX
S. aureus (MR)	Blood, lung, wound, line site	Vancomycin ± rifampin or gentamicin	Teicoplanin, TMP-SMX

Table 10-5 (continued).

Organisms	Common site	Antibiotic of choice	Alternative regimen
S. epidermidis, Enterococcus faecalis (group D Streptococcus)	Blood, line site wound, intra-abdominal sepsis urinary tract endocarditis	Vancomycin Ampicillin Ampicillin/amoxicillin Penicillin G/ampicillin + gentamicin or streptomycin	TMP-SMX + rifampin. Penicillinase-resistant penicillins, imipenem Vancomycin, penicillin + aminoglycoside, imipenem Vancomycin, penicillin + aminoglycoside Vancomycin + gentamicin or streptomycin
Streptococcus pneumoniae (pneumococcus), Alpha-hemolytic streptococci (viridans)	Blood, CNS, blood endocarditis	Penicillin G or V Penicillin G + gentamicin or streptomycin	Cephalosprins, vancomycin, clindamycin, erythromycin
Listeria monocytogenes	Blood, CNS	Ampicillin or penicillin ± gentamicin	TMP-SMX
Corynebacterium	Blood, wound	Penicillin	Erythromycin
Nocardia	Lung, abscess-skin, CNS	TMP-SMX	Imipenem ± amikacin, amikacin ± TMP-SMX

CNS = central nervous system; FGC = first-generation cephalosporin; SGC = second-generation cephalosporin; TGC = third-generation cephalosporin; TMP-SMX = trimethoprim-sulfamethoxazole; MS = methicillin sensitive; MR = methicillin resistant.

Note:
- Aminoglycosides include gentamicin, tobramycin, and amikacin.
- Antipseudomonal penicillins include piperacillin, mezlocillin, and ticarcillin.
- Penicillinase-resistant penicillins include nafcillin, oxacillin, and dicloxacillin.
- First-generation cephalosporins include cefazolin and cephalexin.
- Second-generation cephalosporins include cefuroxime and cefoxitin.
- Third-generation cephalosporins include cefotaxime, ceftazidime, ceftriaxone, and ceftazidime.
- Fluoroquinolones include ciprofloxacin.
- Beta-lactamase inhibitors include ampicillin/sulbactam, amoxicillin/clavulanate, and piperacillin/tazobactam.

is discontinued after 24 hours to minimize the risk of superinfection with resistant bacterial organisms. Ampicillin/sulbactam has activity against some of the urinary tract gram-negative pathogens (*E. coli* and *Klebsiella*), but choosing the precise antimicrobial should be based on institution-specific susceptibility patterns.

Empiric Therapy

In febrile immunosuppressed transplant patients, there may be an understandable temptation to commence empiric antimicrobial therapy. If the patients are hemodynamically and clinically stable, however, it is often safe to await the results of cultures and then to treat accordingly. In patients with suspected bacterial sepsis, a number of antimicrobials can be selected for treatment. Empiric therapy should be guided by the available clinical information, including the suspected anatomic site of infection, the probable bacterial flora and institution-specific susceptibility patterns, any previously administered antimicrobial therapy, the time following transplant, the severity of renal or hepatic dysfunction, and the net state of immunosuppression. Initial empiric therapy should be broad-spectrum. The duration of empiric therapy is based on the resolution of clinical signs and symptoms of bacterial infection, sterilization of infected sites, and tolerance of the agent (adverse reactions). Once a specific pathogen is isolated and sensitivities are available, a narrow-spectrum agent with appropriate antibacterial activity is substituted to avoid the risk of superinfection. Commonly used agents for empiric therapy include broad-spectrum penicillins (piperacillin), third-generation cephalosporins (ceftizoxime), and beta-lactam plus beta-lactamase inhibitor combinations (ampicillin-sulbactam, ticarcillin-clavulanate, or piperacillin-tazobactam) (Tables 10-5 and 10-6).

Specific Therapy

With the isolation of a specific organism, therapy is focused on the specific pathogen to minimize the risk of superinfection. Examples of specific antimicrobial agents used to treat bacterial pathogens are listed in Table 10-5 and their dosage adjustments in Table 10-6. Because nosocomial gram-negative bacteria are associated with an increase in mortality in allograft recipients, these pathogens warrant additional attention. Organisms such as *Enterobacter cloacae* are generally resistant to third-generation cephalosporins; effective therapies for this pathogen include imipenem, ciprofloxacin, TMP-SMX, or piperacillin. Aminoglycosides, although generally active against *E. cloacae* and the majority of other gram-negatives, should be used judiciously in renal allograft recipients due to the risk of increased nephrotoxicity when administered with cyclosporine. When *Pseudomonas aeruginosa* is suspected or cultured, combination therapy using an antipseudomonal penicillin (piperacillin) or ceftazidime plus an aminoglycoside or fluoroquinolone is recommended for synergistic bactericidal activity and the prevention of resistance.

Another potential concern in the renal transplant patient is the reduction of indigenous anaerobic microflora of the colon secondary to overuse of broad-spectrum antimicrobials. *Clostridium difficile* colitis occurs with any of the above agents and subjects the patient to additional fluid and electrolyte disorders, as well as reduces cyclosporine concentrations. Oral vancomycin is the preferred treat-

Table 10-6. Antimicrobial parenteral dosages in renal insufficiency

Antimicrobial agent	Usual adult dosage	CCr 20–50 ml/min	CCr 10–19 ml/min	CCr <10 ml/min	CSF penetration (%)[a]
Acyclovir	5–10 mg/kg q8h[b]	q12h	q24h	2.5 mg/kg q24h	50%
Amikacin	7.5 mg/kg q12h	7.5 mg/kg/q24h	7.5 mg/kg/q24–48h	3.0–4.5 mg/kg/q72h	Low
Ampicillin	2 g q6h	q6–8h	q12h	0.5–1.0 g q12h	25%
Ampicillin/sulbactam	3 g q6h	q8h	q12h	1.5 g q12h	25%
Aztreonam	1 g q8h	Same as usual adult dosage	q12h	0.5–1.0 g q24h	25%
Cefazolin	1 g q8h	q12h	0.5–1.0 g q12h	0.5–1.0 g q24h	Low
Cefoxitin	1 g q6h	q8h	0.75 mg q12–24h	0.5–1.0 g q12–24h	Low
Ceftazidime	1 g q8h	q12h	q24h	0.5–1.0 g q24h	30–40%
Ceftizoxime	1 g q8h	q12h	0.5–1.0 g q12h	0.5–1.0 g q24h	20–30%
Ceftriaxone	1–2 g q24h	Same as usual adult dosage	Same as usual adult dosage	Same as usual adult dosage	10%
Cefuroxime	0.75 g q8h	q12h	0.75 g q24h	0.75 mg q24h	50%
Ciprofloxacin	0.25–0.75 g PO q12h / 0.2–0.4 g IV q12h	Same as usual adult dosage	Same as usual adult dosage	q24h	Low
Clindamycin	0.6 g/q8h	Same as usual adult dosage	Same as usual adult dosage	Same as usual adult dosage	Low
Erythromycin	0.5–1.0 g q6h	0.5–1.0 g q6h	0.5–1.0 g q6h	500 mg q6h	<25%
Fluconazole	0.2–0.4 g PO q24h / 0.2–0.4 g IV q24h	50–200 g q24h	50–100 g q24h	50–100 mg q24–48h	60–90%
Flucytosine	12.5–37.5 mg/kg q6h	q12h	q24h	12.5–25.0 mg/kg q24h	>50%
Ganciclovir	5 mg/kg q12h	2.5 mg/kg q12h	2.5 mg/kg q24h	1.25 mg/kg q24h	25–65%
Gentamicin	1–2 mg/kg q8–12h	1.2–1.5 mg/kg q12–24h	1.5 mg/kg q24–48h	1.0–1.5 mg/kg q48–72h	Low

Imipenem	0.5 g q6–8h	q8–12h	q12h	0.25 mg q12h	10–40%
Metronidazole	0.5 g IV q8–12h; 0.5g PO q8–12h	Same as usual adult dosage	q12h	q12h	100%
Mezlocillin	5 g q8h	4 g q8h	3 mg q8h	2 mg q8h	<20%
Oxacillin	1–2 g q6h	Same as usual adult dosage	Same as usual adult dosage	Same as usual adult dosage	<25%
Penicillin G	1–2 Million U q4h	q6h	q8h	q12h	30–40%
Piperacillin	5 g q8h	4 g q8h	3 mg q8h	2 mg q8h	30%
Piperacillin/tazobactam	4.5–5.625 g q8h	4.5 g q8h	3.375 g q8h	2.25 g q8h	Low
Tobramycin	1–2 mg/kg q8–12h	1–2 mg/kg q12–24h	1 mg/kg q24–48h	1 mg/kg q48–72h	Low
Trimethoprim/sulfamethoxazole	10 mg/kg/day (TMP) q6–12h	5.0–7.5 mg TMP/day q12h	2.5–5.0 mg TMP/kg/day q24h	1.25–2.50 mg TMP/kg/day q24h	>50%
Vancomycin	1 g IV q12h; 0.125 mg PO q6h	10–15 mg/kg q24–48h	10–15 mg/kg q48–72h	10–15 mg/kg every 4–7 days	Low

TMP = trimethoprim.

[a]Reflects percentage of serum concentration.

[b]Dosage for herpesimplex virus; 200 mg PO five times daily or 400 mg PO tid. Dosage for varicella-zoster virus: 12.5–15.0 mg/kg q8h, or 800 mg PO five times daily for 7 days.

[c]Dosage for gram-negative bacillary infection; *Pneumocystis carinii* pneumonia should be treated with total daily dosage of 15–20 mg/kg (TMP).

ment for severe *C. difficile;* orally administered metronidazole can be used in less severe or vancomycin-intolerant cases.

Legionella Infection

Legionella infections have been described in all organ transplant populations. Risk factors for infection increase with the duration of treatment with corticosteroids, the number of days on a ventilator, and persistent contamination of hospital water supplies despite superheating and hyperchlorination. Pneumonia is usually a manifestation of *Legionella micadadei* and *L. pneumophilia,* but extrapulmonary sites of involvement have been reported (renal, hepatic, CNS). Systemic manifestations of *L. pneumophilia* include a nonproductive cough, temperature-pulse dissociation, abnormalities in hepatic enzymes, diarrhea, hyponatremia, myalgias, and confusion. Radiologic findings include alveolar or interstitial infiltrates, frank cavities, pleural effusions, or lobar consolidation.

Specific *Legionella* nucleic acid probes or direct fluorescent antibodies assist in the rapid identification of BAL or sputum specimens. A urinary *Legionella* antigen can be detected that remains positive for some time after the initiation of therapy. IV erythromycin (500–1,000 mg q6h) should be started with the addition of rifampin (RIF) for severe disease. TMP-SMX, ciprofloxacin, doxycycline, and the macrolides (clarithromycin and azithromycin) have demonstrated some efficacy in *Legionella* infections. The macrolides will increase cyclosporine concentrations, necessitating reduction of cyclosporine or tacrolimus doses.

Mycobacterial Infections

Mycobacterial infections can occasionally be a serious problem in renal allograft recipients and can present as early as 1 month following transplantation. The incidence of active tuberculosis (*Mycobacterium tuberculosis*) in this population is estimated to be 1–4% and may increase as a reflection of the overall escalation of tuberculosis reported in the general population and in HIV-infected patients. Unusual presentations of *M. tuberculosis* infection in the transplant population may delay diagnosis and contribute to the overall morbidity. Disseminated disease in kidney transplant recipients is observed in approximately 40% of patients at the time of diagnosis, with involvement of the skin, skeletal system, and CNS. The presence of granulomata in peripheral tissues is suggestive of disseminated disease.

Treatment. Historically, tuberculosis has been effectively treated in kidney transplant patients; however, with the increase in multidrug-resistant strains, appropriate therapy should include a minimum of four antituberculous agents until sensitivities are known Initial drug regimens should include 2 months of oral INH, 300 mg/day; RIF, 600 mg/day; pyrazinamide (PZA), 30 mg/kg/day; and ethambutol (EMB), 15–25 mg/kg/day or IM streptomycin (SM) 15 mg/kg/day. Of these, at least two agents should be continued for an additional 4–10 months according to susceptibility results (e.g., continue only INH and RIF if susceptible). Although there are no controlled clinical trials in kidney transplant recipients to determine the adequacy of a 12-month regimen, treatment should last for a total of 12 months and for at least 6 months after sputum conversion. Adverse effects associated with antituberculous agents include hepatitis (INH, PZA, RIF in descending order of frequency and severity), neuritis and optic neuropathy (INH, EMB), hearing loss, azotemia (SM), and abdominal discomfort (INH, RIF, EMB, PZA).

Both INH and RIF affect the cytochrome P450 enzyme system (see Chap. 4). INH may lead to accumulation of cyclosporine, whereas RIF is an P450 inducer and lowers cyclosporine concentrations, increasing the risk of rejection due to subtherapeutic levels. These interactions are usually predictable and may occur within 1–3 days of initiating antituberculous therapy; appropriate cyclosporine dosage adjustments and monitoring are required. Atypical nontuberculous pathogens have been reported in renal transplant recipients, including virulent forms (*M. kansasii*, *M. chelonae*, and *M. xenopi*), as well as less virulent species (*M. marinum* and *M. haemophilum*). These pathogens involve the lungs, skin, and bone and can disseminate to other sites.

Fungal Infections

Although the incidence of fungal infections in renal transplant recipients is less than that reported for other solid organ transplant populations, the mortality from fungal infections remains high. Predisposing factors for fungal infection include the use of corticosteroids and antibiotics, the overall state of immunosuppression, the use of indwelling catheters, the duration and the number of surgeries, the disruption of intestinal mucosa, vascular complications, and hyperglycemia. In the immediate postoperative period, candidiasis of the oral, vaginal, or intertriginous areas may be seen. From 1 to 6 months, and occasionally later depending on the state of immunosuppression, the following fungal infections can occur: cryptococcosis (meningitis, pneumonia, ocular disease), aspergillosis (pneumonia, invasive, and disseminated forms), coccidioidomycosis (pneumonia, meningitis, musculoskeletal and skin involvement), and pneumocystosis (pneumonia).

The diagnosis of fungal infection remains problematic and often requires invasive diagnostic techniques such as open lung biopsy for confirmation; clinical specimens may be stained with calcofluor to enhance the detection of fungal elements. The majority of fungal infections involve nosocomially acquired pathogens such as *Candida* species, *Aspergillus* species, *Cryptococcus* species, and the endemic mycoses in appropriate geographic settings (*Coccidioides immitis* and *Histoplasma capsulatum*). Other fungal pathogens observed in renal transplant patients include the dermatophytes (*Trichophyton*, *Microsporum*, and *Epidermophyton*) and hyalohyphomycosis (*Fusarium*, *Penicillium*), which may present locally as cutaneous lesions or with disseminated disease.

Treatment

Amphotericin B is the drug of choice for systemic fungal infections, including candidiasis, cryptococcosis, coccidioidomycosis, and aspergillosis. Amphotericin B is often given with flucytosine (5-FC) in cryptococcal disease. For fungal infections due to aspergillosis, amphotericin B should be initiated at high doses (e.g., 1 mg/kg/day). If response is poor, as evidenced by persistent positive cultures or

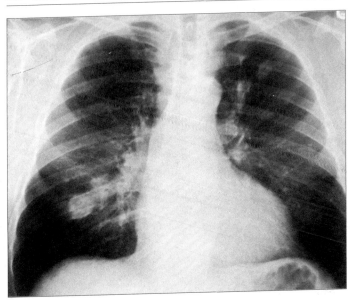

A

Fig. 10-2. Pulmonary apsergillosis following kidney transplantation. Multiple pulmonary nodules with hilar adenopathy are seen on chest radiograph (A). Thoracic computed tomography showing nodules, some with central cavitation (B and C). Chest radiograph showing resolution of pulmonary nodules following amphotericin-intralipid and itraconazole therapy (D).

worsening clinical symptoms, the addition of 5-FC and RIF should be considered based on some evidence for synergy. Adjunctive therapy with macrophage colony-stimulating factor has been attempted for refractory cases of aspergillosis; however, its role in solid organ transplantation remains ill-defined. Figure 10-2 demonstrates the radiologic resolution of invasive pulmonary aspergillosis in a renal transplant recipient using high-dose amphotericin (administered with intralipids) followed by itraconazole therapy. The simultaneous reduction or elimination of immunosuppression should be considered. Ultimately, however, the outcome in kidney transplant patients with disseminated disease is extremely poor regardless of antifungal therapy.

The toxicities of amphotericin are especially concerning in the kidney transplant recipient, and they are often limiting factors in its use. Infusion-related toxicities such as chills, anaphylaxis, hypotension and nausea occur frequently. Nephrotoxic, metabolic, and hematologic abnormalities occur with increased doses or in patients with underlying renal insufficiency. Because of the risk of additive nephrotoxicity, judicious use of amphotericin B is warranted in transplant patients on concomitant nephrotoxic agents such as cyclosporine and tacrolimus. Currently, liposomal encapsulation or incorporation of amphotericin B in a lipid complex (Abelcet) has become a new modality for antifungal therapy with the potential of reducing or delaying toxicity of conventional amphotericin B. Amphotericin B lipid complexes or dispersions

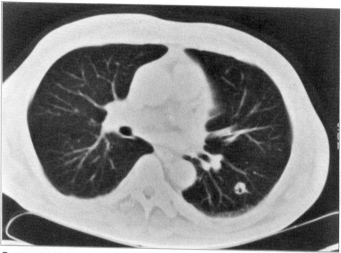

B

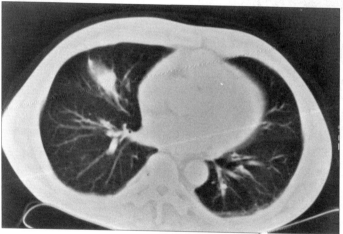

C

are active against *Aspergillus fumigatus, C. albicans, C. guiller-mondi,* and *C. tropicalis,* among other fungal species. The incorporation of amphotericin B into a lipid mixture, however, may affect its functional performance relative to those of non–lipid-associated or unencapsulated drugs. The approved indications for the lipid amphotericin B preparation is invasive aspergillosis—that is, refractory to conventional amphotericin B therapy, or where there is intolerance to conventional amphotericin B therapy. Additional studies will be required in the transplant recipients to determine clinical utility in the treatment or prophylaxis of fungal infections.

Itraconazole can be used in the treatment of histoplasmosis, blastomycosis, sporotrichosis, paracoccidioidomycosis, as well as aspergillo-

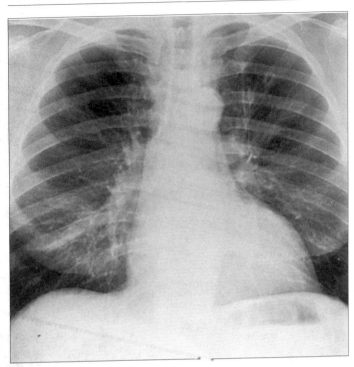

D

Fig. 10-2 *(continued)*.

sis. The activity of itraconazole in vitro appears to be greater than amphotericin B against these pathogens; however, its place in the treatment of immunosuppressed patients remains to be defined. An acid gastric environment is necessary for optimal absorption of itraconazole. Ketoconazole can be used to treat various systemic fungal infections, but due to its variable absorption and toxicity (nausea, vomiting, adrenal suppression, hepatic damage, and drug interactions with cyclosporine), it is less frequently used.

All of the triazole antifungals impair cyclosporine metabolism and increase blood levels (see Chap. 4). This effect is most consistent with ketoconazole; its use may permit a reduction in cyclosporine dose of up to 80%.

Pneumocystosis

P. carinii pneumonia occurs 1–6 months following transplantation. Fever, nonproductive cough, arterial-alveolar mismatching, and diffuse interstitial infiltration or focal air-space consolidation are common manifestations. BAL with transbronchial biopsy is a highly sensitive method for identifying pulmonary disease; a fluorescein-labeled anti-*Pneumocystis* monoclonal antibody improves detectiion in BAL or sputum specimens. First-line treatment is with TMP-SMX at 15–20 mg/kg/day for 14–21 days. Second-line agents include IV pentamidine (3–4 mg/kg/day) and dapsone-trimethoprim (100 mg daily with trimethoprim, 15 mg/kg/day). Adverse effects of trimethoprim include nephrotoxicity, pancreatitis, and marrow suppression; dapsone is associated with hemolytic anemia in G6PD deficiency. Mild to moderate *P. carinii* pneumonia can be treated with atovaquone (750 mg PO tid for 21 days) in patients intolerant to TMP-SMX. Limited data are available with this agent in renal transplant patients. Prophylactic agents in order of efficacy include TMP-SMX (one double-strength tablet bid two times weekly), bimonthly IV pentamidine (4 mg/kg), monthly nebulized pentamidine (300 mg), or dapsone (50–100 mg/day) alone or in combination with trimethoprim (25–50 mg twice weekly).

Viral Infections

Viral infections are a major problem in allograft recipients, particularly between the first to the sixth months post-transplantation. Clinical disease may occur later particularly following intensification of immunosuppression.

Cytomegalovirus

CMV infection occurs primarily after the first month of transplantation, with an estimated incidence of 30–50% depending on the serologic status of the donor and recipient (see Table 10-2). The seronegative recipient of a seropositive donor graft is at the greatest risk, particularly after the use of antilymphocytic preparations, which can reactivate latent infection. CMV causes several clinical syndromes of which fever, often associated with leukopenia, is the most common and pneumonitis, the most serious. Colitis and ulcerative GI lesions, cholecystitis, esophagitis, hepatitis, and retinitis may also occur. CMV is associated with immunomodulatory derangements (e.g., reduced ratio of helper cells to supressor cells) that can lead indirectly to the enhancement of other opportunistic infections and to graft rejection. CMV infection induces antiendothelial cell antibodies, which may be risk factors for both acute and chronic rejection.

   Primary CMV infection represents infection in the previously uninfected seronegative host and may be asymptomatic. **CMV disease** refers to symptomatic CMV infection, which may be further differentiated into the **CMV syndrome** (fever, leukopenia and an increased CMV antigen titer) and **invasive CMV** (e.g., with pneumonitis, hepatitis, and GI involvement proved histologically). **Secondary CMV infection** represents infection in previously infected seropositive hosts caused by either **reactivation** of latent endogenous virus or **reinfection** or **superinfection** with new virus. **Active CMV infection** is a primary or secondary infection that may be asymptomatic or symptomatic and is characterized by viral replication and shedding with a specific immune response to CMV. **Latent CMV infection** represents lifelong persistence of virus without replication in a healthy seropositive host. Immunosuppressive therapy has the capacity to convert latent infection to active infection.

   Factors predisposing to CMV infection include donor CMV seropositive status, recipient CMV seropositive status, the use of blood products from CMV seropositive donors, episodes of acute rejection, the net state of immunosuppression, and the use of antilymphocyte preparations.

Table 10-7. Current diagnosis of cytomegalovirus infection

Method	Description	Comments
Serology	Acute/convalescent CMV IgG or single CMV IgM titer	Serologic response may be slow or absent in primary infection; false positive reactions may occur
Histopathology	Microscopic examination of tissue for inclusion bodies	Insensitive; inclusion bodies may be present only in advanced infection
Other techniques	Polymerase chain reaction and direct culture (shell-vial technique) of bronchoalveolar fluid, buffy coat, tissue material, urine, or throat swab	Detection of CMV from throat swabs, urine, or saliva may not support the presence of CMV disease
	Detection of CMV antigens in tissue (kidney, lung, gastrointestinal tract, blood) by immuno-chemical stain (CMV-labeled monoclonal antibodies)	Immunochemical stains may accelerate detection of CMV antigens in viral culture systems
	Electron microscopic examination of biopsy specimens for CMV	Specialized equipment required

CMV = cytomegalovirus.

Diagnosis. Diagnosis of CMV infection is made by the detection of specific CMV antigens or nucleic acid in tissue or blood specimens (Table 10-7); a monoclonal antibody against early viral antigens can be used to confirm the presence of CMV in cell culture. Serologic detection of specific CMV immunoglobulin G and M by enzyme immunoassay can assist in confirming a CMV infection; an IgG titer equal to or greater than 1:10 is indicative of previous infection, whereas a fourfold increase in IgG or IgM titer that equals or exceeds 1:10 is diagnostic of acute infection. CMV DNA detection by PCR has been attempted in clinical specimens with enhanced sensitivity. Even after successful treatment of symptomatic CMV infection, however, this method may continue to detect CMV DNA despite the disappearance of antigenemia.

Treatment. The availability of effective agents for CMV prophylaxis and treatment has considerably diminished the morbidity and mortality associated with CMV infection. Treatment of active CMV disease includes reduction in the immunosuppressive regimen and administration of intravenous ganciclovir (5 mg/kg bid for 14 days, adjusted for renal dysfunction); an additional period of treatment may be warranted in selected patients. Adverse effects of ganciclovir include reversible dose-related granulocytopenia and thrombocytopenia, fever, rash, seizures, nausea, myalgias, abnormalities in liver enzyme determinations, and, rarely, pancreatitis. Drug interactions include an increased seizure risk when used in combination with acyclovir and imipenem and additive marrow suppression with azathioprine and TMP-SMX. Oral ganciclovir (Cytovene) has become available for suppressive therapy of CMV retinitis in AIDS patients. Ongoing trials in transplant recipients are being conducted to assess its role in primary prophylaxis and suppressive therapy after intravenous therapy.

Experience in treating CMV pneumonitis in bone marrow recipients suggests that the addition of CMV hyperimmune globulin (Cytogam) or IV pooled gammaglobulin may improve the response to ganciclovir. Foscarnet has been used to treat ganciclovir-resistant CMV isolates; however, its use is associated with considerable nephrotoxicity.

Prophylaxis. A rational way to minimize severe CMV infection would be to avoid transplanting CMV-positive kidneys into CMV-negative recipients. Such a policy has been implemented in some transplant centers but has been made largely impractical by the competing need for human leukocyte antigen matching and the shortage of cadaveric kidneys. Several prophylactic regimens have been recommended for the suppression of CMV infection, although none of them are universally accepted. In addition to conflicting data on their effectiveness, their use also depends on economic and logistic considerations.

High-dose oral acyclovir given during the first 3 months post-transplant is moderately effective for CMV prophylaxis in high-risk kidney transplant patients; the efficacy of acyclovir may be increased by adding **CMV hyperimmune globulin**. This preparation has been shown to be of benefit in reducing CMV disease in seronegative recipients of seropositive donor organs. It is not used widely in kidney transplant recipients because of its cost, the logistics of its administration, and the relative infrequency of life-threatening CMV infection in this group. **Preemptive therapy** is the term used to describe the administration of **low-dose IV ganciclovir** (half of the standard treatment dose; see Table 10-6) in high-risk patients during the period of treatment with antilymphocytic preparations. The logic of this approach, which has become popular in many kidney transplant programs, is that antilymphocytic preparations have the capacity to reactivate latent virus, which is then inactivated by the ganciclovir before it becomes clinically manifest.

Herpes Simplex Virus, Varicella-Zoster Virus, Adenovirus, and Epstein-Barr Virus

The most common manifestation of HSV infection in renal transplant patients is herpes labialis, which usually occurs in the first 6 weeks post-transplant. HSV predominates in mucosal surfaces but can, rarely, disseminate to visceral organs. Acyclovir and ganciclovir are active against all herpes viruses in vitro, and both are useful in the treatment or prophylaxis of HSV, with acyclovir as the preferred agent. To treat mucocutaneous infections with HSV, acyclovir can be given IV (5 mg/kg tid for 1 week) or PO (200 mg five times per day, or 400 mg tid). For treatment of encephalitis, acyclovir is given at a higher dosage, 10.0–12.5 mg/kg IV tid for 10 days. IV acyclovir should always be given by slow infusion over several hours to prevent crystallization within the renal tubules; dose adjustment is required in renal insufficiency.

Herpes zoster develops in approximately 10% of organ transplant recipients and may involve two or three adjoining dermatomes. Disseminated VZV, usually as a result of primary VZV infection, is fortunately rare but may cause pneumonia, encephalitis, disseminated intravascular coagulation, and graft dysfunction. Antiviral treatment for VZV includes IV acyclovir, 12.5–15.0 mg/kg tid for 7 days, or 800 mg PO five times daily for 7 days. Ganciclovir and foscarnet are also active against VZV. Famciclovir (500 mg PO tid) can be used for dermatomal zoster.

Adenovirus may cause a self-limiting hemorrhagic cystitis following transplant or may disseminate, causing pneumonia and hepatitis. Treatment options are limited, with the reduction in immunosuppression found to be of some benefit in hemorrhagic cystitis. IV ribavirin has been used experimentally.

EBV infection and its relationship to the development of PTLD is discussed in Chap. 9.

Acute Viral Exposures

Renal transplant recipients who are susceptible to VZV infection are candidates for varicella-zoster immunoglobulin (VZIG) if exposure is considered to be significant (e.g., continuous household or social contact, hospital contact in adjacent beds, prolonged contact with an infectious patient). The complication rate of immunocompromised patients who contract varicella is substantially greater than for healthy individuals. Fortunately, however, at least 90% of adults are seropositive for VZV and are not at risk for primary infection. VZIG is of maximum benefit if administered as soon as possible after the presumed exposure but may be effective given as late as 96 hours after exposure. VZV vaccine is not currently recommended for immunosuppressed patients.

During an outbreak of documented influenza A, vaccination with influenza vaccine and administration with antiviral prophylaxis (rimantadine or amantadine) should follow standard guidelines.

SPECIFIC ORGAN SYSTEM INFECTIONS

The scope of this text does not permit a review of all the potential organ system infections to which the transplant patient is susceptible. Because of their frequency and clinical importance, pneumonitis and urinary tract infection are considered separately.

Pneumonias

Bacterial

Bacterial pneumonias can present at any time post-transplant. Acute onset, cough, productive sputum, and a localized (or occasionally diffuse) pulmonary infiltrate suggest a bacterial process. Pathogens include *Streptococcus pneumoniae, Haemophilus influenzae, Klebsiella pneumoniae,* group A *Streptococcus,* and *Staphylococcus aureus.*

Recently hospitalized and elderly patients are more susceptible to gram-negative pneumonia. *Legionella, Nocardia,* mycobacteria, and

Table 10-8. Pneumonia in the kidney transplant patient

Pathogens	Suggested therapy
Bacteria	
Staphylococcus aureus	Oxacillin, nafcillin, first-generation cephalosporin, vancomycin
Methicillin-resistant *S. aureus*	Vancomycin
Enteric gram-negative bacilli	Third-generation cephalosporin, antipseuodomonal penicillin ± aminoglycoside, ciprofloxacin, imipenem, trimethoprim-sulfamethoxazole
Streptococcus pneumoniae	Penicillin G, first-generation cephalosporin; vancomycin or imipenem may be required for intermediate to penicillin-resistant pneumococci
Legionella pneumophilia	Erythromycin (± rifampin), clarithromycin (mild disease)
Mycobacterial tuberculosis	Isoniazid, rifampin, and pyrazinamide or ethambutol
Nocardia asteroides	Trimethoprim-sulfamethoxazole, sulfisoxazole, minocycline or amikacin and imipenem or third-generation cephalosporin
Fungi	
Cryptococcus neoformans	Amphotericin B ± flucytocine, fluconazole, fluconazole
Aspergillus species	Amphotericin B, itraconazole
Coccidioides immitis	Amphotericin B, fluconazole
Histoplasma capsulatum	Amphotericin B, itraconazole
Candida albicans	Amphotericin B, fluconazole
Non-albicans *Candida* species	Amphotericin B
Pneumoncystis carinii	Trimethoprim-sulfamethoxazole, pentamidine, dapsone + trimethoprim, atovaquone
Viruses	
Cytomegalovirus	Ganciclovir, foscarnet
Herpes group (non-CMV)	Acyclovir, ganciclovir
Varicella-zoster	Acyclovir, famciclovir
Influenza	Amantadine, ramantidine

pneumocystic pneumonia are described above. Therapy is summarized in Table 10-8.

Fungal

Fungal pneumonias in transplant recipients always produce difficult diagnostic and therapeutic dilemmas. *Cryptococcus* infection, *Aspergillus* infection, coccidiodomycosis, and histoplasmosis usually occur after the first post-transplant month. Cryptococcal pneumonia can result from reactivated infection and may produce a unilateral or bilateral interstitial or nodular infiltrate with hilar and mediastinal lymphadenopathy. A respiratory distress syndrome may occur in fulminant cases. BAL, blood, and urine cultures are often positive, and cryptococcal antigen may also be reactive. *Cryptococcus* may disseminate to the skin and CNS. Treatment is with amphotericin B; fluconazole is often added.

Coccidiodomycosis and histoplasmosis are endemic mycoses in the Southwest United States, Midwest, and Mississippi Valley. The diseases may be primary, although reactivation pulmonary disease may occur in heavily immunosuppressed patients. *Histoplasma capsulatum* may be diagnosed histologically or by culture of respiratory, bone, or liver biopsy specimens. Chest radiographic findings range from bilateral patchy infiltrates with hilar adenopathy to miliary infiltrates. *Coccidioides immitis* may be found in pulmonary secretions or at extrapulmonary sites, including the CNS. Chest radiographic findings range from a localized infiltrate with effusion to diffuse bilateral reticulonodular infiltrates.

Aspergillus infection can produce dense and sometimes cavitating pulmonary infiltrates and nodules. Therapy requires high-dose amphotericin followed by itraconazole (see Table 10-8) and reduction of immunosuppression.

Cytomegalovirus

CMV pneumonitis is the most serious complication of CMV infection. The disease typically presents as a nonproductive cough with dyspnea and hypoxemia. CMV can usually be isolated from bronchoalveolar fluid. Bilateral interstitial infiltrates are typically found. Treatment is discussed above.

Urinary Tract Infections

UTIs are most frequent in the early postoperative period but may occur later. Bacteremia or sepsis may result. Catheters, stents, anatomic abnormalities, and neurogenic bladder all predispose to UTIs. The routine post-transplant use of prophylactic antibiotics (TMP-SMX or ciprofloxacin) has reduced the frequency of UTIs to less than 10% and essentially eliminates urosepsis unless urine flow is obstructed. Prophylaxis should start within a few days of the transplant and continue for 3–6 months. The typical pathogens are *E. coli*, *K. pneumoniae*, *Enterobacter* species, *Pseudomonas aeriginosa*, and *Enterococcus*. Pathogens may also reflect hospital-specific nosocomial pathogens such as *Serratia*. UTIs occurring more than 6 months post-transplant often present with pyuria and asymptomatic bacteruria; bacteremia is unusual. Specific therapy is summarized in Tables 10-5 and 10-6.

Perinephric abscesses are unusual; when they occur they are often the result of lymphoceles or other prinephric collections infected by repeated drainage procedures. Fever, graft tenderness, and a typical ultrasound appearance (see Chap. 11) suggest the diagnosis. Common pathogens include staphylococci, enteric gram-negative bacteria, and, rarely, anaerobes or *Candida* species.

SELECTED READINGS

American College of Physicians. *Guide for Adult Immunization* (3rd ed). Philadelphia: American College of Physicians, 1994.

Brayman K. Analysis of infectious complications occurring after solid-organ transplantation. *Arch Surg* 127:38, 1992.

Brown RS, Wake JR, Katzman BA et al. Incidence and significance of *Aspergillus* cultures following liver and kidney transplantation. *Transplantation* 61:666, 1996.

Conti DJ et al. Prophylaxis of primary cytomegalovirus disease in renal transplant recipients, a trial of ganciclovir vs. immunoglobulin. *Arch Surg* 29:443, 1994.

Hibberd PL, Tolkoff-Rubin NE, Conti D et al. Preemptive ganciclovir therapy to prevent cytomegalovirus disease in cytomegalovirus-positive renal transplant recipients. *Ann Intern Med* 123:18, 1995.

Paya CV. Fungal infections in solid-organ transplantation. *Clin Infect Dis* 16:677, 1993.

Rosen HR, Friedman LS, Martin P. Hepatitis C and the renal transplant patient. *Semin Dialysis* 9:39, 1996.

Rubin RH. Infection in the Organ Transplant Patient. In RH Rubin, LS Young (eds), *Clinical Approach to Infection in the Compromised Host.* New York: Plenum, 1994. Pp 629–706.

Rubin RH. Antimicrobial strategies in the care of organ transplant recipients. *Antimicrob Agents Chemother* 37:619, 1993.

Sakhuja V, Vivekanand J, Varma PP et al. The high incidence of tuberculosis among renal transplant recipients in India. *Transplantation* 61:211, 1996.

Tolkoff-Rubin NE, Rubin H. New strategies for the control of viral infection in organ transplantation. *Clin Transplantation* 9:255–259, 1995.

Radiology of Kidney Transplantation

Peter Zimmerman, Nagesh Ragavendra,
Carl K. Hoh, and Zoran L. Barbaric

The clinician evaluating a patient with renal transplant dysfunction
has the choice of a variety of imaging procedures, including ultrasound (US), nuclear medicine studies, computed tomography (CT),
magnetic resonance imaging (MRI), and excretory urography.
Imaging evaluation is usually initiated either with duplex sonography, which provides cross-sectional imaging and physiologic information quickly, noninvasively, and portably; or with nuclear
medicine studies, which provide physiologic information and some
anatomic information. CT provides superb anatomic information,
but it involves the use of iodinated contrast medium and lacks porta-
bility. MRI provides superb anatomic information, can noninvasively image large vessels, and can evaluate function using relatively
non-nephrotoxic contrast medium (gadolinium). MRI, however, is
not portable, is expensive, and currently does not permit guided
interventions or monitoring of critically ill patients. This chapter
emphasizes the use of US and nuclear medicine studies in renal
transplantation, although CT, MRI, and urography may, on occasion, be the optimal imaging modality for certain clinical problems
encountered in renal transplant patients.

RADIOLOGIC EVALUATION OF THE LIVING DONOR

The process of evaluation of a potential living donor is discussed in
Chap. 5. The main reason for subjecting potential living donors to
radiologic investigations is to ensure that, following removal of one
kidney, the donor will be left with an anatomically and functionally
normal kidney, ureter, and lower urinary tract system and to permit
the surgeon to make appropriate technical decisions regarding the
choice of kidney (right or left) and type of vascular anastomosis (see
Chap. 7). The donor radiologic workup has typically consisted of an
intravenous urogram (IVU) followed by angiography.

Helical Computerized Tomography Scan

The helical, or spiral, CT scan followed in the same session by several postcontrast radiographs produces a modified IVU, usually called
a computerized urogram (CTU). This technique is replacing the traditional workup in many centers. The helical CT differs from usual
CT in that IV contrast is injected rapidly (4–5 ml/second), imaging
begins at peak contrast concentration in the aorta (20 seconds after
injection), the beam is collimated to 3 mm, and reconstruction is 2
mm thick. The multitude of images are usually viewed using maximum-intensity projection (MIP). MIP is a computer rendition of all
data made to look like a projectional angiogram that can be rotated
along various planes (Fig. 11-1). The technique of surface shading
renders the surface of the kidney, aorta, and renal arteries totally

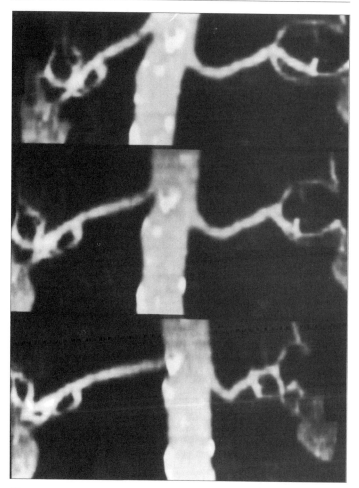

Fig. 11-1. Maximum-intensity projection (MIP) is one of several ways to present a multitude of these axial computed tomography images. An MIP image can be rotated along any axis.

opaque such that is it impossible to see intrarenal details. Artificial shading is applied to give the structures a three-dimensional appearance. Pseudo-cine, or rapid scrolling through a stack of axial images, is probably the cheapest and most accurate method to search for supernumerary renal arteries. The rapid, cine-like mode allows the radiologist to integrate successive images in his or her brain, and the multiple renal arteries are almost always identified. This method may eventually replace renal angiography for the purpose of identifying renal arteries and renal veins in the renal donor evaluation (Fig. 11-2).

The urographic images of the CTU permit an evaluation of the anatomy of the collecting system, ureters, and the bladder. The

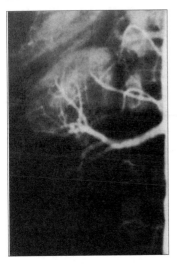 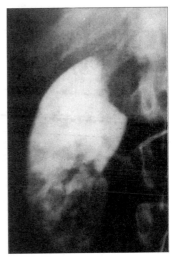

A   B

Fig. 11-2. A. The donor renal angiogram showing a small polar artery. B. Selective renal arteriogram of the main renal artery (nephrogam phase) demonstrates just how much renal parenchyma could be lost if the upper polar artery was ligated during harvest.

entire urinary tract is seen at a glance so that supernumerary ureters, ureteropelvic junction obstruction, papillary necrosis, calyceal diverticula, extrarenal pelves, ureteroceles, urolithiasis, and other abnormalities may be discovered.

RADIOLOGIC TECHNIQUES IN THE EARLY POST-TRANSPLANT PERIOD

The indications for radiologic investigations in the early post-transplant period are discussed in Chap. 8.

Allograft Size

Renal transplant size increases in most acute processes and is thus a nonspecific indicator of renal dysfunction. Some studies have shown that an increase in graft cross-sectional area of more than 10% (measured by US) is suggestive of acute rejection, but the finding is too nonspecific to be clinically reliable. Practical use of allograft size is also limited by the fact that a normally functioning graft may increase in size by up to 30% at 2 months after the time of transplant. The volume of a normal renal transplant usually stabilizes by 6 months.

Collecting System Dilation

Collecting system dilation may be obstructive or nonobstructive in etiology. The degree of dilatation is often expressed via a grading system for US or excretory urography as grades I–IV or as "mild," "moderate," or "severe"; however, both of these systems are subjective. Obstruction of the transplant collecting system may occur sec-

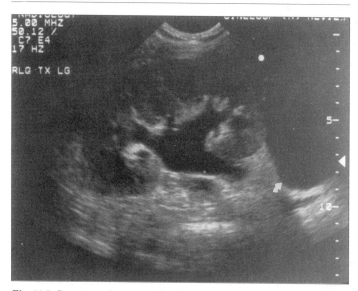

Fig. 11-3. Sonogram demonstrating hydronephrosis secondary to peritransplant fluid collection (arrow).

ondary to extrinsic processes (e.g., peritransplant fluid collection); ureteral stricture (due to vascular insufficiency or rejection); or intraluminal lesions, such as kidney stone, blood clot, or sloughed papilla (Fig. 11-3). A mild, self-limited obstruction may result from early postoperative edema at the ureteroneocystostomy site, and minimal dilation may persist despite resolution of obstruction. Other causes for nonobstructive collecting system dilatation include a full bladder, rejection, infection, and resolved, prior obstruction. This latter cause of nonobstructive dilatation is particularly relevant in the transplanted kidney, since the collecting system is denervated and has no tone.

Use of the resistive index (RI) (see the section on acute rejection) to distinguish obstructive from nonobstructive pyelocaliectasis has been proposed, but data as to its reliability have been inconclusive. The absence of collecting system dilatation does not entirely exclude the possibility of obstruction. The most reliable noninvasive method to diagnose obstruction is progressive collecting system dilatation on serial sonograms. Antegrade pyelography, a mini-nephrostomy, or a Whitaker pressure-flow study may be necessary to determine whether collecting system dilatation is due to an obstructive or nonobstructive etiology. Ureteral obstruction on a nuclear medicine ^{99m}Tc DTPA, ^{99m}Tc MAG 3, or ^{131}I hippurate [131]I (OIH) image (Table 11-1) typically shows normal perfusion and parenchymal uptake but prolonged pelvic retention of activity.

Peritransplant Fluid Collections

Peritransplant fluid collections may be produced by lymphoceles, urinomas, hematomas, and abscesses; all of these may compress the ureter and iliac veins, resulting in hydronephrosis and lower-

Table 11-1. Radiopharmaceuticals used in the evaluation of renal transplants

Isotope carriers	Physiologic property
^{99m}Tc or ^{111}In DTPA (diethylenetriaminepentaacetate)	>95% excreted by glomerular filtration, <5% excreted by tubular secretion, no resorption; therefore, useful for assessing the GFR.
^{51}Cr EDTA (ethyldiaminetetraacetic acid)	>95% excreted by glomerular filtration, however, unable to image due to ^{51}Cr energy; therefore, useful in nonimaging scintillation methods (not available in the United States).
^{131}I or ^{123}I OIH (orthoiodohippurate)	20% excreted by glomerular filtration, 80% excreted by tubular secretion on a first pass; therefore, useful for assessing ERPF. Disadvantage: Increased radiation dose to patient with obstruction or renal failure.
^{99m}Tc MAG 3 (mercaptoacetyltriglycine)	Similar to OIH but labeled with ^{99m}Tc, which is a better isotope for imaging than with ^{131}I.
^{99m}Tc DMSA (dimercaptosuccinate)	Only 7–14% excreted into urine, binds to sulfhydryl groups in perfused renal cortical tubule cells; therefore, useful in imaging regions of functioning versus infarcted renal cortex tissue.
^{99m}Tc GHA (glucoheptonate)	>50% excreted by glomerular filtration, <50% excreted by tubular secretion, 10% bound to tubular cells like DMSA; therefore, useful for assessing a combination of GFR, ERPF, and the amount and shape of functioning renal cortical tissue. Disadvantage: More difficult to accurately estimate GFR or ERPF
^{111}In white blood cell ^{111}In lymphocytes ^{111}In platelets ^{125}I or ^{131}I fibrinogen ^{67}Ga	Localizes in inflammatory tissue; therefore, maybe useful in detecting transplant rejection.

Cr = chromium; Ga = gallium; I = iodine; In = indium; OIH = orthoiodohippurate; Tc = technetium; DMSA = dimercaptosuccinate; GFR = glomerular filtration rate; ERPF = effective renal plasma flow.

extremity edema. They all manifest as fluid collections on cross-sectional imaging studies (US, MRI, CT) or as photopenic regions on scintigrams. Although there are imaging features suggestive of the nature of the fluid collection, their appearance is usually not sufficiently specific; imaging-guided aspiration is often necessary.

Hematomas

Hematomas are common in the immediate postoperative period, may be extrarenal or subcapsular in location, and usually resolve spontaneously. They may also occur after a biopsy or are due to rupture of a graft pseudoaneurysm. On occasion, the hematoma may be large enough to obstruct the ureter. The sonographic appearance of a hematoma varies with time, being echogenic in the acute phase and decreasing in echogenicity as clot lysis occurs. An acute hematoma is of high attenuation on CT and also decreases with time. The signal intensity of a hematoma on MRI is quite variable.

Urinomas

Urinomas due to extravasation of urine from the renal pelvis, ureter, or ureteroneocystostomy usually occur in the first 1–3 weeks following transplantation and may be due to disruption of the ureterovesical anastomosis, incomplete bladder closure, ischemia of the collecting system, postbiopsy injury, or severe obstruction.

Ultrasonography reveals a nonspecific, usually nonseptated, fluid collection, often adjacent to the lower pole of the transplant. The CT appearance of a urinoma is a peritransplant fluid collection that may contain contrast opacified fluid that is isodense to collecting system fluid if the leak is active at the time of the scan. MRI reveals a fluid collection that has identical signal characteristics to urine in the bladder. The leak may be extraperitoneal, intraperitoneal, or both, and in the latter circumstance, ascites may also be present. Characterization of the fluid can be achieved by obtaining a sample via US-guided aspiration and then determining the creatinine concentration (see Chap. 8).

Cystography is the examination of choice to confirm or exclude the bladder as the source of leak. If the bladder is not the source, the extravasation must be from above the ureterovesical anastomosis. If kidney function is adequate, a nuclear medicine study or a urogram may visualize the urinoma, although the precise location of the leak may be difficult to identify. The nuclear medicine images typically show abnormal accumulations of activity outside of the collection system (Fig. 11-4). Occasionally, this finding may be confused with ureteral stasis, in which case, the abnormal accumulation will resolve when the patient voids or is given IV furosemide. Antegrade pyelography is the most accurate and definitive method for determining the extravasation site.

Lymphoceles

Lymphoceles are the most common type of peritransplant fluid collection and are the product of extraperitoneal or renal lymphatic disruption at surgery or during graft harvesting (see Chap. 7). They usually occur several weeks to months after surgery. Small lymphoceles are common and are usually asymptomatic, but larger ones may cause obstruction.

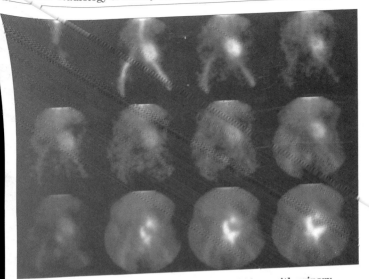

Fig. 11-4. ⁹⁹ᵐTc DTPA images of a transplanted kidney with urinary extravasation seen as an enlarging irregular activity between the kidney and urinary bladder.

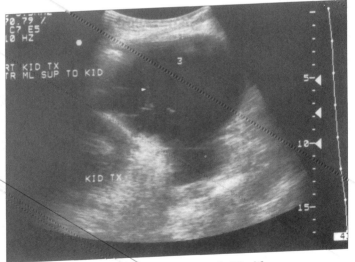

Fig. 11-5. Sonogram demonstrating lymphocele (3) with septations (arrowhead).

The typical sonographic appearance of a lymphocele is a fluid collection inferior and medial to the transplant that often contains septations and low-level echoes (Fig. 11-5). The MRI signal characteristics of a lymphocele tend to be low-signal intensity on T1-weighted images, and high-signal on T2-weighted images.

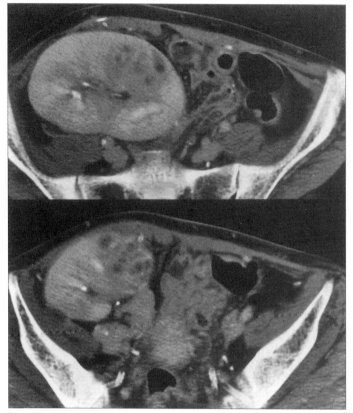

Fig. 11-6. Abscess in a renal allograft. There is a heterogeneous mass on contrast-enhanced computed tomography. Many small compartments preclude percutaneous drainage. Renal function was surprisingly well-preserved. Abscess resolved after intensive antibiotic therapy.

Abscesses

A peritransplant abscess is usually secondary to infection of a preexisting fluid collection and generally occurs 4–5 weeks after transplantation. The sonographic appearance is a fluid collection that contains debris, low-level echoes, and occasionally gas, the latter of which is manifest as mobile, nondependent, echogenic foci with "dirty" shadowing or "ring-down" artifact.

The CT appearance is a heterogeneous fluid attenuation lesion (Fig. 11-6) that may contain gas. In the acute setting, cross-sectional imaging techniques (US, CT) allow rapid diagnosis and potential treatment of a suspected abscess by providing guidance for aspiration and drainage. The absence of any imaging features suggestive of an abscess does not exclude the presence of infection.

Radiopharmaceutical agents such as indium 111-white blood cells (^{111}In WBC), ^{111}In lymphocytes, ^{111}In platelets, iodine 131-fibrinogen, (^{131}I fibrinogen), or gallium 67 (^{67}Ga) localize in inflamma-

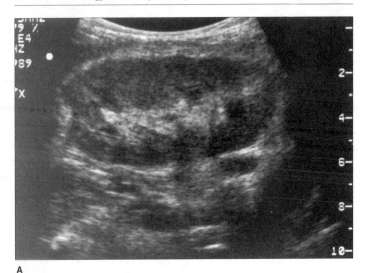

A

Fig. 11-7. A. Sonogram of normal transplant kidney. B. Sonogram of
transplant undergoing rejection reveals graft enlargement, decreased
echogenicity of renal sinus (compare to echogenic sinus in A), and
obscured corticomedullary delineation. Margins of graft marked by
arrows.

tory tissue and may be helpful in detecting a renal or perirenal
abscess; a rejecting transplant, however, may also "light up." With
these nuclear medicine techniques, the radiopharmaceutical is
injected and allowed to accumulate. Images are acquired at 1–2
days for ^{111}In-labeled blood products and up to 3 days postinjection
for [67]Ga.

Acute Rejection

A variety of morphologic alterations may occur with acute rejection. All of these abnormalities may be seen with other medical
complications of transplantation. Many of them are very subjective; therefore, these findings are not sufficiently sensitive or
specific to definitively diagnose rejection and obviate the need for
biopsy. These sonographic abnormalities include graft enlargement, obscured corticomedullary definition, decreased echogenicity of the renal sinus, thickened urothelium, prominent
hypoechoic medullary pyramids, increased or decreased cortical
echogenicity, and scattered heterogeneous areas of increased
echogenicity, the latter probably representing foci of hemorrhage
(Fig. 11-7A and 11-7B).

With the advent of duplex sonography (combining gray-scale
imaging with Doppler capability), it was hoped that the physiologic parameters that could be measured with this technique
would be diagnostic of rejection. The major parameter studied
was vascular resistance (impedance), which is quantified by the
resistive index (RI = peak systolic velocity minus end diastolic
velocity divided by peak systolic velocity) or the **pulsatility index**
(PI = peak systolic velocity minus end diastolic velocity divided

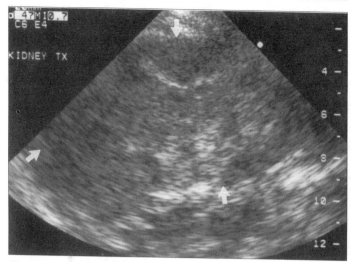

B

by the mean velocity). These indices are indeed often elevated in rejection (Fig. 11-8), but since any cause of renal dysfunction may increase vascular resistance in the kidney, the finding of an elevated RI is nonspecific. Elevation of the RI (greater than 0.9) has been reported in rejection, severe acute tubular necrosis (ATN), renal vein obstruction, pyelonephritis, extrarenal compression, obstruction, and cyclosporin toxicity.

Duplex Sonography

Duplex sonography combines a two-dimensional image with flow information, the latter being in the form of color or **pulsed Doppler.** This technique employs the same sound waves as real-time imaging but processes frequency shifts in the returning echoes to measure the velocity of blood flow within the vessels. Color Doppler sonography provides an estimate of the mean velocity of flow within vessel by color-coding the information and displaying it superimposed on the gray-scale image. Pulsed Doppler allows a sampling volume to be positioned in a vessel visualized on the gray-scale image and provides a spectrum, or graph, of velocities of blood within the gate plotted as a function of time. A readout of absolute velocities and calculation of the RI and PI are obtained using a spectrum from pulsed Doppler. It should be noted that since the Doppler equation uses the angle between the beam axis and the vessel to calculate the velocity (performed by the machine software) and that since this angle is estimated by the sonologist, incorrect angle correction can yield spurious velocities.

Nuclear Medicine Evaluation of Graft Dysfunction

Transplant dysfunction can be evaluated with filtered or tubular-secreted radiopharmaceuticals using a three-phase approach. The first phase assesses the perfusion and is also known as the angiographic phase or the first-pass study. The second phase is the

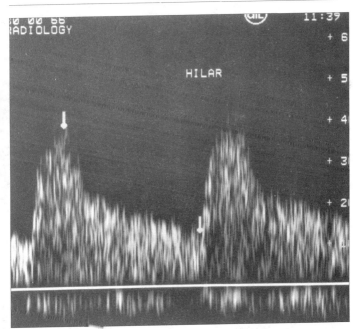

A

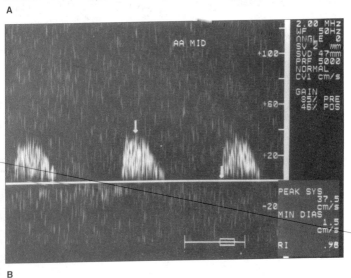

B

Fig. 11-8. A. Normal pulsed-gate Doppler spectrum from kidney transplant with considerable flow throughout diastole and normal RI (0.65). B. Doppler spectrum of graft undergoing acute rejection with no diastolic flow (RI = 1). This is a nonspecific indicator of graft dysfunction.

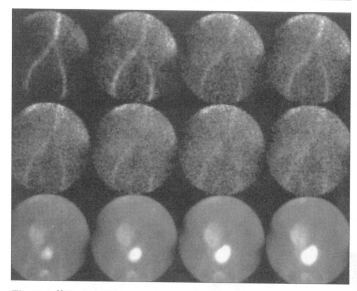

Fig. 11-9. ^{99m}Tc MAG3 images of a transplanted kidney with severe acute rejection. Note the poor perfusion to the transplant (delayed renal visualization) in the initial images. Overall reduction in glomerular filtration is represented by the high surrounding background tissue activity, poor parenchymal washout of accumulated tracer in the tubules, and reduced collecting system or urinary bladder activity.

parenchymal phase, during which the accumulation of tracer in the renal parenchyma reflects the physiologic mode of clearance of that radiopharmaceutical (i.e., filtered or secreted). The third phase is the excretory phase, which reflects the glomerular filtration rate (GFR) and permits an assessment of the integrity of the ureteral system.

Typically, acute rejection appears on nuclear medicine ^{99m}Tc DTPA, ^{99m}Tc MAG 3, or ^{131}I OIH scans as delayed transplant visualization (decreased perfusion) on the first-pass renal scintangiography phase, with poor parenchymal uptake and high background activity (poor renal function and clearance) in the second and third phases (Fig. 11-9). Transplant rejection may also be detected by several static imaging techniques. Increased uptake can be seen with ^{67}Ga, ^{131}I- or ^{125}I-labeled fibrinogen, ^{99m}Tc sulfur colloid, or ^{111}In-labeled blood components. Unfortunately, the low specificity of uptake of these agents prevents them from being of much value in the differential diagnosis of graft dysfunction.

Acute Tubular Necrosis

On nuclear medicine imaging studies, ATN typically shows good renal perfusion on the first-pass phase with ^{99m}Tc DTPA, ^{99m}Tc MAG 3, or ^{131}I OIH. On the second and third phases, ^{99m}Tc DTPA shows poor parenchymal accumulation and washout of the radiotracer due to decreased glomerular filtration (Fig. 11-10). In addition, high surrounding tissue background activity is seen due to

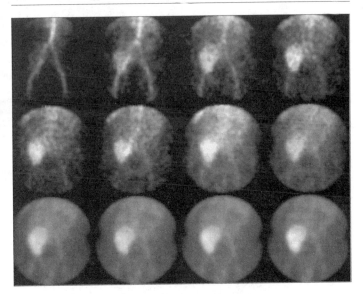

Fig. 11-10. ⁹⁹ᵐTc DTPA images of a transplanted kidney with acute tubular necrosis. Note the well-preserved perfusion to the transplant (prompt renal visualization) in the initial stages. Overall reduction in glomerular filtration is represented by the high surrounding background tissue activity, poor parenchymal washout of accumulated tracer in the tubules, and no collecting system or urinary bladder activity. A similar pattern is seen with ⁹⁹ᵐTc MAG3 in acute tubular necrosis.

poor overall plasma clearance of the radiotracer. With ⁹⁹ᵐ Tc MAG 3 and ¹³¹I OIH radiopharmaceuticals, preserved parenchymal accumulation is seen in the second phase due to relatively preserved renal blood flow and tubular secretion. In the third phase, however, there is a similar poor washout of the accumulated renal parenchymal activity due to diminished glomerular filtration. These findings are consistent with the pathophysiology of ATN, in which renal blood flow is preserved relative to glomerular filtration.

Post-Transplant Vascular Complications

Arterial Thrombosis

Renal arterial thrombosis is an uncommon complication of transplantation and usually occurs in the early postoperative period. The most common causes are faulty surgical anastomoses, severe acute rejection, and progression of a stenosis to thrombosis. The findings in color and pulsed Doppler imaging consist of absent arterial and venous blood flow within the graft. There is some controversy regarding the necessity of further imaging to confirm this diagnosis, as there are several reported cases in which no flow was demonstrated by Doppler but digital subtraction angiography revealed patent vessels.

The ⁹⁹ᵐTc DTPA flow scan shows lack of perfusion, absent visualization of the transplanted kidney, poor background clearance of activity, and sometimes a photopenic space in the transplant bed

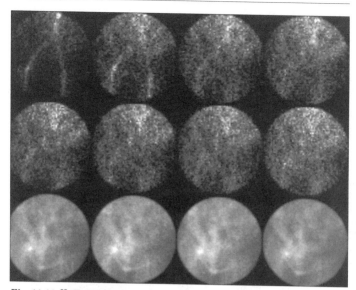

Fig. 11-11. ^{99m}Tc DTPA images of a transplanted kidney with renal artery thrombosis. Note the absence of renal blood flow (nonvisualization of the transplant in the images) and absence of filtration (no collecting system activity and high background tissue activity).

(Fig. 11-11). Renal vein thrombosis, acute cortical necrosis, and hyperacute rejection may all have similar scintigraphic findings.

Infarction

Acute segmental infarction may be diagnosed with Doppler sonography by demonstration of lack of flow to the infarcted parenchymal region. This diagnosis is facilitated by use of color Doppler, which provides a global evaluation of flow to the organ and helps identify segmental arteries, which can then be interrogated individually with pulsed Doppler.

Segmental renal infarction on a ^{99m}Tc DMSA, ^{99m}TcMAG3, or ^{99m}Tc GHA scan (see Table 11-1) appears as a wedge-shaped, "cold" defect. DMSA radiopharmaceutical binds to sulfhydryl groups in perfused renal cortical tubule cells, allowing the visualization of the mass of functioning renal tissue.

Renal Vein Thrombosis

Renal vein thrombosis is an uncommon complication of transplantation that usually occurs in the first postoperative week. The sonographic diagnosis is mainly dependent on the Doppler portion of the examination, as the gray-scale diagnosis is limited by the difficulty of direct visualization of the anechoic or hypoechoic acute thrombus and the nonspecificity of the frequently associated graft swelling and hypoechogenicity. The combination of Doppler findings of very high impedance renal arterial waveforms with reversed, prolonged diastolic flow, a spike-like systolic component, and no detectable venous flow in the graft is highly suggestive of renal vein thrombosis (Fig. 11-12). It

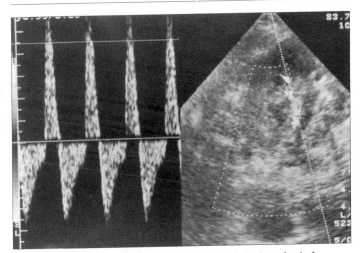

Fig. 11-12. Duplex sonogram of transplant renal vein thrombosis demonstrates reversed flow in diastole and a spike-like systolic peak. No venous flow was detectable in the kidney, renal hilum, or location of renal vein.

should be noted that reversal of diastolic flow per se is a nonspecific finding that is reflective of increased arterial impedance in the graft. It may also be seen in ATN, acute rejection, and severe obstruction.

Chronic Rejection

In chronic rejection, there is gradual deterioration of kidney function, and the allograft is usually decreased in size. Angiographic findings include decreased blood flow and reduction of the number of arteries, which may be narrow and irregular. The nephrogram is patchy. Sonographic findings include decreased size of kidney, cortical thinning, and altered cortical echogenicity, often with increased echogenicity. Doppler sonography may show a nonspecific elevation in resistive index.

Renal Artery Stenosis

Renal scintangiography may be very useful in the diagnosis of renal artery stenosis (RAS) in a native kidney because the contralateral kidney acts as a control for comparison. In the transplanted kidney with RAS, there may be a delayed blush on scanning, but in the absence of a paired kidney, this finding is too nonspecific to be diagnostically reliable.

The diagnosis of RAS by Doppler sonography is made by demonstration of a focal, segmental region of flow abnormality, characterized by elevated peak systolic velocities and turbulent flow (Fig. 11-13). Various threshold values for peak systolic velocity have been proposed for optimal detection of RAS, ranging from 100 cm/second to 190 cm/second; reported sensitivities and specificities range from fair to excellent. The accurate calculation of velocity by the machine's software, however, is highly dependent on the accuracy of the operator's estimate of the angle of insonation, and errors in this regard can yield spuriously elevated velocities. The accuracy of this estimate

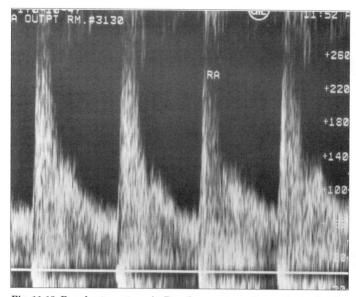

Fig. 11-13. Renal artery stenosis. Doppler spectrum demonstrates focal elevated peak systolic velocity (faster than 260 cm/second) with mild spectral broadening at the anastamosis.

("angle correction") is dependent on the adequacy of delineation of the course of the renal artery, which is often small and tortuous and also may course in a plane not demonstrable by the two-dimensional color Doppler image. Color Doppler, by providing a map of the vascular anatomy, is very helpful in tracing a vessel and therefore in determining the appropriate angle. A confident diagnosis of RAS using Doppler sonography can be made if the characteristic findings occur in a well-delineated vessel, allowing accurate angle correction. Conversely, high velocities without associated turbulence in a region where the accuracy of angle correction is equivocal must be viewed with skepticism. Angiography remains the gold standard for diagnosis of RAS, and the threshold for performance of this study remains a matter of clinical judgment (see Chaps. 7 and 9). CO_2 angiography provides a useful alternative to nephrotoxic iodinated contrast agents.

Arteriovenous Fistulas

Postbiopsy arteriovenous fistulas most often resolve spontaneously but can produce persistent hematuria or hypertension. Grayscale sonography cannot identify these small vascular communications, but they are readily demonstrated on color Doppler as an area of artifactual color assignment in the renal parenchyma (Plate 2). This finding is believed to be due to high-velocity flow in the fistula, which results in localized turbulence and vessel wall vibrations that are transmitted to the perivascular tissues. The vibrating interfaces in the perivascular tissue produce phase shifts in the reflected sound wave and result in random color assignment in this region. This phenomenon is

essentially the Doppler equivalent of a bruit. Once an area of suspicion is identified, the fistulized vessels may be visualized on
color Doppler by virtue of their high-velocity flow. Confirmation of
the presence of an arteriovenous fistula is achieved by performing
waveform analysis with pulsed Doppler and by demonstrating
high-velocity, low-resistance flow in the supplying artery and arterialization (highly pulsatile flow) of the waveform in the draining
vein. A focal, intrarenal arterial stenosis can produce high-velocity flow and tissue vibration, thereby mimicking a fistula, but no
changes in the venous waveform should occur.

Doppler sonography is readily able to demonstrate many fistulas and should be the initial, primary imaging modality. If no fistula can be demonstrated sonographically in a patient with
persistent gross hematuria and hypertension, angiography may
be necessary. Angiography is the examination of choice for defining the extent of the fistula and for treatment planning.
Superselective occlusion of the segmental or interlobar branches
is possible using a variety of occlusive devices, including steel
coils and detachable balloons.

Pseudoaneurysms

Pseudoaneurysms in a renal transplant may be intrarenal, usually secondary to a biopsy, or less commonly, extrarenal, usually
due to faulty surgical anastomosis or perianastomotic infection.
Extrarenal pseudoaneurysms have a much higher risk of spontaneous rupture and are therefore treated as a relative surgical
emergency. Arteriovenous fistulas may be associated with pseudoaneurysms. The sonographic findings are the same for intrarenal
and extrarenal pseudoaneurysms and consist of a spherical fluid
collection that may or may not contain thrombus. Color Doppler
reveals swirling internal flow (Plate 3) and occasionally adjacent
tissue vibrations.

Measurement of Glomerular Filtration Rate

Clinicians generally rely on the serum creatinine level as a marker
of graft function, and although this simple test is indisputably
invaluable in transplant management, its accuracy as a marker of
GFR is inconsistent. In chronic renal failure with proteinuria, tubular secretion of creatinine may form a significant percentage of total
creatinine excretion and overestimation of GFR results.
Radiolabeled DTPA, EDTA, and iothalamate are all accurate filtration markers that, like inulin, reach the urine by filtration but without any element of tubular secretion or reabsorption. The
clearances of these compounds are equivalent to the "classic" chemical inulin clearance. They are more convenient to use than inulin,
since their plasma and urine levels can be measured with a scintilla-
tion counter.

The best isotopic techniques for measuring GFR are true clearance techniques during which, after intravenous injection and
bladder emptying, serial blood and urine samples are taken over
several hours and GFR is calculated from the standard clearance
formula. GFR can also be extrapolated from the disappearance
curve of the plasma isotope concentration, the so-called plasma
clearance.

SELECTED READINGS

Bude RO, Rubin JM. Detection of renal artery stenosis with Doppler sonography: It is more complicated than originally thought. *Radiology* 196:612, 1995.

Budihna NV, Milcinski M, Kajtna-Koselj M, Malovrh M. Relevance of ^{99m}Tc DMSA scintigraphy in renal transplant parenchymal imaging. *Clin Nucl Med* 19:782, 1994.

Grant EG, Perrella RR. Wishing won't make it so: Duplex Doppler sonography in the evaluation of renal transplant dysfunction. *AJR Am J Roentgenol* 153:538, 1990.

Grenier N, Douws C, Morel D et al. Detection of vascular complications in renal allografts with color Doppler flow imaging. *Radiology* 178:217, 1991.

Griffin JF, McNicholas MMJ. Morphological appearance of renal allografts in transplant failure. *J Clin Ultrasound* 20:529, 1992.

Harrison KL, Nghiem HV, Coldwell DM, Davis CL. Renal dysfunction due to arteriovenous fistula in a transplant recipient. *J Am Soc Neph* 5:1300, 1994.

Kuo PC, Peterson J, Semba C et al. CO_2 angiography—A technique for vascular imaging in renal allograft dysfunction. *Transplantation* 61:652, 1996.

Middleton WD, Kellman GM, Melson GL et al. Post biopsy renal transplant arteriovenous fistulas: Color Doppler US characteristics. *Radiology* 171:253, 1989.

Phillips AO, Deane C, O'Donnell P et al. Evaluation of Doppler ultrasound in primary non-function of renal transplants. *Clin Transplantation* 8:83, 1994.

Rigg HM, Proud G, Taylor RM. Urological complications following renal transplantation: A study of 1016 consecutive transplants from a single centre. *Transpl Int* 7:120, 1994.

Rubin GD, Alfrey EJ, Dake MD et al. Assessment of living renal donors with spiral CT. *Radiology* 195:457, 1995.

Swierzewski SJ III, Konnak JW, Ellis JH. Treatment of renal transplant ureteral complications by percutaneous techniques. *J Urol* 150:1115, 1993.

Pathology of Kidney Transplantation

Cynthia C. Nast and Arthur H. Cohen

Structural abnormalities in the transplanted kidney may be assessed by either of two methods: standard tissue histopathology of a biopsy or transplant nephrectomy or cytologic evaluation of cells aspirated from the graft using a thin needle (Table 12-1). The core biopsy typically is regarded as the "gold standard," whereas aspiration cytology, while clinically valuable and quite accurate in experienced hands, is somewhat limited as a procedure by the lack of trained individuals to interpret the material. In this chapter, these techniques are considered separately, although the information obtained from them is often complementary and certain important concepts and actual lesions described for one method bear directly on an understanding of the other.

KIDNEY TRANSPLANT HISTOPATHOLOGY

Core Needle Biopsy

Indications and Technique

Kidney transplant biopsies are performed at times of graft dysfunction when the etiology cannot be accurately elucidated by clinical or noninvasive techniques. More precise indications for biopsy are reviewed in Chaps. 8 and 9. Transplant programs vary in their reliance on biopsies and the clinical setting in which biopsies are performed.

Preparations for transplant biopsy are similar to those for biopsy of the native kidney. Informed consent is required from patients, who should be specifically warned of the risk of bleeding and occasional damage to the graft (see the section on complications of core needle biopsy). Before biopsy, coagulation studies are usually performed, although in the absence of liver disease, thrombocytopenia, or a clinical history of bleeding, these may not be necessary. The blood pressure should be controlled to less than 160/100 mm Hg.

The locations of the graft and biopsy site can be determined by palpation or by ultrasound guidance. A small pillow or towel roll in the small of the patient's back may facilitate palpation. Ultrasound offers the advantage of more precise localization of the graft and its depth and may reduce the frequency of inadequate specimens. Ultrasound may detect perinephric fluid collections or hydronephrosis. It is unwise to biopsy through a fluid collection because of the inability to adequately tamponade the biopsy site. Significant hydronephrosis should be relieved before the biopsy is performed, since it may be the cause of the graft dysfunction; a small blood clot after the biopsy may exaggerate the degree of obstruction. Generally, the upper or lower poles of the transplant are sought, depending on which is more easily palpated or near the surface. Disposable automatic spring-loaded needles (18-gauge is usually adequate) have largely replaced the traditional modified 14-gauge VIM-Silverman needle and may be less traumatic to the kidney. The site chosen for the biopsy is locally anesthetized with 1% lidocaine, and a small stab

Table 12-1. Diagnostic capabilities of histologic and cytologic techniques for evaluation of kidney transplants

Lesion	Fine-needle aspiration	Core biopsy
Acute cellular rejection	Yes	Yes
Acute vascular rejection	No	Yes
Acute cyclosporine toxicity	Yes	Yes
Acute tubular necrosis	Yes	Yes
Viral infection	Yes	No
Allograft rupture	No	No
Bacterial infection	Yes	Yes
Infarction	Yes	Yes
Chronic transplant rejection	No	Yes
Chronic cyclosporine toxicity	No	Yes
Glomerular lesions	No	Yes
Recurrent nonglomerular disorders	No	Yes

wound in the skin is made to facilitate the passage of the needle. Precise instructions for use of the newer needles are provided in the package inserts. The needles are advanced up to the depth assigned by ultrasound or until an increase in resistance is felt as the needle makes contact with the kidney. When the automatic needles are used, it may be advisable to withdraw the needle slightly before taking the sample to avoid excessive depth.

Two biopsy cores should be adequate. It is advisable to inspect the specimen immediately with a stereomicroscope to ensure adequacy. As soon as the needle is withdrawn, hemostasis should be augmented by manual compression or with a sandbag. Postbiopsy orders should include observation of the patient's vital signs every 15 minutes for at least 2 hours and then hourly for several hours. Patients initially should be immobile; in the absence of macroscopic hematuria, ambulation can begin after 6–8 hours. Many transplant centers permit outpatients to go home the same day as the biopsy.

Complications of Core Needle Biopsy

Core needle biopsy is an invasive technique and is not risk-free; these risks must be weighed against the benefit gained from the information obtained from the procedure. Careful assessment of potential risks and benefits must precede every decision to subject a patient to a biopsy.

All major complications following needle biopsy manifest themselves as perinephric or urinary bleeding. Transient macroscopic hematuria is common and is of little clinical significance. Macroscopic hematuria follows approximately 3% of biopsies and may prolong hospitalization or lead to blood transfusion or placement of a bladder catheter for clot drainage. Ureteral obstruction occasionally occurs, requiring placement of a percutaneous nephrostomy; massive hemorrhage necessitating surgical exploration, graft nephrectomy, or angiographic embolization is rare. Postbiopsy arteriovenous fistulas may sometimes be detected by Doppler ultrasound and can usually be treated expectantly. Angiographic embolization may occasionally be required, and graft loss has been reported.

Specimen Handling

Detailed methods for handling tissue specimens are beyond the scope of this chapter. For all specimens, portions are obtained for each of the three traditional methods of evaluating renal parenchyma: light microscopy, electron microscopy, and immunofluorescence. For the initial biopsy, all methods should be used; for subsequent biopsies, electron and immunoflourescent microscopies are performed only if indicated. This approach allows the pathologist to obtain maximal diagnostic and prognostic information. In selected instances, rapid processing or frozen sections can be performed on the tissue placed in fixative for light microscopy when an immediate assessment of the changes in the graft is necessary for initiating or modifying therapy.

Transplant Rejection

Traditionally, three major forms of rejection are recognized: **hyperacute**, **acute**, and **chronic**. Each has reasonably distinctive changes, although acute and chronic rejection may be present simultaneously, resulting in a mixture of histopathologic features. Pathologic findings in the major lesions responsible for functional impairment of the graft are shown in Table 12-2.

Hyperacute Rejection

Hyperacute rejection is produced by preformed cytotoxic antibodies and is an infrequent event as long as the pretransplant crossmatch is negative (see Chaps. 0 and 5) It becomes manifested shortly after vascular anastomoses are established. It is characterized by rapid and widespread vascular thrombosis, predominantly affecting arteries, arterioles, and glomeruli, often with polymorphonuclear leukocytes incorporated in the thrombi. The kidney is usually cyanotic, slightly edematous, and flaccid, and urine production suddenly ceases or does not begin at all. If the kidney is not removed immediately, extensive cellular necrosis ensues, followed after 24 hours by numerous cortical and medullary infarcts. Immunofluorescence may disclose capillary and arterial wall IgG or IgM, C3, and fibrin, with fibrin also in the thrombi. Electron microscopy in the early lesions indicates degeneration and early necrosis of vascular endothelium.

Hyperacute rejection needs to be differentiated from other circumstances in which extensive vascular thrombi occur. The differential diagnoses include physical perfusion-related injury to vascular endothelium and injury caused by cold-reacting IgM antibodies against blood cells. Both of these conditions rarely may be manifested in the immediate post-transplant period and may produce entrapment of leukocytes in thrombi. It is only in hyperacute rejection, however, that polymorphonuclear leukocytes are typically and regularly incorporated in the thrombi. Recurrent hemolytic-uremic syndrome and a thrombotic microangiopathy associated with cyclosporine administration are discussed below and characterized by thrombi usually without leukocytes and generally are later occurring lesions.

Acute Rejection

There are two immunopathologic mechanisms responsible for acute rejection: **cell-mediated immunity** and **humoral (antibody) immunity**.

Table 12-2. Histopathologic findings in the major causes of allograft dysfunction

Type	Interstitium	Tubules	Glomeruli	Arteries
Acute cellular rejection	Edema, lymphocytes	Lymphocytes, cell degeneration	Capillary lymphocytes	Swollen endothelium, lymphocytes, foam cells
Acute humoral rejection	Hemorrhage, zonal necrosis (infarction)	Necrosis	Neutrophils, thrombosis	Necrosis, neutrophils, thrombosis
Acute tubular necrosis	Edema	Cell degeneration, necrosis, mitotic figures	Normal	Normal
Acute cyclosporine toxicity	Edema	Isometric vacuoles		
Chronic rejection	Fibrosis, lymphocytes	Atrophy, dropout	Normal Chronic transplant glomerulopathy	Normal Fibrosis, lymphocytes, narrowed lumina
Chronic cyclosporine toxicity	Striped fibrosis	Atrophy	Ischemic collapse	Arteriolopathy, hyalinazation

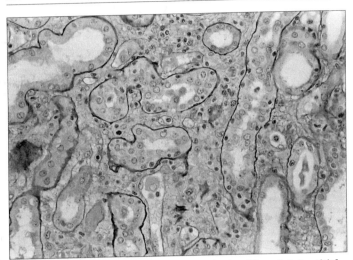

Fig. 12-1. Acute cell-mediated interstitial rejection. There is interstitial edema with lymphocytes in both the interstitium and tubular walls in association with tubular cell degeneration. (Periodic acid-methenamine silver ×200.)

Cell-Mediated Acute Rejection. Cell-mediated acute rejection is the most common form of early rejection. Light microscopy represents the major diagnostic procedure, although at times immunofluorescence and electron microscopic evaluation may be helpful for differential diagnosis. The major lesion is in the interstitium, which is diffusely edematous and infiltrated by numerous leukocytes, the vast majority of which are mature and transformed lymphocytes (T4, T8) with fewer monocytes and plasma cells (Fig. 12-1). Eosinophils are either absent or are found focally in small numbers; polymorphonuclear leukocytes are not a regular feature. Peritubular capillaries are dilated and filled with lymphocytes that may be seen migrating into the interstitium. A characteristic lesion called **tubulitis** occurs, whereby lymphocytes and monocytes extend into the walls and lumina of tubules with associated degenerative changes of epithelial cells. The cells and basement membranes of tubular walls may be damaged and discontinuous. When this lesion affects cast-containing distal tubules, cast matrix (Tamm-Horsfall protein) may be found in the interstitium and occasionally in peritubular capillaries and small veins. For tubulitis to have diagnostic significance, the inflammation should be documented in normal (nonatrophic) tubules. The significance of tubulitis in atrophied tubules only is not known. **Acute transplant glomerulopathy** is a form of glomerular cell–mediated rejection in which lymphocytes and monocytes accumulate in glomerular capillary lumina and mesangial regions (Fig. 12-2). Endothelial and mesangial cells are swollen, and capillary walls display subendothelial lucencies, with occasional segmental peripheral mesangial migration and interposition on ultrastructural examination. In **cell-mediated vascular rejection**, lymphocytes, monocytes, and foam cells may undermine arterial endothelium but rarely extend into the muscularis (Fig. 12-3). The endothelial cells are

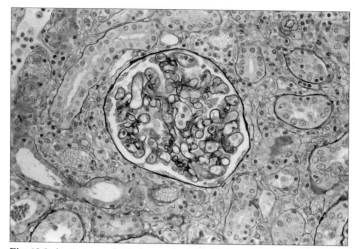

Fig. 12-2. Acute transplant glomerulopathy. Glomerular capillary lumina contain monocytes and lymphocytes. There are also lymphocytes in tubular walls and interstitial rejection with interstitial edema and inflammation. (Periodic acid-methenamine silver ×200.)

swollen and often vacuolated, but arterial wall necrosis is not a feature of this type of acute rejection. When acute cellular rejection is treated successfully, the interstitial inflammatory infiltrate diminishes, whereas edema, tubular inflammation, and tubular cell damage may persist for some time. Immunofluorescence typically discloses fibrin in the interstitium; segmental linear or granular IgM, C3, and fibrin may be found in glomerular capillary walls in acute transplant glomerulopathy. Ultrastructural examination usually confirms the light microscopic findings and provides additional diagnostic information only for the glomerular lesion.

Antibody-Mediated Acute Rejection. Antibody-mediated acute rejection is an uncommon form of rejection and is characterized primarily by **necrotizing arteritis**, with mural "fibrinoid" necrosis and variable inflammation, including a proliferation of lymphocytes, monocytes, and neutrophils (Fig. 12-4). Endothelial cells are severely damaged or absent, and luminal thrombosis is common. This lesion typically results in cortical infarction with focal interstitial hemorrhage. Immunofluorescence discloses IgG and sometimes IgM accompanied by C3 in the walls of arteries. In these structures, fibrin may be intramural and intraluminal and may also be in the interstitium when hemorrhage is present. Some investigators consider intimal arterial lymphocytic infiltration, described above for cell-mediated rejection, to be a part of the vascular pathology of antibody-mediated rejection. At the present time, it is believed that the two forms of arterial inflammation are distinct and unrelated to one another. **Vascular rejection** is therefore an imprecise term in current usage that signifies merely inflammation of arteries, which can result either from cell-mediated or humoral-mediated immunity. When arterial inflammation is present, it should be further categorized to indicate the etiologic mechanism. The humoral form is

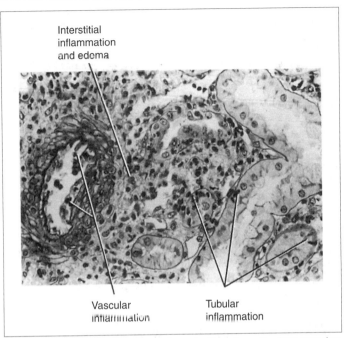

Interstitial
inflammation
and edema

Vascular
inflammation

Tubular
inflammation

Fig. 12-3. Acute cell-mediated vascular rejection. A small artery contains lymphocytes in the lumen and in the intima beneath swollen endothelial cells. Note the interstitial edema and infiltration by lymphocytes, which are also in the walls of tubules. (Periodic acid-Schiff ×220.)

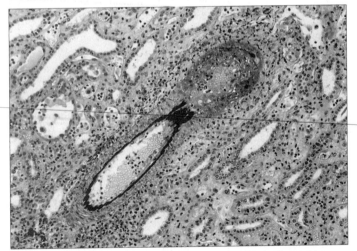

Fig. 12-4. Acute humoral rejection. The arterial wall is infiltrated by neutrophils and lymphocytes and has segmental fibrinoid necrosis. There are edema and inflammation in the adjacent interstitium. (Elastic-van Gieson ×200.)

characterized by arterial mural necrosis, neutrophilic infiltrate, and luminal thrombosis and represents a more severe lesion that is poorly responsive to therapy.

Differential Diagnosis of Acute Cell-Mediated Rejection. Other forms of acute interstitial nephritis may have many of the same structural lesions as acute rejection, including infectious interstitial nephritis (viral, bacterial) and drug-induced acute hypersensitivity interstitial nephritis. Certain viral and bacterial interstitial nephritides may be characterized by a mononuclear, rather than polymorphonuclear, infiltrate, thereby simulating rejection. Glomerular inflammation and arterial inflammation, when present, indicate rejection. Because of the negligible role of polymorphonuclear leukocytes in acute cellular rejection, their presence should be taken to signify acute infection, especially when antibody-mediated rejection with fresh infarction is excluded. Acute hypersensitivity lesions induced by drugs may have a prominent component of eosinophils and sometimes granulomas. Some biopsies with cyclosporine toxicity may have small focal interstitial lymphocytic infiltrates that do not extend into tubules. These infiltrates are not usually associated with diffuse edema. A morphologic pattern of acute cell-mediated rejection may occur in up to 30% of patients without clinical signs or symptoms of rejection or following apparently successful treatment of rejection. The significance of this asymptomatic inflammatory process relative to short- or long-term renal function is not yet known.

Differential Diagnosis of Antibody-Mediated Rejection. The arterial inflammation may be indistinguishable from a systemic necrotizing arteritis, but recurrence of vasculitic lesions in the transplant is very rare. The effects of vascular occlusion, infarction, and parenchymal hemorrhage may be manifestations not only of arteritis, but of arterial occlusion from other causes, including surgical ligation of a large artery and emboli of any nature.

Chronic Rejection (Chronic Allograft Nephropathy)

Chronic rejection is characterized by chronic changes in arteries, tubules, interstitium, and glomeruli. The pathogenesis is uncertain; it may be the result of repeated episodes of overt or covert acute rejection exaggerated by nonimmunologic factors (see Chap. 9). Because many of the chronic changes may be evident in several different forms of chronic injury to the transplant, including chronic rejection, chronic cyclosporine toxicity, nephrosclerosis, and obstruction/reflux, chronic infection, or both, the umbrella term **chronic allograft nephropathy** has been coined. In chronic rejection, the changes are primarily cortical. There is patchy interstitial fibrosis with infiltrates of lymphocytes, plasma cells, and mast cells associated with tubular atrophy or dropout. The walls of arteries are thickened with intimal and sometimes medial fibrosis, variable mononuclear leukocyte inflammation including foam cells, and disruption and duplication of the internal elastic lamina, all resulting in luminal narrowing (Fig. 12-5). Immunofluorescence may document IgG, IgM, C3, and fibrin in the walls of arteries. In addition, juxtaglomerular apparatus hyperplasia may be present and is indicative of large artery involvement. The glomeruli are often abnormal and exhibit a variety of changes, many of which constitute the lesion of **chronic transplant glomerulopathy**, which may occur as early as 4 months post-transplant (see

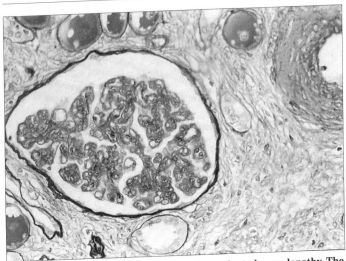

Fig. 12-5. Chronic rejection with chronic transplant glomerulopathy. The arterial wall is thickened and lumen is narrowed due to intimal fibrosis. Glomerular capillary walls often display "double contours," and monocytes are within widened mesangial regions and few capillary lumina. (Periodic acid-methenamine silver ×200.)

Fig. 12-5). This abnormality probably represents chronic glomerular rejection, most likely evolves from acute transplant glomerulopathy, and occurs in approximately 7% of patients engrafted for more than 1 year and in 25% of grafts after 10 years. Capillary walls are thickened with a double-contoured appearance; mesangial matrix, mesangial cells, or both are increased. The glomeruli may have a lobular appearance, and segmental sclerosis can occur. Mesangiolysis, or dissolution of mesangial matrix with resulting capillary microaneurysms, is seen uncommonly. Immunofluorescence usually discloses mesangial and capillary wall granular deposits of IgM, C1q, and C3 with linear fibrin along capillary walls. When segmental sclerosis also is present, these same immune reactants are in a segmental distribution in a coarsely granular-to-amorphous pattern. Electron microscopy reveals a variety of abnormalities, including peripheral migration of mesangium, subendothelial new basement membrane formation, subendothelial flocculent material, and, infrequently, subendothelial and mesangial electron-dense deposits. The basement membranes of peritubular capillaries are often thickened and multilayered; this change has been correlated with the presence of chronic transplant glomerulopathy. As with other forms of chronic renal parenchymal diseases, acquired cystic disease has been documented in the chronically rejected transplant.

Differential Diagnosis. As noted above, the parenchymal changes of chronic rejection need to be differentiated from those of hypertension and chronic cyclosporine toxicity. The presence of transplant glomerulopathy and arterial fibrosis with or without inflammation suggests chronic rejection. In the absence of these findings, these lesions may be difficult to differentiate from one another.

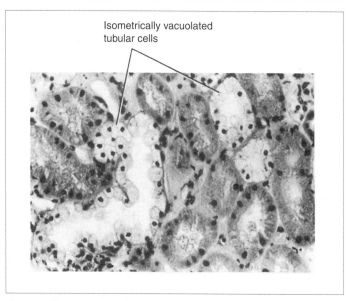

Fig. 12-6. Cyclosporine toxicity with tubular cell isometric vacuoles. The cells of the lighter staining tubules contain numerous closely packed uniform vacuoles. Note the lack of interstitial edema or inflammation. (Hematoxylin & eosin ×200.)

Cyclosporine Nephrotoxicity

Cyclosporine has a variety of renal structural and functional effects. The functional effects are considered in Chap. 4.

Acute Toxicity

Few structural abnormalities are evident in acute cyclosporine toxicity; the dysfunction likely relates to cyclosporine-induced alterations in renal blood flow. There may be tubular dilatation, tubular cell flattening, and occasional individual tubular cell necrosis, all with little or no interstitial edema or inflammation. Giant mitochondria and focal tubular calcification are also present. Unlike the lesions of acute rejection, lymphocytes, when present, are usually restricted to peritubular capillaries and small foci in the interstitium. They are rarely observed in tubules and are not in any other vascular location. Uniform, clear **isometric vacuoles** may be seen in a variable number of proximal tubular cells (Fig. 12-6).

Vascular Effects

A number of structural lesions of the vasculature are ascribed to cyclosporine.

Arteriolopathy. Arteriolopathy is composed of a variety of abnormalities that occur separately or together. There is necrosis of individual myocytes, often with massive accumulation of plasma protein precipitates; these insudates (**"hyalinization"**) are characteristically on the adventitial aspect of arteriolar walls (Fig. 12-7).

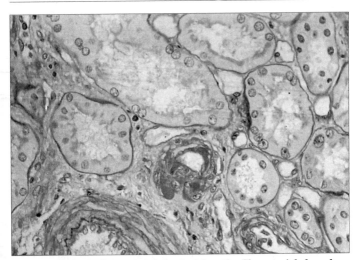

Fig. 12-7. Cyclosporine-associated arteriolopathy. The arteriole has plasma protein insudates ("hyalinization") along the outer aspect of the hypertrophied muscularis. There is no significant edema or inflammation in the interstitium. (Periodic acid-Schiff ×285.)

In contrast, in hypertension and diabetes mellitus, the insudative lesions more typically are subendothelial or within the muscularis. Cessation of or reduction in cyclosporine administration has resulted in amelioration or clearing of the arteriolopathy in some patients.

Thrombotic Microangiopathy. Thrombotic microangiopathy is an infrequent complication of cyclosporine administration. In its mildest form, bland thrombi are present within lumina of arterioles and glomerular capillaries. This lesion is rarely widespread or associated with extensive tissue necrosis. If severe and prolonged, however, thrombotic microangiopathy may result in more severe arterial and arteriolar alterations with extensive cortical necrosis similar to that observed in the hemolytic-uremic syndrome. In patients whose original disease is hemolytic-uremic syndrome, it may be impossible to differentiate between these two lesions. The pronounced intimal changes ("onion skin" lesions) of interlobular arteries seen in the hemolytic-uremic syndrome are not regular features of the cyclosporine-associated process.

Chronic Toxicity

The changes of chronic cyclosporine toxicity are similar to chronic renal ischemia. In their purest form, they consist of focal fibrosis, or so-called **striped interstitial fibrosis,** and tubular atrophy without inflammation. Glomerular ischemic collapse or complete sclerosis is also present. These features appear not to be a consequence of intrarenal arterial narrowing, for the arteries are largely unremarkable; therefore, the combination of normal arteries with a vascular pattern of parenchymal fibrosis is highly suggestive of chronic cyclosporine nephrotoxicity. Juxtaglomerular apparatus hyperplasia may be quite pronounced. It should be noted that the morphologic features of chronic toxicity from tacrolimus therapy are very similar to those of cyclosporine. These include arteriolopathy, juxtaglomerular apparatus hyperplasia, and striped fibrosis. The mechanism of injury is discussed in Chap. 4.

Differential Diagnosis. The differentiation of chronic rejection, nephrosclerosis, and chronic cyclosporine nephrotoxicity may be difficult. Perhaps the most salient feature permitting this distinction in ideal circumstances is the status of the arteries (interlobular, arcuate), which are often fortuitously included in the biopsy. Normal arteries usually indicate chronic cyclosporine nephrotoxicity. Intimal and medial fibrosis of arteries, often with lymphocytic infiltrates, is diagnostic for chronic rejection. If the arteries disclose the usual features of hypertension, nephrosclerosis is likely. These three lesions may coexist and cloud the picture. In addition, characteristic findings may be present in large (large arcuate and interlobar) arteries only and may not be included in a core biopsy specimen, further causing diagnostic difficulty.

Other Pathologic Transplant Lesions

Acute Tubular Necrosis

Acute tubular necrosis in transplants is similar histologically to the lesion found in native kidneys, although there may be more overt necrosis of epithelial cells and sloughing of nonpyknotic epithelium into tubular lumina (Fig. 12-8). It is most often encountered in a biopsy performed within the first month or so following transplantation because of delayed graft function (see Chap. 8). In addition to the usual changes of tubular necrosis, focal interstitial lymphocytic infiltrates may be present.

Infections

While the transplanted kidney may be the site of various infections, it may be difficult to diagnose them on the basis of tissue examination. This is not the case for usual forms of acute bacterial interstitial nephritis (acute pyelonephritis), in which the predominant interstitial and tubular infiltrating cells are polymorphonuclear leukocytes. Some uncommon, nonsuppurative, bacterial infections, however, are characterized by mononuclear leukocytic tubular and interstitial infiltrates. It is extremely difficult to histologically diagnose viral infections such as cytomegalovirus because typical intranuclear or cytoplasmic inclusions are rare.

De Novo Glomerulopathies

De novo membranous glomerulonephritis is found in up to 10% of kidneys in place for more than 1 year, and the capillary wall deposits are not infrequently combined with lesions of chronic transplant glomerulopathy. Other forms of de novo glomerulonephritis are infrequent. Membranous glomerulonephritis is often clinically silent or mild and is usually detected as an incidental finding. The most reliable manner in which to diagnose this lesion is with immunofluorescence and electron microscopy, as the

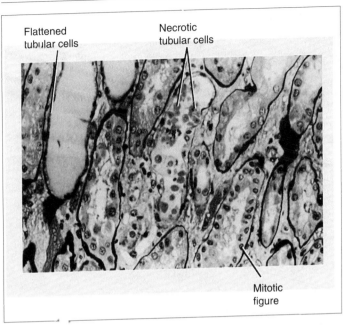

Fig. 12-8. Acute tubular necrosis. The tubule in the center is incompletely lined by epithelial cells; sloughed cells and cellular debris are in the lumen. There is mild interstitial edema with few accompanying lymphocytes. (Periodic acid-methenamine silver ×175.)

deposits and basement membrane changes are often not readily visible by light microscopy or are overshadowed by transplant glomerulopathy.

Recurrent Lesions

Glomerular Lesions. Although many glomerulonephritides may recur, the recurrences are most often of immunopathologic rather than clinical significance and may not appreciably affect graft survival or function (see Chap. 9). These lesions include IgA nephropathy, membranoproliferative glomerulonephritis type II (dense deposit disease), and, occasionally, membranous glomerulonephritis. Focal and segmental glomerulosclerosis, however, may recur early after engraftment and may be responsible for loss of the transplanted kidney. Anti-glomerular basement membrane disease rarely recurs but can arise in a normal kidney transplanted into a patient with Alport's syndrome (see Chap. 6).

Other Lesions. Metabolic diseases, such as amyloidosis, multiple myeloma, light chain deposit disease, and oxalosis, can recur, often with significant graft dysfunction. The structural changes of diabetic nephropathy have been noted to recur in the transplanted kidney but are rarely responsible for graft loss (see Chap. 13). Nodular glomerulosclerosis and arteriolar "hyalinization" are the usual morphologic manifestations of the recurrent lesion.

Table 12-3. Selected features of the Banff classification

Grade	Criteria
Acute rejection	
1 (mild)	Interstitial inflammation (>25% of paren-chyma) tubulitis (>4 lymphocytes/tubular cross section)
2 (moderate)	Interstitial inflammation (as above) tubulitis (>10 lymphocytes/tubular cross section) and/or mild-to-moderate intimal arteritis
3 (severe)	Severe intimal arteritis and/or transmural arteritis with necrosis infarction, hemorrhage
Chronic rejection (includes chronic vascular and glomerular changes)	
1 (mild)	Mild interstitial fibrosis and tubular atrophy
2 (moderate)	Moderate interstitial fibrosis and tubular atrophy
3 (severe)	Severe interstitial fibrosis and tubular atrophy or drop-out

Classification Schema

In an attempt to develop an organized and consistent approach to the classification and grading of the various structural lesions in the transplanted kidney, a conference was held in Banff, Canada. The resulting schema, known as the **Banff classification**, defines the abnormalities and assigns them a numerical score. There are two parts to the schema: (1) the diagnostic classifications and (2) grading of each pathologic component in the tissue sample. The latter is somewhat cumbersome and involves assigning a degree of severity to changes affecting the tubules, interstitium, vessels, and glomeruli. The diagnostic categories include a borderline lesion; mild (see Fig. 12-1), moderate (see Fig. 12-3), and severe (see Fig. 12-4) acute rejection; acute tubular necrosis; acute cyclosporine toxicity; mild, moderate, and severe chronic rejection (chronic nephropathy); and other lesions (e.g., infection, glomerulonephritides, post-transplant lymphoproliferative disorder). A summary of the important aspects of the Banff classification is provided in Table 12-3. It should be noted that, according to the Banff classification, mild interstitial edema, patchy lymphocytic infiltration, and mild tubulitis in the absence of arterial intimal inflammation are not deemed indicative of acute rejection but together are considered a "**borderline lesion**." There remains some controversy regarding the significance of the borderline lesion; some studies have shown this lesion to be associated with treatment-responsive clinical acute rejection. The grade III rejection criteria do, however, appear to correlate with more severe clinical rejections, which may be unresponsive to treatment with high-dose steroids alone (see Chap. 4). Further work is required to clarify the clinical usefulness of the Banff classification. Other scoring systems for assessing acute rejection also have been developed, including one used in the National Institutes of Health (NIH)–funded Cooperative Clinical Trials in Transplantation. The diagnostic criteria for acute rejection differ somewhat between the Banff and NIH schemata. All classification schemata with specific quantifiable criteria require further validation in clinical studies.

FINE-NEEDLE ASPIRATION CYTOLOGY

Aspiration cytology is a relatively new technique for assessing intrarenal events in allografts with a qualitative and quantitative comparison of the cells within the graft and peripheral blood. Transplant aspiration was first used clinically by Hayry and von Willebrand as a minimally invasive procedure for monitoring immunologic processes in renal allografts. There is little morbidity associated with aspiration, and it may be performed daily on an outpatient basis. It allows for close monitoring of the immunologic status of the graft and its response to therapeutic interventions. Aspiration cytology is a valuable tool for the investigation of transplant biology, providing intragraft cells for culture or characterization by immunohistochemistry and in situ hybridization.

Indications

Aspiration is usually performed within the first several months posttransplant for episodes of acute graft dysfunction. The procedure is best used in a serial fashion to follow changes in the graft cell population, and a baseline sampling performed within the first post transplant week is useful for comparison with subsequent aspirates. It may be done successfully up to 6–12 months following transplantation. After this time, fibrosis in the interstitium tends to prevent adequate numbers of cells from being aspirated, and inadequate samples are frequently obtained.

Diagnostic Uses

Aspiration cytology may be used in the assessment of graft dysfunction due to acute cellular (interstitial) rejection, acute tubular necrosis, acute cyclosporine nephrotoxicity, bacterial infections (pyelonephritis), viral infection, or renal infarction. Aspirate material can also be obtained in a serial manner for following response to therapy by evaluation of the numbers and types of intragraft cells.

Diagnostic Limitations

Several renal allograft abnormalities cannot be diagnosed with aspiration. Vascular inflammation cannot be assessed because the anatomic location of the aspirated inflammatory cells is not ascertainable. Chronic rejection and chronic cyclosporine nephrotoxicity are fibrotic processes and usually result in inadequate specimens, since cells within scar tissue cannot be aspirated. Graft rupture, intraparenchymal hemorrhage, and obstruction result in inadequate aspirates that mimic blood contamination of the sample. Glomeruli are infrequently obtained and, when present, are not interpretable in the usual cytologic preparations. Their presence merely serves to prove the cortical location of the aspirate.

Aspirate Handling and Interpretation

Technique

The patient is supine and rotated contralaterally to the allograft, with the contralateral knee bent and the ipsilateral knee straight. This position tends to make the graft more prominent. After sterile preparation, a 25-gauge spinal needle is inserted into the graft, the trocar removed, and the needle attached to a 10-ml syringe containing 4 ml of tissue culture medium, which is fitted into an aspiration gun. Suction is then applied, the needle is rotated and removed quickly, and the sample and medium expressed through the needle into a culture tube. The procedure is repeated two to four times, each aspirate being placed into a separate tube. A finger-stick blood sample is obtained simultaneously and placed separately in 2 ml of medium. All samples must be immediately refrigerated and processed within 24 hours to prevent cellular degeneration. Routine preaspiration coagulation studies are not required, and the patient may ambulate immediately after the procedure.

Processing

The aspirate and blood specimens are handled similarly. Samples are centrifuged, resuspended in medium, and cytocentrifuged onto glass slides. Aspirates containing similar quantities of blood contamination are pooled before cytocentrifugation to allow preparation of the maximum number of slides. The cytospin preparations are air dried and stained with May-Grünwald-Giemsa or stored in a desiccator for additional staining procedures.

Interpretation

Qualitative and quantitative assessments of aspirate leukocytes, parenchymal cells, and blood leukocytes are performed for routine evaluation of the specimens.

Leukocytes. The entire aspirate cytospin preparation is screened to assess the total number of T and B cell immunoblasts and plasma cells. A 100-cell differential count is then performed separately on the aspirate and peripheral blood samples. The peripheral blood count is subtracted from the aspirate count, resulting in increments for each type of leukocyte observed; negative increments are not included. Immunoblasts and plasma cells observed in the peripheral blood differential count are added to those in the aspirate, rather than subtracted, to give a higher blast increment. The increments are multiplied by correction factors, which give added weight to those cell types more strongly associated with acute rejection (Table 12-4). The corrected increments are then added to give the **total corrected increment (TCI)**. The TCI and total immunoblast and plasma cells count are used to evaluate the status of immune activation in the graft.

Parenchymal Cells. Tubular and endothelial cells are assessed to determine parenchymal injury in the graft and to determine **aspirate adequacy**, which is defined as a minimum of seven parenchymal cells per 100 leukocytes. Endothelial cells may be either normal or swollen. Tubular cells may appear normal, swollen, irregularly vacuolated, isometrically vacuolated, phagocytic, degenerated, or necrotic, in increasing order of injury. Phagocytosis is an in vitro

Table 12-4. Correction factors for leukocytes within aspirate preparations*

Leukocyte	Correction factor
Immunoblast	1.0
Plasma cell	1.0
Macrophage	1.0
Activated lymphocyte	0.5
Large granular lymphocyte	0.2
Monocyte	0.2
Lymphocyte	0.1
Neutrophil	0.1
Basophil	0.1
Eosinophil	0.1

*Used for calculation of the total corrected increment (TCI) (see text).

event occurring in the test tube following aspiration wherein injured tubular cells ingest erythrocytes or leukocytes. Parenchymal cells are often artifactually smashed; only intact cells are evaluated qualitatively, although all parenchymal cells are used for adequacy determination.

Acute Cellular (Interstitial) Rejection

May-Grünwald-Giemsa Stain

Immune activation is defined as more than four immunoblasts, plasma cells, or both in the aspirate; a TCI of more than 3; or both. The degree of activation often correlates with the amount of inflammation observed in corresponding core biopsy specimens. Tubular cells may be swollen, irregularly vacuolated, phagocytic, and degenerated. Severe rejection is associated with high TCI and blast counts and the presence of intragraft macrophages and peripheral blood immunoblasts (Fig. 12-9 and Table 12-5). Resolution of rejection is reflected by fewer immunoblasts, a decreasing TCI, and less tubular cell injury and can be evaluated by serial aspiration during and following antirejection therapy.

Immunochemical Stains

In acute rejection, there is upregulation of tubular cell major histocompatibility complex (MHC) class II antigens that are not constitutively expressed. This can be used to improve diagnostic sensitivity of aspiration by immunostaining aspirate samples for class II antigens; they are found in 30% or more of tubular cells following the onset of acute rejection. This staining decreases incrementally following successful treatment of rejection but may not disappear for up to 2 weeks after therapy.

Differential Diagnosis

Aspirate immune activation may be observed in other circumstances. In viral infections, the TCI and blast count are increased, with additional elevation of the numbers of large granular lymphocytes in the aspirate and peripheral blood as described in the section on viral infection. In acute rejection, however, it is only in the aspi-

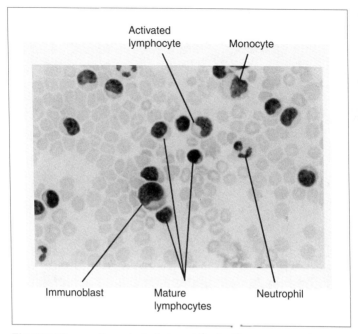

Fig. 12-9. Fine-needle aspirate from a patient with severe acute intersti-tial (cellular) rejection. There are many mononuclear leukocytes, includ-ing immunoblasts, activated lymphocytes, and mature lymphocytes, with relatively few neutrophils. (May-Grünwald-Giemsa ×400.)

Table 12-5. Fine-needle aspirate findings in the major causes of acute renal allograft dysfunction

	Acute rejection	Acute tub-ular necrosis	Acute cyclo-sporine toxicity
Increased TCI	Yes	No	Variable
Increased immuno-blasts	Yes	No	No
Tubular cell necrosis	Variable	Yes	Variable
Tubular cell isometric vacuoles	No	No	Yes

TCI = total corrected increment.

rate that there are increased numbers of large granular lympho-cytes. In the first few days post-transplantation, mononuclear leuko-cytes may infiltrate the graft in response to surgical manipulation. If aspiration is repeated 1 week after transplantation, the periopera-tive inflammation is noted to subside. Cyclosporine use is occasional-ly associated with focal intragraft lymphocyte collections, which will seem to indicate immune activation if aspirated; however, there is no increase in immunoblasts. Lymphoceles adjacent to the allograft are infrequently aspirated; the fluid appears yellow as opposed to the clear or blood-tinged normal aspirates and normal and reactive mesothelial cells may be present. If the needle also passed through the kidney, there may be immunoblasts, lymphocytes, and, rarely, tubular cells. Clinical correlation is required to assess the likelihood of sampling a lymphocele.

In all instances, after the first 2–3 postoperative days, elevated tubular cell MCH class II antigen expression is related to acute rejection and can be used to aid in determining the etiology of immune activation.

Infection

Viral Infection

In viral infections, there is aspirate immune activation, with increased numbers of immunoblasts and particularly plasma cells, and a TCI of more than 3. The aspirate and peripheral blood samples often have the elevated numbers and size of large granular lymphocytes, the peripheral blood increase representing a specific host response observed in viral infections. The peripheral blood may also have atypical mononuclear cells and increased numbers of blasts out of proportion to the degree of graft activation. Tubular cell injury is variable, ranging from swelling to necrosis; intracellular inclusions are not observed. Cytomegalovirus (CMV) infection has been extensively studied with immunostaining for the early CMV nuclear protein; antigen can be demonstrated in more than 35% of tubular cells in the face of active CMV disease. Increased numbers of tubular cells with MHC class II antigen expression are generally not present unless there is a recent prior or concurrent acute rejection episode. In situ hybridization techniques may be used to detect viral genomes (including CMV, herpesvirus, and Epstein-Barr virus) in tubular or endothelial cells.

Differential Diagnosis. As described, the increase in size and number of peripheral blood large granular lymphocytes, the presence of viral genome or protein, and the absence of MHC class II antigen aid in distinguishing viral infection from acute rejection. Increases in immunoblasts and the TCI may accompany tubular injury in the first few postoperative days but then subside.

Bacterial and Fungal Infections

There is typically an increase in the number of intragraft neutrophils relative to the peripheral blood. There is no immune activation, and tubular cell damage is variable, ranging from swelling to necrosis. Organisms may be observed extracellularly and within neutrophil cytoplasm. Because the aspirate is obtained using sterile medium, it may also be used for culture.

If organisms are not evident, if the neutrophil increase is small, and if there is substantial tubular cell injury, it may be impossible to distinguish infection from tubular necrosis. When no organisms are observed and there is modest tubular cell damage, the lack of immune activation may simulate the aspirate from a well-functioning graft.

Acute Tubular Necrosis

In acute tubular necrosis, tubular cells range from swollen and irregularly vacuolated to phagocytic, degenerated, and necrotic (Fig. 12-10).

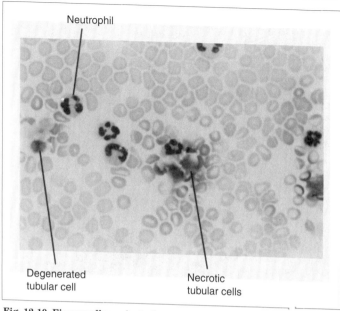

Fig. 12-10. Fine-needle aspirate demonstrating acute tubular necrosis. There are degenerated and necrotic tubular cells, with occasional neutrophils. No increase in mononuclear leukocytes is evident. (May-Grünwald-Giemsa ×400.)

Endothelial cells may be normal or swollen. There is no immune activation, the TCI is less than 3, and there are four or fewer immunoblasts and plasma cells. Mitotic figures, presumably in tubular epithelial cells, may be observed. The degree of tubular cell injury tends to correlate with the clinical course, and serial aspiration demonstrates diminishing tubular cell injury as renal function improves. Acute cyclosporine toxicity may mimic acute tubular necrosis, as the characteristic isometric vacuoles are not always observed.

Acute Cyclosporine Nephrotoxicity

In acute cyclosporine nephrotoxicity, there are small, cytoplasmic **isometric vacuoles** in more than 50% of the tubular cell population (Fig. 12-11). Similar vacuoles may be seen in endothelial cells and aspirate leukocytes, particularly neutrophils. Vacuoles are not present in peripheral blood leukocytes. Tubular cells also may display phagocytosis, degeneration, and necrosis. The TCI is less than 3 or may be slightly increased because of elevated numbers of intragraft lymphocytes from the focal interstitial infiltrates that may occur with cyclosporine use. There is no elevation of the immunoblast and plasma cell count.

Some patients with cyclosporine nephrotoxicity have tubular degeneration with scant isometric vacuoles, mimicking tubular necrosis. The vacuolated tubular cells occur focally in proximal tubules, so repeat aspiration may yield vacuolated cells and a definitive diagnosis. Isometric vacuoles and tubular necrosis are observed

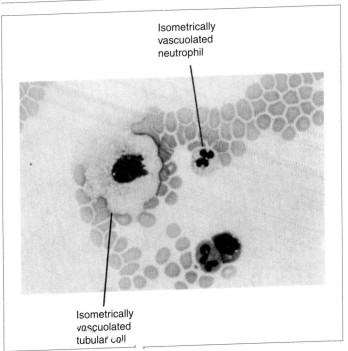

Isometrically
vascuolated
neutrophil

Isometrically
vascuolated
tubular cell

Fig. 12-11. Aspirate preparation from a patient with acute cyclosporine toxicity. Small uniform (isometric) vacuoles are in the cytoplasm of the tubular cell and a neutrophil. (May-Grünwald-Giemsa ×450)

in occasional aspirates performed within the first 3–4 days following transplantation in the absence of cyclosporine toxicity; they do not persist beyond the first week. Acute tacrolimus toxicity is also associated with uniform tubular cell vacuoles, although they are somewhat larger than those observed in cyclosporine toxicity.

SELECTED READINGS

Alexofoulos E, Leontsini M, Daniilidis M et al. Differentiation between renal allograft rejection and cyclosporine toxicity: A clinicopathological study. *Am J Kidney Dis* 18:108, 1991.

Chung WY, Nast CC, Ettenger RB et al. Acquired cystic disease in chronically rejected renal transplant. *J Am Soc Nephrol* 2:1298, 1992.

Colvin RB. Kidney. In RB Colvin, AK Bhan, RT McClusky (eds), *Diagnostic Immunopathology*. New York: Raven, 1995, Pp 329–365.

Curtis JJ, Julian BA, Sanders CE. Dilemmas in renal transplantation: When the clinical course and histologic findings differ. *Am J Kidney Dis* 27:435, 1996.

Danovitch GM, Nast CC, Wilkinson A. Evaluation of fine-needle aspiration biopsy in the diagnosis of renal transplant dysfunction. *Am J Kidney Dis* 17:206, 1991.

Davis CL, Chandler WL. Thromboelastography for the prediction of bleeding after transplant renal biopsy. *J Am Soc Nephrol* 6:1250, 1995.

Dixon TK, Bowman JS, Sago AL et al. A safer renal allograft needle biopsy. *Clin Transplant* 5:126, 1991.

Gaber LW, Moore LW, Alloway RR et al. Correlation between Banff classification, acute renal rejection scores and reversal of rejection. *Kidney Int* 49:481, 1996.

Gudat F, Mihatsch MJ, Ryffel B et al. Cyclosporine Nephropathy. In CC Tisher, BM Brenner (eds), *Renal Pathology*. Philadelphia: Lippincott, 1994.

Habib R, Zurowska A, Hinglais N et al. A specific glomerular lesion of the graft: Allograft glomerulopathy. *Kidney Int* 44(Suppl):104S, 1993.

Hayry P, Lautenschlager I. Fine-needle aspiration biopsy in transplantation pathology. *Semin Diagn Pathol* 9:232, 1992.

Kasiske B, Kalil RS, Lee HS. Histopathologic findings associated with a chronic progressive decline in renal allograft function. *Kidney Int* 40:514, 1991.

Myers BD, Newton L. Cyclosporine-induced chronic nephropathy: An obliterative microvascular renal injury. *J Am Soc Nephrol* 2:545, 1991.

Nast CC, Wilkinson A, Rosenthal T et al. Differentiation of cytomegalovirus infection from acute rejection using renal allograft fine needle aspirates. *J Am Soc Nephrol* 1:1204, 1991.

Neumayer HH, Kienbaum M, Graf S et al. Prevalence and long-term outcome of glomerulonephritis in renal allografts. *Am J Kidney Dis* 22:320, 1993.

Solez K, Axelsen RA, Benediktsson H et al. International standardization of nomenclature and criteria for the histologic diagnosis of renal allograft rejection: The Banff working classification of kidney transplant pathology. *Kidney Int* 44:411, 1993.

Solez K, Benediktsson H, Cavallo T. Final report on the Third Banff Conference on Allograft Pathology (July 20–24, 1995) on classification and lesion scoring in renal allograft pathology. *Transplant Proc* 28:441, 1996.

Solez K, Racusen LC, Marcussen N et al. Morphology of ischemic acute renal failure, normal function, and cyclosporine toxicity in cyclosporine-treated renal allograft recipients. *Kidney Int* 43:1058, 1993.

Kidney and Kidney-Pancreas Transplantation in Diabetics

John D. Pirsch and Hans W. Sollinger

Insulin-dependent diabetes mellitus is the leading cause of end-stage renal disease (ESRD), accounting for approximately one-third of new ESRD patients each year and approximately 20% of kidney transplants performed annually. Although the incidence of diabetic nephropathy in patients with insulin-dependent diabetes mellitus appears to be falling, this diagnosis remains the one that most commonly leads to kidney transplantation in adult whites, Asians, and Native Americans.

There is little question that kidney transplantation, alone or with a pancreas transplantation, is the treatment of choice for end-stage diabetic nephropathy. In the University of Wisconsin transplant program, living-related kidney transplantation in diabetic recipients is associated with a survival advantage compared with cadaveric transplantation (8-year patient survival is 78% versus 63%, respectively); however, both forms of transplantation offer a pronounced survival advantage over chronic dialysis (5-year patient survival is 17%). These patient groups, however, are not strictly comparable, since the patients with the least severe morbid manifestations of diabetes are more likely to select, or be selected for, transplantation. Controlled studies have been performed that evaluate the quality of life benefits of these treatment modalities and have clearly illustrated the benefits of transplantation over dialysis for patients with diabetes. Although all forms of kidney replacement therapy can stabilize or slow some of the secondary complications of diabetes, successful transplantation with correction of uremia and control of blood pressure can stabilize or improve complications, such as neuropathy, diabetic gastroparesis, and retinopathy.

This chapter considers the management issues associated with kidney and pancreas transplantation in diabetics and the pros and cons of the different forms of pancreas transplantation.

KIDNEY TRANSPLANTATION

Preoperative Assessment

The preoperative evaluation of potential kidney transplant recipients is discussed in Chap. 6. The following section considers issues particularly relevant to diabetic patients.

Coronary Artery Disease

Approximately one-third of potential diabetic transplant recipients have significant coronary artery disease. The majority of these patients are asymptomatic, so the possibility of covert coronary artery disease should be considered in every diabetic transplant candidate. In many transplant programs, all diabetics undergo screening with an exercise stress test to help determine which patients should undergo further evaluation with cardiac catheterization. The stress test is usually supplemented with thallium or sestamibi scintography or echocardiography to increase its specificity. Many diabetic patients with kidney failure, however, have poor functional capacity or are physically unable to exercise adequately to reach a target heart rate. In some centers, such patients undergo an oral or intravenous dipyridamole-thallium stress test or a dobutamine stress echocardiogram designed to simulate the effect of exercise on the heart. The reliability of these tests is disputed, so recipients with multiple risk factors or a positive or inadequate stress test should undergo cardiac catheterization before transplantation. Patients with coronary lesions amenable to bypass or angioplasty should be treated before transplantation. Patients with significant coronary artery disease who are not candidates for intervention may not be transplant candidates, although centers differ in their approach to such patients.

In an attempt to avoid an expensive and invasive workup in all diabetic patients, attempts have been made to determine which diabetic candidates are most unlikely to suffer covert coronary artery disease. Asymptomatic patients younger than age 45 who have had diabetes for fewer than 25 years, who have not smoked for more than 5 "pack-years," and who have a totally normal electrocardiogram have a very low incidence of covert coronary artery disease; therefore, further workup may be unnecessary. Diabetic patients who wait for prolonged periods on the cadaveric transplant waiting list should have their cardiac status reassessed at intervals. An algorithm for screening diabetic transplant candidates for coronary artery disease is shown in Fig. 13-1.

Infections

Patients should be free of significant infections such as peritonitis, osteomyelitis, or unhealed foot ulcerations at the time of transplantation. Should a patient develop these complications while awaiting a transplant, his or her candidacy should be placed on hold until the problem is resolved.

Predialysis Transplantation

In patients with diabetic nephropathy, transplantation should be strongly considered before the initiation of dialysis (creatinine clearance of approximately 20 ml/min or a creatinine level of 4–5 mg/dl). Early transplantation can obviate the need for dialysis access, can prevent episodes of congestive heart failure and volume overload, and can correct hypertension, which may contribute to loss of vision. Early transplantation may slow retinopathy and correct neuropathy secondary to uremia, which can exacerbate diabetic neuropathy. The development of diabetic complications on dialysis may impair the rehabilitation potential of transplantation.

Predialysis diabetic transplant candidates who require coronary angiography risk precipitation of dialysis by contrast nephropathy. This risk needs to be carefully weighed against the risks of delaying transplantation or leaving coronary artery disease undiagnosed. Predialysis transplantation is also discussed in Chap. 6.

Post-Transplant Insulin Requirements

By the time many diabetic patients develop advanced nephropathy or the need for dialysis, their insulin requirements have often dimin-

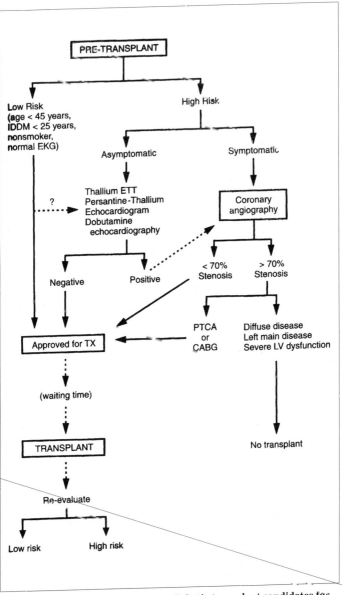

Fig. 13-1. Algorithm for screening of diabetic transplant candidates for coronary artery disease based on data that suggest that noninvasive evaluation of low-risk patients may be unnecessary. (From ME Williams. Management of the diabetic transplant recipient. *Kidney Int* 48:1660, 1995.)

ished or their diabetes may be controlled by oral agents or diet alone. Following transplantation, the carbohydrate intolerance induced by corticosteroids, cyclosporine, and tacrolimus (see Chap. 4) may lead to increased insulin requirements and make non–insulin-dependent diabetics require insulin. Patients should be forewarned.

Preoperative Preparation

In patients with severe gastroparesis, a nasogastric tube may need to be placed. Use of the microemulsified form of cyclosporine (Neoral) may obviate the need for intravenous cyclosporine, since this preparation is very well absorbed. Slow resumption of bowel function may follow transplantation, and, occasionally, nasogastric suction may be required in cases of prolonged ileus. In the immediate preoperative period when the patient is receiving nothing by mouth, half the normal dose of insulin should be given. Blood glucose levels should be monitored every 4 hours, and a sliding scale used for dosing regular insulin. Patients should be dialyzed if there is significant evidence of volume overload or congestive heart failure.

The immunosuppressive protocol used does not differ in diabetic transplant recipients. Some programs prefer sequential protocols using OKT3 or polyclonal antibodies (see Chap. 4) to lessen the reliance on corticosteroids, to prevent early postoperative rejection, and to help decrease the incidence of cyclosporine toxicity.

Postoperative Complications

Several studies have shown no significant difference in major postoperative complications in diabetics versus nondiabetics, especially with regard to wound complications. Postoperative ileus, nausea, and vomiting are more common, however, secondary to diabetic enteropathy. Because of the use of high-dose corticosteroids, frequent blood sugar monitoring is essential, and an insulin drip may be necessary in the first 24–48 hours post-transplant. All patients should receive instruction in blood sugar self-monitoring and in using sliding scale administration of regular insulin for the control of episodes of hyperglycemia. Long-acting insulin, such as NPH, should be used in a twice-a-day regimen. Occasionally, dividing the prednisone dose into a morning and afternoon dose will help control postprednisone hyperglycemia.

Graft Dysfunction

Rejection. The incidence of rejection and cyclosporine toxicity in diabetics is not different from that in nondiabetics. When possible, a kidney biopsy should be employed to determine the cause of graft dysfunction to prevent unnecessary immunosuppression in this high-risk population. Therapy with high-dose corticosteroids is frequently accompanied by poor blood sugar control and requires close monitoring.

Pseudorejection.   In patients with poor blood sugar control, hypovolemia can cause elevations in the blood urea nitrogen and creatinine levels and mimic a rejection episode. Careful review of the previous blood sugar record as well as a careful assessment of volume status is usually sufficient to make this diagnosis. Occasionally, functional obstruction secondary to neurogenic bladder will also simulate rejection. This condition is usually diagnosed by ultrasound or renal scan, which shows a large distended bladder and a prominent renal pelvis. The volume of the postvoid residual may be more than 500 ml, and Foley catheter drainage with a fall in creatinine level confirms the diagnosis.

Urinary Tract Infection.   Urinary tract infections are more common in diabetic recipients because of the higher incidence of neurogenic bladder. Prophylaxis with daily double-strength trimethoprim-sulfamethoxazole is recommended.

Long-Term Complications

Peripheral Vascular Disease

Although successful kidney transplantation is a solution for the nephropathy associated with insulin-dependent diabetes mellitus, many other diabetic manifestations, including peripheral vascular disease, continue to progress. Up to 30% of patients have been reported to have undergone at least one amputation within 3 years of transplantation. Meticulous foot care is essential to help prevent amputations. Although many ischemic ulcers are secondary to microvascular disease, macrovascular occlusion secondary to atherosclerotic plaquing is not uncommon. Angiography should be employed when indicated to identify patients with peripheral vascular lesions that are amenable to bypass grafting.

Retinopathy

Stabilization of retinopathy is common following transplantation, with the majority of patients experiencing no change in visual acuity or showing some improvement. Recipients with severely impaired vision may note some improvement, although some patients will progress to blindness.

Neuropathy

Neuropathy shows initial improvement with the correction of uremia; however, there is slow deterioration with the progression of the diabetes.

Diabetic Gastropathy.   Diabetic gastropathy is common, and gastroparesis is best treated with metoclopramide, 10 mg qid, or cisapride, 10 mg qid before meals. Side effects associated with metoclopramide include mental confusion and a Parkinson-like syndrome with cogwheel rigidity, which is an indication to decrease the dose or discontinue the medication. Many patients who require metoclopramide before transplant may discontinue it post-transplant. Diabetic diarrhea can be treated with oral or transdermal clonidine.

Neurogenic Bladder   Neurogenic bladder is a frequent complicating factor following transplantation. Bethanechol chloride, 10–25 mg qid, may improve bladder emptying, but cholinergic side effects may limit its use. Intermittent self-catheterization may be necessary in some patients.

Orthostatic Hypotension   Orthostatic hypotension with supine hypertension is common secondary to autonomic neuropathy and may be transiently exacerbated after successful transplantation, particularly if the patient was in a fluid-positive state prior to transplantation. Treatment includes fludrocortisone acetate (Florinef), 0.1–0.3 mg daily, or sodium chloride tablets if the patient is not edematous. Clonidine has been shown to improve orthostatic hypotension, probably by a peripheral venoconstricting effect. Orthostatic hypotension typically resolves as the hematocrit rises; this process can be expedited with erythropoietin injections if necessary.

Hypertension

Hypertension is frequent following transplantation and may be due to the effects of cyclosporine, retained native kidneys, or rarely, renal artery stenosis (see Chap. 9). Agents useful in treatment include the spectrum of antihypertensives; however, diuretics and beta blockers should be used with caution. Diuretics may impair glucose control or increase cholesterol levels; beta blockers may block the hypoglycemic response to norepinephrine and epinephrine and predispose the patient to severe hypoglycemic episodes. Calcium channel blockers are effective; however, verapamil and diltiazem increase cyclosporine levels. Close monitoring of cyclosporine levels is necessary if these agents are used. Nifedipine, which does not interfere with cyclosporine metabolism, is very effective in controlling post-transplant hypertension. The long-acting preparation is preferred. Alpha blockers are also effective, especially oral or transdermal clonidine, but side effects at higher doses may limit their use. Angiotensin-converting enzyme inhibitors are effective; however, kidney function may decline, especially in undiagnosed renal artery stenosis or chronic rejection.

Hyperlipidemia

Hyperlipidemia is very common in recipients of transplants, especially patients with diabetes, and it should be treated aggressively. Dietary treatment alone is usually ineffective; lovastatin or other HMG-CoA inhibitors, given in low doses with careful monitoring of muscle and liver enzymes, is often required (see Chap. 9). There is little experience with other lipid-lowering drugs in this situation.

Recurrent Diabetic Nephropathy

Pathologic changes in the allograft consistent with diabetic nephropathy are common following transplantation; graft loss secondary to recurrent diabetic nephropathy, however, is unusual. In the future, with longer survival of transplant patients, recurrent diabetic nephropathy may become a more significant problem.

Pregnancy

Pregnancy in transplant recipients is discussed in Chap. 9. Pregnant diabetic transplant patients represent a particularly high-risk group; a limited number of successful pregnancies have been reported. Prematurity is universal, and deterioration of graft function is common. These factors, together with the potentially limited maternal life span, should be considered in the decision to proceed with the pregnancy.

Table 13-1. Pancreas transplantation options

	Pro	Con
Preuremic pancreas alone	Good surgical risk Complications at early stage	Major surgical procedure Side effects of immunosuppressive therapy may outweigh potential benefits of pancreas transplants Mediocre results
Pancreas after kidney transplantation	Patient already immunosuppressed	Surgical procedure Advanced diabetic complications Mediocre results
Simultaneous kidney and pancreas transplantation	Only one surgical procedure Same immunosuppression Good results	Advanced diabetic complications

KIDNEY-PANCREAS TRANSPLANTATION

Surgical Options

At present, in order to provide the pancreatic islets needed to produce insulin and cure diabetes, it is necessary to transplant both the exocrine and endocrine pancreas. This situation will change if pancreatic islet transplantation becomes available (see the section on transplantation of pancreatic islets). Three patient groups can be considered for whole organ pancreas transplantation: **pancreas alone (PA)**, for patients who have not yet developed advanced kidney disease; **simultaneous pancreas-kidney (SPK) transplantation**, for patients with renal failure; and **pancreas-after-kidney (PAK) transplantation**, for patients who have previously received a successful kidney transplant. There are advantages and disadvantages in each of these approaches, and they must be considered when determining the indications for pancreas transplantation (Table 13-1).

Much of the success of all types of cadaveric pancreas transplantation depends on meticulous attention to the technical aspects of donor selection, organ harvesting, and back-table preparation. Detailed discussion of these issues is beyond the scope of this text, and the reader is referred to the article by SS Mizrahi et al. (see Selected Readings).

Preuremic Pancreas Transplantation

Some centers offer PA transplantation as a therapeutic alternative for recurrently ketotic "brittle" patients and for patients with hypoglycemic unawareness. The prolonged normoglycemia that follows the successful procedure does not, unfortunately, lead to resolution of established nephropathy or retinopathy. For the great majority of diabetic patients, the risk-to-benefit ratio for PA transplantation is unfavorable, since a pancreas transplant exposes them both to the risks of surgery and to the long-term side effects of immunosuppressive therapy.

Transplantation of the Pancreas After the Kidney

In PAK transplantation, immunosuppressive therapy is not a major concern. In the long-term, the drug therapy the patients are already receiving for their kidney transplant is not significantly changed after the addition of a pancreatic transplant. The significant risks for these patients are the risk of the surgical procedure itself and the short-term risk of a temporary postoperative boost in their immuno-suppressive therapy. Unfortunately, these patients have already suffered significant secondary diabetic complications, and it is uncertain whether a well-functioning pancreas transplant will accomplish more than rendering these patients insulin-independent. The results of PAK transplantation are significantly worse than those in SPK transplantation, possibly because there are two separate sources of foreign histocompatibility antigens.

Simultaneous Kidney-Pancreas Transplantation

SPK transplantation is the preferred type of pancreas transplant. It has the advantage that only one surgical procedure is required and there is only one source of foreign histocompatibility antigens. Immunosuppressive therapy is similar to the therapy that these patients would receive with a kidney transplant alone. As in PAK transplantation, however, many patients have already suffered substantial secondary diabetic complications, and the extent to which these complications will reverse or stabilize is uncertain (see the section on the effect of pancreas transplantation on secondary diabetic complications). Nevertheless, many centers now consider SPK transplantation to be established as a therapeutic and effective procedure; substantial improvement in the quality of life as compared with kidney transplantation alone has been documented by several centers (see the section on SPK versus kidney transplant alone).

Outcome of Pancreas Transplantation

Approximately 85% of pancreas transplants performed in the United States between 1987 and 1996 were SPK transplants. Data reported to the United Network for Organ Sharing and in individual reports show an overall 1-year pancreas graft survival rate of 75% and patient survival rate of at least 90% (1-year patient survival for diabetic recipients of a kidney transplant alone is similar). Pancreas transplantation does not adversely affect 1-year kidney graft survival, which is approximately 80% for SPK and for diabetic recipients of kidney transplant alone. One-year graft survival for PAK and PA recipients is worse than for SPK recipients and is reported to be approximately 50%. Accurate comparison of survival statistics for SPK versus kidney transplant alone for diabetics is difficult because the SPK recipients tend to be younger, with less vascular disease. In fact, the mortality of SPK has been reported to increase considerably if patients with heart disease are not excluded as candidates.

Surgical Techniques

Much of the controversy with respect to the optimal surgical technique for pancreas transplantation has been focused on the handling of the exocrine pancreatic secretions. Three surgical techniques have been used by centers around the world.

Enteric Drainage of Exocrine Secretions

Enteric drainage of exocrine secretions requires either a segmental pancreatic graft drained end-to-end into a roux-en-Y loop or, preferably, a whole pancreas transplantation with side-to-side anastomosis of a duodenal segment into the small bowel (**primary enteric drainage**). The former technique has been abandoned in favor of the latter, which is associated with fewer septic complications from bowel contamination. A prospective, randomized trial will be required to judge whether enteric drainage is as good as bladder drainage (see below).

Duct Injection

Pretransplantation injection of the pancreatic duct with polymeric solutions such as neoprene, latex, or prolamine serves to obliterate the ductal system and obviates a surgical drainage procedure. Unfortunately, this technique is associated with a high incidence of vascular thrombosis and fistula formation. Nevertheless, the surgical complication rate after duct injection is smaller than that reported after enteric drainage.

Bladder Drainage

At the current time, at least 90% of all centers worldwide have chosen bladder drainage as their procedure of choice. Whole pancreatic grafts are used with a side-to-side pancreaticoduodenocystostomy (Fig. 13-2). The advantages of bladder drainage include a lower surgical complication rate and the use of urinary amylase for monitoring rejections (see the section on the diagnosis of rejection). The pancreas is placed contralaterally to the simultaneously performed kidney transplant. The disadvantages of bladder drainage are discussed below and have led some centers to return to the enteric drainage technique.

Complications

Significant surgical complications after pancreas transplantation with bladder drainage occur in approximately 25% of patients (Table 13-2). Even in centers with the best results, the rate of early reoperation and the length of hospital stay are considerably greater for SPK transplantation than for kidney transplantation alone.

Approximately 20% of bladder-drained pancreas transplants eventually need **enteric conversion** by removing the pancreas with its duodenal segment from the bladder and reanastomosing it to a loop of small bowel. If possible, the conversion is delayed until at least 6 months post-transplant, at which time the risk of acute rejection is small and the doses of immunosuppressants are relatively low.

Urine Leak

Leakage of urine from the duodenal segment is most often encountered within the first 3 months after transplantation and is the most frequent serious postoperative complication. Patients present with sudden onset of abdominal pain and significantly elevated serum amylase. In most cases, a cystogram or computed tomography scan confirms the diagnosis, and re-exploration is required, with closure

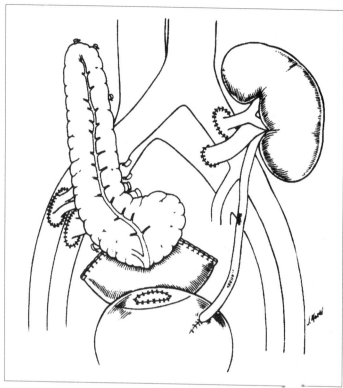

Fig. 13-2. Schematic diagram of the bladder drainage technique for simultaneous kidney and pancreas transplant. Note side-to-side pancreaticoduodenocystostomy.

Table 13-2. Urologic complications related to pancreas transplant

Complication	Number of patients (%)
Hematuria	33 (15.7)
Bladder/duodenal segment leak	30 (14.2)
Reflux pancreatitis	24 (11.4)
Recurrent urinary tract infection	22 (10.4)
Urethritis	7 (3.3)
Urethral stricture/disruption	6 (2.8)

Source: Reproduced with permission from HW Sollinger, EM Messing, DE Eckhoff et al. Urological complications in 210 consecutive simultaneous pancreas-kidney transplants with bladder drainage. *Ann Surg* 208:561, 1993

of the leak or enteric conversion. In some patients with very small leaks, conservative therapy consisting of placement of a Foley catheter for several weeks is adequate. Small leaks may be difficult to detect radiologically and are suggested by recurrence of pain following removal of the Foley.

Graft Pancreatitis

Pancreatitis of the allograft is a common postoperative complication and can occur in a variety of settings. In the immediate postoperative period, the effects of preservation and handling of the pancreas may induce a transient mild hyperamylasemia without significant clinical consequence. Pancreas rejection may also be heralded by an increase in serum amylase levels, which may be an important marker of rejection in PAK or PA transplantation. Urine leaks may also cause hyperamylasemia.

Reflux pancreatitis has generally been believed to be due to the irritant effects of refluxing urine on the pancreas. It is most frequent in patients with distended neurogenic bladders. It is managed by Foley drainage, often followed by self-catheterization to avoid high urinary residuals; alpha$_1$-adrenoceptor blocking agents such as terazosin (Hytrin) may be useful. Enteric conversion may be required.

Vascular Thrombosis

Vascular thrombosis, a complication described by many groups after pancreas transplantation, is more frequent with segmental grafts, and some groups advocate systemic anticoagulation or dextran infusions for several days after transplantation. Vascular thrombosis of the pancreas can be caused by either arterial or venous thrombosis. In the case of arterial thrombosis, which is rare, the pancreas on reexploration will appear soft and pale. In contrast, venous thrombosis is characterized by a large, engorged, and dark blue discolored pancreatic graft. Thrombosed pancreatic grafts have to be removed immediately, as they constitute a focus of infection and toxemia.

Intra-Abdominal Abscess

Serious infections are more common after pancreas transplantation than after kidney transplant alone, and in most series they are the most common cause of death. The most feared complication is the formation of intra-abdominal abscesses or infected peripancreatic fluid collections. In most instances, conservative therapy with antibiotics and percutaneously inserted drains are helpful; if the patient does not respond or infection persists, however, abdominal exploration and possible pancreatectomy should be considered early on. A late complication of peripancreatic infections is the development of a mycotic aneurysm at the site of the arterial anastomosis, resulting in life-threatening bleeding. If the diagnosis of a mycotic aneurysm is suspected, it must be confirmed by angiography, and the pancreas must be removed.

Urinary Tract Infections

Urinary tract infections occur with a high frequency after pancreas transplantation with bladder drainage. In some cases, persistent urinary tract infections are caused by sutures protruding from the anastomotic site; these sutures have to be removed through a cystoscope. In some cases, stone formation around retained sutures is noted. Use of absorbable sutures may prevent this problem.

Hematuria

Hematuria after pancreas transplantation with bladder drainage can be divided into acute postoperative hematuria and chronic hematuria. Whereas acute postoperative hematuria is usually due to a bleeding vessel, either from the suture line or from the duodenal segment, chronic hematuria may be due to an ulcer in the duodenal segment or granulation tissue at the suture line. In acute cases, cystoscopy, clot evacuation, and cauterization of the bleeding point will be sufficient. In cases of chronic hematuria, excision of the inflammatory focus, removal of sutures, or conversion of bladder drainage into enteric drainage can be considered.

Urethritis

Sterile urethritis with dysuria and balanitis occurs after bladder-drained pancreas transplantation because of the irritant effect of pancreatic enzymes on the lower urinary tract mucosa; urethral strictures sometimes result. It can usually be treated conservatively by Foley drainage or suprapubic cystostomy; enteric conversion is sometimes required.

Metabolic Abnormalities

In the bladder-drained pancreas transplantation, complications can arise from the loss of large quantities of alkaline, enzyme-rich pancreatic fluid via the urinary tract. Metabolic acidosis, hyponatremia, and extracellular fluid volume depletion may develop, and oral and sometimes intravenous sodium chloride and bicarbonate supplementation are required. If patients are receiving tacrolimus (see the section on immunosuppressive therapy), the bicarbonate should be administered at least 2 hours before or after the dose to avoid impaired tacrolimus absorption.

Carbohydrate metabolism in bladder-drained pancreas recipients is similar to immunosuppressed nondiabetic kidney transplant recipients. It should be remembered that, in these patients, the delivery of insulin is into the systemic circulation, which may lead to peripheral hyperinsulinemia and make the patients more susceptible to hypoglycemic symptoms. In the enterically drained pancreas, the delivery of insulin is into the portal circulation and is thus more "physiologic"; lipoprotein metabolism is improved in enteric drainage compared to bladder drainage.

Immunosuppressive Therapy

Immunosuppressive therapy for all forms of whole organ pancreas transplantation is the same in principle as for kidney transplantation alone and is discussed in detail in Chap. 4. Because of the frequency of acute rejection episodes in SPK transplantation, there is a tendency to use more aggressive immunosuppressive protocols; most centers use induction protocols with OKT3 or antithymocyte globulin. All centers use cyclosporine- or tacrolimus-based protocols, although the latter is gaining in popularity. It may be wise to maintain somewhat higher than usual cyclosporine or tacrolimus levels in the early postoperative period.

Diagnosis of Rejection

The diagnosis of rejection after pancreas transplantation may be extremely difficult. This difficulty can be explained by the histologic sequence of events, which is characterized by a cellular infiltrate first involving the exocrine pancreatic tissues. In the initial phases of the rejection process, the islets are spared, and serum glucose remains normal. Only at the later stages of rejection, when fibrosis, inflammation, and destruction of the islets occur, does the patient become hyperglycemic. At this stage, rejection is usually irreversible. Rejection must be recognized early, before the development of hyperglycemia, to prevent complete destruction of islet tissues.

In SPK transplantation, the kidney allograft is usually involved first in the rejection process, and a significant elevation of serum creatinine or a kidney biopsy will permit the diagnosis of rejection to be made. Treating the kidney allograft rejection usually adequately treats the concomitant pancreas rejection. The timely diagnosis of pancreas rejection in PAK and PA transplantation is much more difficult, which may partially explain their inferior results. For the bladder-drained SPK transplant, the determination of the **urinary amylase** has proved to be a very useful marker of pancreas rejection. Amylase excretion is usually measured in a 4-hour morning urine collection and is expressed as units per hour; the well-functioning pancreas excretes several thousand units per hour. The excretion level drops during the initial phases of the rejection process, when only the exocrine gland is involved. During this stage, the reduced perfusion of the pancreas as determined by technetium nuclear scan can also be used as a confirmatory test. Some investigators also believe that an elevation of serum amylase is associated with rejection. More recently, the determination of serum anodal trypsinogen levels has been demonstrated to be an extremely early and sensitive parameter of pancreas allograft rejection, although the assay is not widely available. Serum levels of tumor necrosis factor, interleukin-2, and interleukin-2 receptors and urinary cytology may also be useful. Invasive techniques include transcystoscopic biopsy of the head of the pancreas and percutaneous biopsy using an 18-gauge disposable automatic needle (see Chap. 12), both of which carry a small risk of bleeding and fistula formation.

Effect of Pancreas Transplantation on Secondary Diabetic Complications

The purpose of pancreas transplantation is to improve the quality of life of patients with end-stage diabetic nephropathy over and above that which can be achieved by kidney transplant alone. This is achieved by normalization of carbohydrate metabolism, which frees the patients from years of insulin therapy and dietary constraint, and by arresting, preventing, and even reversing secondary diabetic complications. Although there is no question that a successful procedure makes the patient insulin-independent, the impact on secondary manifestations of diabetes is less clear-cut and is the subject of ongoing research and controversy

Nephropathy

When renal allografts from nondiabetic donors are placed into a diabetic recipient, morphologic signs of diabetic nephropathy in the form of thickening of the glomerular basement membrane appear as early as 2 years after transplantation. No microscopic evidence of diabetic nephropathy is seen up to 4 years after SPK transplantation. Mesangial and glomerular volume and basement membrane thickness are less after SPK transplantation than after kidney transplantation alone. Whereas changes of diabetic nephropathy can often be seen on biopsies of kidneys transplanted alone into diabetics, loss of grafts to diabetic nephropathy is unusual, although renal function is better maintained in recipients of SPK transplants. Within the time frame of follow-up presently available, the benefit of SPK transplantation in diabetic nephropathy is more evident histologically rather than clinically.

Neuropathy

Pancreas transplantation alone in preuremic patients has been shown to result in significant improvement in motor and sensory nerve conduction velocity. Subjective and objective improvement of established neuropathy occurs after both SPK and kidney transplantation alone, although a variety of markers of autonomic function has been shown to improve more after SPK transplantation. It is difficult to differentiate between the improvement in the uremic and diabetic components of neuropathy, and the added benefit of SPK transplantation may take months or years to manifest clinically.

Retinopathy

Pancreas transplantation either prior to or simultaneous with kidney transplantation has not been shown to produce a greater improvement in retinopathy than kidney transplantation alone. It is possible that this disappointing failure to show benefit may relate to the relatively short period of follow-up. Preliminary studies have observed a trend in favor of pancreas transplantation during follow-up of at least 3–4 years.

Microcirculation

Using thermography, muscle oxygen tension measurements, and laser Doppler determination, SPK transplantation has been shown to have a beneficial effect on the microcirculation that is greater than with kidney transplantation alone. This objective determination is strengthened by the clinical observation that SPK transplant recipients suffer fewer amputations and diabetic ulcers of the lower extremities than diabetic patients receiving kidney transplantation alone.

Coronary Artery Disease

Many centers apply more stringent criteria to rule out significant coronary artery disease in candidates for SPK transplantation than in candidates for a kidney transplant alone. Such a policy prevents comparative evaluation of the impact of the pancreas transplant on the progress of the coronary artery disease. As greater confidence with SPK transplantation has developed, some centers are accepting patients at greater cardiac risk, and comparative groups have shown that the risk of early cardiac-related mortality is equal or greater in the SPK transplant patients.

Quality of Life

After the first few months following a successful SPK transplant, patients generally report a better quality of life than that of recipients of kidney transplants alone. SPK transplant recipients have been reported to require less sickness pension, have more full-time employment, and have fewer lost workdays. It is difficult to quantitate the sense of liberation felt by lifetime diabetics who no longer must self-inject insulin and monitor every morsel they eat.

Choice of Procedure

Patients and their physician advocates may be faced with a difficult dilemma when choosing between a kidney transplant alone and an SPK transplant. This dilemma is reflected in the ongoing discussions on this topic in the medical and transplant literature. SPK transplantation is associated with increased early morbidity but may offer better long-term quality of life and the greater potential for stabilization or improvement of diabetic complications. Most centers recommend kidney transplantation alone when a live donor is available because this option offers the best long-term patient and graft survival. Patients choosing between SPK and cadaveric kidney transplantation must be well-informed regarding the comparative risks and benefits of the two procedures. The morbidity and mortality rates for diabetics on chronic dialysis is high, and in many centers, patients are swayed toward SPK transplantation because the waiting time for the combined procedure is less than for kidney transplantation alone.

TRANSPLANTATION OF PANCREATIC ISLETS

The capacity to successfully and consistently transplant pancreatic islets would represent a quantum leap in the management of diabetes mellitus and would relegate our present efforts at whole organ transplantation to the history books. The main appeal of islet transplantation, either as a purified graft or in the form of dispersed pancreatic tissue, is that morbidity of the procedure is very low compared with whole organ transplantation. The goal will be to transplant nonimmunogenic or immunoprotected islets soon after presentation of insulin-dependent diabetes, before the development of diabetic complications.

A normal human pancreas contains approximately 1 million islets; it has been estimated that more than half a million (approximately 10,000/kg) are required for normal carbohydrate tolerance. Isolation of sufficient islets from a single cadaveric donor has proved difficult, and multiple pancreases may be required. Although islet transplantation has been successful in rodent models, only 11 fully documented cases of insulin independence have occurred out of 139 reported attempts at clinical islet transplantation since 1974. In most of these cases, the islets have been injected intraportally to simulate the normal release of insulin into the portal circulation, and all of the patients have required standard immunosuppression.

The problems preventing the stable engraftment of a sufficient number of islets to achieve a state of insulin independence can be broadly classified into four categories: (1) transplantation of an insufficient mass of viable islets, (2) immune-mediated destruction of transplanted islet tissue, (3) drug toxicity (both cyclosporine and tacrolimus are islet toxic), and (4) metabolic "exhaustion" due to the foreign microenvironment.

Transplantation of an insufficient mass of islets can be overcome by the use of multiple donors. The disadvantage of this approach is that several donor pancreases are required that could otherwise have been used for whole organ transplantation. Because of the isolated nature of the foreign antigen, immune-mediated destruction of the transplanted islet tissue is vigorous; multiple donors may also make the pancreas even more immunogenic. There are no reliable markers of early islet rejection, and institution of antirejection therapy is often delayed. There have been some preliminary reports of success with single donors, but long-term success has not been achieved.

Even well-functioning islets may deteriorate with time even in the absence of immune attack, a phenomenon ascribed to **metabolic exhaustion.** Islets removed by separation procedures from their natural environment in the exocrine pancreas may lack growth factors necessary for vascularization and growth. It is possible that the addition of growth factors may overcome this problem, but preliminary attempts have not been encouraging.

Attempts are being made to make islets less immunogenic by culturing them prior to transplant or by immunoprotecting them with membranes or capsules. If pancreatic islet transplantation is to become a therapeutic reality for all diabetics rather than the minority that reach ESRD, nonhuman sources will be required, and the barriers of xenotransplantation will need to be crossed. For all of the above reasons, it appears unlikely that islet transplantation will become a practical clinical reality in the near future.

SELECTED READINGS

Douzdian V, Rice JC, Gugliuzza KK. Renal allograft and patient outcome after transplantation: Pancreas-kidney versus kidney-alone transplants in type 1 diabetic patients versus kidney-alone transplants in nondiabetic patients. *Am J Kidney Dis* 27:106, 1996.

El-Gebely S, Hathaway DK, Elmer DS et al. An analysis of renal function in pancreas-kidney and diabetic kidney-alone recipients at two years following transplantation. *Transplantation* 59:1410, 1995.

Esmatjes E, Ricart MJ, Fernandez-Crua L. Quality of life after successful pancreas-kidney transplantation. *Clin Transplantation* 8:75, 1994.

Gaber AO, El-Gebely S, Sugathan P. Early improvement in cardiac function occurs for pancreas-kidney but not diabetic kidney-alone transplant recipients. *Transplantation* 59:1105, 1995.

Hathaway D, Abell T, Cardoso S et al. Improvement in autonomic function following pancreas-kidney versus kidney-alone transplantation and correlation with quality of life. *Transplantation* 57:816, 1994.

London NJM, Robertson GSM, Chadwick DR et al. Human pancreatic islet isolation and transplantation. *Clin Transplantation* 8(Suppl):421S, 1994.

Manske CL, Wang Y, Thomas W. Mortality of cadaveric kidney transplantation versus combined kidney pancreas transplantation in diabetic patients. *Lancet* 346:1658, 1995.

Manske CL, Thomas W, Yang W et al. Screening diabetic patients for coronary artery disease: identification of a low risk subgroup. *Kidney Int* 44:617, 1993.

Mizrahi SS, Jones JW, Bentley FR. Preparing for pancreas transplantation: Donor selection, retrieval technique, preservation, and basic table preparation. *Transplantation Rev* 10:1, 1996.

Pirsch JD, Andrews C, Hricik DE et al. Pancreas transplantation for diabetes mellitus. *Am J Kidney Dis* 27:444, 1996.

Remuzzi G, Ruggenenti P, Mauer SM. Pancreas and kidney-pancreas transplants: Experimental medicine or real improvement? *Lancet* 343:27, 1994.

Robertson RR. Pancreatic and islet transplantation for diabetes—Cures or curiosities? *N Engl J Med* 327:1861, 1992.

Sollinger HW, Messing EM, Eckhoff DE et al. Urologic complications in 210 consecutive simultaneous pancreas-kidney transplants with bladder drainage. *Ann Surg* 208:561, 1993.

Williams ME. Management of the diabetic transplant recipient. *Kidney Int* 48:1600, 1995.

Kidney Transplantation in Children

Robert B. Ettenger

Despite significant advances in dialysis technology, kidney transplantation is accepted today as the optimal available treatment for end-stage renal disease (ESRD) in children and adolescents. A well-functioning kidney transplant can improve the physical, social, and psychological quality of life of a child more than any form of dialysis. Children are constantly growing, developing, and changing. Each developmental stage presents a unique series of challenges that must be recognized and addressed by the medical team if a truly successful graft outcome and rehabilitation are to be achieved.

INCIDENCE AND ETIOLOGY OF END-STAGE RENAL DISEASE AND RESULTS OF KIDNEY TRANSPLANTATION IN CHILDREN

Incidence

In the United States, the incidence of ESRD in children has remained generally constant over the past decade at approximately 11 children per million child population. The point prevalence of ESRD in the pediatric population is 55 per million child population. The rate of ESRD incidence increases with age such that approximately 75% of pediatric patients are between the ages of 10 and 19 years. In infants younger than 1 year of age, the incidence approaches 0.2 per million. There are geographic variations in incidence related to specific disease entities (e.g., hemolytic-uremic syndrome in Argentina, congenital nephrotic syndrome in Finland).

Etiology

Table 14-1 lists the primary renal diseases of children receiving kidney transplants in the United States during the 8-year period between January 1987 and January 1995. The etiology of ESRD in children varies significantly with age; in Table 14-2 the frequency of major diagnostic categories is broken down by age grouping. The major differences in ESRD etiology between children and adults (see Chap. 1) are both the greater incidence of urologic, congenital, and hereditary diseases and the rarity of diabetic nephropathy in children.

Frequency and Demographics of Pediatric Candidacy and Transplantation

Data from the United Network for Organ Sharing (UNOS) show that in the period between October 1987 and January 1994, 3,809 kidney transplants were performed in the United States in children younger than 18 years of age (6.4% of the total transplants during the same period). The donor source for pediatric recipients was evenly split between cadaveric and living donors. This compares with an approximately 5:1 ratio of cadaveric to living donor transplants in adults. The number of pediatric patients awaiting cadaveric transplants has remained stable in recent years, although the percentage

Table 14-1. Renal diagnosis of children in the United States transplanted between January 1987 and January 1995*

Diagnosis	Number	Percentage of total
Obstructive uropathy	605	16.5
Aplasia, hypoplasia, or dysplasia	603	16.4
Focal and segmental glomerulosclerosis	425	11.6
Reflux nephropathy	209	5.7
Systemic immunologic disease	174	4.7
Chronic glomerulonephritis	160	4.4
Prune-belly syndrome	112	3.0
Congenital nephrotic syndrome	103	2.8
Hemolytic uremic syndrome	101	2.7
Polycystic kidney disease	100	2.7
Medullary cystic disease/juvenile nephronophthisis	94	2.6
Cystinosis	92	2.5
Pyelonephritis/interstitial nephritis	84	2.3
Membranoproliferative glomerulonephritis type 1	84	2.3

*Only diagnoses representing more than 2% of the total are listed.

Table 14-2. Cause of end-stage renal disease in children of different ages undergoing kidney transplantation (Percentage of total)

	Age in years			
	0–1	2–5	6–12	13–17
Aplastic, hypoplastic, or dysplastic kidneys	29	24	17	11
Obstructive uropathy	20	20	17	14
Focal glomerulosclerosis	0	8	14	13
Other	51	48	51	61

of the total waiting list that children represent is falling (currently 2.5%) as the adult waiting list inexorably expands (see Chap. 1).

Data from the North American Pediatric Renal Transplant Cooperative Study (NAPRTCS) detail the age distribution of children receiving transplants from 1987 to 1994. Approximately 6% were younger than 2 years of age; 16% were between 2 and 6 years of age; 35% were between 6 and 12 years of age, and 40% were between 13 and 18 years of age.

Patient and Allograft Survival

Short-Term Results

Data from the NAPRTCS report 2-year patient survival rates of 96% and 93.5%, respectively, for recipients of live-related and cadaveric donor transplants. At 1, 2, and 5 years, post-transplant actuarial graft survival rates were 89.5%, 85%, and 75%, respectively, for live-related transplants and 76%, 71%, and 61.5% for cadaveric transplants. When results of first cadaveric transplants in children are compared to those in adults, children of all ages have significantly poorer rates of graft survival, although there has been a trend toward improvement. The youngest children (0–5 years of age) have the poorest graft survival rates, because of a high rate of graft loss in the first 3 months post-transplant.

Long-Term Results

Reports dealing with patient and graft survival for more than 10 years are few and describe transplants that were mostly performed before the availability of cyclosporine. In these studies, patient survival was 80–90% and graft survival was 50–60% for 1-haplotype–matched donors and up to 90% for 2-haplotype–matched donors. Long-term patient survival for first cadaveric recipients was reported to be approximately 60% and graft survival 40–50%.

Current long-term patient survival appears to be improving. The 5-year patient survival rate for recipients of living donor grafts and cadaveric grafts is reported to be 94% and 90%, respectively. When long-term graft outcome is expressed as graft half-life, a figure of 7.4 years has been estimated for children between 6–18 years of age; this figure is only marginally lower than that estimated for adults.

PRETRANSPLANT PREPARATION

Workup of the Potential Living Donor

The evaluation and preparation of a living donor for a child is essentially the same as for an adult (see Chap. 5). As a general rule, it is possible to consider an adult donor of almost any size for a child, no matter how young. Live donation from siblings is usually restricted to donors who have reached their eighteenth birthday, although the courts have given permission for younger children to donate under extraordinary circumstances. Ethical issues related to young donors are discussed in Chap. 16.

Histocompatibility matching considerations are not different for pediatric recipients of kidneys from live donors. Human leukocyte antigen (HLA)–identical transplants are optimal and enable the lowest amount of immunosuppression to be used, thereby minimizing steroid and other side effects. The first live donor for a child is most frequently a 1-haplotype–matched parent; there are no significant differences in outcome between transplants from a maternal or paternal donor. Siblings may become donors when they reach the age of consent. Second-degree relatives and 0-haplotype–matched siblings may also be considered as donors.

Pretransplant Recipient Workup

The workup of the potential pediatric transplant recipient is similar to that performed in adults (see Chap. 6), but because certain problems occur with more frequency in children, the emphasis may be different. It is important to establish the precise cause for ESRD in children whenever possible. Surgical correction may be required for certain structural abnormalities prior to transplantation (see the section on urologic problems). The precise cause of metabolic or glomerular disease should also be established if possible because of the propensity for post-transplant recurrence. Discussion of common medical, surgical, and psychiatric issues in pediatric transplant candidates follows.

Neurologic Development

Infants. Infants with ESRD during the first year of life frequently suffer neurologic abnormalities, including alterations in mental function; microcephaly; and involuntary motor phenomena, such as myoclonus, cerebellar ataxia, tremors, seizures, and hypotonia. The pathogenesis is unclear, although a number of lines of evidence incriminate aluminum toxicity. To help ameliorate this problem, some authors have suggested preemptive kidney transplantation, whereas others have advocated institution of dialysis at the very earliest sign of a reduction in head circumference growth rate, developmental delay, or both. Studies describe an improvement in psychomotor development in many infants who have undergone successful transplantation; a significant percentage of infants who have undergone successful transplantation regain normal developmental milestones. Tests of global intelligence show increased rates of improvement after successful transplantation.

Older Children. It is often difficult to assess to what extent uremia contributes to cognitive delay and impairment in older children. Uremia has an adverse, but often reversible, effect on a child's mental functioning and may often cause psychological depression. It may be necessary to institute dialysis and improve the uremic symptomatology before making a precise assessment of the child's mental function. Initiation of dialysis often clarifies the picture and permits progression to transplantation in situations in which it might otherwise have not seemed feasible. Severely retarded children, on the other hand, respond poorly to the constraints of ESRD care. A child with a very low IQ cannot comprehend the need for procedures that are often confusing and uncomfortable. In this situation, the family must be involved and supported in the decision to embark on a treatment course that does not include chronic dialysis or transplantation.

Seizures. A seizure disorder requiring anticonvulsant medication may be present in up to 10% of young pediatric transplant candidates. Whenever possible, prior to transplant, seizures should be controlled with drugs that do not interfere with cyclosporine or prednisone metabolism (see Chap. 4). Benzodiazepines are a good choice when circumstances permit. Carbamazepine does reduce cyclosporine and prednisone levels, but its effect is not as strong as phenytoin or barbiturates. Should it prove necessary to use one of the latter drugs for seizure control, moderately augmented doses of prednisone are given twice daily. Cyclosporine (Sandimmune) is administered three times a day with careful monitoring of trough blood levels. The use of cyclosporine in the newer Neoral formulation, with its improved gastrointestinal absorption (see Chap. 4), may reduce the requirement for tid dosing.

Psychoemotional Status

Psychiatric and emotional disorders are not by themselves contraindications to dialysis and transplantation; however, the involvement of health care professionals skilled in the care of affected children is mandatory. Primary psychiatric problems may be amenable to therapy and should not exclude children from consideration for transplantation.

Noncompliance is prevalent in adolescent transplant recipients. Patterns of medication and dialysis compliance should be established as part of the transplant evaluation. Psychiatric evaluation should be performed in high-risk cases (see Chap. 15). If noncompliance is identified or anticipated, behavior modification programs or other interventions should be in place before transplantation.

Cardiovascular Disease

Children and adolescents are unlikely to have overt atherosclerotic cardiovascular disease that requires invasive diagnostic workup. Hypertension and chronic fluid overload during dialysis may predispose to left ventricular hypertrophy, and severe hypertensive cardiomyopathy may supervene. Even at this relatively late stage, kidney transplantation may be beneficial to cardiac function. The importance of hypertension control in children with ESRD cannot be overemphasized, and bilateral nephrectomy is occasionally required.

Infection

Common Bacterial Pathogens. Urinary tract infections and infections related to peritoneal dialysis are the most common sources of bacterial infection in children with ESRD. Aggressive antibiotic therapy and prophylaxis of urinary tract infections in children may effectively suppress infections, although pretransplant nephrectomy is occasionally required for recalcitrant infections in children with reflux. Peritonitis and related infections with peritoneal dialysis are discussed below.

Cytomegalovirus. The incidence of cytomegalovirus (CMV) infection increases with age; young children are unlikely to have developed CMV seropositivity. This factor may dictate specific drug prophylactic strategies when contemplating transplanting a CMV-seronegative child with an organ from a seropositive donor (see the section on post-transplantation infections in children and Chap. 10).

Epstein-Barr Virus. It is important to establish the Epstein-Barr virus (EBV) antibody status of the child before transplant. As with CMV, the incidence of EBV infections and resultant seropositivity increase with age. There is some suggestion that a primary EBV infection, in the context of intensive immunosuppressive therapy, may predispose to a particularly aggressive form of post-transplant lymphoproliferative disease (PTLD).

Immunization Status. Whenever possible, immunizations should be brought up to date while the patient is still requiring dialysis. This is particularly true with respect to live vaccines, the use of which may be contraindicated in immunosuppressed patients.

Urologic Problems

Obstructive uropathy accounts for approximately 20% of ESRD in young children and needs to be fully evaluated before transplant. Cystoscopy, voiding cystourethrography, and urodynamic studies may be required. Intractable urinary tract infection in the presence of hydronephrosis or severe reflux may require nephrectomy prior to transplantation. Nephrectomy should be avoided if possible, since leaving the kidneys in situ may facilitate fluid management during dialysis, an important consideration for small children, in whom fluid balance may be tenuous.

The presence of an abnormal lower urinary tract is not a contraindication to transplantation. Some studies have reported an inferior outcome in patients with obstructive uropathy; however, no significant difference in outcome has been detected in the NAPRTCS database. Recipients with an abnormal bladder may have an increased incidence of post-transplant urologic complications and urinary tract infections. Malformations and voiding abnormalities (e.g., neurogenic bladder, bladder dyssynergia, remnant posterior urethral valves, urethral strictures) should be identified and repaired if possible. Excellent results have been reported using a previously defunctioned bladder; bladders that have not been used for an extended period of time can be hydrodilated and assessed for adequacy.

If the bladder is unusable, it can be augmented with a segment of stomach, ileum, or native ureter before transplantation. Continent internal urinary diversions have also been quite successful when the bladder has been rudimentary or absent. If a child has a neurogenic bladder or other voiding abnormality, it may be possible to teach self-catheterization safely and successfully. Urinary tract infections may occur when catheterization technique is poor, however, and noncompliance may lead to partial obstruction.

Renal Osteodystrophy

Aggressive diagnosis and treatment of hyperparathyroidism, osteomalacia, and aluminum bone disease are important in the pretransplant period. Control of hyperparathyroidism with vitamin D analogues or even parathyroidectomy may be required before transplantation. Failure to do so may both predispose to post transplant hypercalcemia and limit the growth potential of a successful transplant recipient.

Children on Peritoneal Dialysis

Children on peritoneal dialysis have graft and patient survival rates that are similar to those of children receiving hemodialysis. Typically, the extraperitoneal placement of the transplant allows for continued peritoneal dialysis post-transplant in the event of delayed graft function. Intraperitoneal graft placement is not an absolute contraindication to peritoneal dialysis.

A recent episode of peritonitis in a child awaiting a transplant does not preclude transplantation. Potential transplant recipients should be appropriately treated for 10–14 days and have a negative peritoneal fluid culture off antibiotic treatment before transplantation is contemplated. In addition, the preoperative peritoneal cell count should not suggest peritonitis. If there is a chronic exit site infection present at the time of surgery, the catheter should be removed and appropriate parenteral antibiotics administered. An overt tunnel infection should be treated before transplantation. The incidence of post-transplant peritoneal dialysis-related infections is low. Such infections typically respond to appropriate antibiotic therapy, although catheter removal may be necessary for recurrent infections. In the absence of infections, the peritoneal catheter may be left in place until good graft function has been established for approximately 4 weeks, though earlier removal may be appropriate.

Nephrotic Syndrome

In children with glomerular diseases, proteinuria usually diminishes as kidney function deteriorates and ESRD ensues. Occasionally, florid nephrotic syndrome may persist, particularly in children with focal glomerulosclerosis or congential nephrotic syndrome. Controlling heavy proteinuria before transplantation is important and can sometimes be achieved with nonsteroidal anti-inflammatory drugs and/or angiotensin-converting enzyme inhibitors. Renal embolization or bilateral nephrectomy may be required.

Portal Hypertension

Portal hypertension may occur in certain forms of ESRD that are common in children, such as autosomal recessive polycystic kidney disease. Its manifestations must be controlled. Esophageal varices require portal-systemic shunting or sclerotherapy. If neutropenia and thrombocytopenia are present as a result of hypersplenism, partial splenectomy or splenic embolization may be required before transplantation.

Prior Malignancy

Wilms' tumor is the principal malignancy producing ESRD in children. A disease-free period of 1 year should be observed before considering transplantation, since earlier transplantation has been associated with development of recurrent or metastatic disease in nearly 50% of reported cases. Premature transplantation in this setting has also been associated with overwhelming sepsis, which may be related to chemotherapy for the tumor. The presence of a primary nonrenal malignancy is not an absolute contraindication to transplantation, although an appropriate waiting time must be observed between tumor extirpation and transplantation (see Chap. 6).

Predialysis Transplantation

More children are receiving transplants before commencing dialysis; preemptive transplants now account for 24% of all pediatric transplants. Nearly 75% of these transplants are from living donors. A preemptive transplant protects a child from the physical and emotional stress of dialysis, although it has been suggested that medication noncompliance may be more common when a child has not received prior dialysis. The 1-year graft survival statistics are not influenced by pretransplant dialysis.

FACTORS AFFECTING PEDIATRIC TRANSPLANT OUTCOME

Donor Source

As noted above, graft and patient survival rates are clearly better in children when kidneys from living-related donors are used, although with the advent of new immunosuppressive agents, the gap in results between live-related and cadaveric transplants has closed considerably. At some centers, the short-term results of cadaveric transplantation in children are identical to those found in live-related transplantation, although UNOS registry data continue to show that the long-term outcome is better in live-related transplant recipients. The importance of HLA matching in cadaveric kidney distribution in children is not different from that in adults (see Chap. 3).

Donor Age

In pediatric transplantation, it was originally thought to be wise to use kidneys from young donors for young recipients. There is now considerable evidence to indicate that this logic is flawed. Both ethical considerations and the high incidence of vascular thrombosis and increased incidence of urinary tract malformations make anencephalic newborns poor candidates as kidney donors. Kidneys from donors younger than 18 months of age often fail because of a high incidence of primary nonfunction and graft thrombosis.

The use of pediatric donors younger than 10 years of age is controversial. In the past, young donors had provided a large proportion of the cadaveric kidneys for pediatric recipients, and the young transplanted kidney has been shown to grow with time. Nevertheless, a large body of experience supports the conclusion that kidneys from donors younger than 6 years of age have graft survival rates 20–40% lower than those from adolescents or adults. In the early 1990s, UNOS revised the national sharing algorithm for kidneys (see Chap. 3) to facilitate pediatric access to adult kidneys. Subsequently, there has been a 9% improvement in 1-year graft survival for children. While the change in allocation strategy was probably not the sole reason for this improvement, this experience supports the move to transplant larger kidneys whenever possible (see the section on nephron dose, Chap. 3). The impact of allograft size and function on growth is discussed in the section on determinants of post-transplant growth.

Recipient Age

The age at the time of transplantation influences the results of graft and patient survival. NAPRTCS data from 1987 to 1995 show that 3-year cadaveric graft survival for infants younger than 2 years old is only 51%, compared with 66–69% for older age groups. Better results can be obtained in infant recipients when grafts from adult live-related donors are used; however, a recipient age of younger than 2 years is associated with a 3-year live-related graft survival of 77%, compared with 81–86% in older children, depending on age. Children 2–6 years of age historically have had poorer graft survival than children older than 6 years of age, but graft survival in the 2- to 6-year-old age group has been rapidly improving with attention to the factors discussed below.

Cyclosporine Metabolism

In its original Sandimmune formulation, cyclosporine is metabolized more rapidly and absorbed less well by children than adults. As a result, it may be more difficult to achieve target blood concentrations. Estimation of dose based on body surface area is more likely to result in therapeutic blood levels. Administration of cyclosporine using a three times a day regimen may serve to maximize the "area under the curve" (AUC) of the administered drug (see Chap. 4). The Neoral formulation improves the bioavailability and AUC of cyclosporine, particularly in younger children, though the clinical impact of this improvement has not yet been proved.

Technical Considerations

Small children present unique technical challenges. Long reanastomosis time and resultant early allograft dysfunction with acute tubular necrosis (ATN) significantly reduce allograft survival and impair long-term allograft function. The 3-year graft survival rates for pediatric patients with and without ATN are 52% and 74%, respectively, for cadaveric grafts and 55% and 87% for grafts from living donors. The small vessels and anatomy of the uremic child make vascular anastomosis more time-consuming and thus increase the chances for impaired graft outcome, particularly when cyclosporine is used from the outset. The placement of relatively large kidneys in small children may result in improved graft survival and kidney function but may present a formidable technical challenge (see Chap. 7). Generally, extraperitoneal graft placement is preferred in all children, particularly in those who are undergoing peritoneal dialysis. In the child who weighs less than 20 kg, the kidney may be placed intraperitoneally. The aorta and vena cava are frequently used for vascular anastomosis in smaller children to ensure adequate blood flow.

Immunologic Considerations

There is evidence that young children have heightened immunologic reactivity. Adult dialysis patients may manifest defects of immunologic function that have not been observed in children. Children younger than 6 years of age have higher indices of nonspecific cellular immune responsiveness than do older children or young adults. These indices include spontaneous blastogenesis; increased numbers of CD4+ helper T cells, B cells, and immature activated T cells; as well as an increased CD4-to-CD8 (helper-to-suppressor) T cell ratio. Following OKT3 treatment, young children may show a faster reappearance of CD3+ cells and higher rate of anti-OKT3 antibody generation than adults (see Chap. 4). All these findings suggest that young children may be at a higher risk for graft rejection than older children and may require more intensive immunosuppression. A significantly greater percentage of children younger than 6 years of age suffer graft failure after their first rejection episode than do older recipients.

Presensitization

Presensitization is as vexing a problem in children as it is in adults (see Chap. 3). Children tolerate anemia poorly and may be transfused frequently, with resultant broad anti-HLA sensitization. In the NAPRTCS database, children who had received more than five pretransplant blood transfusions had a poorer graft outcome. Younger children are also more likely to develop anti-HLA antigens in response to transfusions. Sensitization is often particularly troublesome in the child who has rejected a previous transplant. Highly sensitized children may wait inordinately long periods for a crossmatch-negative transplant; this wait can represent a particularly onerous problem for small children, who often tolerate dialysis poorly. The availability of human recombinant erythropoietin allows for a reduced transfusion requirement and a subsequent reduction in the level of sensitization.

Recurrence of Primary Kidney Disease

Recurrence of disease as a cause of graft dysfunction and failure is discussed in Chaps. 6 and 9. In adults, recurrent disease accounts for less than 2% of all graft failure, whereas in children it may account for 7% or more. The two main categories of kidney disease that can potentially involve the graft are inherited metabolic disease and glomerulonephritis. Discussion of the most common causes of recurrence in pediatric transplants follows.

Inherited Metabolic Disease

Oxalosis. Type 1 primary hyperoxaluria is an autosomal, recessively inherited inborn error of metabolism due to the deficiency of the hepatic enzyme peroxisomal alanine glyoxylate aminotransferase (AGT). Children with oxalosis have long been regarded as unsuitable candidates for transplantation because recurrence of devastating renal oxalate deposition during periods of graft insufficiency has led to almost invariable graft failure. While some reports have suggested that short-term success may be possible with renal transplantation alone, the long-term results remain poor. In children with ESRD and documented AGT deficiency, combined kidney and liver transplantation may be the most effective option, since the transplanted liver provides the deficient enzyme. In patients with high plasma oxalate levels (e.g., >50 mg/ml), intensive preoperative reduction of plasma oxalate levels by hemodialysis is required together with immediate postoperative diuresis to minimize oxalate deposition in the graft. Post-transplant management should include the administration of pyridoxine, neutral phosphate, magnesium, and noncalciuric diuretic therapy, as well as the avoidance of infection and graft dysfunction due to ATN or rejection. Reported results of combined organ transplantation in this condition have been encouraging.

Nephropathic Cystinosis. Recurrence of Fanconi's syndrome and precipitous deterioration of renal function have not been described after transplantation in children with cystinosis, although cystine crystals have been described in the graft interstitium as a result of the elevated cystine content of host leukocytes that infiltrate the transplanted organ. There is no accumulation of cystine in the renal tubular or glomerular epithelial cells, since the donor kidney cells contain normal transport mechanisms. Other extrarenal manifestations of cystinosis continue to progress after transplantation, including loss of vision, photophobia, hypothyroidism, and, occasionally, significant central nervous system symptomatology.

Recurrent Glomerular Disease

Focal and Segmental Glomerulosclerosis. Focal and segmental glomerulosclerosis (FSGS) is the most common glomerular disease to cause ESRD in children and is reported as the cause of renal failure in nearly 12% of the patients in the NAPRTCS database. It recurs in up to 40% of transplants in children and is the cause of graft failure in half of these cases. Recurrence is usually characterized by persistent and sometimes massive proteinuria, which may develop precipitously immediately post-transplant or insidiously weeks or months later.

Children older than 6 years of age, yet still in the childhood age range, whose initial disease led to ESRD in less than 3 years are at greatest risk for graft recurrence of FSGS. The finding of mesangial proliferation in the native kidney may also predispose to recurrence.

If FSGS causes the loss of the first transplant, it will recur in 80% of subsequent transplants.

There is no definitive treatment for recurrence of FSGS. Patients deemed to be at high risk of recurrence should be monitored compulsively in the first few post-transplant months for the appearance of proteinuria. The patient should then have a biopsy to confirm the diagnosis. Early use of plasmapheresis and high-dose cyclosporine therapy has been associated with complete or partial remission. There have also been reports of remission following cyclophosphamide treatment and the use of extracorporeal perfusion through *Staphylococcus* protein A columns. Recurrence of FSGS appears to be associated with high serum levels of an as yet undefined factor that increases glomerular permeability to albumin ($P_{albumin}$) in isolated rat glomeruli. The factor has an apparent molecular mass of about 50 kD. $P_{albumin}$ is reduced by cyclosporine, a finding that presumably explains its therapeutic effectiveness.

Membranoproliferative Glomerulonephritis. Histologic evidence of recurrence occurs commonly in both membranoproliferative glomerulonephritis (MPGN) type I and type II in children. Clinically significant recurrence is less frequent. The recurrence rate of MPGN type I ranges from 30% to 70%, with graft loss in up to 30% of these cases in some series. Histologic recurrence of MPGN type II is present in almost all patients. Its clinical impact is usually benign, although some centers report graft loss in up to 50% of cases. The presence of crescentic changes in the native kidneys with either form of MPGN increases the changes of significant recurrence.

Henoch-Schönlein Purpura and IgA Nephropathy. Histologic recurrence with IgA deposits is noted frequently but rarely leads to graft loss. When recurrence is clinically significant, it can be severe, with crescentic glomerular disease, nephrotic syndrome, and precipitous graft failure. In cases of Henoch-Schönlein purpura, it has been recommended that transplantation be deferred until 6–12 months after the last episode of purpura.

Hemolytic-Uremic Syndrome. Hemolytic-uremic syndrome (HUS) is the most common cause of primary acute kidney failure in children. When strict diagnostic criteria have been applied, up to 50% recurrence has been reported, although this figure is probably a considerable overestimate. HUS presents clinically in two forms: the more frequently occurring so-called "typical" diarrhea associated HUS and the less frequently occurring "atypical" HUS, in which there is no diarrheal prodrome. It has been suggested that recurrence of HUS may be related to the use of cyclosporine or antilymphocyte globulin. Although this may well be true for the atypical variety of HUS, these drugs can be used successfully for typical HUS. Transplantation should be delayed until all systemic manifestations of HUS have been quiescent for at least 12 months.

Congenital Nephrotic Syndrome. As a general rule, nephrotic syndrome does not recur in this disease, although occasional instances have been reported. The nephrotic syndrome also does not recur in familial steroid-resistant nephrotic syndrome with focal sclerosis or in the nephrotic syndrome associated with the Drash syndrome.

TRANSPLANT IMMUNOSUPPRESSION IN CHILDREN

The immunosuppressive agents used in pediatric kidney transplantation are the same as those used in adults (see Chap. 4). There are subtle, yet critical, nuances in the use of these drugs in children.

Corticosteroids and Azathioprine

The familiar side effects of corticosteroids are common to both adults and children (see Table 4-2). Growth retardation is a crucial concern in children; its relationship to steroid dose is discussed below (see the section on growth). Alternate-day prednisone protocols may improve growth velocity, hypertension, obesity, acne, and other side effects. Some centers, however, have reported an increased incidence of acute rejection episodes with alternate-day regimens and thus prefer a low-dose daily regimen. Discontinuation of corticosteroids in growing children has been advocated by some centers, and noncontrolled studies suggest that this may be possible in up to half the patients. An increased incidence of both early and late rejection may result, however, and the ensuing graft dysfunction may significantly impair growth. Steroid discontinuation protocols should still be regarded as experimental. The usual daily dose of prednisone for children 2-3 years post-transplant is 0.17–0.19 mg/kg/day.

Corticosteroids, like cyclosporine, are metabolized by the hepatic P450 enzyme system. Enzyme induction by anticonvulsant medications may accelerate steroid metabolism; therefore, higher doses or more frequent dosing intervals are required in patients on anticonvulsant drug therapy. Unfortunately, since there is no readily available drug assay, dose adjustments are made empirically in these patients (e.g., by giving the standard prednisone dose twice daily).

Azathioprine is given to most children as adjunctive immunosuppression in triple-therapy regimens (see Chap. 4). The daily dose varies from 1 mg/kg to 2 mg/kg and may need to be reduced in the presence of neutropenia or hepatic enzyme elevations. The concurrent administration of corticosteroids tends to boost the neutrophil count; if they are discontinued, a reduction of the azathioprine dosage may be required.

Cyclosporine

Cyclosporine is the backbone of immunosuppressive regimens in children and is used for most transplants. There are some important differences between the use of cyclosporine in adults and children.

Metabolism in Children

Children metabolize cyclosporine more rapidly than adults. The half-life of cyclosporine is age-dependent, so young children metabolize the drug much more rapidly than older children. Children may thus require higher doses on a milligram-per-kilogram basis or shorter dosing intervals to achieve therapeutic AUCs and blood levels. In addition, the pharmacokinetics of cyclosporine are highly variable in children, so frequent blood level monitoring is required. Periodic pharmacokinetic studies have been advocated to expeditiously and safely achieve appropriate therapeutic levels. Young children may be strong immunologic responders, and the requirement for adequate cyclosporine doses and blood levels is compelling.

The intestinal absorption of cyclosporine may be relatively impaired in young or growth-retarded children. Cyclosporine absorption is dependent on the length of the small intestine, so smaller children or children with disproportionately short small intestines may have difficulty achieving therapeutic blood levels on doses normally prescribed for adults. The mean cyclosporine dose in milligrams per kilograms required to achieve a therapeutic target is significantly higher in young children than in adolescents.

The development of the Neoral formulation of cyclosporine is potentially an important advance for children. Intestinal absorption is improved, particularly in young children, who may be poor absorbers of Sandimmune. The milligram-per-kilogram dose of Neoral in children is the same as that of adolescents to achieve comparable AUCs. There is also less variability in the pharmacokinetic profile.

Cyclosporine drug interactions are discussed in detail in Chap. 4. Because of concurrent medical problems, pediatric transplant recipients often receive multiple medications, so potential interactions must always be considered. Anticonvulsant medications, particularly barbiturates and phenytoin, are potent activators of the P450 hepatic enzyme system. If their use is mandatory, higher doses of cyclosporine will be required, together with more frequent dosing intervals and assiduous attention to therapeutic blood levels. The use of Neoral may facilitate dosing in these patients.

Toxicity in Children

Nephrotoxicity.   The nephrotoxic potential of cyclosporine is exaggerated in the presence of early graft dysfunction. The administration of cyclosporine in the early post-transplant period in the presence of graft dysfunction may result in a suboptimal GFR, which may, in turn, have a negative impact on growth and impair long-term graft survival. In children, as in adults, it is unclear what precise level and dosage of cyclosporine is required for long-term maintenance therapy, although higher levels may result in better long-term function by forestalling acute rejection episodes and blunting chronic rejection.

Cosmetic Side Effects.   Attention to cosmetic side effects is particularly important in children because of the emotional distress they produce and because of the temptation for children not to comply with the therapeutic regimen. A characteristic facial appearance has been described in children receiving cyclosporine involving a coarsening of facial features and prognathism. This finding occurs frequently and is due to a shortening of the posterior facial height and a lengthening of the anterior facial height (Fig. 14-1). Its severity appears to diminish with time.

Children appear particularly prone to developing gingival hypertrophy, particularly if they are also receiving the antihypertensive agent nifedipine. Hypertrichosis is particularly burdensome in adolescent females and Hispanic and black children. Facial depilatories and bleaching of excess hair can be quite effective. Experience with the use of tacrolimus in children is limited, but the cosmetic side effects of this drug are less marked (see Chap. 4).

Convulsions.   Seizures have been described in children receiving cyclosporine and may occur more commonly than in adults taking the medication. They have usually been ascribed to hypertension, although a direct neurotoxic effect has been suggested. Hypo-

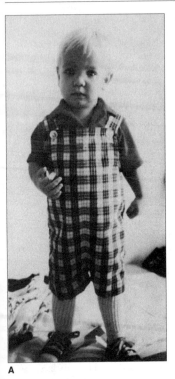 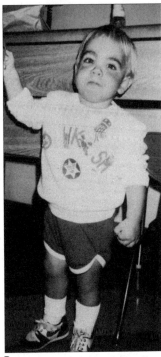

A   B

Fig. 14-1. A. An 18-month-old child with renal dysplasia. B. The child is 8 months older and 2 months post-transplant. Note the cushingoid facies and truncal weight gain typical of prednisone use and the prominent brow and eyebrow hair typical of cyclosporine use.

magnesemia, due to magnesuria or increased intracellular magnesium concentration, may also lower the seizure threshold. Oral magnesium supplements may be needed in the first few post-transplant months when the cyclosporine dose tends to be higher.

Mycophenolate Mofetil

Mycophenolate mofetil (MMF) is discussed in detail in Chap. 4. It was approved for the prophylaxis of acute rejection in mid-1995; in many transplant programs, it has been introduced into routine use with cyclosporine and prednisone, replacing azathioprine. Experience with MMF in children is limited, but preliminary results suggest that its use may halve the incidence of acute rejection episodes from the rate of 50–67% reported by NAPRTCS. The dose used in children has been extrapolated from the doses used in the adult clinical trials and is approximately 20 mg/kg bid. There is some evidence that the dosing in children should be calculated based on body surface area. MMF is generally well-tolerated by children with an adverse event profile similar to that reported for adults.

Table 14-3. Sequential immunosuppressive protocol for pediatric kidney transplantation at UCLA

Pretransplant (6–12 hr)
Cyclosporine: 10 mg/kg PO if ATG is to be used[a]; 4 mg/kg PO if OKT3 is to be used, or if donor procurement history suggests an increased likelihood of acute tubular necrosis

Induction therapy
1. ATG at 15 mg/kg/day or OKT3 1 mg for 2 days then 2.5 mg for body weight <30 kg and 5 mg for >30 kg
Continue until serum creatinine $\leq$ 2 mg/dl or 10 days
2. Azathioprine 1–2 mg/kg/day
3. Methylprednisolone 10 mg/kg IV intraoperatively and 1–3 hours prior to OKT3 dose for days 1–3; then prednisone 0.5 mg/kg/day (minimum dose: 20 mg)
4. If OKT3 is to be used, give cyclosporine 6 mg/kg PO divided bid to reduce the formation of anti-OKT3 antibodies; dose increased when serum creatinine $\leq$ 2 mg/dl; cyclosporine unnecessary with ATG

Maintenance therapy
1. Cyclosporine: 12 mg/kg/day divided bid or tid for children $\leq$ 6 yrs; give 500 mg/m^2/day divided bid or tid[b]
2. Cyclosporine dosage is adjusted to achieve target levels (see Table 14-4) using the lower range if the child has not achieved a serum creatinine of less than 2 mg/dl by the 10 days that the anti–T cell preparation must be concluded
3. Azathioprine: 1–2 mg/kg/day
4. Prednisone: Taper to approximately 0.15 mg/kg/day at 6 mos

ATG = antithymocyte globulin.
[a]ATG and OKT3 are described in detail in Chap. 4.
[b]The cyclosporine and monoclonal or polyclonal antibody preparations should be overlapped for 1–3 days until therapeutic levels of cyclosporine are achieved.

Pediatric Immunosuppressive Protocols

The logic behind the design of immunosuppressive protocols in children is essentially the same as that in adults and is discussed in Chap. 4. The various protocol options available in adults are applicable to children. The fact that children may be strong immunologic responders and may be particularly susceptible to early cyclosporine nephrotoxicity, however, supports the use of induction therapy with an antilymphocytic agent. In such a protocol, cyclosporine is withheld or given in low doses in the early postoperative period. A polyclonal or monoclonal antibody preparation is given until graft function begins to improve or 10–12 days have elapsed.

Table 14-3 describes the sequential immunosuppressive protocol presently used at the UCLA Pediatric Transplant Program. Using this protocol, the actuarial graft survival results at 1 and 3 years in primary pediatric cadaveric transplantation have been 92% and 83%, respectively.

Most programs employ triple therapy (cyclosporine, prednisone, and azathioprine) for immunosuppression maintenance (see Chap. 4). The therapeutic target cyclosporine levels and prednisone and azathioprine doses are listed in Table 14-4. MMF will likely replace azathioprine in the future. Table 14-5 summarizes the cyclosporine doses prescribed by the UCLA Pediatric Transplant Program to

Table 14-4. Therapeutic targets for sequential immunosuppressive regimen at UCLA Pediatric Transplant Program

	12-hr cyclosporine whole blood trough levels*			
Weeks after transplantation	Polyclonal TDx (ng/ml)	HPLC (ng/ml)	Prednisone dosage (mg/kg/day)	Azathioprine dosage (mg/kg/day)
0–4	500–750	150–200	0.5 (minimum 20 kg)	2
4–8	350–500	125–175	0.33	2
8–12	300–450	100–150	0.25	2
12–16	250–350	80–125	0.18–0.20	2
16–26	200–300	75–100	0.13–0.18	2

*See Chap. 4 for discussion of cyclosporine monitoring techniques.

Table 14-5. Mean total daily cyclosporine dose* at UCLA in relation to patient age

	Months after transplantation				
Age (yr)	1	3	6	12	24
2–12	16.6 ± 7.1	12.2 ± 7.3	10.6 ± 6.7	9.2 ± 6.6	6.2 ± 2.4
13–21	10.8 + 4.2	7.5 ± 2.7	6.3 ± 2.5	6.0 ± 2.1	5.1 ± 2.0

*mg/kg body weight ± standard deviation.

achieve target levels at different time intervals post-transplant in younger and older children. These doses may need to be modified with the introduction of Neoral.

TRANSPLANT MANAGEMENT PROBLEMS IN CHILDREN

Perioperative Fluid and Electrolyte Management

Preoperative Dialysis

Children, like adults, should be adequately dialyzed before transplantation. For the child on hemodialysis, a complete dialysis treatment should be performed within 24 hours of the surgery. If electrolyte values are within acceptable limits, it is often not necessary to dialyze immediately before transplantation. Chronic peritoneal dialysis patients rarely require additional dialysis before transplantation, although the peritoneal cavity should be emptied of fluid. When performing pretransplant dialysis of whatever type, aggressive fluid removal should be avoided in an attempt to minimize post-transplant delayed graft function. Similarly, the polyuric child should receive appropriate hydration before surgery.

Intraoperative Fluid Management

Precise intraoperative fluid management and maintenance of adequate vascular volume are essential to minimize post-transplant delayed graft function. Fluid management is particularly crucial when placing an adult kidney in a relatively small child. An adult donor kidney may sequester as much as 150–250 ml of blood. To prevent hypotension, this amount of fluid should be administered as isotonic crystalloid and colloid solutions before the renal vessels are unclamped. The central venous pressure (CVP) and arterial blood pressure should be closely monitored during surgery. The intraoperative CVP should be maintained at 10–14 cm H_2O and the mean arterial pressure maintained above 70 mm Hg before vascular clamps are removed.

Aggressive fluid therapy may be insufficient to optimize the blood pressure, particularly in children whose myocardial function is suboptimal. If the mean arterial blood pressure is relatively low despite an adequate CVP, a low-dose dopamine infusion may elevate blood pressure and facilitate renal vasodilatation. Some programs routinely institute intravenous dopamine infusions at 2–4 mg/kg/minute at the start of surgery. If mean arterial blood pressure is inadequate to effect good renal perfusion (e.g., less than 60 mm Hg) to adult donor organs, the dopamine infusion rate can be raised to as high as 9 mg/kg/minute, with excellent results. Furosemide (2–4 mg/kg) and mannitol (0.5–1.0 g/kg) may be given during creation of the vascular anastomosis to facilitate urine output. When these drugs are administered, however, the urine output must be replaced to prevent hypovolemia.

Postoperative Fluid Management

The principles of post-transplant fluid management are discussed in Chap. 8. It is particularly important that small patients receiving relatively large kidneys maintain intravascular volumes and blood pressure. The CVP should be maintained in the range of 6–10 cm H_2O, and mean arterial blood pressure should remain above 70 mm Hg. Insensible fluid losses should be calculated and administered as 5% dextrose (either 400 ml/m^2 body surface area or 40 ml/100 kcal metabolized). The urine output should be replaced "milliliter-for-milliliter" with 0.33% or 0.45% saline. Because urine volume can be prodigious after transplant, the dextrose is omitted from the urine replacement to avoid hyperglycemia. Supplemental fluid boluses (10 ml/kg of normal saline or 5% albumin solutions in saline) may be required to support blood pressure, reestablish an acceptable CVP, and restore urine output. Augmentation of fluid therapy and inotropic support may be required to keep mean arterial pressures at acceptable levels (i.e., above 70 mm Hg). If the child is fluid overloaded, it may be appropriate to replace only a portion of the urine output for a few hours until the CVP is reestablished at a desired level.

Early initiation of dialysis may be appropriate for the child with delayed graft function, congestive heart failure, or electrolyte abnormalities. Either hemodialysis or peritoneal dialysis may be performed safely. It is important to avoid overly aggressive ultrafiltration and fluid removal, since this can exacerbate ATN.

Acute Transplant Dysfunction in Young Children

In children, as in adults, the principal causes of early acute allograft dysfunction are acute rejection, ATN, cyclosporine nephrotoxicity, prerenal azotemia, obstructive uropathy, urine leak, renal artery stenosis, and viral and bacterial infections. The differential diagnosis is discussed in detail in Chap. 8. In children, there may be subtle differences in the presentation of graft dysfunction. In small children who receive large kidneys and in whom the baseline serum creatinine level is less than 1.0 mg/dl, a small rise in the serum creatinine levels (e.g., 0.2–0.3 mg/dl) can reflect a significant diminution in allograft function. Since the muscle mass and creatinine production of a child are small, there may be no recognizable rise in the serum creatinine level despite graft dysfunction; the most sensitive indicator of rejection in small children is the development of hypertension with or without accompanying fever. Even a modest elevation in serum creatinine, particularly in the context of a low-grade fever, should be presumed to be rejection until proved otherwise.

Because of the higher incidence of CMV seropositivity in adults, the use of kidneys from adult donors, although preferable because of enhanced graft outcome, results in a greater incidence of primary CMV infection in young children. The use of sequential induction immunosuppressive strategies also makes it more likely that severe CMV disease will appear. The aggressive anti-CMV prophylactic therapies now employed in many centers (see Chap. 10) may attenuate the typical disease course, however, and CMV infection may manifest as only modest fever and a minimal rise in the serum creatinine level. Urinary tract infections in young children may be clinically indistinguishable from acute rejection; therefore, urine culture and urinalysis must not be omitted in cases of fever and graft dysfunction.

The diagnostic tools for the evaluation of graft dysfunction do not differ between children and adults. Ultrasound and radionuclide scanning are discussed in Chap. 11. Fine needle aspiration biopsy and core biopsy are discussed in Chap. 12.

Treatment of Acute Rejection in Children

Pulse Steroids

High-dose corticosteroid pulses are the mainstay of treatment of acute rejection in children, as they are in adults (see Chap. 4). Doses at different centers range from 5–10 mg/kg/day of methylprednisolone IV for 3–5 days. Following pulse treatment, the maintenance corticosteroid dose is usually resumed at the prerejection level or recycled back down from the high levels that were used posttransplant. Some centers prefer oral prednisone pulses, in which case 3–5 mg/kg is given for 3 days followed by tapering the dose back to baseline levels over 2–3 days. It may be advisable to give furosemide (0.5-1.0 mg/kg) either PO or IV during high-dose steroid therapy to minimize fluid retention and hypertension.

OKT3

Approximately 20–30% of rejection episodes will not respond to high-dose steroids, but up to 90% of these can be reversed by OKT3. OKT3 is discussed in detail in Chap. 4 and the pediatric protocol for OKT3 administration shown in Table 14-6. In children, as in adults, OKT3 can be administered on an outpatient basis after the first few doses. Before completion of the OKT3 course, the cyclosporine dose should be increased by 1 mg/kg/day over the pre-OKT3 level so that blood levels are somewhat higher than they were prior to treatment; this regimen reduces the incidence of rebound rejections. When rebound rejections do occur, they may be amenable to high-dose steroids.

Table 14-6. Treatment protocol for children receiving OKT3*

Before initiating therapy
Chest x-ray to show no evidence of fluid overload
If weight is more than 3% above dry weight, start dialysis or vigorous
diuresis to attain dry weight
Prior to first and second doses of OKT3
Acetaminophen, 250 mg PO
Diphenhydramine hydrochloride (Benadryl), 0.5–1.0 mg/kg IV
Methylprednisolone, 10 mg/kg IV 1–3 hours before OKT3
Dose of OKT3
Body weight <30 kg = 2.5 mg OKT3
Body weight >30 kg = 5 mg OKT3
Cyclosporine to be continued at half previous dose during course
Prednisone at maintenance dose levels after second dose of OKT3

*See also Chap. 4.

It is wise to monitor the effectiveness of OKT3 by following the levels of CD3+ T cells. Immunologic monitoring is mandatory during a second course of OKT3, since the development of OKT3 antibodies may abrogate the effectiveness of the drug. Children may regenerate the CD3/T cell receptor complex more rapidly than adults, so twice daily dosing of OKT3 is occasionally necessary to effect successful rejection reversal. Following a first course of OKT3, up to 35% of children may develop anti-OKT3 antibodies. The titer of antibodies is usually low and can be overcome by increasing the OKT3 dose; however, approximately 15% of children develop high titers of antibody, preventing further use.

The side effects of OKT3 are similar in children and adults. Children must be euvolemic before administration of the first dose to prevent pulmonary edema. Fever is nearly universal; diarrhea and vomiting occur in nearly half of all children treated. Severe headache is common and may represent a mild form of aseptic meningitis. There have been occasional fatalities associated with OKT3-mediated cerebral edema.

Tacrolimus and Mycophenolate Mofetil

Both of these new agents have been used successfully to reverse episodes of acute rejection that are refractory to treatment with corticosteroids and OKT3 (see Chap. 4). Most of the published experience has been in adults, although each agent has been used successfully in children and adolescents. Further intensification of immunosuppression in patients who are already heavily immunosuppressed demands caution because of the ever present dangers of opportunistic infection and lymphoproliferative disorders. The danger is particularly great in children who are prone to develop primary EBV infection.

Noncompliance

Psychosocial and emotional problems in children and adolescents undergoing dialysis and transplantation frequently manifest themselves as noncompliance with the therapeutic regimen. The importance of this problem cannot be overemphasized.

Frequency

Approximately 50% of pediatric cadaveric transplant recipients demonstrate significant noncompliance in the post-transplant period. This figure exceeds 60% in adolescents. Noncompliance has been estimated to be the principal cause of graft loss in 10–15% of all pediatric kidney transplant recipients; in pediatric recipients of retransplants, this figure may exceed 25%. Reversible and irreversible episodes of graft dysfunction related to noncompliance occur in up to 40% of adolescents and are somewhat less frequent in younger children.

Prognostication and Recognition

It is difficult to predict in the pretransplant period who will not comply post-transplant. A disorganized family structure, female sex, adolescence, and a history of previous graft loss due to noncompliance are all significant risk factors. Personality problems related to low self-esteem and poor social adjustment are found with higher frequency in noncompliant patients.

Noncompliance in children must be suspected when any of the following are observed: diminution in cushingoid features, sudden unexplained weight loss, and unexplained swings in the patient's kidney function or cyclosporine trough blood level. After an acute rejection episode is reversed, psychological support is of the utmost importance if long-term graft function is to be salvaged.

Management

Prospective introduction of behavior modification programs and other forms of psychological intervention have had moderate success in improving compliance. In the pretransplant period, an ongoing program of counseling should be undertaken in high-risk patients. Clearly defined therapeutic goals should be set while the patient is on dialysis, and family problems that are recognized in the pretransplant period should be addressed prior to activation on the transplant list. The presence of at least one highly motivated caretaker is a helpful factor in long-term graft success.

Adolescence brings with it rapid behavioral and bodily changes. The adolescent's strong desire to be normal conflicts with the continued reminder of chronic disease that the taking of medication engenders; this tendency is particularly true when medications are taken many times a day and alter the physical appearance. Ambivalence between the desire for parental protection and autonomy, combined with the adolescent's "magical" belief in his or her invulnerability, sets the stage for experimentation with noncompliance. Adolescents with psychological or developmental problems may use impulsive noncompliance during self-destructive episodes. The transplant teams must be aware of these developmental issues so that they can initiate appropriate psychological intervention before the onset of significant noncompliant behavior. Cadaveric transplant outcome in adolescents is comparable with that reported for other pediatric age groups. With careful follow-up and appropriate attention to the particular developmental needs of adolescents, destructive noncompliance can be avoided.

Growth

Impaired statural growth frequently accompanies renal insufficiency in children and is improved little by dialysis. In general, the earlier in life ESRD occurs, the greater the lifelong growth retardation; when the onset of ESRD is in infancy, growth retardation is most severe. Potential etiologic factors for this growth failure include renal osteodystrophy, metabolic acidosis and other electrolyte disturbances, the accumulation of uremic toxins, anemia, anorexia resulting from protein and calorie malnutrition, and specific effects of the primary disease.

Estimation of Growth Impairment

Growth in children with chronic illness is best expressed by comparing their height with that of unaffected children. This comparison is made by using a so-called **standard deviation score (SDS)** for age, which expresses a patient's height in terms of standard deviations above (positive value) or below (negative value) the median (fiftieth percentile) for normal controls.

At the time of transplantation, the mean height deficit for all pediatric patients is –2.16 and is somewhat greater for boys than girls. Younger patients and those with prior transplants have substantially greater deficits. For such children to attain normal or near normal adult height, the post-transplant growth must improve at least +1 SDS. Unfortunately, overall mean height scores tend to remain relatively constant in the post-transplant period.

Determinants of Post-Transplant Growth

Although growth after kidney transplant is superior to growth during dialysis, a normal growth pattern is not always attained. There seem to be at least three important factors affecting post-transplant growth.

Age at Transplant. Young children exhibit the best growth improvement after transplantation. Children at or below the ages of 7–9 years fare better than older children, often with an improvement of SDS of more than one unit. By 1–2 years post transplant, children younger than 6 years of age have gained an average of close to 1 SDS. Children between the ages of 6 and 12 years gain only approximately 0.1 SDS; over the age of 13 years, there may be no mean increase. While children with a bone age of more than 12 years tend to grow minimally, growth may continue well into puberty in some patients. The pubertal growth spurt, however, is blunted or lost.

The fact that younger children benefit the most in statural growth from early transplantation provides a strong argument for expedited transplantation in an attempt to optimize and perhaps normalize stature. In addition, earlier transplantation allows less time for growth failure on dialysis and therefore less requirement for catch-up growth.

Corticosteroid Dose. If kidney function remains good (see the section on allograft function), post-transplant growth is largely dependent on the corticosteroid dose, although the exact mechanism by which corticosteroids impair growth is unknown. Steroids may reduce the release of growth hormone, reduce insulin-like growth factor (IGF) activity, directly impair growth cartilage, decrease calcium absorption, or increase renal phosphate wasting. Each of these factors may impair growth.

Growth may be improved in pediatric kidney transplant recipients by using low-dose daily steroids, by shifting to an alternate-day steroid dosage schedule, or by tapering steroids to discontinuation. There is evidence that alternate-day steroid regimens significantly improve growth compared with daily steroids; however, the studies illustrating this benefit have not been randomized and may tend to favor children with better allograft function, fewer rejections, and better compliance. To achieve optimal growth, steroid therapy must still be individualized.

If a low-dose daily steroid protocol is to be used, the target dose should be 0.25 mg/kg or less of prednisone. Daily doses as low as 0.12–0.15 mg/kg are achievable (see Table 14-5). If daily dose is based on surface area, the target is 4 mg/m². If an alternate-day protocol is used, twice the daily dose is given on the alternate day, with no prednisone given on the intervening day. In some centers, this regimen is reached by gradually increasing the dose on one day and decreasing it the next. Steroid discontinuation is experimental and should not be started until graft function has been stable for at least several months. Recurrent rejections are a contraindication to steroid discontinuation. Some centers have succeeded in stopping prednisone in up to 50% of pediatric patients, with resulting catch-up growth. Patients who cannot tolerate steroid discontinuation and experience rejection episodes may suffer reduction in function and growth retardation.

Allograft Function. An allograft GFR of less than 60 ml/minute/1.73 m² is associated with poor growth and low IGF levels; optimal growth occurs with a GFR of more than 90 ml/minute/1.73 m². Graft function is the most important factor after high corticosteroid dosage in the genesis of post-transplant growth failure. The immunosuppressive properties of corticosteroids needed to control rejection and preserve kidney function need to be balanced against the need to minimize steroids to maximize growth. Thus, an excessive steroid dose will lead to impairment of growth, an inadequate dose to impairment of graft function. Administration of high-dose recombinant human growth hormone may induce acceleration of growth even in the presence of chronic graft dysfunction. Definitive studies on the use of growth hormone in the post-transplant period are not yet available. There is some suggestion, however, that in some patients such therapy may further impair graft function and may induce episodes of rejection in patients who have suffered recent rejection episodes

Post-Transplant Sexual Maturation

Restoration of kidney function by transplantation improves pubertal development. This occurs most likely by normalization of gonadotropin physiology. Elevated gonadotropin levels and reduced gonadotropin pulsatility are found in patients with chronic renal failure, whereas children with successful kidney transplants demonstrate a higher nocturnal rise and increased amplitude of gonadotropin pulsatility.

Female patients who are pubertal before transplantation typically become amenorrheic during the course of chronic renal failure. Menses with ovulatory cycles usually return within 6 months to a year after transplantation, so potentially sexually active adolescent patients should be given appropriate contraceptive information (see Chap. 9).

Adolescent female transplant recipients receiving cyclosporine, prednisone, and azathioprine have successfully borne children; the only consistently reported neonatal abnormality has been an increased incidence of prematurity. Adolescent boys should be made aware that they can successfully father children. No consistent pattern of abnormalities has been reported in their offspring.

Post-Transplant Infections in Children

Infection in the immunosuppressed transplant patient is discussed in Chap. 10. In children, the spectrum of infections and their presentation may differ somewhat from adults. Infection in the immuno-compromised child remains the major cause of morbidity and mortality post-transplant.

Bacterial Infections

Pneumonia and urinary tract infections are the most common post-transplant bacterial infections. Urinary tract infection can progress rapidly to urosepsis and may be confused with episodes of acute rejection. Opportunistic infections usually do not occur until after the first post-transplant month.

Viral Infections

The herpes group viruses (CMV, herpesvirus, varicella-zoster virus, and EBV) pose a special problem in view of their common occurrence in children. Many young children have not yet been exposed to these viruses, and because they lack protective immunity, their predisposition for serious primary infection is high.

Cytomegalovirus. The incidence of CMV seropositivity is approximately 30% in children older than 5 years of age and rises to approximately 60% in teenagers. Thus, the younger the child, the greater is the potential for serious infection when a CMV-positive donor kidney is transplanted. CMV infection tends to be less severe in children than in adults; however, in heavily immunosuppressed children, it may have the same impact on the course of pediatric transplantation as on adult transplantation (see Chap. 10). Various strategies have been proposed to minimize this impact. It has been suggested that seronegative children receive only kidneys from seronegative donors; however, given the frequency of seropositivity in the adult population, this restriction would penalize seronegative children by prolonging their wait for a transplant. CMV hyperimmune globulin, high-dose standard immune globulin, high-dose oral acyclovir, and so-called "preemptive" intravenous ganciclovir (see Chap. 10) are all potentially valuable options for CMV disease prevention. Ganciclovir is effective therapy for proved CMV infection in children, as in adults.

Varicella-Zoster. The most commonly seen manifestation of varicella-zoster infection in older pediatric transplant recipients is dermatome-restricted herpes zoster. In younger children who have received a transplant, however, primary varicella infection (chickenpox) can result in a rapidly progressive and overwhelming infection, with encephalitis, pneumonitis, hepatic failure, pancreatitis, and disseminated intravascular coagulation. It is important to know a child's varicella-zoster antibody status because seronegative children require prophylactic varicella-zoster immune globulin (VZIG) within 72 hours of accidental exposure. VZIG is effective in favorably modifying the disease in 75% of cases. All seronegative children on dialysis should receive the new varicella vaccine. Since it is a live, attenuated vaccine, it is regarded as inadvisable to administer it post-transplant.

A child with a kidney transplant who develops chickenpox should begin receiving parenteral acyclovir without delay; with zoster infection there is less of a threat for dissemination, although acyclovir should also be used. In both situations, it is wise to discontinue azathioprine administration until 2 days after the last new crop of vesicles has dried. The dose of other immunosuppressive agents will depend on the clinical situation and response to therapy.

Epstein-Barr Virus. Approximately 50% of the pediatric population is seronegative for EBV, and infection will occur in approximately 75% of these patients. Even in immunosuppressed patients, most EBV infections are clinically silent. PTLD has been reported in children and may be related to EBV infection in the presence of vigorous immunosuppression (see Chap. 9). PTLD is likely to be particularly aggressive if the EBV infection is primary.

Herpes Simplex. The typical perioral herpetic ulcerations are common in immunosuppressed children and will usually respond to oral acyclovir therapy. The diagnosis and treatment of disseminated herpes infections is discussed in Chap. 10.

Post Transplant Antibiotic Prophylaxis in Children

Protocols for post-transplant antibiotic prophylaxis in children vary from center to center. Most centers use an intravenous cephalosporin for the first 48 hours post-transplant to reduce infection from graft contamination and the transplant incision. The use of nightly or twice-weekly trimethoprim-sulfamethoxazole for the first 3–6 months post-transplant serves as prophylaxis against *Pneumocystis carinii* pneumonia and urinary tract infections. Prophylactic oral nystatin minimizes oral and gastrointestinal fungal infections. CMV prophylaxis has been discussed. Children who have undergone splenectomy should be immunized with pneumococcal vaccine and should receive postoperative prophylaxis for both gram-positive and gram-negative organisms, both of which may cause overwhelming sepsis.

Post-Transplant Hypertension and Cardiovascular Disease in Children

Persistent post-transplant hypertension is a serious problem in children, as it is in adults. Between 50% (children with transplants from living-related donors) and 70% (children with transplants from cadaveric donors) of recipients require antihypertensive medications; many children require multiple medications for adequate blood pressure control. The differential diagnosis and treatment of post-transplant hypertension are discussed in Chap. 9. Calcium channel blockers are generally well-tolerated in children over 1 year of age and are the agents of choice for blood pressure management.

Concern regarding long-term post-transplant cardiovascular morbidity and mortality has generally been directed toward the adult post-transplant population (see Chap. 9). Risk factors should also be addressed in children who will, it is hoped, grow to adulthood with their transplants. Serum cholesterol levels are frequently higher than the 185 mg/dl "at-risk" level for children with transplants. Dietary measures are appropriate to reduce hyperlipidemia. There are currently insufficient data to make firm recommendations for the use of pharmacologic measures in children.

Post-Transplant Malignancy

In the NAPRTCS database, the incidence of post-transplant malignancy in children has been reported to be 1.4%. Of these, 60% were PTLDs and lymphomas.

Rehabilitation of Children Receiving Transplants

Within a year of successful transplantation, the social and emotional functioning of the child and the child's family appears to return to pre-illness levels. Pretransplant personality disorders, however, continue to manifest themselves. Within 1 year after transplantation, at least 90% of children attend school, and at least 90% are involved in vocational or education programs. Three-year follow-up shows that nearly 90% of children are in appropriate school or job placement. Surveys of 10-year survivors of pediatric kidney transplants report that the overwhelming majority of patients consider their health to be good; engage in appropriate social, educational, and sexual activities; and experience a very good or excellent quality of life.

SELECTED READINGS

Avner ED, Chavers B, Sullivan EK et al. Renal transplantation and chronic dialysis in children: The 1993 annual report of the North American Pediatric Renal Transplant Cooperative Study. *Pediatr Nephrol* 0:C1, 1995.

Brodehl J. Consensus statement on the optimal use of cyclosporine in pediatric patients. *Transplant Proc* 26:2759, 1994.

Conley SB, Al-Uzri A, So S et al. Prevention of rejection and graft loss with an aggressive quadruple immunosuppressive therapy regimen in children and adolescents. *Transplantation* 57:540, 1994.

Ettenger RB, Rosenthal JT, Marik J et al. Long term results with cyclosporine immunosuppression in pediatric cadaver renal transplantation. *Transplant Proc* 23:1011, 1991.

Ettenger RB. Improving the utilization of cadaver kidneys in children. *Kidney Int* 44(Suppl):S99, 1993.

Harmon WE. Treatment of children with chronic renal failure. *Kidney Int* 47:951, 1995.

Hokken-Koelega AC, Stijnen T, DeJong RC et al. A placebo-controlled, double-blind trial of growth hormone treatment in prepubertal children after renal transplant. *Kidney Int* 49:S128, 1996.

Jabs K, Sullivan K, Avner ED et al. Alternate-day steroid dosing improves growth without adversely affecting graft survival or long-term graft function. *Transplantation* 61:31, 1996.

Johnson RW, Webb JA, Lewis MA, et al. Outcome of pediatric cadaveric renal transplantation: A 10-year study. *Kidney Int* 49:S72, 1996.

Morel P, Almond PS, Matas AJ et al. Long-term quality of life after kidney transplantation in children. *Transplantation* 52:47, 1991.

Matas AJ, Chavers BM, Nevins TE et al. Recipient evaluation, preparation, and care in pediatric transplantation: The University of Minnesota protocols. *Kidney Int* 49:S99, 1996.

Penn I. De novo malignancy in pediatric organ transplant recipients. *J Pediatr Surg* 29:221, 1994.

Rosenthal JT, Ettenger RB, Ehrlich RM et al. Technical factors contributing to successful kidney transplantation in small children. *J Urol* 144:116, 1990.

Savin VJ, Sharma R, Sharma M et al. Circulating factor associated with increased glomerular permeability to albumin in recurrent focal segmental glomerulosclerosis. *N Engl J Med* 334:878, 1996.

Tejani A, Costes L, Sullivan EK. A longitudinal study of the natural history of growth post-transplantation. *Kidney Int* 49:S103, 1996.

Tejani A, Sullivan EK, Fine RN et al. Steady improvement in renal allograft survival among North American children: A five year appraisal by the North American Pediatric Renal Transplant Cooperative Study. *Kidney Int* 48:551, 1995.

Psychiatric Aspects of Kidney Transplantation

Deane L. Wolcott and Thomas B. Strouse

The major clinical advantages of routine pretransplant psychiatric and psychosocial assessment of transplant candidates lie in the capacity to use the information obtained to develop individualized management plans to minimize adverse psychiatric, psychosocial, and behavioral outcomes post-transplant. Achieving this goal requires active participation of the team psychiatrist, psychologist, or social worker in patient selection meetings, as well as active collaboration between the team surgeons, nephrologists, coordinators, and mental health professionals in pre- and post-transplant patient care. Pretransplant psychiatric assessment and the mutual patient-psychiatrist understanding and trust that arise from the assessment contribute to the effectiveness of post-transplant psychiatric care.

This chapter considers the rationale and goals of pretransplant psychiatric assessment of potential kidney transplant recipients and of living kidney donor candidates. Early post-transplant psychiatric problems and their management and the long term adaptation of kidney recipients are also discussed.

PRETRANSPLANT PSYCHIATRIC ASSESSMENT

The goals of pretransplant psychiatric assessment of kidney transplant candidates include determination of psychiatric suitability for transplantation and development of an individualized psychiatric and behavioral management plan for each candidate. Such a management plan includes determination of the optimal timing of transplantation from a psychiatric perspective, as well as acquisition of a psychiatric baseline assessment, which facilitates psychiatric management of post-transplant psychiatric and behavioral problems.

The use of pretransplant psychiatric assessment of candidates for purposes of making selection decisions remains controversial. The fundamental rationale for using such assessment in selection decisions is that certain post-transplant psychiatric or behavioral outcomes are unacceptable and can be predicted with some degree of accuracy by pretransplant psychiatric assessment. Strong psychiatric contraindications to acceptance for kidney transplantation are listed in Table 15-1.

Critical unacceptable post-transplant psychiatric and behavioral outcomes include treatment regimen noncompliance resulting in graft loss or premature patient death, and the new onset or exacerbation of severe acute psychiatric disorders that are poorly responsive to treatment. Undesirable post-transplant psychosocial outcomes include continued vocational dysfunction with personal or family economic catastrophe, severe marital or family disruption, and participation in substance abuse or other health-related behaviors that threaten long-term graft or patient survival.

Table 15-1. Strong psychiatric and psychosocial contraindications to acceptance for kidney transplantation*

Current functional psychosis (psychotic depression, manic episode, schizophrenia, other)

Past severe acute psychiatric disorder with marked psychiatric treatment, regimen noncompliance, and/or very malignant psychiatric course

Active psychoactive substance abuse (alcohol, illicit psychoactive substance, or prescribed psychoactive substance)

Severe personality disorder

Severe intellectual deficits or severe dementia with inadequate social support to ensure compliance with the treatment regimen

Residential instability

Lack of adequate social support and personally inadequate illness coping behavior (e.g., regimen noncompliance)

Ongoing significant medical treatment regimen noncompliance predicted to continue post-transplant

Continuing ambivalence about or reluctance to undergo transplant

Highly conflicted and negative relationship with transplant team members

Confidently predicted unacceptable psychiatric or psychosocial outcome post-transplant despite maximal possible psychiatric or psychosocial treatment and interventions

*These criteria are based on the relevant available literature and the authors' experience and should not be assumed to be absolute or authoritative. Further collective experience and research is needed to document psychiatric and psychosocial contraindications to kidney transplantation.

Noncompliance Prediction

Serious, persistent post-transplant treatment regimen noncompliance (most critically with immunosuppressive medications) is widely considered to be an unacceptable transplant outcome. Factors that have been associated with risk for noncompliance in chronically ill, dialysis, and organ transplant patient populations are listed in Table 15-2. Noncompliance is itself a complex behavioral variable that is the result of the interaction of multiple enduring and short-term psychiatric and psychosocial factors. In spite of the many complexities involved in accurate assessment and prediction of treatment regimen noncompliance, clinical experience indicates that such predictions can be made with some degree of reliability. Many candidates who are judged to be psychiatrically unacceptable at one point in time may later be acceptable (e.g., after demonstrating improved compliance with their current medical treatment regimen or participating in a substance abuse treatment program). An extended evaluation process for certain psychiatrically marginal candidates often facilitates optimal decisions about their candidacy.

Timing of Transplant

Psychiatric considerations in the timing of acceptance for kidney transplantation are important. Examples of clinical problems that may indicate that the candidate's acceptance for transplant would best be delayed are listed in Table 15-3. Pretransplant psychiatric or psychological care and support may be needed to increase the likelihood of

Table 15-2. Risk factors for treatment regimen noncompliance in kidney transplant recipients*

Sociodemographic factors
    Age—adolescent or young adult
    Living alone
    Not in committed relationship with partner
    Less medical sophistication
    More dysfunctional family unit—greater family conflict
Personality factors
    Narcissistic personality
    Histrionic personality
    Passive dependent or aggressive personality
    Impulsive, undisciplined, chaotic
    Helpless or hopeless illness responses
    Less realistic understanding of illness and treatment alternatives
Psychiatric disorders
    Major affective disorder
    Cognitive impairment or organic mental disorder
    Substance abuse disorder
    Significant personality disorder
    Functional psychotic disorder
    Post-traumatic stress disorder
Other psychological factors
    Less effective illness coping behavior
    Less mature psychologically
    Undesirable health beliefs
    Secondary gains from illness
    Phobic avoidance of hospital or medical team
    Ambivalence about undergoing transplant
    Passive desire to die or active suicidal intent
    Persistent regrets about having undergone transplant
    Possibly low socioeconomic status
Historical factors
    History of dialysis and other treatment regimen noncompliance
    Interval of greater than 6 mos since transplant
Situational factors
    Away from home or medication unavailable
    Other priorities—work
    Major stressful life events
    Great distance from transplant unit
Financial factors
    Cost of medications and medical treatment
    General economic hardship
Patient-team relationship factors
    Feeling abandoned or angry toward team
    Inadequate or conflicting communication with team
    Negative or defiant pattern of relationships with health care
      providers
    Transplant team unavailable
    Living at great distance from the transplant center

Table 15-2 (continued).

Regimen or illness factors
    Increased regimen complexity
    Increased regimen duration
    Regimen side effects
    Lack of perceived benefit from regimen
    Lack of immediate adverse consequences from noncompliance
    Nausea or vomiting

*These factors are derived from the general literature on compliance with medical treatment, the transplantation literature, and personal experience

Table 15-3. Psychiatric indications for delay in transplant candidacy

Inadequate information about transplantation and post-transplant regimen
Ambivalence about undergoing transplantation
Severe acute psychiatric disorders (e.g., anxiety, depression)
Unrealistic expectations of post-transplant quality of life
Phobias interfering with management (e.g., needle or catheter phobias)
Recent significant substance abuse
Morbid, intractable obesity
Major acute life disruption (e.g., divorce, bereavement)

long-term graft survival and successful patient outcome. Consideration of psychiatric factors in selection decisions and transplant timing must always occur in conjunction with consideration of medical issues that may mandate early rather than delayed transplantation.

Enhancement of quality of life is a major goal of transplantation. Restoration of vocational function is a related goal that is facilitated by minimizing the time the transplant candidate spends on dialysis prior to transplant. From a psychiatric standpoint, many patients with approaching end-stage renal disease (ESRD) are appropriate candidates for a kidney transplant after minimal or no time on dialysis. Some psychologically vulnerable candidates are judged on clinical psychiatric grounds to have a better prognosis for optimal long-term psychiatric and treatment regimen compliance outcome if they have experienced successful adaptation to dialysis prior to transplant.

Cadaveric or Living Transplant Donor?

From the psychiatric perspective, most potential candidates are acceptable for either a cadaveric or living kidney donor transplant. Some candidates, however, have strongly ambivalent or negative relationships with their potential living donor and may be vulnerable to acting out these relationship conflicts or resentments by being noncompliant with the treatment regimen, thereby destroying the donor's gift of the kidney. This recipient-donor relationship-specific risk factor for noncompliance or for psychological damage to their relationship can be lowered by pretransplant individual psychotherapy with the recipient or by brief conjoint psychotherapy that includes the recipient and the donor.

The psychological problems that occur in the relationship between the recipient and living donor tend to be centered around issues of guilt or obligation. In the situation of the parent donor and child recipient, there may be particular psychological and relationship risks related to the normal developmental tasks of individuation and separation from the parent.

High-Risk Candidate Populations

Children and adolescent candidates pose special pretransplant psychiatric or psychological assessment problems. Depending on the pediatric candidate's age and intellectual and emotional maturity, the decision-making process regarding the transplant option may rest primarily with the parents, the child, or both. This may pose special problems, particularly when there is major strain or dissolution of the parental unit; major child-parent conflict; or major socioeconomic, language, or cultural barriers to effective communication and decision-making between the child, parent, and the transplant team.

Preadolescent and adolescent transplant candidates are at great risk for post-transplant treatment regimen noncompliance, which commonly results in acute graft rejection episodes and may result in premature graft loss. Pediatric and adolescent kidney transplant programs should psychiatrically assess all pediatric candidates and their families and have active programs to prevent, identify, and intervene in post-transplant treatment regimen noncompliance.

Physical, psychological, social, educational, and vocational maturity are all commonly delayed in pediatric ESRD patients. Successful kidney transplantation may help relieve some of these problems, but side effects of the immunosuppressive medications may contribute to problems of body image and self-esteem. Routine support groups and other educational and psychologically supportive interventions should be available to the pediatric population to facilitate optimal graft function and overall successful development and adaptation.

Some adult transplant candidates with a history of onset of diabetes mellitus in the pediatric age range are at greater risk for post-transplant adverse psychological and regimen noncompliance. Many diabetic patients have multiple end-organ damage by the time of development of ESRD. Some have never fully accepted themselves with their disease and have a history of poor compliance with their diabetic regimen, poor self-esteem, self-destructive behavior, and psychiatric disorders. Some have been highly disciplined in following their diabetic regimen but develop pronounced depression, anger, and demoralization with the deterioration of their independence and quality of life secondary to progressive end-organ damage. A significant minority of candidates with a history of pediatric-onset diabetes require psychotherapeutic support pre- and post-transplant to help them cope with the special and often severe health problems they experience. These problems are often minimally improved by medically successful transplantation.

LIVING KIDNEY DONORS

Living kidney donation is associated with generally positive donor and donor-recipient relationship psychological and psychiatric outcomes. Most living donors are biologically related, although donation by biologically unrelated donors is increasing in frequency largely in response to the shortage of cadaveric donors and the excellent results that have been achieved (see Chap. 5). It is generally accepted that biologically unrelated donors should have a clearly definable emotional bond; the term *emotionally-related donor* is a wise one.

Examples of such relationships are spouses, fiancees, adopted parents or siblings, or close personal friends.

Living kidney donors usually demonstrate sustained improved self-esteem and lowered levels of depressive mood post-transplant. At least 90% of donors indicate that they would donate again if they had the choice. Generally, the donor-recipient relationship is improved or unchanged post-transplant. Donors whose recipient experiences early graft failure are somewhat more likely to report regret over having donated and poorer relationships with their recipient. Adverse psychological outcomes that have been reported in small numbers of donors include onset of depression and other psychiatric disorders and onset of chronic physical symptoms that reflect somatization. Donation may add additional stress to already troubled marriages (especially if the spouse is opposed to the donation) and may contribute to postdonation divorce in some cases. Some donors experience significant unreimbursed financial costs associated with the donation.

All potential donors should be psychiatrically assessed before the donation. Fundamental psychological and ethical considerations in live-related kidney donation include the following:

1. Adequacy and completeness of the donor's understanding of the potential personal benefits and risks associated with donation
2. The voluntary nature and stability of the donation decision in a donor who is in every way capable of making such a decision
3. The absence of financial or material gain as an incentive for donation
4. The absence of predominant psychologically unhealthy conscious or unconscious motives to donate
5. The absence of predictors of elevated postdonation risk for onset or exacerbation of psychiatric disorder
6. The absence of predictors of elevated risk for post-transplant adverse donor-recipient relationship outcomes

Certain groups of donors pose special psychiatric and ethical concerns. These groups include potential donors who are younger than age 18 years, are intellectually or cognitively handicapped, are incarcerated, have a history of significant psychiatric disorder, or have a history of significant conflict with the potential recipient or other nuclear family members (the negatively valued family deviant, or "black sheep"). Living donation in which the relationship between the donor and the potential recipient is potentially coercive (e.g., the donor is employed by the recipient) should be evaluated with particular care.

The cornerstones of an optimal program to prevent adverse donor psychological and psychiatric outcomes are appropriate psychiatric assessment and pretransplant education with psychological preparation, donor-recipient relationship assessment, and psychological interventions as needed. Postdonation reinforcement and psychological support of the donor should also be available. Greater efforts by transplant programs and by society at large to honor and support donors post-transplant are desirable.

EARLY POST-TRANSPLANT PSYCHIATRIC ISSUES

Delirium

One of the most common problems seen immediately after transplant is delirium. Patients exhibit confusion, fluctuating consciousness, hallucinations, delusions, and agitated behavior. Delirium usually indi-

Table 15-4. Organic causes of post-transplant delirium

Acute graft failure with elevated central nervous system pressure
Intracerebral hemorrhage
Hypoxia
Central nervous system infection or other significant infections
Metabolic encephalopathy
Uremic encephalopathy
Drug toxicity (cyclosporine, tacrolimus, steroids, OKT3, antibiotics)
Intraoperative cerebral ischemia
Sleep deprivation
Alcohol or other central nervous system depressant drug-withdrawal
    syndromes
Psychotropic drug intoxication (prescribed or nonprescribed)

cates the existence of an organic problem affecting the central nervous system (CNS), and the patient should be fully evaluated for possible etiologies (Table 15-4).

When symptoms of delirium become apparent, psychiatric consultation with careful mental status examination is indicated. It is critical to rule out infectious and metabolic etiologies of delirium as well as the possibility of withdrawal from CNS depressant substances (e.g., alcohol) or toxicity from prescribed medications, including immunosuppressants. Neurologic evaluation may be needed to rule out CNS infection, bleeding, or space-occupying lesion. At the same time, all nonessential medications should be eliminated and dosages of essential ones reevaluated. If the patient is very agitated and needs to be calmed to prevent pulling out intravenous lines, a high-potency neuroleptic such as haloperidol or droperidol (IM or IV) can be used. Lorazepam might also be used, especially if the patient has insomnia that is not helped by a neuroleptic. Oversedation should be avoided.

Several medications commonly used in the post-transplant period deserve special consideration as possible etiologies for delirium. Both cyclosporine and tacrolimus, particularly the latter, can cause a number of neurologic and psychiatric symptoms, including seizures, drowsiness, confusion, headaches, paresthesia, tremors, aphasia, depression, cerebellar dysfunction, and visual hallucinations. White matter changes can be seen on magnetic resonance imaging, but these changes and the neuropsychiatric symptoms are generally reversible after discontinuation or significant reduction in dose or switching from one agent to the other. Hypomagnesemia, high steroid doses, and aluminum overload are all associated with an increase in neurotoxicity. OKT3 can cause delirium, especially during the first few treatments. Other medications commonly used after transplantation, such as antibiotics in high doses (penicillin, gentamicin, and ganciclovir), can cause delirium.

Depression

Depression may be seen immediately following a transplant and can be due to both organic or purely psychological causes. Patients exhibit depressed mood, feelings of hopelessness, somatic complaints, sleep disturbances, and decreased appetite. Organic etiologies include infection, medications (particularly steroids), electrolyte imbalance, and poor graft function. In general, depression due to organic causes improves with stabilization of the physical condition of the patient. Patients may also become depressed as they adjust to the transplant, especially if the graft fails. A mental health specialist should see the patient to help delineate the nature of the depression and determine if an organic etiology is likely. Even if the etiology is organic, the symptoms may be so severe that psychiatric treatment is needed before stabilization of the medical condition can be achieved. Sometimes supportive psychotherapy is sufficient, but antidepressants may be needed. In cases of psychotic or life threatening depression, electroconvulsive therapy (ECT) should be considered.

Anxiety

As with depression, anxiety in the post-transplant patient can be the result of organic causes or adjustment to post-transplant conditions. Organic etiologies such as pulmonary embolus, hypoxemia, arrhythmias, electrolyte disturbances, infections, organ rejection, and medication toxicity should be evaluated. Patients may also have a history of anxiety disorder that becomes apparent after the transplant, or they may become anxious about the survival of the graft. Some patients become particularly anxious during ward placement changes or just before discharge. Nonpharmaceutical techniques such as relaxation therapy may be used initially, but if they fail or the anxiety is too severe, short-acting benzodiazepines such as lorazepam or oxazepam may be used to decrease the anxiety. If they are used for prolonged periods, they must be tapered to avoid withdrawal symptoms.

Uncooperative Behavior or Agitation

Sometimes uncooperative behavior or agitation may indicate a manic episode or other psychiatric problem such as anxiety, depression, or delirium. It may be seen in patients who are accustomed to control over their affairs; their lack of cooperation represents an attempt to establish control in their medical treatment. Reassurance, listening to the patient's complaints, and allowing the patient some role in medical decisions is usually sufficient to establish cooperation. When a patient exhibits dangerous behavior, however, firm limits must be established. Completed suicide has been reported in patients with functioning grafts.

PSYCHIATRIC INTERVENTIONS IN KIDNEY TRANSPLANTATION CANDIDATES AND RECIPIENTS

Psychotherapeutic Interventions

During the pretransplant period, general education about the procedure and what to expect postoperatively can often prevent anxiety and depression and can sometimes improve patient compliance. The patient's family or support system should be involved before and after the transplant. One of the most difficult periods for patients is the pretransplant period, when many become depressed or anxious while awaiting the surgery.

Post-transplant patients should be assessed for supportive therapy. They should also be encouraged to discuss with the medical team their fears and complaints. Cognitive behavioral and relaxation techniques are especially helpful for depressed and anxious patients.

Group psychotherapy and visits by previous transplant recipients can prove extremely helpful, not only for psychological support, but also for education about post-transplant issues. Exercise can be useful in bolstering the patient's self-confidence and sense of improvement.

Psychopharmacologic Interventions

It may sometimes be necessary to use psychotropic medications in kidney transplant patients, either because they were taking them prior to the transplant or because symptoms arise after the transplant that necessitate their use.

If the antidepressants are used, it is important to use those without significant side effects. Hydroxylated metabolites of tricyclic antidepressants (TCAs) can cause cardiac arrhythmias and CNS toxicity and may accumulate in patients with renal insufficiency. These metabolites possess approximately 50% of the reuptake inhibition effect of the parent drug, possibly explaining both the therapeutic benefits and side effects observed at lower than expected doses. TCA serum levels do not measure the hydroxymetabolites. The newer selective serotonic reuptake inhibitor antidepressant medications (e.g. fluoxetine, paroxetine, sertraline) appear to have a generally more favorable side effect profile than the older TCAs, although some patients may suffer significant nausea, insomnia, agitation, and sedation. Kinetic studies of fluoxetine in patients with chronic renal failure (CRF) have shown no delay in its clearance or that of its major metabolite, norfluoxetine. Elevated levels of paroxetine, venlaxatine, and trazodone have been reported in CRF, and the clearance of bupropion may be delayed by up to 50% with the accumulation of metabolites, which may cause delirium, seizure disorder, and movement disorder. Stimulants such as methylphenidate are an effective alternative for short-term depressive symptoms and pose little cardiac or seizure risk. Monoamine oxidase inhibitors should be avoided because they can complicate anesthesia and may have dangerous interactions with pressor agents and meperidine. ECT should be considered in patients with severe, life-threatening depression in which immediate results are needed.

Patients who are on lithium before the transplant may require an increase in dose if the graft functions; therefore, levels should be checked immediately post-transplant. Cyclosporine may decrease lithium excretion, and levels need to be followed closely. Lithium use may be problematic if the patient has massive fluid and electrolyte shifts, and it is important to remember that lithium can cause polyuria and renal dysfunction due to interstitial fibrosis, which is similar to the pathologic lesion produced by cyclosporine.

In the early post-transplant period, neuroleptics are often needed to control agitated patients, particularly those with delirium. In such cases, high-potency neuroleptics such as haloperidol or droperidol can be useful. Both have fewer cardiac side effects than other neuroleptics and can be given parenterally. Droperidol is especially useful, due to its short half-life and more rapid clearance.

Benzodiazepines do not present any special problems in kidney transplant patients with good graft function, but they should be used only when clearly needed. Shorter-acting ones such as lorazepam and oxazepam are preferable, but care should be taken not to oversedate the patient. If used for a long period, they must be tapered to prevent withdrawal effects. Table 15-5 provides dosage

Table 15-5. Guidelines for commonly used psychopharmacologic agents in the post-transplant period

Class/agent	Indications	Usual total 24-hour dose range[a] (mg/day)	Half-life	Dosage adjustment for decreased renal function
Benzodiazepines[b]				
Oxazepam (Serax)	Anxiety, insomnia	30–120	Medium	Probably
Lorazepam (Ativan)	Anxiety, insomnia	2–6	Medium	Probably
Flurazepam (Dalmane)	Insomnia	15–30	Long	Yes
Triazolam (Halcion)	Insomnia	0.125–0.500	Short	No
Diazepam (Valium)	Anxiety, insomnia	10–30	Long	Yes
Neuroleptics[c]				
Haloperidol (Haldol)	Delirium, severe anxiety, severe emotional or behavioral liability	1–10	Long	No
Droperidol (Inapsine)	Delirium, severe anxiety, severe emotional or behavioral liability	1–10	Short	No
Perphenazine (Trilafon)	Delirium, severe anxiety, severe emotional or behavioral liability	4–16	Long	No
Fluphenazine (Prolixin)	Delirium, severe anxiety, severe emotional or behavioral liability	2–10	Long	No
Lithium carbonate[d]	Prophylaxis of bipolar affective disorder, manic episode	600–1,200	Related to function	Yes
Antidepressants[e]				
Amitriptyline (Elavil)	Major depressive episode, severe organic depressive syndrome	150	Long	Probably

Imipramine (Tofranil)	Major depressive episode, severe organic depressive syndrome	150	Long	Probably
Trazodone (Desyrel)	Major depressive episode, severe organic depressive syndrome	400	Long	Probably
Sertraline (Zoloft)	Major depressive episode, severe organic depressive syndrome	50–100	Long	No
Fluoxetine (Prozac)	Major depressive episode, severe organic depressive syndrome	20	Long	Probably
Doxepin (Sinequan)	Major depressive episode, severe organic depressive syndrome	150	Long	Probably
Nortriptyline (Pamelor)	Major depressive episode, severe organic depressive syndrome	100	Long	Probably

[a]Benzodiazepines, neuroleptics, and lithium carbonate usually given in 2–4 divided doses/day. Antidepressants given 1–3 doses/day. All dose ranges are for healthy adults younger than 65 years of age and are for the specified indications. Higher doses may be used after psychiatric consultation.

[b]Regular, higher dose, and/or chronic use beyond a few weeks can be associated with risk for dependence and development of a withdrawal syndrome with sudden discontinuation. Do not stop suddenly, especially early post-transplant.

[c]Psychiatric consultation recommended when indications for neuroleptics exist. Behavioral and psychotherapeutic interventions often combined with neuroleptics. Acute extrapyramidal syndromes may develop.

[d]Psychiatric consultation *essential* for management of pretransplant patients with major affective disorder or who develop manic psychosis post-transplant. Lithium carbonate is the drug of choice. Lithium carbonate should be used very cautiously in patients with impaired renal function. Lithium dosage guided by serum levels. Narrow toxic-therapeutic ratio.

[e]Psychiatric consultation strongly recommended for patients with severe depression and/or those being treated with antidepressants pretransplant. Many post-transplant depressed patients do not require antidepressants.

guidelines for commonly used pharmacologic agents in the early post-transplant period.

LONG-TERM ADAPTATION OF KIDNEY TRANSPLANT RECIPIENTS

Treatment Regimen Noncompliance

Whereas early studies indicated very low rates of treatment regimen noncompliance and noncompliance-associated graft loss, more recent studies using better methods indicate that as many as 20% of graft losses after 6 months are secondary to known noncompliance. Noncompliance is probably the third leading cause of late graft loss (see Chap. 9). Missed clinic appointments and immunosuppressant noncompliance are often associated. Major immunosuppressant noncompliance (see Table 15-2) occurs in about 5% of recipients, usually later than 6 months post-transplant, and has been associated with a patient age of less than 20 years, ethnicity (probably a proxy measure for lower socioeconomic status), more immunosuppressant medication side effects, greater pretransplant dialysis noncompliance, more immunosuppressant physical side effects, and living farther than 150 miles from the transplant institution. Up to 13% of recipients have been reported to admit missing one to two immunosuppressant medication doses per month, and about 7% to admit missing three or more doses per month. Studies in other groups of organ transplant recipients have suggested that personality disorder and history of psychoactive substance abuse are also risk factors for post-transplant regimen noncompliance.

Quality of Life Outcome

Accumulated evidence clearly shows that successful kidney transplant recipients as a group have a better quality of life than hemodialysis patients and peritoneal dialysis patients. While patient selection has not been ruled out as the basis for these findings, it seems evident that successful transplantation is associated with improved quality of life for the majority of recipients. Vocational rehabilitation rates in transplant recipients are not as high as would be desirable, but this outcome reflects multiple factors other than the success of the transplant itself.

A fundamental unresolved question concerns the pretransplant predictors of post-transplant quality of life. Determination of the factors that predict very poor post-transplant quality of life and rehabilitation could be used to develop specific intervention programs for such high-risk candidates and might play a role in making optimal candidate selection decisions.

SELECTED READINGS

Craven J, Rodin GJ. Introduction. In J Craven, GJ Rodin (eds), *Psychiatry Aspects of Organ Transplantation*. New York: Oxford University Press, 1992. Pp 1–5.

De Geest S, Borgermans L, Gemoets H et al. Incidence, determinants, and consequences of subclinical noncompliance with immunosuppressive therapy in renal transplant recipients. *Transplantation* 59:340, 1995.

Freeman A, Davies L, Libb JW et al. Assessment of Transplant Candidates and Prediction of Outcome. In J Craven, GJ Rodin (eds),

Psychiatric Aspects of Organ Transplantation. New York: Oxford University Press, 1992. Pp 9–19.

Garcia LL, Agueru AE, Cavalli J et al. Kidney transplantation: Absolute and relative psychologic contraindications. *Transplant Proc* 23:1344, 1991.

Kiley DJ, Lam CS, Pollack R. A study of treatment compliance following kidney transplantation. *Transplantation* 55:51, 1993.

Trzepacz PT, DiMartini A, Tringali R. Psychopharmacologic issues in organ transplantation. Part I: Pharmacokinetics in organ failure and psychiatric aspects of immunosuppressants and anti-infectious agents. *Psychosomatics* 34:199, 1993.

Trzepacz PT, DiMartini A, Tringali R. Psychopharmacologic issues in organ transplantation. Part II: Psychopharmacologic medications. *Psychosomatics* 34:290, 1993.

Twillman RK, Manetto C, Wolcott DL. The transplant evaluation scale: A revision of the psychosocial levels system for evaluating organ transplant candidates. *Psychosomatics* 34:144, 1993.

Ethical and Legal Issues in Kidney Transplantation

Leslie Steven Rothenberg

Medicine and surgery in the late twentieth century are filled with ethical dilemmas; the field of kidney transplantation is no exception. Questions inevitably involve the underlying ethical principles of respecting the self-determination of patients with decision-making capacity (sometimes called **autonomy**), acting to protect the patient's well-being (sometimes called **beneficence**), and acting in a manner that promotes fairness and equity to all involved (sometimes called **justice**).

The applications of these principles with regard to kidney transplantation are explored in this chapter with reference to the donation and procurement of organs, the selection of patients for transplantation, and the place of kidney transplantation in the allocation of health care resources and the development of national priorities.

DONATION AND PROCUREMENT OF ORGANS

Current Shortage of Cadaveric Organs

The United Network for Organ Sharing (UNOS) reported that as of January 31, 1996, 31,022 people on its national patient list were waiting for a kidney. Kidney transplants are being performed in the United States at a rate of approximately 10,000 per year for the last several years; the extent of the scarcity of donor kidneys for transplants is so great that it would take almost the entire combined total of transplants performed in the last 3 years to meet the need of patients waiting. Furthermore, in recent years the kidney donor supply has remained fairly constant despite national and local efforts to increase donations. The reported average waiting time for a cadaveric kidney transplant is approaching 2 years, and there are thousands of patients who, using hemodialysis as a backup, have been waiting longer than 3 years for such a transplant.

The existing kidney organ supply, therefore, is clearly inadequate to meet the current and future needs in this country. Donor kidneys are a genuinely scarce resource, and questions of fairness in their procurement and distribution are inevitable. It is speculative to presume that increased educational programs, new legal approaches, or financial or other incentives can increase the supply of cadaveric organs.

Determination of Death

Acceptance of organ procurement and transplantation depends, in large part, on public confidence that cadaveric organs, including kidneys, are being taken from people who are truly dead in the public's understanding of that term. In other words, the often-quoted truism that the determination of death is a medical decision hides the reality that the concept of death, while given both a medical and legal rationale, is fundamentally a social and not a scientific concept, informed by cultural and religious beliefs.

The medical criteria for whole brain death were authoritatively defined by a U.S. presidential commission in 1981 (see Chap. 5). The major principles are the following:

1. Both cerebral and brain stem functions must be absent.
2. The cause(s) of this total lack of brain functioning must have been identified and determined to be irreversible.
3. The absence of all brain function must have persisted during a period of treatment and observation.

The **Uniform Determination of Death Act** (1981) provided the legal framework by stating that "an individual is dead if there is irreversible cessation of circulatory and respiratory functions or if there is irreversible cessation of all brain functions of the entire brain, including the brain stem." This statutory definition has been adopted by an overwhelming majority of U.S. state legislatures. In other states, courts have upheld these "brain death" criteria in judicial rulings.

Yet difficulties persist. The very phrase *brain death* connotes to some the existence of two types of death, *regular death* and *brain death*. This distinction is aided by the perception that the death of patients who lose cardiac and respiratory functions and who are not on ventilator support is different than the death of patients on ventilators.

It might be helpful to stop using the phrase *brain death* and use only the single word *death* for persons on or off the ventilator, no matter how the determination of that death was made. Yet, the phrase *brain death* is used precisely to explain how this breathing person with a heartbeat could be said to be dead.

Efforts to broaden the category of what constitutes death in humans, including suggestions that babies with anencephaly and patients in persistent vegetative states be treated as though dead for purposes of organ donation, have met with significant public and professional resistance.

Altruism Versus Duty or Payment for Organs

Use of Live Donors

Approximately 25% of the kidney transplants performed in the United States involve living donors. Living donors are usually defined in three categories:

1. **Living-related donors** (such as parents, siblings, or children), who are genetically related to the recipient.
2. **Living emotionally related donors** (such as spouses, "significant others," and close friends), who are genetically unrelated.
3. **Living-unrelated donors**, who are strangers to the recipient and who may or may not be compensated for their donated kidney.

Although living donors do well after donating a single kidney, there was initial resistance in some circles to using such donors in kidney transplantation. The rare death of a living kidney donor, the potential morbidity risks for those who survive, and the uncertainty as to the degree of improvement in recipient and graft survival compared with cadaveric organs seemed to militate against their use. The continuing shortage of cadaveric organs, however, pushed in the other direction.

Organ donation by living donors brings into focus perplexing ethical problems because of the dangers of coercion and external as well as self-generated pressures on the donor. While wishing to respect the freely made decisions of prospective donors with decision-making capacity and while valuing the life-saving potential of this gift to the recipients and the satisfaction of donors, transplant teams have been forced to evaluate the motives, capacities, and emotional feelings of prospective donors in a variety of factual contexts. They have also struggled with the question as to what level of informed consent can be obtained in such situations and the role of altruism in such decisions.

The following three clinical vignettes illustrate some of the ethical dilemmas that using such donors may generate:

Susan, a 30-year-old divorcee, suffered from chronic nephritis and hypertension, as well as systemic lupus erythematosus. She was evaluated as a kidney transplant candidate. Susan's parents, ages 63 and 56 years, and four of her adult siblings were tested as possible donors, and the best match was her 23-year-old brother, Marvin. Marvin is healthy but has a severe developmental disability, Down's syndrome, and the mental age of a 3- or 4-year-old. Thus, Marvin does not have the capacity to make the decision to donate his organ, although he states that he wants to help his sister. His sister, in turn, has offered to take care of Marvin after their parents' deaths. The family has agreed that Marvin should be the donor. How should the risks and benefits to Marvin and Susan be evaluated?

Diane and Dione are identical twins born 12 years ago. Dione is now suffering from hemolytic-uremic syndrome and needs a kidney transplant. Both parents were ruled out as donors on medical grounds. No other related donors are available, leaving her sister, Diane, who being an identical twin, would be an ideal donor. Diane is fond of her sister and says she would like to help her. How should the risks and benefits to Diane and Dione be evaluated?

Mrs. P., a middle-aged woman with diabetic nephropathy and progressive retinopathy, is doing poorly on dialysis. She has 70% panel reactive antibodies and has been on a cadaveric waiting list for 2 years. She is a patient of a nephrologist, Dr. N., who has encouraged her to discuss the possibility of living-related donation with her siblings. She tells Dr. N. that her sister has volunteered to donate a kidney to her. Dr. N. arranges for testing but then receives a call from the potential donor's husband, who relates that his wife has a strong ambivalence about being a donor, coupled with a fear of having to face her sister with a negative decision. Dr. N. next meets with the potential donor, who repeatedly asks him about the risks involved in the donation, is very tense throughout the conversation, and says at one point, "Is the kidney machine really that bad for her?" The tissue typing shows that the patient's sister is a 2-haplotype–match to her and all crossmatching is negative. Dr. N. has real doubts about her willingness to give the kidney freely, yet he realizes that Mrs. P. has a poor prognosis on dialysis and may have to wait a long time for a cadaveric kidney. How should he handle this situation?

These scenarios highlight but a few of the ethical questions. Can families, such as Marvin's, be trusted in making gifts of one child's kidney to save the life of (or remove from hemodialysis) another child, such as Susan? Should Marvin's developmental disability be viewed as an absolute contraindication to his being considered as a donor? How does one weigh the potential for coercion or feelings of obligation implicit in the offer of a potential recipient to take future care of the would-be donor?

Courts hearing such cases have often permitted parents to donate kidneys or bone marrow from their minor children as long as an argument could be made that the donor children will "benefit" from the donation. The concept of benefit here is usually the satisfaction that the donor has helped, or saved the life of, a relative. This judicial standard clearly favors such donations, since this abstract concept of a positive benefit, especially if voiced by the would-be donor, is far easier to grasp and endorse than is an understanding of the more negative medical risks for living donors.

The duty or obligation to make a gift of a kidney can also be present in the mind of the donor, even if never articulated. In the examples given above, Diane may feel such an obligation to her sister, Dione, in addition to her love for her. Mrs. P.'s sister, on the other hand, may be unable to express her opposition to or fear of donating a kidney to Mrs. P. and may resent the pressure to do so.

For these reasons, various national guidelines have emphasized limiting living donation to people who are either genetically or emotionally related to the recipient, whose motives seem altruistic and not based on duty or coercion, and who can make informed decisions with a clear understanding of the risks and benefits involved. It is also required that potential donors not receive any economic reward other than payment of reasonable medical expenses and lost income. This guideline clearly excludes almost all living-unrelated donors (in contrast with living emotionally related donors). The case of Mrs. P. illustrates the importance of donor advocacy. It must be clear to all parties that donors are not to be sacrificed for recipients. Dr. N. would have been wise to have asked a colleague to evaluate the potential donor (see Chap. 5).

Sale of Organs and Rewarded Gifting

The use of living-unrelated kidney donors may have begun, albeit unwittingly, in 1971 at the Christian Medical College in Vellore, India, when the surgeon, Dr. Mohan Rao, discovered that the donor, introduced to Dr. Rao as the recipient's "cousin," was, in fact, a paid stranger.

There is a tradition in India of paying living-related donors. Media advertisements by both kidney donors and would-be recipients have been commonplace, as well as efforts to control the brokering of kidneys by carefully monitored programs in individual transplant centers. The argument is made that this practice is ethically acceptable given the inability to provide dialysis for more than a small percentage of Indian patients with end-stage renal disease (ESRD) and the social acceptance in India of paid donors as an alternative to the deaths of recipients. Others have said that there is greater public sympathy in India for kidney donors in need of the money than for the hospitals and medical teams, who are viewed as exploitative.

There is evidence to suggest that wealthy recipients from the Middle East who have gone to India or other countries in the Third World for living-unrelated transplants have received inferior medical care, have sustained higher than normal complication rates, and have been financially exploited along with their donors. Such commercialized programs may inhibit the development of local transplant programs involving cadaveric donors because families of prospective donors see no reason to authorize the removal of organs if such organs are available elsewhere for purchase.

Western nations have been quick to condemn such practices. The **National Organ Transplantation Act** of 1984 in the United States makes the buying and selling of human organs illegal. Britain passed a similar law in 1989 after a scandal in which four paid Turkish donors hired by an organ broker was publicized. In 1990, three British physicians were disciplined for their role in those transplants.

Yet, in the United States, donors of sperm and blood plasma are legally paid for their donations. It has been argued that, given the chronic shortage of both cadaveric and even living-related and living emotionally related donors, there should be a program of **rewarded gifting** for kidneys just as there is for sperm and plasma.

Those arguing for such a program claim that, even among related donors and recipients, money or some other reward is often secretly exchanged. Moreover, they suggest that people should have the right to sell organs or tissues under controlled circumstances, and the benefit to recipients should be matched by a benefit to donors beyond abstract altruistic joy.

Those who argue most strenuously for a rewarded gifting program would exclude brokers and direct payment from recipients or transplant programs. They would change the nature of the reward from money to tax rebates or credits, burial grants, insurance policies, future medical coverage, or tuition subsidies for children. They would introduce a carefully regulated system in which both living-related and living-unrelated donors would be evaluated by transplant centers under uniform medical and ethical guidelines with a third party, such as the government, independently handling the rewards after the transplant was completed.

Those opposed claim that such programs, even with the limits contemplated, will jeopardize public support for organ transplantation, particularly for cadaveric organ donation. They claim that programs will be costly and are unjustified without greater educational efforts to encourage donation. Some even argue that the use of living donors is increasingly unjustified in the face of improved techniques for cadaveric organ transplantation and a failure to maximize the retrieval of cadaveric organs.

Anencephalic and Xenograft Organs

Human kidney transplants using anencephalic organ donors have been reported in the United States, Europe, and Japan. Xenograft organs have also been used, although largely in research on animals. Space does not permit a review of the ethical issues involving anencephalic and xenograft transplants, but there are concerns about the functional usefulness of the transplanted organs, the application of brain death standards in the case of anencephalic donors, the animal rights debate in the context of xenograft organs, and the currently unmet need each year for nearly 600 children in the United States who require kidney transplants.

The U.S. center with the greatest experience in seeking anencephalic organ donors, Loma Linda University Medical Center, California, concluded in 1989, after a research effort involving 12 infants and no successful transplants, that "it is usually not feasible, with the restrictions of current [US] law [regarding the determination of death], to procure solid organs from anencephalic infants."

Allocation of Organs Among Transplant Centers

In the United States, the national organ procurement and transplantation network is privately operated under governmental supervision. The National Organ Transplant Act (Public Law 98-507), passed by Congress in 1984, called for such a network to be established and administered by a nonprofit entity under contract to the U.S. Department of Health and Human Services. UNOS (see Chap. 3) was created as a legal entity in 1984 as an outgrowth of the South-Eastern Organ Procurement Foundation (SEOPF) of Richmond, Virginia, which had been established in 1975 by several transplant centers as a means of sharing transplant information and protocols and creating a shared computer registry system. Other U.S. transplant centers sought to join this computer registry, and, in the late 1970s and early 1980s, a loosely formed national network was created with the SEOPF offices and computers as its center.

UNOS created a system for distributing cadaveric kidneys, based on a scoring approach developed at the University of Pittsburgh by Dr. Thomas Starzl. Beginning in 1987, with refinements in 1995, the UNOS system assigns points to each patient on the transplant waiting list. Three major criteria are used: the quality of the tissue match, the time waiting for the kidney, and the level of preformed antibodies. The system is applied uniformly across the United States. "Zero antigen mismatch" kidneys, however, must be shared nationally, and less well-matched kidneys are shared on a regional basis with variances approved by UNOS to take into account local needs and circumstances (see Chap. 3).

Family Veto of Organ Donor Cards

The National Kidney Foundation and state motor vehicle departments seeking potential organ donors have sought to portray the decision to donate organs as solely within the control of the would-be donor. Transplant programs, however, have routinely permitted family members to veto such decisions. Even though properly signed organ donor cards were in the possession of kidney transplant teams and although the **Uniform Anatomical Gift Act** (the model law written in 1968 to provide a legal basis for such gifts in advance of the death of the donor and adopted in all of the states and the District of Columbia) authorized such gifts by any person older than 18 years of age with decision-making capacity, transplant teams have routinely refused to honor such cards when family members objected, reportedly for public relations reasons.

The mere fact that family members are even asked for their consent in the presence of a properly signed donor card suggests that the donor card process is misleadingly presented as a donor decision process. No warning is given to the donor card signer of the power of the family to veto his or her decision to donate. It is, in fact, a family or next-of-kin decision rather than a donor decision. The ability of the family to veto raises ethical questions about campaigns to obtain signed donor cards.

As of early 1996, 21 states (Arkansas, California, Connecticut, Hawaii, Idaho, Indiana, Iowa, Minnesota, Montana, Nevada, New Mexico, North Dakota, Ohio, Oregon, Pennsylvania, Rhode Island, Utah, Vermont, Virginia, Washington, and Wisconsin) had adopted a revised Uniform Anatomical Gift Act that specifically provides that next of kin need *not* consent to organ donations if the document making the gift is given to the donor's attending physician. The new law also removes the previous legal requirements for a witness's signature on the donor card or other document.

Required Request Laws

In the mid-1980s, many U.S. state legislatures began adopting laws requiring hospitals to develop policies that facilitated the possibility of organ donation. These policies required the identification as possible donors all patients determined to be, or anticipated to soon become, "brain dead," and the offering to the legal next of kin or other authorized person for such patients an opportunity to donate the patient's organs.

Almost all U.S. states have now adopted varying forms of such "routine inquiry/required request" laws; federal law now mandates that all hospitals receiving Medicare or Medicaid funds make such donor inquiries. The theory behind this legal approach was that it would generate more kidneys and other organs available for transplantation, but that theory remains to be proved. Although organ donations have increased in some states and referrals to organ procurement agencies of potential donors have increased in all states, the actual number of available kidneys has remained the same nationally for 4 years.

This result has prompted some commentators to suggest that the problem is not a legal one but a psychological one on the part of attending physicians and nurses who do not wish either to be involved in or to see families "stressed" by organ donation requests at the time a loved one has died. Others, perhaps more pragmatic, have suggested that the better approach is to adopt **presumed consent** laws similar to those adopted in a number of U.S. states that permit the removal of pituitary glands and corneas from eligible cadavers unless the patient objected in writing prior to death or the family objected at the time of death. This approach assumes, of course, that public as well as judicial reaction will be equally tolerant to the removal of kidneys without explicit consent.

There appears to be a deeply felt preference among physicians for the organ procurement process to be a voluntary one. In France, which has "presumed consent" laws, physicians, for public relations reasons, seek family consent despite the laws and refuse to take organs when families object. It has been suggested that routine inquiry about organ donation in the event of sudden death should become part of the standard medical history.

SELECTION OF PATIENTS FOR TRANSPLANTATION

Equitable Selection and Access

The system of distribution of cadaveric kidneys is theoretically blind to the possibility of discrimination based on age, race, gender, and socioeconomic status. In practice, this equity has not always proved to be the case, and unanticipated distortions in the allocation of donor organs may occur. There is evidence to suggest that women, blacks, and low-income patients do not receive transplants at the same rate as white men with high incomes.

A patient must pass through several stages before actually receiving a transplant. First, he or she must be appropriately informed as to available treatment options (see Chap. 1). The patient is then referred for transplant evaluation (see Chap. 6). The transplant team, following a favorable consideration of objective medical factors, then offers the transplantation option to the patients they have helped educate. If the patient accepts, he or she is placed on the cadaveric waiting list both locally and nationally. When a suitable kidney eventually becomes available, the patient must have priority over other patients based on the scoring system described above (see Chap. 3).

Such a complex system is inevitably prone to distortion. Are all patients with ESRD equivalently educated as to their options? Do all dialysis units refer patients for evaluation expeditiously? Do all transplant programs distribute kidneys fairly? Similarly, we must quantitate the medical and biologic factors (e.g., high levels of antibodies in multiparous women, excess of blood group O in blacks) that may have an impact on organ distribution.

Role of Perceived Noncompliance in Selection

One exclusionary factor that is not widely understood is the role of perceived or past noncompliance with medical regimens. This psychosocial issue affords great opportunity for discrimination, since it can be used to deny access if used too loosely. Noncompliance is perhaps best measured by looking to objective criteria such as the patient's past record of keeping medical appointments, taking prescribed drugs in the proper regimen, stopping substance abuse (smoking, alcohol, and drugs) with professional assistance and maintaining abstinence, and obtaining psychological or psychiatric therapy for diagnosed mental health problems (see Chap. 15).

A social support system in the form of friends or family is obviously crucial and can help a patient overcome physical and learning disabilities. On the contrary, the absence of a support network and the inability of the patient to understand or comply with the demands of a lifelong treatment regimen and to make medical appointments can be a legitimate reason for denying a transplant to a patient.

Foreign Nationals as Potential Recipients

Press reports during the 1980s of foreign nationals "buying their way to the front of the line" for kidney transplants raised the issue as to whether organs donated by U.S. citizens and residents ought to be restricted to U.S. recipients. In 1985, some 300 of the approximately 6,000 cadaveric kidneys transplanted in the United States went to nonresident patients who came to the United States for the procedures. There was a suggestion that in communities with extensive publicity about foreign patients receiving transplanted kidneys, cadaveric donations fell below previous levels.

While some argued that humanitarian considerations precluded the use of national citizenship as a criterion for acceptance as a recipient, others suggested that the donated organs are a national resource and that U.S. citizens and residents should at least have priority over foreign nationals. Others proposed a ceiling, or cap, on the number of nonresident aliens on any one program's waiting list, but then treating all on the list equally.

In response to this concern, the American Society of Transplant Surgeons adopted guidelines in 1986 limiting the transplantation of kidneys into foreign nationals to an average of "5% per year of the organs transplanted at any single center" and mandating that the charges for such transplants be on the same basis as the charges to U.S. citizens. The UNOS board in 1988 adopted a somewhat similar policy that provided for the potential review by a UNOS committee of any program's transplants involving foreign nationals and the automatic review of any UNOS member center that has foreign nationals constituting more than 10% of its recipients. In 1994, the UNOS board changed the percentage figure to 5%. The UNOS policy also requires that all patients accepted for kidney transplants be treated equally under UNOS guidelines for the distribution of organs.

RESOURCE ALLOCATION ISSUES

Future of End-Stage Renal Disease Program

There are congressional concerns about the dollar costs of the End-Stage Renal Disease Program under Medicare as part of the federal health care budget, and there are ongoing controversies within medicine as to which activities should take funding and programmatic priority.

Kidney transplantation is unlike any other solid organ transplantation effort in that it usually has hemodialysis as a long-term fallback modality. Heart, liver, and lung transplant recipients have no similar treatment mechanism. Thus, while kidney transplantation led the way and remains the volume leader in the transplantation community, there is a potential source of tension among the various organ transplant teams.

This competitiveness was observed vividly when organ procurement teams jockeyed for position as to which organs were to be removed first. Collegial collaboration was mixed with a sense of a "pecking order" in which heart and liver teams were placed before kidney teams, partly because of their claim of a life-and-death time struggle and partly because of their greater recent media publicity. Fortunately, the technical aspects of multiorgan donation have been resolved, and the capacity to store organs for longer periods has helped defuse a potential source of tension. There may remain a sense of inequity over the full Medicare funding of kidney transplants in contrast to the more limited federal funding of liver and heart transplants.

We stand on the verge of significant technological breakthroughs in clinical medicine that may radically alter the distribution of our resources. Human gene therapy has begun in closely monitored research trials at the National Institutes of Health and elsewhere. Those involved in the exploration of the human genome predict not only the identification of most of the genes, but also the development of techniques to engineer proteins that can optimize gene functioning or even create new gene functions for particular kinds of organs. Cellular transplantation may replace surgical transplants.

Thus, it may be possible to address ESRD as a disease process by totally different medical treatment approaches in the next century without the use of either hemodialysis or kidney transplantation, at least for some patients. Will we then, as a society, be willing to invest the large sums of money required to produce and clinically apply such treatment modalities? If the funding mechanism for health care is correctly perceived as a national combination of public and private funds, who will determine these priorities? Which diseases will get the greatest attention and funding? Will transplantation be as exciting as the new gene therapy approaches in the next several decades?

There remains the possibility that those in a position to influence these decisions (as much political and business decisions as they are medical and scientific) may decide that primary or preventive care treatment should take precedence over acute care programs, such as organ transplantation, and thus receive funding priority and greater patient access. These resource allocation or rationing decisions, as they are sometimes labeled, are going to become particularly difficult when those arguing for funding pit diseases with larger patient populations against those that are rarer, those with greater mortality against those with lesser morbidity, those that affect majority populations against those that only affect specific races or ethnic groups, and the like. Hospitals threatened with financial ruin may find in the future that transplant programs, currently a significant "revenue enhancer," are less attractive if funding patterns change or if patient populations shift.

With health care spending spiraling ever higher and many patients and providers fighting for their share of that health care funding pie, these issues will have to be faced, and they have enormous ethical implications. This all assumes, however, that the health care portion of the societal budget maintains its present significant percentage and growth pattern.

Future of Health Care Expenditures

In the United States, the seeming primacy of health care costs over other governmental expenses is being increasingly questioned. The relevant statistics offer some insight. Recently published data show that overall health care costs in the United States have passed the $600 billion figure, seven times higher than the 1970 cost, and now represent almost 12% of the gross national product.

Public Law 92-603, the law passed by Congress in 1972 to fund all ESRD care, through Medicare, has been the basis for federal expenditures for ESRD costs that amounted to $242 million in 1974 and that now exceed several billion dollars annually. No other potentially lethal chronic disease involving high treatment costs, including hemophilia, has been granted this across-the-board, categorical coverage under Medicare. Recent reports highlight concern in Congress over the increasing costs of the ESRD Program.

As talk of rationing and cost containment becomes more fashionable, particularly in a context of national economic budgetary constraints, it will be interesting to see whether the U.S. public will continue to support such priorities for health care over potentially competing claims for law enforcement and prisons, education, and social welfare (to mention only three). Medicare budget cuts, even without a public debate about health care priorities, may reduce the ESRD Program under Medicare or, at the very least, prevent its expansion to treat new patients. The ESRD Program has had an average annual growth in recent years of 15%.

Some commentators suggest that, while Congress may have passed Medicare funding for ESRD in 1972 because it believed that saving life should take priority over other values, including cost and cost-effectiveness, the federal government's values may have shifted to place cost containment higher than individual survival. If that is a correct assessment, future kidney transplantation programs in the United States will have to cope with the same issues of funding and insurance coverage that all other solid organ and bone marrow transplantation programs have been facing.

SELECTED READINGS

Arisi L. Quality of life in kidney donors. *Nephrol Dial Transplant* 9:733, 1994.

Bonomini V. Ethical aspects of living donation. *Transplant Proc* 23:2497, 1991.

Childress JF. Ethical criteria for procuring and distributing organs for transplantation. *J Health Polit Policy Law* 14:87, 1989.

Chugh KS, Jha V. Commerce in transplantation in Third World countries. *Kidney Int* 49:1181, 1996.

First International Congress on Ethics, Justice, and Commerce in Transplantation: A global view. Proceedings. *Transplant Proc* 22:891, 1990.

Gokol R. Cadaveric transplantation. *J Postgrad Med* 39:105, 1993.

Granvik A. Ethical dilemmas in organ donation and transplantation. *Crit Care Med* 16:1012, 1988.

Halasz NA. Medicine and ethics: How to allocate transplantable organs. *Transplantation* 52:43, 1991.

Kilner JF. *Who Lives? Who Dies?: Ethical Criteria in Patient Selection.* New Haven, CT: Yale University Press, 1990.

Kittur DS, Hagan MM, Thukral VK et al. Incentives for organ donation? *Lancet* 338:1441, 1991.

Kjellstrand CM, Dosseter JB (eds). *Ethical Problems in Dialysis and Transplantation.* Dordrecht, The Netherlands: Kluwer Academic, 1992.

Moskop JC. Organ transplantation in children: Ethical issues. *J Pediatr* 110:175, 1987.

Qunibi W, Abulrub D, Shaheen F et al. Attitudes of commercial renal transplant recipients toward renal transplantation in India. *Clin Transplantation* 9:317, 1995.

Ramos EL, Kasiske BL, Alexander SR et al. The evaluation of candidates for renal transplantation: The current practices of U.S. transplant centres. *Transplantation* 57:490, 1994.

Salahudeen AK, Woods HF, Pingle A et al. High mortality among recipients of bought living-unrelated donor kidney. *Lancet* 336:725, 1990.

Sever MS, Ecder T, Aydin AE et al. Living unrelated (paid) kidney transplantion in Third-World countries. *Nephrol Dial Transplant* 9:530, 1994.

Simmons RG, Abess L. Ethics in Organ Transplantation. In CG Cerilli (ed), *Organ Transplantation and Replacement.* Philadelphia: Lippincott, 1988, Pp 691–702.

Singer PA. A review of public policies to procure and distribute kidneys for transplantation. *Arch Intern Med* 150:523, 1990.

Spital A. The shortage of organs for transplantation: Where do we go from here? *N Engl J Med* 325:1243, 1991.

Spital A. The ethics of unconventional living organ donation. *Clin Transplantation* 5:322, 1991.

Takemoto S, Terasaki PI, Gjertson DW et al. Equitable allocation of HLA-compatible kidneys for local pools and minorities. *N Engl J Med* 331:760, 1994.

Veatch RM. *Case Studies in Medical Ethics.* Cambridge, MA: Harvard University Press, 1977. Pp 222–227.

Veatch RM. Routine inquiry about organ donation—An alternative to presumed consent. *N Engl J Med* 325:1246, 1991.

Nutrition in the Kidney Transplant Recipient

Susan E. Weil

The nutritional management of the renal transplant recipient is an important adjunct to the optimization of outcome. Diet can be used to both prevent and ameliorate many transplant-related complications, although the precise nutrient requirements of kidney transplant recipients continue to be incompletely defined. The following recommendations, which are based on available studies in the transplant population and extrapolated data in comparable settings, provide a guide to nutrition care management in the pretransplant, acute post-transplant, and long-term post-transplant periods.

PRETRANSPLANT NUTRITION MANAGEMENT

Major Concerns

In the pretransplant period, a multidisciplinary approach should incorporate diet, lifestyle changes, and use of medications to aid in the correction or improvement of malnutrition, dyslipidemia, obesity, renal osteodystrophy, and hypertension. To varying degrees, the presence of these comorbidities in the pretransplant patient are predictors of related complications in the post-transplant period. Although the etiology of these problems is multifactorial, it is reasonable to presume that aggressive nutritional management in the pretransplant period may help minimize post-transplant morbid events.

Malnutrition

The primary nutritional focus of the pretransplant period is the prevention and treatment of malnutrition, which is clearly related to dialysis morbidity and mortality. At times, optimization of protein and calorie nutrition may seem to be at cross purposes with other nutrition goals such as phosphate restriction. Some element of malnutrition has been identified in up to 70% percent of the dialysis population. Low serum albumin levels are powerful predictors of mortality risk in the dialysis population. Inadequate dialysis may compound the impact of malnutrition on dialysis mortality.

It is unclear how these findings specifically affect transplant outcome. Low serum albumin levels and other nutritional assessment parameters are predictors of surgical risk, and severely malnourished patients may be deemed inappropriate transplant candidates. Aggressive treatment of malnutrition with various forms of nutritional supplementation as well as careful attention to adequacy of dialysis and a thorough evaluation of intervening causes of poor intake (e.g., medications, intercurrent illness, psychosocial issues) may improve transplant outcome and allow transplantation to be an option for patients who may otherwise have been excluded.

Obesity

Operative risk and wound healing can be negatively influenced by the presence of obesity, conveniently defined in terms of ideal body weight (>130%) or body mass index (>30 kg/m^2). Obesity is a defined risk factor for failure of both kidney transplants and kidney-pancreas transplants (see Chaps. 6 and 13). Aside from surgical risk, obesity is associated with increased mortality, while weight levels greater than 120% of ideal have been associated with increased morbidity. In the obese patient, attempts should be made to approach ideal body weight before surgery, although this is often easier to propose than achieve, particularly in patients with limited exercise tolerance.

Dyslipidemia

End-stage renal disease (ESRD) is associated with dyslipidemia, as evidenced by moderate hypertriglyceridemia with a normal total cholesterol, normal or increased triglyceride-rich low-density lipoprotein (LDL), decreased high-density lipoprotein (HDL), and increased cholesterol-rich very-low-density lipoprotein (VLDL). In addition, decreased apoprotein AI, AII, or both and normal or increased apoprotein B levels have been described. These abnormalities are considered potential risk factors for atherosclerosis and may be particularly important in diabetic patients, who are susceptible to coronary artery disease and peripheral vascular disease. Independent of its role in surgical risk, atherosclerotic cardiovascular disease remains the major cause of death in the ESRD population. Dyslipidemia should be treated in the pretransplant candidate either by diet or by a combination of diet, exercise, and lipid-lowering agents.

Assessment of Nutritional Status

Assessment of nutritional status by a renal dietitian specialist should, ideally, be incorporated as part of the transplant candidate selection process with a view to identifying the transplant candidate in need of more intensive nutritional support and monitoring. Typical parameters of assessment may be unreliable or of limited value in the patient with renal disease. Evaluation parameters include the following:

Diet History

The history includes discussion of appetite, usual food intake, and previous diet modifications; information about food preparation; physical, emotional, or psychosocial impediments to eating; information about usual body weight and weight changes; medications that may interfere with nutrient intake, absorption, or metabolism; concomitant illnesses including gastrointestinal disorders, febrile illnesses, diabetes, and hypertension; food allergies; activity level; and educational needs. Use of over-the-counter medications, vitamin or mineral supplements, and herbal preparations should also be reviewed.

Physical Examination

The fluid status of the patient is assessed by examination. Physical signs of malnutrition such as temporal wasting and signs of vitamin and mineral deficiency should be sought. Serial anthropometric measurements can be used to assess somatic protein and fat stores. Parameters include height, weight, body mass index, ideal or rela-

Table 17-1. Degree of malnutrition assessed from height and weight

	Mild (%)	Moderate (%)	Severe (%)
Ideal body weight	80–90	70–79	<70
Usual body weight	85–95	75–84	<75
Recent weight loss	≥5 over 1 mo	≥7.5 over 3 mos	≥10 over 6 mos

tive body weight, weight changes, triceps skinfold thickness, and mid-arm muscle circumference. In patients on dialysis, skinfold thickness and mid-arm muscle circumference should be measured postdialysis, as results are influenced by hydration state. Unintentional weight loss and an actual weight of less than 90% of ideal body weight, or a body mass index of less than 20, may indicate protein and calorie malnutrition and the need for nutritional support. Table 17-1 provides guidelines devised and adapted to indicate degrees of malnutrition based on height and weight information.

Laboratory Data

1. In the absence of proteinuria, volume overload or depletion, catabolic stress, or hepatic synthetic dysfunction, the albumin concentration is considered a reliable indicator of protein nutrition in the stable renal patient. Transferrin levels are of limited value in assessing protein nutriture in the presence of iron deficiency or iron overload. Prealbumin and retinol-binding proteins, acute-phase proteins used to assess protein nutriture in patients without renal failure, may also be of limited use because levels are elevated in chronic renal failure, independent of nutritional status. In the immediate post-transplant period, these values are unreliable. Hypoalbuminemia has been shown to be a strong independent risk factor for all causes of mortality after renal transplantation.
2. Phosphorus, calcium, and parathyroid hormone levels help to assess the need for phosphate modification, calcium supplementation, vitamin D therapy, and, less commonly, parathyroidectomy.
3. Other laboratory data, including measurements of serum potassium and other electrolytes, creatinine, blood urea nitrogen (BUN), lipid profile, as well as urine measurements for urea and protein, help determine additional nutrient requirements.
4. Hemoglobin, hematocrit, mean corpuscular volume, ferritin, iron, and total iron-binding capacity help to monitor the need for iron supplementation or erythropoietin therapy. Folic acid and B_{12} deficiencies should be considered.
5. Creatinine/height index and 3-methylhistidine levels are not reliable indicators of protein status in patients with renal disease.
6. Delayed hypersensitivity to skin test antigens, a measurement of immunocompetence, is difficult to use as an assessment tool in chronic renal failure because anergy may be present as a result of the disease process alone and because of the post-transplant use of immunosuppressive agents.
7. A decreased total lymphocyte count may be indicative of malnutrition in the setting of renal failure in conjunction with other diagnostic parameters, although it may also be influenced by immunosuppressive agents.

8. Nitrogen balance can be assessed by calculating the urea nitrogen appearance in the stable predialysis patient. Urea kinetic modeling for patients on dialysis assesses both protein catabolic rate and dialysis adequacy.

ACUTE POST-TRANSPLANTATION NUTRITION MANAGEMENT

In the post-transplant period, appropriate macro- and micronutrients need to be provided as for any surgical patient. Ideally, nutrition can be optimized preoperatively in the kidney transplant candidate to minimize nutrition-related complications postoperatively. The acute post-transplant period generally refers to the 4- to 6-week period after surgery.

Major Concerns

Protein Catabolism

The stress of surgery combined with the use of high-dose corticosteroids can lead to severe protein catabolism, particularly in the patient with underlying malnutrition. Severe protein catabolism contributes to poor wound healing and an increased susceptibility to infection. The degree of protein catabolism can be assessed by the measurement of urea nitrogen appearance, although in the routine, uncomplicated patient, this assessment may not be warranted.

Fluid and Electrolyte Balance

During the postoperative period, fluid and electrolyte requirements vary depending on the level of renal function, volume status, and drug-nutrient interactions. Needs are reassessed daily, and routine ordering of a standard diet in the acute period should be avoided. Specific guidelines are discussed in the section on acute post-transplant nutrient requirements.

Drug-Nutrient Interactions

Drug-nutrient interactions, important in the long-term management of the transplant patient, should also be considered in the acute period. Table 17-2 lists both short- and long-term interactions with immunosuppressive agents.

Cyclosporine Administration.   Capsules are the most common form of cyclosporine administration, although liquid cyclosporine continues to be available and has specific administration recommendations. It can be effectively taken with a variety of beverages (juices or milk), provided the beverages are not heated, excessively chilled, or carbonated. Liquid cyclosporine should be mixed and taken in a glass container rather than in a container made of foam, paper, or plastic, which adsorbs the medication. Patients are advised to be consistent in choice of beverage, proximity to eating, and timing of taking cyclosporine so that fluctuations in absorption can be avoided. The Neoral formulation of cyclosporine improves absorption characteristics and pharmacokinetic consistency.

Grapefruit juice contains a substance that inhibits the metabolism of cyclosporine and other substances in the liver by the P450 enzyme system (see Chap. 4). The peak blood levels of cyclosporine

Table 17-2. Drug/nutrient interactions of immunosuppressive agents

Immunosuppressive agent	Interaction
Corticosteroids	Polyphagia, glucose intolerance, hyperlipidemia, osteoporosis, gastritis and peptic ulcer disease, fluid retention, hypertension
Cyclosporine	Hypertension, glucose intolerance, hyperlipidemia, hyperkalemia, hypomagnesemia, hyperuricemia
Azathioprine	Leukopenia, thrombocytopenia, megaloblastic anemia, nausea and vomiting, pancreatitis
Antithymocyte globulin	Leukopenia, thrombocytopenia, hypotension, hyperglycemia (rare), diarrhea, nausea, vomiting
OKT3	Hypertension, pulmonary edema, nausea, vomiting, diarrhea
Tacrolimus	Anemia, leukocytosis, hypertension, hyperglycemia, hyperkalemia or hypokalemia, hyperuricemia, hypomagnesemia, nausea, abdominal pain, gas, vomiting, anorexia, constipation, diarrhea, leukopenia
Mycophenolate mofetil	Anorexia, nausea, epigastric pain, gas, diarrhea, abdominal pain

may increase if grapefruit juice is taken in close proximity to the cyclosporine dose.

Acute Post-Transplantation Nutrient Requirements

For many patients, a successful kidney transplant represents a long-awaited opportunity to be liberated from the stringent dietary restrictions required of them while on dialysis. When providing dietary instruction, this need for "liberation" should be recognized and respected and directed in a manner that will permit the patient a well-deserved sense of dietary freedom without potentially morbid dietary indiscretion. For some patients, it is hard to "loosen up" from years of compulsive dietary control, but dietary instruction serves to provide the confidence needed to allow them to enjoy their newly won freedom.

In the following section, the recommendations listed as "per kilogram of body weight" should be based on actual body weight or body weight adjusted for obesity.

Protein

In the acute postoperative period, protein requirements are generally accepted to be 1.3–1.5 g/kg body weight. These levels are compatible with neutral or positive nitrogen balance, provided caloric intake is adequate. In patients who continue to require dialysis, these levels of protein intake have been demonstrated not to result in an increased dialysis requirement, and therefore are used in both the functioning and nonfunctioning graft. In the postoperative patient on peritoneal dialysis or with evidence of protein depletion, protein is provided at the upper end of the recommended range.

Calories

For the uncomplicated patient, caloric requirements are 30–35 kcal/kg. This level appears to be compatible with maintaining or achieving neutral or positive nitrogen balance. Calorie needs may increase in the presence of fever, infection, or increased surgical or traumatic stress. In the stressed patient requiring nutritional support, caloric requirements can also be calculated using the Harris-Benedict equation to determine basal energy requirements with a stress factor of 1.5; however, its usefulness has not been well studied in the renal transplant recipient.

Carbohydrates

Limitation of simple sugars and overall restriction of carbohydrates in combination with a high-protein diet may lessen cosmetic steroid side effects in the 3- to 4-week period post-transplantation. The level of carbohydrate restriction used in one early study was 1 g carbohydrate/kg body weight. It is unclear if less severe levels of restriction combined with a high protein intake have similar benefit. The side effects reported to improve are cushingoid facies and development of fat deposition patterns commonly seen with use of high-dose corticosteroids. Other effects, such as the development of steroid diabetes, do not correlate with dietary manipulation. It should be noted that the use of a low-carbohydrate diet necessitates concurrent use of a high-fat diet to make the diet calorically adequate. This modification may be contraindicated or impractical, although it is unlikely that the short-term use of a high-fat diet will have any lasting impact on the lipid profile of a given patient. These guidelines may also be impractical for the diabetic patient because of the potential for hypoglycemia despite high doses of steroids.

Fat

Treatment of hyperlipidemia is a critically important issue in the long-term management of the transplant patient. In the short-term period after surgery, however, manipulations in fat content or composition are unlikely to affect patient outcome. For the purpose of patient education, it is reasonable at this time to begin dietary fat and cholesterol guidelines as discussed in the section on nutrition requirements for the stable post-transplant patient.

Sodium

Post-transplant hypertension, often exaggerated by cyclosporine use, is a common problem in the immediate post-transplant period. Cyclosporine-related hypertension is, in part, salt-dependent (see Chap. 9). Control of sodium intake to 2 g/day is appropriate in this context or in the presence of volume overload. Normotensive patients who are edema-free do not require strict sodium restriction.

Potassium

Hyperkalemia is often seen in the post-transplant period and may be exaggerated by the use of cyclosporine or tacrolimus. If serum potassium levels exceed 6 mEq/liter, restriction of potassium intake to the level of 70 mEq daily may be warranted, and dialysis may be

Table 17-3. Selected phosphorus and magnesium supplements

Product	Form	Mineral content
K-Phos Neutral	Tablet	250 mg phosphorus, 45 mg (1.1 mEq) potassium, 298 mg (13 mEq) sodium
K-Phos Original	Tablet	114 mg phosphorus, 144 mg (3.7 mEq) potassium
K-Phos M.F.	Tablet	125.6 mg phosphorus, 44.5 mg (1.1 mEq) potassium, 67 mg (2.9 mEq) sodium
K-Phos No. 2	Tablet	250 mg phosphorus, 88 mg (2.3 mEq) potassium, 134 mg (5.8 mEq) sodium
Neutra-Phos	Powder	250 mg phosphorus, 278 mg (7.13 mEq) potassium, 164 mg (7.13 mEq) sodium
Uro-Mag	Capsule	140 mg magnesium oxide, 84.5 mg (6.93 mEq) elemental magnesium
Mag-Ox 400	Tablet	400 mg magnesium oxide, 241.3 mg (19.86 mEq) elemental magnesium
Magtab SR	Caplet	84 mg (7 mEq) elemental magnesium as magnesium lactate

required for patients with delayed graft function. Adequate protein intake, however, should not be compromised in an attempt to control potassium intake. Other causes of hyperkalemia should be considered, including the use of medications, such as beta-adrenergic blocking agents, angiotensin-converting enzyme inhibitors, and nonsteroidal anti-inflammatory agents.

Phosphorus

Hypophosphatemia is a common finding post-transplant, primarily as a result of increased urinary excretion of phosphate both mediated by and independent of residual secondary hyperparathyroidism. In addition, glucocorticoid-induced gluconeogenesis in the renal proximal tubule contributes to phosphaturia. Increased intake of high-phosphorus foods may not be sufficient for repletion, and oral replacement is often necessary. Table 17-3 lists some available phosphate supplements, all of which contain potassium, sodium, or a combination of both.

With a nonfunctioning graft, the use of phosphate-binding antacids and modification of phosphorus intake to less than 1,000 mg/day may be temporarily warranted but is discontinued as renal function improves to avoid severe hypophosphatemia.

Magnesium

Hypomagnesemia is a common finding postoperatively secondary to cyclosporine-induced hypermagnesuria. Dietary replacement of magnesium is likely to be inadequate, necessitating the use of magnesium supplements. Table 17-3 lists some available oral supplements.

Fluid

Early post-transplant fluid management is discussed in detail in Chap. 8. With a well-functioning graft and a normovolemic state, a reasonable minimum fluid intake is 2,000 ml/day. In the oliguric patient, a fluid volume should be provided to equal urine output plus a minimum of 500–750 ml to cover insensible losses. Variations should be determined by volume status and blood pressure, typically erring on the positive side, as urine output increases.

Vitamins

If dialysis treatments continue to be temporarily necessary, water-soluble vitamin replacement is continued. The efficacy of routine supplementation of water-soluble vitamins once the patient no longer requires dialysis has not been well studied. 1,25-dihydroxyvitamin D_3 replacement may continue to be warranted in the immediate postoperative period if the patient is hypocalcemic.

Trace Minerals

Iron. A transferrin saturation rate (iron/total iron-binding capacity) of less than 20% or a plasma ferritin level of less than 100 ng/ml is indicative of iron deficiency. A baseline evaluation of iron status should be performed preoperatively, as iron deficiency is commonly found in the dialysis population in conjunction with erythropoietin therapy. If oral iron replacement is warranted, intake should be scheduled so that it does not coincide with antacid therapy to avoid interference with iron absorption.

Other Trace Minerals. Post-transplant trace mineral requirements have not been well investigated in this setting. Although increased zincuria has been associated with steroid therapy, its clinical significance is not well substantiated. Routine supplementation of trace minerals is not indicated in the uncomplicated postoperative patient on an oral diet.

NUTRITIONAL SUPPORT IN THE POST-TRANSPLANT PERIOD

In nutritionally high-risk patients, early nutritional support is indicated. Use of aggressive nutritional support in patients with ESRD and septic complications, including post-transplant patients, has been shown to reduce mortality rates.

In the course of a typical post-transplant patient, progression to oral intake and solid foods usually occurs within 2–3 postoperative days. The length of hospitalization may be less than a week, and aggressive nutritional support is rarely necessary. The following guidelines, however, can be used for either recent or long-term transplant recipients who may be at high nutritional risk or may be undergoing additional major surgical procedures. Guidelines also may be pertinent for the combined kidney-pancreas transplant recipients who may not be able to tolerate oral nutrition for prolonged periods (see Chap. 13).

Indications for Aggressive Nutritional Intervention

Delayed Oral Intake

Nutritional support in the form of parenteral nutrition may be warranted if postoperative oral intake is delayed for more than 5 days because of complications such as protracted ileus or intractable nausea and vomiting. The decision to begin nutritional support requires consideration of the overall nutritional status of the patient, as evidenced by anthropometric and laboratory data. Nutritional support may be necessary even in patients who are adequately nourished before transplant surgery, who will become catabolic with the combination of high-dose corticosteroids and surgery.

Inadequate Intake

Any patient unable to sustain adequate intake to meet protein and calorie needs after the fourth or fifth postoperative day is considered a potential candidate for some type of nutritional intervention. The decision to intervene will again depend on the nutritional status of the patient, degree of catabolism (either measured by urea generation rate or estimated by type and degree of surgical or medical complication), amount of intake deficit, and assessment of the cost-benefit risks of initiating support.

Choice of Feeding Modality

Oral Supplements

Supplements are considered after 4–5 days postoperation in any patient in whom protein and calorie needs are not being met on a standard diet. Correctable reasons for inadequate oral intake should be assessed, such as overly restrictive diet; unnecessarily slow progression to a full diet; and interference with meals by dialysis, scheduled tests, and procedures.

Tube Feeding

Tube feeding is considered in the postoperative period in any patient with a functional gastrointestinal tract who, by 7 days after surgery, is unable to maintain adequate protein and calorie nutriture with the use of diet or oral supplements. Tube feeding is rarely required after kidney transplantation but may be more commonly indicated after combined kidney-pancreas transplantation. Small bowel access and use of continuous feeding are preferred when tube feeding is indicated in this setting.

Tube feeding is preferred over parenteral nutrition because of a decreased risk of infection related to the avoidance of central line use and because of the production of secretory immunoglobulins, which help to prevent adverse bacterial growth in the intestinal mucosal lining. The maintenance of normal intestinal function and integrity, a decreased potential for electrolyte imbalance, and cost savings are other benefits of enteral feeding.

A wide variety of oral and enteral products are commercially available to meet the needs of the transplant recipient (see Selected Readings).

Total Parenteral Nutrition

A mixture of both essential and nonessential amino acids, fat, and dextrose should provide a daily intake of 1.5 g protein/kg and 30–35 kcal/kg. Ideally, calorie requirements are assessed by indirect calorimetry.

Dietary Considerations During Acute Rejection Episodes

In acute rejection, provision of optimal protein and calorie intake is the primary nutritional concern. High-dose steroids produce a dose-related increase in protein catabolic rate, and, with rising creatinine and BUN levels, there is a common inclination to restrict protein intake. Protein restriction in this setting leads to severe catabolism, and a daily protein intake in the range of 1.3–1.5 g/kg is appropriate. Minimum daily calorie requirements during rejection therapy are 33–35 kcal/kg.

Special Considerations for the Combined Kidney-Pancreas Recipient

In the well-functioning combined kidney-pancreas transplant, nutritional guidelines are essentially the same as with solitary kidney transplants except with regard to fluid and electrolyte intake. In the typical bladder-drained pancreas transplant, persistent exocrine pancreatic drainage into the bladder results in sizable urinary losses of sodium chloride and sodium bicarbonate (see Chap. 13). Extracellular fluid volume contraction and metabolic acidosis may ensue. Sodium and bicarbonate intake often needs to be supplemented.

LONG-TERM NUTRITION MANAGEMENT

Major Concerns

Hyperlipidemia

Accelerated atherosclerosis is commonly seen in transplant patients and remains the main cause of long-term mortality in the transplant population. Hyperlipidemia, a known risk factor for atherosclerotic disease, is associated with numerous factors in the post-transplant patient, including diabetes and glucose intolerance, use of glucocorticoids and cyclosporine, obesity, genetic predisposition, use of certain diuretics and beta-adrenergic blocking agents, nephrotic syndrome, hypothyroidism, ovarian failure of menopause, and inappropriate diet. Progression of renal disease in the transplanted kidney may also be enhanced by the presence of hyperlipidemia.

Transplant recipients treated with corticosteroids and azathioprine typically present with elevated VLDL cholesterol levels and elevated LDL levels. HDL levels are typically normal or elevated. In patients receiving cyclosporine, VLDL levels are often normal or only slightly elevated except in the presence of diabetes. The LDL cholesterol level tends to be elevated, with a normal or elevated HDL cholesterol level. The effect of transplantation and immunosuppressive agents on atherogenic lipoprotein(a) levels is unclear.

Diet therapy and exercise may be at least partially effective in lipid reduction in the post-transplant patient and should be attempted as first-line therapy prior to trial of lipid-lowering agents. Before considering pharmacologic measures, it is appropriate, in most patients, to allow a 3-month trial of diet therapy, which should include regular dietitian follow-up.

Obesity and Weight Gain

Hyperphagia associated with steroid therapy, together with a sense of liberation from the dietary constraints of dialysis and an increased sense of well-being, contribute to the propensity for weight gain in the post-transplant patient. If obesity ensues, it may contribute to the development or exacerbation of hypertension, hyperlipidemia, cardiovascular disease, and, in some series, steroid-induced diabetes.

Obesity has also been associated with increased graft loss related to both acute and chronic rejection.

The reported prevalence of obesity varies considerably. The degree of weight gain does not appear to correlate with corticosteroid dose, donor source, rejection history, preexisting obesity, length of time on dialysis before transplantation, and post-transplant renal function. Demographic factors such as young age and black race have been associated with the most weight gain in the first post-transplant year. Male and female patients have comparable weight gains in the first year, though women continue to gain weight thereafter. The average weight gain in the first year is approximately 10% of body weight.

Management of Obesity.   In addition to limitation of caloric intake, management of post-transplant obesity includes behavior modification and an aerobic exercise program. Frequent follow-up by members of the health care team, including a physician, dietitian, and nurse, along with group support techniques, may optimize adherence to weight management programs. The serotonergic agent fenfluramine (Pondimin) and the noradrenergic agent phentermine (Fastin) have been used successfully, in combination, to produce impressive weight loss in obese transplant recipients.

Bone Disease

Diet plays both a palliative and preventive role in certain post-transplant bone abnormalities. Osteoporosis has been associated with long-term glucocorticoid use in part as a result of decreased intestinal absorption of calcium. In addition, hyperparathyroidism may persist long after transplantation and may influence the severity of bone loss. Provision of adequate calcium and phosphorus intake may attenuate these problems. A low-purine diet may be useful for patients with gout or severe hyperuricemia. Additional manifestations of transplant-related bone disease are reviewed in Chap. 9 and are not clearly related to nutritional factors.

Hypertension

The prevalence of hypertension is reported in most series to be approximately 50% in the transplant population. Hypertension is an important risk factor for cardiovascular disease as well as for graft survival. Although post-transplant hypertension is multifactorial in origin, cyclosporine-related hypertension is a common contributing component (see Chap. 9). Sodium sensitivity is a hallmark of cyclosporine-related hypertension; however, weight control or weight loss in the obese hypertensive patient may play at least as important a role as sodium restriction in its treatment. Exercise provides a beneficial adjuvant. The beneficial effect of other nonpharmacologic influences such as calcium, potassium, and magnesium intake, and avoidance of alcohol use have not been well defined.

Post-Transplant Diabetes Mellitus

The prevalence of post-transplant diabetes mellitus is probably in the range of 5–20%, with risk factors including advanced age, obesity, glucocorticoid and cyclosporine use, certain human leukocyte antigen types (A30 and Bw42 antigens), and cadaveric donor source (see Chap. 9).

Corticosteroids have been shown to produce a peripheral insulin resistance as well as cause an alteration in pancreatic beta cell insulin secretion. Cyclosporine also appears to alter peripheral insulin sensitivity and to diminish islet cell function. Percentage weight gain is not clearly associated with the development of glucose intolerance. The presence of post-transplant diabetes appears to be associated with poor graft survival and is a risk factor for the development of cardiovascular disease.

Diet, weight loss if appropriate, and exercise, along with decreased dosing of corticosteroids and cyclosporine when possible, provide the basis for initial management. Oral hypoglycemics may be warranted; approximately half of those diagnosed will eventually require insulin.

Progression of Renal Disease in Kidney Transplants

The role of diet in the progression of renal disease in the transplanted kidney requires further study. The potential deleterious effect of excess protein on the kidney versus the known effect of protein wasting from chronic corticosteroid therapy suggest conflicting recommendations. In the patient with chronic rejection and a glomerular filtration rate below 40 ml/minute, some degree of protein restriction may be appropriate, though there is no clearcut evidence that protein restriction delays the progression of chronic rejection. Evidence of continued protein wasting has been described even with low dosages of corticosteroids, necessitating ongoing assessment of nutritional status. Control of hyperlipidemia may play a role in the prevention of progression of chronic rejection.

Food-Borne Infectious Complications

Even the non-nutritionally compromised transplant patient may be susceptible to an increased incidence of infection (see Chap. 10). Infectious complications in the renal transplant recipient have been reported to occur at a level 10 times higher than anticipated in the presence of malnutrition, defined as a serum albumin less than 2.8 g/dl. An awareness of potentially pathogenic organisms commonly found in food may provide an often ignored, relatively simple, preventive measure. Providing education on safe and sensible food habits may help minimize the morbidity associated with certain post-transplant infectious disease complications.

Food vehicles for *Listeria monocytogenes* include raw milk, soft cheeses, and hot dogs. Pasteurization and proper food handling technique may help minimize the risk of contamination. *Nocardia asteroides*, although ubiquitous in the environment and not uncommonly nosocomially acquired, can be present in decaying vegetables. *Salmonella* infections are associated with undercooked, contaminated meat, poultry and eggs, as well as raw milk. Raw seafood and raw fruits and vegetables also present an increased risk. Prevention includes proper food handling, preparation, and pasteurization. The potential for *Legionella* infection exists in areas with a contaminated or unsafe water supply.

Nutrient Recommendations for the Stable Post-Transplant Patient

Protein and Calories

Protein requirements in the stable post-transplant patient are ill-defined, with muscle wasting identified even at corticosteroid

Table 17-4. Nutrient recommendations for cholesterol control

Nutrient	Recommended intake
Total fat	≤30% total kcal[a]
Saturated fatty acids	8–10% total kcal[b]
	<7% total kcal if not responsive to initial diet
Polyunsaturated fatty acids	Up to 10% kcal[b]
Monounsaturated fatty acids	Up to 15% kcal[c]
Cholesterol	<300 mg
	<200 mg if not responsive to initial diet
Total calories	Individualized level to achieve or maintain ideal body weight

[a]60 g/day on an 1,800-kcal diet.
[b]20 g/day on an 1,800-kcal diet.
[c]20–30 g/day on an 1,800-kcal diet.

doses of 0.20 mg/kg/day. A daily protein intake ranging from 0.55 to 1.0 g/kg has been recommended for the stable post-transplant patient. Negative nitrogen balance has been reported in short-term studies of protein intake levels of 0.6 g/kg/day unless calorie intake is maintained above 25 kcal/kg/day. These levels may be difficult to achieve even in "compliant" patients. A daily protein intake approaching 1 g/kg combined with exercise and adequate calorie intake appear to be compatible with neutral or positive nitrogen balance.

For the stable transplant patient requiring weight reduction, a daily calorie intake of 25 kcal/kg ideal body weight is a reasonable starting point. Caloric restriction should be combined with exercise, behavior modification techniques, and regular team follow-up.

Fat

Given the incidence of post-transplant hypercholesterolemia, the propensity toward weight gain, and the potential contribution of lipids to decreased graft survival, a reduced fat and reduced cholesterol diet is appropriate for the majority of long-term patients.

The recommendations of the National Cholesterol Education Program (NCEP) seem to be of some benefit for lipid control in this group. For patients who ultimately require pharmacologic management for control of hypercholesterolemia, diet guidelines should continue to be encouraged as adjunctive therapy. NCEP guidelines are listed in Table 17-4.

Fish Oil

Further studies are needed to clarify and evaluate the effect of n-3 fatty acids, in the form of fish oil, as an adjunct to immunosuppressive therapy. Supplemental fish oil in the amounts of 3–6 g/day may have a positive impact on glomerular filtration rate, effective renal plasma flow, and blood pressure in cyclosporine-treated patients. The incidence of acute rejection and 1-year graft survival, however, has not been shown to be significantly improved.

Sodium

Sodium restriction to 2–3 g/day is warranted in cyclosporine-treated patients with hypertension. In the normotensive, nonedematous patient, strict sodium restriction is not warranted and may be of little benefit in hypertensive transplant patients not receiving cyclosporine.

Potassium

Hyperkalemia, associated with the use of cyclosporine and tacrolimus, may continue to be observed in the otherwise stable transplant patient. Guidelines as discussed in the section on acute post-transplant management continue to apply in this situation. Potassium levels up to 5.5 mEq/liter are common and are rarely a source of concern in stable patients.

Calcium, Phosphorus, and Vitamin D

In the absence of hypercalcemia, calcium should be provided at the level of 1,000–1,500 mg/day by diet, supplements, or both. If hypocalcemia or evidence of secondary hyperparathyroidism persists, vitamin D therapy in the form of active 1,25-dihydroxyvitamin D_3 is instituted. Hypophosphatemia may persist into this period, necessitating phosphate supplementation. Hypercalcemia may persist in as much as a third of patients in the first year and subsequently in as many as 10% after 1 year as a result of secondary hyperparathyroidism. When related to secondary hyperparathyroidism, hypercalcemia may respond to judiciously monitored 1,25-dihydroxyvitamin D_3 therapy.

Magnesium

Hypomagnesemia may persist into the long-term post-transplant period, and magnesium supplements are often prescribed (see Table 17-3). Magnesium supplementation may favorably influence the blood lipid profile, primarily by increasing HDL cholesterol levels. The role of magnesium in controlling blood pressure in this population remains equivocal.

Vitamins and Trace Minerals

To ensure adequate intake of vitamins and trace minerals, water-soluble vitamin supplementation is warranted for patients on diets restricting protein (to less than 60 g/day), potassium, or calories (to less than 1,200 kcal/day). Supplementation is not otherwise routinely warranted. Vitamin A levels are typically elevated in kidney transplant recipients, so vitamin A is not supplemented. A daily intake of vitamin C of more than 100 mg should be avoided to minimize the possibility of oxalate deposition in the transplanted kidney. Iron supplementation may be appropriate. Zinc supplementation may be warranted with the long-term use of corticosteroids, although specific needs have not been determined.

Alcohol

Conflicting studies are available as to the effect of alcohol consumption on cyclosporine metabolism. Data suggest that excessive alcohol intake increases the absorption and therefore potential toxicity of cyclosporine, although moderate amounts may be tolerated without a marked effect on absorption. Other nonroutine medications should be screened for drug and alcohol interactions. Alcohol intake should be discouraged in patients with poorly controlled hypertension, and used with caution in the diabetic patient to avoid severe hypoglycemia.

Exercise

Physical training appears to be of benefit in transplant recipients in attenuating some of the side effects of immunosuppressive therapy such as protein catabolism and muscle wasting, hyperlipidemia, obesity, hypertension, and osteoporosis. The patient's sense of well-being may also improve markedly.

SELECTED READINGS

Bergstrom J. Nutrition and mortality in hemodialysis. *J Am Soc Nephrol* 6:1329, 1995.

Cabelof DC. Preventing infection from foodborne pathogens in liver transplant recipients. *J Am Diet Assoc* 94:1140, 1994.

De Caterina R, Endres S, Kristenson SD, Schmidt EB. N-3 fatty acids and renal diseases. *Am J Kidney Dis* 24:397, 1994.

Gottschlich MM, Matarese LE, Shronts EP (eds). *Nutrition Support Dietetics Core Curriculum* (2nd ed). Gaithersburg, MD: Aspen, 1993.

Guijarro C, Massy ZA, Kasiske BL. Clinical correlation between renal allograft failure and hyperlipidemia. *Kidney Int* 48:S56, 1995.

Guijarro C, Massy ZA, Weiderker MR et al. Serum albumin and mortality after renal transplantation. *Am J Kidney Dis* 27:117, 1996.

Jaggers HJ, Allman MA, Chan M. Changes in clinical profile and dietary considerations after renal transplantion. *J Renal Nutr* 6:12, 1996.

Johnson CP, Gallagher-Lepak S, Zhu Y et al. Factors influencing weight gain after renal transplantation. *Transplantation* 56:822, 1993.

Julian BA, Quarles LD, Niemann KMW. Musculoskeletal complications after renal transplantation: Pathogenesis and treatment. *Am J Kidney Dis* 19:99, 1992.

Khan M, Lum CT, Rao V. Successful appetite suppression therapy with fenfluramine and phentermine in the obese diabetic patient. *Transplant Proc* 27:975, 1995.

Kiberd BA. The effect of routine magnesium supplementation on blood pressure and blood lipids in cyclosporine-treated renal allograft recipients. *J Renal Nutr* 3:135, 1993.

Luke RG. Pathophysiology and treatment of post-transplant hypertension. *J Am Soc Neph* 2(Suppl 1):37S, 1991.

Markell MS, Armenti V, Danovitch G et al. Hyperlipidemia and glucose intolerance in the post-renal transplant patient. *J Am Soc Neph* 4(Suppl 1):37S, 1994.

Moore LW, Gaber AO. Patterns of early weight change after renal transplantation. *J Renal Nutr* 6:21, 1996.

Owen WF, Lew NL, Liu Y et al. The urea reduction ratio and serum albumin concentration as predictors of mortality in patients undergoing hemodialysis. *N Engl J Med* 329:1001, 1993.

Pirsch JD, Armbrust MJ, Knechtle SJ et al. Obesity as a risk factor following renal transplantation. *Transplantation* 59:631, 1995.

Pruchno CJ, Hunsicker LG. Nutritional Requirements of Renal Transplant Patients. In WE Mitch, S Klahr (eds), *Nutrition and the Kidney*. Boston: Little, Brown, 1993.

Windus DW, Lacson S, Delmez JA. The short-term effects of a low-protein diet in stable renal transplant recipients. *Am J Kidney Dis* 17:693, 1991.

Index

watch
thiazide diuretics / warfarin /
can ↑ levels / digital   PRISCILLA

Handbook of Psychiatric   MERRILL
Drug Therapy   FNP
by Leonard

Hilton (Dover)   Psych + ER meds

Valproate - lithium bipolar (p. 174) blood
control p (22)   dyscrasias

Fourth Edition

If asthma / COPD / elderly
use metoprolol   ⟨| W9-BPK-819

Ø use if ↓BP ²⁰/₆₀ or HR < 55

★ clonidine   α₂ adrenergic agonist ↓
(Catapres) (HTN -
anx / mania / neuroleptic akathisia / OD / drug
Haldol - Tourette)

TCA's - p 91 - 10 mg imipramine q hs

Pref. SSRI - elderly ~ venlafaxine (Effexor)
(p 93)   150 mg id - ↑ severe
melancholic
Lithium - ✓ thyroid
watch levels / intracran

★ Remeron = hs - (mertazapine)

Ritalin to perk ↑ - 5 mg AM boost
very old - ★ .25 bid -   appetite

Remeron ↓ dose
sedating
nice for elderly
hs

Handbook of Psychiatric Drug Therapy

Fourth Edition

George W. Arana, M.D.
Associate Dean for Graduate Medical Education
Vice Chair & Professor, Department of Psychiatry
    and Behavioral Medicine
College of Medicine, MUSC
Director, Mental Health Service
Ralph H. Johnson VA Medical Center
Charleston, South Carolina

Jerrold F. Rosenbaum, M.D.
Professor of Psychiatry
Harvard Medical School;
Associate Chief of Psychiatry
Massachusetts General Hospital
Boston, Massachusetts

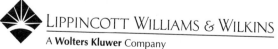 LIPPINCOTT WILLIAMS & WILKINS

A **Wolters Kluwer** Company

Philadelphia · Baltimore · New York · London
Buenos Aires · Hong Kong · Sydney · Tokyo

Acquisitions Editor: Charley Mitchell
Developmental Editor: Michael Standen
Production Editor: Aureliano Vázquez, Jr.
Manufacturing Manager: Kevin Watt
Cover Designer: Mark Lerner

Library of Congress Cataloging-in-Publication Data

Arana, George W.
    Handbook of psychiatric drug therapy / George W. Arana, Jerrold F.
Rosenbaum.— 4th ed.
        p. ; cm.
    Includes bibliographical references and index.
    ISBN 0-7817-1609-8
    1. Mental illness—Chemotherapy--Handbooks, manuals, etc.
    2. Psychopharmacology—Handbooks, manuals, etc.   I. Rosenbaum, J.F.
(Jerrold F.) II. Title.
        [DNLM: 1. Mental Disorders—drug therapy.   2. Psychotropic
Drugs—pharmacology.
WM 402 A662h 2000]
RC483 .A73 2000
616.89′18—dc21   00-025396

Contents

Disease-Specific Table of Contents

This table provides the reader with easy access to major places in the book that discuss the indications for medications in specific disorders or clinical situations. The major chapters in which a disorder is discussed are given in bold. This table does not refer to every citation; that purpose is served by the index.

Preface

This handbook is a practical guide to the use of the various categories of modern psychiatric drugs. It is written in a way that should be useful for psychiatrists but easily accessible to generalists and to other health professionals who are involved in the management of patients with psychiatric disorders. We have avoided the encyclopedic approach and focused on the major classes of drugs used in clinical practice. In the interest of brevity and practicality, we have excluded those agents whose use is primarily of historic interest (e.g., some of the older sedative-hypnotics). We have attempted to delineate what is known on the basis of controlled clinical trials, but in the areas where there is little systematic evidence to guide clinical practice, we have tried not to allow pedantry to interfere with practicality and clinical need.

GWA
JFR

Handbook of Psychiatric Drug Therapy

Fourth Edition

1

Introduction to Psychopharmacology

The practice of psychopharmacology can be extremely challenging. Psychiatric disorders frequently have unpredictable courses, complicating comorbid psychiatric or medical disorders are common, and symptoms of psychiatric disorders may interfere with compliance (e.g., denial of illness in mania, suspiciousness in many psychotic disorders, and a pattern of interpersonal turmoil in certain personality disorders that does not spare caregivers). Additionally, medications are not fully effective in many patients. Although in some illnesses, such as major depression, bipolar disorder, and panic disorder, available therapies help the majority of patients, many patients respond only incompletely, and a substantial minority prove to be treatment refractory. For other disorders, such as schizophrenia, the current treatments are only palliative, leaving the patient with many disabling symptoms. It takes great skill for the practitioner to maintain the right balance between pharmacologic and psychological approaches to therapy. Skilled use of the psychiatric drugs currently available can result in good outcomes for many patients who would otherwise suffer severe morbidity or even death.

Although pharmacologic interventions are the most effective treatments for many psychiatric disorders (e.g., bipolar disorder, panic attacks, and major depression), cognitive and behavior therapy or other psychotherapies also should be initiated if indicated. For many patients, the benefits of medical treatment and psychotherapy are additive or synergistic. For example, some patients who have panic disorder with agoraphobia may recover from their panic attacks with drug therapy but remain disabled by agoraphobia unless they participate in behavior therapy. Major depression responds well to pharmacotherapy, but many patients are optimally treated when medication and psychotherapy are combined to treat all aspects of their problem. On the other hand, there are situations, such as acute mania, in which psychotherapy might be counterproductive, until the acute symptoms abate.

In general, an ideologic preference for either pharmacologic or psychosocial treatment, as opposed to reliance on the best available information derived from controlled studies, has no place in successful psychiatric practice. An ideologic preference for one form of treatment over another—which may be caricatured as "Here is the treatment, now tell me the problem"—serves patients' needs poorly. The standard of care for psychiatric disorders requires a careful diagnostic assessment prior to the introduction of therapy, and the therapy chosen must have documented efficacy for the patient's condition. This standard leaves much room for clinical judgment. The clinician must recognize that available controlled studies are as yet an incomplete guide to actual clinical situations. Subjects eligible for clinical

1

studies are a small subset of patients requiring treatment. They are typically relatively young, on no other medications, lacking serious comorbidity, and willing to be on a placebo for several weeks. Furthermore, clinical research trials that fully establish efficacy often lag behind clinical observation and practice by several years.

A case in point not so many years ago was the International Psychopharmacology Algorithm Project, where clinician researchers met to draft decision trees to provide prescribing practices for psychiatric disorders. From the outset it was clear that solid scientific data were barely available beyond the first node of the algorithm. Few existing studies addressed the approach to initial treatment failures, poor responders, or those discontinuing treatment due to side effects. For panic disorder, for example, the most extensive data available at that time supported the use of imipramine as the initial treatment of choice. The consensus among the assembled experts, however, was that selective serotonin reuptake inhibitors had become their clinical choice, despite the fact that controlled trials had not yet been completed at that time. The panel agreed to construct the algorithm to reflect their actual preferred clinical choices but qualified their choices with descriptions indicating the quality of available supporting evidence: A for replicated controlled studies, B for open trials and pilot studies, and C for clinical observations and anecdotes. This compromise is consistent with the philosophy of this book: to present state-of-the-art clinical psychopharmacology emphasizing clinical practice as informed by clinical science.

In the spirit of practicality, we offer certain principles that have guided our treatment of major psychiatric illnesses and that we believe have general merit in psychiatric drug therapy.

BEFORE INITIATING MEDICATIONS

1. Before prescribing psychotropic medication, it is important to be clear as to the diagnosis. If the diagnosis has not been determined, a clear set of diagnostic hypotheses should be established, and a systematic approach to clarifying the diagnosis should be outlined. For example, depressive, psychotic, or catatonic states may result from medical or psychiatric illness or from drug abuse, or they may represent an adverse reaction to antipsychotic drugs.

2. Before prescribing psychotropic medications, it is important to be aware of medical problems or drug interactions that could (a) be responsible for the patient's psychiatric symptoms, (b) increase the toxicity of prescribed drugs (e.g., diuretics or nonsteroidal antiinflammatory agents may increase lithium levels), or (c) decrease the effectiveness of the planned therapy (e.g., carbamazepine could hasten the metabolism of certain tricyclic antidepressants).

3. Be aware of the possibility of alcohol or drug abuse, which might confound treatment. It is recommended that patients first be detoxified from alcohol or drugs rather than attempting treatment of a presumed psychiatric disorder (e.g., depression) during ongoing substance abuse.

4. Before prescribing a psychiatric medication, it is imperative to identify **target symptoms** (e.g., sleep disturbance, panic attacks, or hallucinations) that can be followed during the course of therapy to monitor the success of treatment. It is also important to monitor changes in the patient's quality of life (e.g., satisfaction with home and family life, functioning at work, and overall sense of well-being). An alternative for patients who cannot report their own symptoms (e.g., demented or psychotic patients) is to ask the patient's family to rate behavior (e.g., a simple daily rating on a scale of 1–10 points). The use of identified target symptoms and quality of life assessment is especially important when the medication is being given as an **empirical trial** in a patient whose diagnosis is unclear.

5. Principles of optimal drug selection are presented throughout this manual. However, if a medication was previously effective and very well tolerated by a patient, it is a reasonable clinical judgment to use that medication again even if newer drugs are now available for the patient's condition.

6. When there is doubt about the correct diagnosis or therapy, consultation should be sought. The clinician's response to the consultant's recommendations (including agreement or disagreement) should be documented.

ADMINISTRATION OF MEDICATIONS

1. Once a drug is chosen, **administer a full trial with adequate doses and duration of treatment** so that if the target symptoms do not improve, there will be no need to return to that agent. **Inadequate dosing and duration are the main reasons for failure of antidepressant trials in well-diagnosed patients.**

2. Be aware of side effects, and warn patients in advance if appropriate (e.g., about sedation early in the course of daytime benzodiazepine use, or dry mouth or blurred vision with tricyclic antidepressants). Develop a clear idea of which toxicities require reassurance (e.g., dry mouth), treatment (e.g., neuroleptic-induced parkinsonism), or drug discontinuation (e.g., lithium-induced interstitial nephritis). Examine patients when appropriate (e.g., for rigidity or oral dyskinesia). Recall that the side effects of some psychotropic agents may mimic symptoms of the disorder being treated (e.g., neuroleptic-induced akathisia may present as agitation; neuroleptic-induced akinesia may be indistinguishable from catatonia due to the illness).

3. When possible, keep regimens simple both to improve compliance and to avoid additive toxicity. Compliance is often enhanced if regimens and dosing schedules are kept simple (e.g., lithium one or twice daily instead of three or four times daily), if patients are engaged in a dialog about the time course of expected improvement, and if complaints about side effects are taken seriously. Patients who are psychotic, demented, or retarded may need careful supervision from family to maintain compliance.

4. Readjust the dosage of medication to determine the lowest effective dose for the particular stage of the patient's illness because, for psychotic disorders in particular, dosage require-

ments often change over time. For example, in schizophrenia, the dosage of antipsychotic medication that is needed to treat acute exacerbations is generally higher than for long-term maintenance.

5. In the elderly, it is prudent to initiate treatment with lower doses of medication. Dosage changes should be less frequent in the elderly than in younger patients because the time required for drugs to achieve steady-state levels is often prolonged.

6. Follow-up care includes evaluating efficacy of treatment; monitoring and managing side effects, treatment-relevant inter-current life events, and comorbid medical and psychiatric conditions; obtaining and evaluating appropriate laboratory data; and, when necessary, planning changes in the treatment regimen. These elements of care require the budgeting of adequate time. We generally budget 15 to 30 minutes for a follow-up visit with a relatively stable patient.

DISCONTINUATION OF MEDICATIONS

1. All too often ineffective medications are continued indefinitely and multiple medications accumulate in the patient's regimen, leading to unnecessary costs and side effects. Adjunctive and combination therapies may be appropriate for certain conditions; however, when medications no longer prove useful to the treatment regimen, it is critical to discontinue them. It may be difficult to determine that a medication has failed unless the physician has kept track of objective target symptoms from the beginning of the trial.

2. Even after apparent therapeutic success, criteria for discontinuation of psychotropic drugs in most clinical situations are ill-defined. When discontinuing psychotropic medications, it is best to taper dosages slowly, which can help prevent rebound or withdrawal symptoms. Because they have different therapeutic implications, it is important to distinguish among temporary symptom **rebound** (as frequently occurs after discontinuing short-acting benzodiazepines), which is brief and transient, but can be severe; **recurrence** of the disorder, in which original symptoms return long-term; and **withdrawal,** in which new symptoms characteristic of withdrawal from the particular drug appear. In general, conditions that have been chronic before treatment, recurrent, or have emerged late in life are more likely to require long-term maintenance treatment.

OTHER ISSUES IN PSYCHOPHARMACOLOGY

1. To optimize clinical management of complicated illnesses, it is important to **document** observations of the patient (including mental status at baseline and changes with treatment), clinical reasoning, and side effects. Particular attention should be given to documenting risk of suicide or violence and risk of serious side effects such as tardive dyskinesia. It is also important for the record to indicate that the patient understands the reason for treatment, its risks and benefits, alternative treatments, and the risks of no treatment. If the competence of the patient to make his or her own decisions fluctuates or is questionable, the clinician should obtain the patient's permission to include the family in important treatment decisions. If the patient is clearly not

competent to make decisions, a formal legal mechanism for substituted judgment must be used.

2. Many of the drugs discussed in this book have not yet been approved by the U.S. Food and Drug Administration for the particular indication discussed (e.g., fluoxetine for panic disorder). However, a physician is free to choose any approved drug for nonapproved indications. The record should reflect the basis for this clinical decision, which ideally should reflect appreciation and understanding of the available evidence.

3. The cost of therapeutic drugs is an important issue in treatment selection. For clinicians, cost effectiveness should be a factor in guiding drug choice. A drug which appears to be more cost effective initially may ultimately prove to be the least cost effective if suboptimal clinical outcome, diminished quality of life, and costs due to side effects offset the initial savings. If compliance and safety are enhanced and risk of relapse diminished, an initially more costly drug may ultimately prove to be the most cost-effective choice. Thus, a narrow focus on drug costs alone is not good practice. On the other hand, where drugs are equally safe and effective, cost is a valid basis for selection.

2

Antipsychotic Drugs

The antipsychotic drugs are the cornerstone of treatment for schizophrenia and other psychotic disorders, such as schizoaffective disorder. Antipsychotic drugs have been in clinical use since the 1950s, when chlorpromazine, a phenothiazine derivative, was synthesized in France. Although developed as a potential antihistamine, chlorpromazine was noted to have antipsychotic properties in clinical use. Chlorpromazine provided a model for the development of a wide variety of chemically distinct compounds effective for the psychoses, but all of these first-generation compounds (with the exception of clozapine) had a liability for causing extrapyramidal symptoms (EPS) by virtue of their major shared property, potent antagonism of the D_2 dopamine receptor. In addition to their antipsychotic properties, these drugs have had other uses based on their ability to block D_2 dopamine receptors (e.g., as antiemetics and in palliation of some movement disorders characterized by excessive movement). The D_2 antagonist antipsychotic drugs were called *typical* to contrast them with clozapine and with newer *atypical* drugs that have a reduced liability for EPS. The EPS burden also led to use of the term *neuroleptic* for these older, typical drugs because these drugs could literally produce a neurologic disorder. In addition, long-term use of these drugs, as typically required in schizophrenia, posed a high risk of a permanent movement disorder, tardive dyskinesia (TD). Even in the short term, in addition to producing parkinsonian symptoms, typical antipsychotic drugs produce side effects (e.g., akathisia or akinesia) that could mimic or exacerbate the symptoms for which the drugs were originally prescribed. In short, these older, typical antipsychotic drugs were effective, and indeed critically important in the treatment of psychotic disorders for more than 40 years, but at the price of serious motor system problems that could limit therapy.

The past 5 years have witnessed a new era in the treatment of psychotic illnesses with the introduction and widespread adoption of a group of compounds with a much reduced liability for producing EPS. Ironically, clozapine, the drug with the lowest EPS liability and the greatest efficacy in schizophrenia, is the oldest of the atypical drugs. However, over the years, it was underused because it carried a risk of agranulocytosis, necessitating cumbersome and expensive weekly monitoring of white blood cell counts. In addition, clozapine has its own troublesome side effects (including sedation, weight gain, and a reduction in seizure threshold). However, the benefits of clozapine have been demonstrated to outweigh its risks for many individuals with schizophrenia who respond poorly to other treatments. More recently, several newer atypical compounds—risperidone, olanzapine, quetiapine, and ziprasidone [likely to be approved soon by the U.S. Food and Drug Administration (FDA)]—have been shown to be effective for schizophrenia and other psychoses, and useful for mania as well. Because these drugs have reduced EPS liability, a generally milder side effect profile than clozapine, and do not pose a risk of agranulocytosis, they have rapidly become the first-line drugs for the treatment of psychotic disorders. As a group, these drugs have been shown in well-controlled trials of over 4 to 20 weeks' duration to be at least as effective as the older typical antipsychotic drugs, although they have not convincingly shown the degree of efficacy of clozapine in the most resistant cases.

A high affinity for D_2 dopamine receptors among the older compounds is clearly associated with their liability for producing EPS. However, the decreased liability for EPS in the newer compounds appears to reflect diverse mechanisms and is still not fully understood. The atypical drug risperidone has high affinity for the D_2 receptor, like haloperidol (Table 2.1), but its high affinity for the serotonin 5-hydroxytryptamine 2A (5-HT$_{2A}$) receptor appears to mitigate its EPS liability when it is given at lower doses (<6 mg/day). In contrast, the atypical drug quetiapine has a lower affinity for the 5-HT$_{2A}$ receptor than does haloperidol, but also has a lower affinity for the D_2 dopamine receptor. Clozapine has a relatively low D_2 receptor affinity and a high affinity for the 5-HT$_{2A}$ receptor, but interacts with so many receptors (Table 2.1) that the basis of its efficacy and atypical side effect profile remains unclear.

CHEMISTRY

Phenothiazines, the first chemical class of antipsychotic drugs developed, are tricyclic molecules. Three subtypes of phenothiazines are available: aliphatics, piperidines, and piperazines. Those phenothiazines with **aliphatic** side chains (e.g., chlorpromazine) tend to be low-potency compounds (i.e., higher doses are needed to achieve therapeutic effectiveness). **Piperidine** substitutions impart anticholinergic properties and a lower incidence of extrapyramidal symptoms (e.g., thioridazine, mesoridazine). **Piperazine** phenothiazines (e.g., perphenazine, trifluoperazine, fluphenazine) are among the most potent antipsychotic molecules.

The **thioxanthene** class of antipsychotic drugs is chemically similar to the phenothiazines. The **butyrophenones** represent a class of extremely potent antipsychotic drugs. Of these, only haloperidol is currently approved for psychiatric use in the United States. Droperidol, a shorter-acting butyrophenone, is approved for use as a preanesthetic agent.

Several other compounds of varied chemical structures have been approved for the treatment of psychotic and other illnesses in the United States. Pimozide, a **diphenylbutylpiperidine** approved for Gilles de la Tourette syndrome, is also a potent antipsychotic drug with a very long half-life (several days). Also, there are compounds closely resembling the tricyclic antidepressants with a seven-member central ring and a piperazine substitution called **dibenzodiazepines;** this class of antipsychotic drug is represented by the typical antipsychotic drug loxapine, as well as by the atypical drug clozapine. Risperidone is a

Table 2.1. Receptor affinities of atypical antipsychotic drugs compared with haloperidol

	D_1	D_2	D_3	D_4	$5\text{-}HT_{2A}$	$5\text{-}HT_{2C}$	α	H_1	ACh
Haloperidol	210	1	2	3	45	>10,000	6	440	5,500
Clozapine	85	160	170	50	16	10	7	1	2
Olanzapine	31	44	50	50	5	11	19	3	2
Quetiapine	460	580	940	1,900	300	5,100	7	11	>1,000
Risperidone	430	2	10	10	0.5	25	1	20	>1,000
Ziprasidone	525	4	7	32	0.4	1	10	50	>1,000

The affinities (dissociation constants) are expressed in nanomolar. The lower the number, the higher the affinity (i.e., the lower concentration to produce half saturation of the receptor).
Reprinted with permission from Tamminga CA. Principles of the pharmacotherapy of schizophrenia. In: Charney DS, Nestler EJ, Bunney BS, eds. *Neurobiology of mental illness*. New York: Oxford University Press, 1999:274.

benzisoxazole derivative that combines high affinity for D_2 dopamine receptors and 5-HT_2 serotonin receptors. Olanzapine is a **thienobenzodiazepine** agent with greater affinity for the serotonin 5-HT_2 receptors than for dopamine receptors and which, compared with other atypicals, is most like clozapine in its receptor affinities. Quetiapine is a **dibenzothiazepine** derivative with low affinity for serotonin receptors but weaker activity at dopamine receptors and multiple other receptors.

PHARMACOLOGY

Potency Versus Efficacy

The distinction between potency and efficacy is helpful to an understanding of the pharmacology of antipsychotic drugs. **Efficacy** refers to the therapeutic benefits that can be achieved by a drug, whereas **potency** describes the amount of the drug needed to achieve the therapeutic effect. All of the typical antipsychotic drugs are equivalent in efficacy, meaning that at an optimal dosage, which differs for each drug (Table 2.2), each of the older, typical drugs has been found to be equally efficacious in treating psychotic disorders. A useful generalization about the older typical antipsychotic drugs is that those with low potency (which must therefore be given in higher doses), tend to be more sedating, more anticholinergic, and cause more postural hypotension than the high-potency drugs. The high-potency drugs tend to cause more extrapyramidal symptoms.

Clozapine is the only drug that unquestionably has greater efficacy than the older typical drugs, although there are hints in clinical trials that other atypical drugs may be somewhat more efficacious than haloperidol in a subset of treatment-refractory patients. A trial conducted in patients with schizophrenia who had been unresponsive to at least two different antipsychotic drugs found significant improvement in 30% of 126 patients treated with clozapine for 6 weeks compared with only 5% of 141 patients treated with chlorpromazine (Kane et al., 1988). Clinical experience and meta-analyses have amply confirmed the results of this well-designed trial; that is, clozapine may effectively treat patients who do not respond to other antipsychotic drugs.

Absorption and Distribution

Traditional antipsychotic drugs are available for both oral and parenteral use, whereas atypical drugs have until recently only been available for oral use, but new parenteral formulations of atypical drugs are becoming available (e.g., risperidone and ziprasidone) (Table 2.3). Among the typical drugs, their pharmacokinetics are well understood only for a few, especially chlorpromazine, thioridazine, and haloperidol, because of the complexity of active and inactive metabolites. Taken orally, the drugs are absorbed adequately, although somewhat variably. Food or antacids may decrease absorption. Liquid preparations are absorbed more rapidly and reliably than tablets. There is a marked first-pass effect through the liver with oral administration (i.e., a high percentage of the drug is metabolized as it passes through the hepatic portal circulation). The peak effect of an oral dose generally occurs within 2 to 4 hours.

Table 2.2. Typical antipsychotic drugs: relative potencies and side effect profiles

Drug	Approximate Dose Equivalent (mg)	Sedative Effect	Hypotensive Effect	Anticholinergic Effect	Extrapyramidal Effect
Phenothiazines					
Aliphatic					
Chlorpromazine (Thorazine)	100	High	High	Medium	Low
Piperidines					
Mesoridazine (Serentil)	50	Medium	Medium	Medium	Medium
Thioridazine (Mellaril)	95	High	High	High	Low
Piperazines					
Fluphenazine (Prolixin, Permitil)	2	Medium	Low	Low	High
Perphenazine (Trilafon)	8	Low	Low	Low	High
Trifluoperazine (Stelazine)	5	Medium	Low	Low	High

Thioxanthene						
Thiothixene (Navane)	5	Low	Medium	Low	Low	High
Dibenzodiazepines						
Loxapine (Loxitane, Daxolin)	10	Medium	Medium	Medium	Medium	High
Benzisoxazole						
Risperidone (Risperdal)	1–2	Low	Low	Medium	Low	Low
Butyrophenones						
Droperidol (Inapsine—injection only)	1	Low	Low	Low	Low	High
Haloperidol (Haldol)	2	Low	Low	Low	Low	High
Indolone						
Molindone (Moban)	10	Medium	Medium	Low	Medium	High
Diphenylbutylpiperidine						
Pimozide (Orap)	1	Low	Low	Low	Low	High

Table 2.3. Available preparations of antipsychotic drugs

Drug	Tablets (mg)	Capsules (mg)	Sustained-release Forms (mg)	Liquid Concentrate[a]	Liquid Suspension[a] or Elixir	Syrup[a] (mg/5 mL)	Injection[b]
Phenothiazines							
Aliphatics							
Chlorpromazine (Thorazine, generics)	10, 25, 50, 100, 200		30, 75, 150, 200, 300	30 mg/mL, 100 mg/mL		10 mg/5 mL	25 mg/mL, 10 mg/mL
Piperidines							
Mesoridazine (Serentil)	10, 25, 50, 100		25 mg/mL				25 mg/mL
Thioridazine (Mellaril, generics)	10, 15, 25, 50, 100, 150, 200			30 mg/mL, 100 mg/mL	25 mg/5 ml, 100 mg/5 mL		
Piperazines							
Fluphenazine HCl (Proloxin, Permitil, generics)	1, 2.5, 5, 10			5 mg/mL	0.5 mg/1 mL, 2.5 mg/5 mL		2.5 mg/mL
Fluphenazine enanthate, decanoate (Prolixin)							25 mg/mL
Perphenazine (Trilafon, generics)	2, 4, 8, 16			16 mg/5 mL			5 mg/mL
Trifluoperazine (Stelazine, generics)	1, 2, 5, 10			10 mg/mL			2 mg/mL

Thioxanthene			
Thiothixene (Navane, generics)	1, 2, 5, 10, 20	5 mg/mL	2 mg/mL, 5 mg/mL
Dibenzodiazepines			
Loxapine (Loxitane, generics)	5, 10, 25, 50	25 mg/mL	50 mg/mL
Clozapine (Clozaril)	25, 100		
Benzisoxazole			
Risperidone (Risperdal)	1, 2, 3, 4		
Butyrophenone			
Haloperidol (Haldol, generics)	0.5, 1, 2, 5, 10, 20	2 mg/mL	5 mg/mL
Thienobenzodiazepine			
Olanzapine (Zyprexa)	2.5, 5, 7.5, 10		
Dibenzothiazepine			
Quetiapine (Seroquel)	25, 100, 200		
Haloperidol decanoate (Haldol)			50 mg/mL, 100 mg/mL
Indolone			
Molindone (Moban)	5, 10, 25, 50, 100	20 mg/mL	
Diphenylbutylpiperidine			
Pimozide (Orap)	2		

[a]Liquid form for oral use.
[b]Parenteral form, which is packaged in either vial or ampule.

Parenterally administered antipsychotics are rapidly and reliably absorbed. Drug effect is usually apparent within 15 to 20 minutes after intramuscular (i.m.) injection, with peak effect occurring within 30 to 60 minutes. With intravenous (i.v.) administration, some drug effect is apparent within minutes, and peak effect occurs within 20 to 30 minutes. (Intravenous administration of antipsychotic drugs has not been approved by the FDA. The haloperidol-like drug droperidol is approved for i.v. use, although it is not marketed as an antipsychotic drug.) Because parenteral administration bypasses the first pass through the portal circulation, it results in a significantly higher serum level of the parent drug than equivalent oral dosages.

Antipsychotic drugs are generally highly protein bound (85%–90%). Clinicians have traditionally been cautioned when concomitantly treating with other medications that are highly protein bound (e.g., warfarin, digoxin) because of the expectation that displacement and competition for these binding sites could increase concentrations of free or unbound antipsychotics and other drugs. Antipsychotics are also highly lipophilic; thus, they readily cross the blood–brain barrier and attain high concentrations in the brain. Indeed, concentrations in the brain appear to be greater than those in blood. Given their high degree of protein and tissue binding, these drugs are not removed efficiently by dialysis.

Metabolism and Elimination

Many antipsychotic drugs are metabolized in the liver to demethylated and hydroxylated forms. These are more water soluble than the parent compounds and thus more readily excreted by the kidneys. The hydroxylated metabolites often are further metabolized by conjugation with glucuronic acid. Many of the hydroxyl and desmethyl metabolites of phenothiazines are active as dopamine receptor antagonists. The hydroxyl metabolite of the butyrophenone antipsychotic drug haloperidol (hydroxyhaloperidol) does not appear to be active. Much remains unknown about the metabolites of other chemical classes of antipsychotics.

The elimination **half-life** of most of the typical antipsychotic drugs is 18 to 40 hours, but numerous factors, such as genetically determined metabolic rates, age, and the coadministration of other hepatically metabolized drugs, affect the half-life to such a degree that plasma levels may vary among individuals by 10- to 20-fold.

Long-Acting Preparations

Long-acting preparations of typical antipsychotic drugs in which the active drug is esterified to a lipid side chain are available. The drug is given as an i.m. injection in an oily vehicle that slows absorption. The only depot preparations currently available in the United States are the decanoate ester of fluphenazine and the decanoate ester of haloperidol. Fluphenazine decanoate has a half-life of 7 to 10 days, allowing administration approximately every 2 weeks. Haloperidol decanoate has a longer half-life, allowing dosing intervals of 3 to 6 weeks, depending on the individual. Long-acting preparations of atypical drugs (e.g., risperidone) are in development.

Blood Levels

Given the marked interindividual differences in plasma levels produced by a given oral dose and the concerns about the consequences of noncompliance among psychotic patients, it would be useful to have some objective measure of drug level to aid in optimizing efficacy and clinical improvement. Specifically, it has been hoped that a range of therapeutic blood levels could be determined for the various antipsychotic drugs. Unfortunately, the measurement of blood levels by various chromatographic techniques and mass spectroscopy has not correlated well with clinical response. This problem reflects, at least partly, the presence of many active metabolites. Some antipsychotic drugs have so many active metabolites (e.g., thioridazine) that measurement to assess dose–response relationships is impractical. Thus, clinical observation and documentation of specific symptom changes over time remain the mainstays of assessment of drug efficacy.

MECHANISM OF ACTION

The therapeutic mechanism of action of the antipsychotic drugs is only partly understood. The typical (e.g., haloperidol-like) antipsychotic drugs and the atypical drugs risperidone and ziprasidone are all potent antagonists of D_2 dopamine receptors. On the other hand, clozapine and quetiapine are weak D_2 antagonists, and by positron emission tomography show significantly lower levels of D_2 receptor occupancy at effective doses, compared with the haloperidol-like drugs. A common property of atypical antipsychotic drugs is the ability to block serotonin 5-HT_{2A} receptors. Olanzapine, risperidone, and ziprasidone do so with high affinity; quetiapine has relatively lower affinity for all its receptor targets (Table 2.1). The atypical drugs interact with a variety of other serotonin receptors, but not with any obvious pattern. All but quetiapine have high affinity for 5-HT_{2C} receptors; all but risperidone have high affinity for 5-HT_6 receptors; risperidone has a particularly high affinity for the 5-HT_7 receptor. All of the atypical antipsychotics interact with α_1-adrenergic receptors and histamine H_1 receptors, which may contribute to side effects. Both clozapine and olanzapine are strongly anticholinergic.

This welter of receptor binding properties makes it difficult to pinpoint the mechanism of action. D_2 receptor antagonism correlates well with both efficacy and with EPS liability for the typical (haloperidol-like) antipsychotic drugs. In addition, blockade of 5-HT_{2A} receptors appears to correlate with diminished EPS liability. Given the high ratio of D_4 antagonism to D_2 antagonism exhibited by clozapine, there was much excitement about a possible role for D_4 antagonists as antipsychotic drugs. However, relatively selective D_4 antagonists, as well as a mixed $D_4/5$-HT_{2A} antagonist (fananserin), have shown no antipsychotic efficacy.

To date it appears that blockade of D_2 receptors in mesolimbic and mesocortical projections are responsible for initiating the therapeutic actions of typical antipsychotic drugs and may contribute to the efficacy of clozapine-like drugs that exhibit lower D_2 affinity. D_2 blockade in the striatum is responsible for the extrapyramidal effects of the typical antipsychotic drugs (Fig. 2.1). In addition to these mid-brain dopamine systems, there is a dopamine projection in the tuberoinfundibular system of the hypothalamus. In this system, dopamine acts as an inhibitor of the synthesis and release of prolactin by pituitary lactotrophs. By antagonizing dopamine in this system, antipsychotic drugs with strong D_2 antagonist properties often produce hyperprolactinemia. The key to the increased efficacy of clozapine remains unknown.

The full therapeutic effects of all antipsychotic drugs take weeks to appear (similar to the antidepressants) and are far slower than the time required to block central nervous system (CNS) receptors or, in most cases, to achieve steady-state plasma levels of the drug. Similarly, behavioral effects in patients can last long after serum levels are no longer detectable. Such observations suggest that the therapeutic response to antipsychotic drugs is a secondary or adaptive response to receptor blockade with a time course characterized by slower onset and offset than would be predicted by serum or even brain levels. (D_2 receptor occupancy in the human brain may now be inferred experimentally from positron emission tomography.) Inasmuch as some initially responsive patients relapse even with apparently adequate serum levels of drugs, other types of adaptations may occur in the brain, reflecting such factors as primary alterations in the disease process, changes in the psychosocial circumstances of the patient's life, intercurrent psychiatric or physical

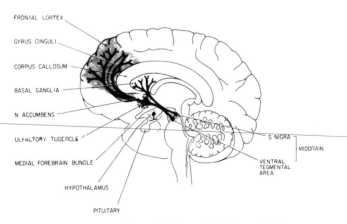

Figure 2.1.   Dopamine projections of the human brain.
Cells in the substantia nigra project to the basal ganglia;
cells in the ventral tegmental area of the mid-brain
project to the frontal cortex and limbic areas.
Hypothalamic dopamine neurons project to the pituitary.

illness, or drug tolerance. The therapeutically relevant delayed-onset neurobiologic effects of antipsychotic drugs remain unknown, but are believed to reflect drug-activated changes in gene expression, protein synthesis, and subsequent synaptic reorganization.

In addition to their effects on dopamine receptors, antipsychotic drugs may cause side effects by binding to a variety of other neurotransmitter receptors. For example, low-potency typical antipsychotic drugs are potent antagonists of muscarinic cholinergic receptors with a highest relative affinity for thioridazine followed by chlorpromazine and mesoridazine. (Mesoridazine is a metabolite of thioridazine as well as a marketed antipsychotic in its own right.) Among the atypicals, clozapine and olanzapine also have substantial anticholinergic potency. As a result, these drugs can produce side effects such as dry mouth and constipation. Postural hypotension is produced by antagonism of α_1-adrenergic receptors. Antipsychotic drugs with substantial affinity for this receptor include all atypical compounds and especially mesoridazine, chlorpromazine, and thioridazine among typical drugs. Sedation appears to result from antagonism of several neurotransmitter receptors, including α_1-adrenergic, muscarinic, and histamine H_1 receptors. Because of substantial affinity for these receptor types, low-potency antipsychotics, such as chlorpromazine and thioridazine, and all the atypical drugs can be sedating (particularly clozapine and quetiapine). Additionally, many antipsychotic drugs block certain calcium channels on neurons, cardiac muscle, and smooth muscle.

INDICATIONS

Overview

Occasionally antipsychotic drugs have been referred to as antischizophrenic drugs, but they are effective in a wide variety of disorders (Table 2.4). Indeed, given their broad spectrum of effectiveness, a patient's response to these agents is not helpful in making a diagnosis (e.g., a history of response is not diagnostic of schizophrenia). In addition to their antipsychotic action, these drugs have nonspecific sedating effects. Because of their extrapyramidal effects and especially the risk of TD, the long-term use of typical antipsychotic drugs is generally limited to treatment of psychoses and refractory bipolar disorders, for which they have proven to be uniquely effective. Although clozapine does not appear to cause EPS or TD, its own troubling side effects, and particularly the risk of agranulocytosis, requiring weekly or biweekly blood drawing, limit its utility.

In addition to their use in psychiatric disorders, the D_2 antagonist drugs are potent antiemetics; for example, prochlorperazine, a phenothiazine not used for psychosis, is marketed for that indication. In addition, the short-acting, extremely potent butyrophenone droperidol is used as a preanesthetic drug but also can be useful in the treatment of acute psychoses. Finally, these drugs, by virtue of their dopamine receptor antagonism, can be used to control severe choreoathetoid movements arising in such conditions as Huntington's disease or hemiballismus.

Table 2.4.   Indications for use of antipsychotic drugs

Short-term use (<3mo)
  Effective
    Exacerbations of schizophrenia
    Acute mania
    Depression with psychotic features (combined with
      antidepressant)
    Other acute psychoses (e.g., schizophreniform psychoses)
    Acute deliria and organic psychoses
    Drug-induced psychoses due to hallucinogens and
      psychostimulants (not phencyclidine)
    Nonpsychiatric uses: nausea and vomiting; movement
      disorders
  Possibly effective
    Brief use for episodes of severe dyscontrol or apparent
      psychosis in some personality disorders
Long-term use (>3 mo)
  Effective
    Schizophrenia
    Tourette syndrome
    Treatment-resistant bipolar disorder
    Huntington's disease and other movement disorders
    Chronic organic psychoses
  Possibly effective
    Paranoid disorders
    Childhood psychoses

Schizophrenia

Schizophrenia is a chronic illness in which psychotic symptoms are prominent (e.g., hallucinations, delusions, ideas of reference, or thought disorder). Although the course may be punctuated by acute exacerbations followed by periods of less florid psychosis, the course of this illness over years involves deterioration to a diminished plateau of function and generally an inability to maintain an active and productive life.

Multiple clinical trials have shown that antipsychotic drugs are effective both for acute exacerbations of schizophrenia and for long-term maintenance. Rigorous studies of clozapine have shown that it may be of particular benefit in chronic schizophrenia refractory to other antipsychotic drugs; case series and anecdotal reports suggest that it also may be effective in refractory atypical psychoses, such as schizoaffective disorder. Trials are now underway to determine whether some of the new atypical drugs have efficacy advantages to match their advantages over older drugs in side effect burden.

Symptoms of schizophrenia are often divided into positive symptoms (i.e., symptoms that are not present in normal human cognitions, perceptions, or affect, such as hallucinations, delusions, and thought disorder) and negative or deficit symptoms (i.e., loss of qualities normally present in healthy individuals, such as impoverishment of thought, deficits of attention, blunted affect, and lack of initiative). It often has been stated that traditional antipsychotic drugs are more effective in treating positive than negative symptoms. However, when examined carefully, this generalization is not entirely accurate in that those negative symptoms that occur during an acute exacerbation of schizophrenia often respond well to antipsychotic drugs. Moreover, many patients continue to have some positive symptoms, such as hallucinations and delusions, despite antipsychotic medication. The expectation that all positive symptoms should respond to antipsychotic therapy has led to the use of excessive doses in some patients. Negative symptoms that characterize the patient's chronic course (i.e., negative symptoms that are present even at times when positive symptoms are minimal) tend to be relatively refractory to typical antipsychotic drug treatment and appear somewhat more responsive to clozapine. The relative efficacy of newer atypical drugs in this domain remains to be fully established.

It is also important to recall that side effects of traditional antipsychotic drugs can mimic both positive and negative features of schizophrenia. Akathisia can be indistinguishable from agitation and anxiety (positive symptoms), and EPS effects of antipsychotics (e.g., bradykinesia, akinesia, and masked facies) can masquerade as negative symptoms of the disorder. Indeed the D_2 dopamine receptor antagonism of typical antipsychotic drugs, by causing even subtle akinesia, may create a therapeutic ceiling effect vis-à-vis negative symptoms in some patients.

Acute Exacerbations of Schizophrenia

When a patient with known or suspected schizophrenia develops an exacerbation of psychotic symptoms, it is important to consider all possible causes. These include worsening course of illness (despite medication), noncompliance with medication, a superimposed medical disorder, a superimposed mood disorder, drug abuse, psychosocial crises, or toxic effects of the antipsychotic drugs (especially akathisia or neuroleptic-induced catatonia). If the exacerbation involves florid psychotic symptoms, the treatment is the same as that for acute psychosis (see later section on Therapeutic Usage).

Identification, if possible, of the cause for the exacerbation is both helpful in treatment of acute relapse and necessary for long-term planning. If noncompliance is the problem, it is often helpful for the physician to explore with the patient the reasons for avoiding medication. If the physician and patient agree that compliance could be improved with injectable drug preparations, the use of long-acting depot preparations may be indicated. If drug abuse or an intercurrent medical or psychiatric illness (such as depression) is to blame, disorder-specific treatment is necessary. Failure to address psychosocial factors in relapse (e.g., family problems or lack of an adequate living situation) will predispose the patient to further difficulties.

Long-Term Treatment of Schizophrenia

Many studies have proven that long-term treatment with antipsychotic drugs increases the time between exacerbations among schizophrenic patients who respond to short-term treatment. The relapse rate for schizophrenic patients who are not on maintenance antipsychotic drugs may be as high as 50% at 6 months and 65% to 80% at 12 months, whereas for those maintained on antipsychotic drugs, the relapse rate may be 10% to 15% at 6 months and no higher than 25% at 12 months. Given the disorder's morbidity, most patients with well diagnosed schizophrenia will have net benefit from long-term treatment. Because long-term treatment with typical antipsychotic drugs brings with it the risk of TD, the clinician should carefully consider the risks and benefits of using the older drugs over time with each patient.

Some patients with refractory symptoms have been treated with high antipsychotic doses (more than the equivalent of 20 mg/day of haloperidol), often more reflective of physician frustration than appropriate therapy. There is no evidence of extra benefit at very high doses of antipsychotic drugs, although side effects are clearly worsened. Currently, for patients who have failed to respond to adequate doses of several antipsychotic drugs, including atypical drugs, a trial of clozapine is indicated. As described previously, clozapine is the only antipsychotic drug that has been found to be effective for substantial numbers of patients with schizophrenia who have proved refractory to other antipsychotic drugs.

Manic Episodes

Although lithium or the anticonvulsant valproic acid may be the first choice for the treatment of mania (see Chapter 4), antipsychotic drugs often play an important role in the acute phase of manic episodes and may be required for prevention of recurrences in some cases.

Acute Mania

Although mild episodes of mania can usually be treated with lithium or valproate alone or in combination, such drugs may not be effective for 10 to 14 days or more. Thus, when mania is accompanied by disruptive or dangerous behavior requiring rapid treatment, antipsychotic drugs may prove useful. Severe manic presentations with marked agitation and florid psychotic symptoms are optimally treated as an acute psychosis (see later section on Therapeutic Usage) with antipsychotic drugs and often the concomitant use of a benzodiazepine such as lorazepam or clonazepam, while also obtaining laboratory tests and initiating lithium or other mood stabilizers. Once the patient is on therapeutic doses of a mood stabilizer such as lithium (serum level 1.0–1.2 mEq/L for acute episodes) or an anticonvulsant, and there is marked symptomatic improvement, the antipsychotic drug can be slowly tapered. Should symptoms reemerge during the tapering phase, the antipsychotic drug can be increased or restarted if necessary. Although the use of typical antipsychotic drugs in acute mania is well established, there is now evidence that atypical drugs such as risperidone or olanzapine are also effective with milder side effects.

Long-Term Treatment of Mania

Lithium and valproate are the first-line agents for the long-term treatment of bipolar disorder. Long-term use of antipsychotic drugs for prophylaxis of bipolar illness has generally not been recommended because patients with mood disorders appear to have heightened susceptibility to TD. Bipolar patients, however, clearly benefit from antipsychotic drugs when break-through symptoms of mania emerge despite prophylaxis with mood stabilizers, and patients with unremitting or rapidly cycling manic symptoms (despite other treatments) have stabilized with antipsychotic medication. Given the lower risk of EPS and the possibility that atypical drugs may cause less TD (unproven in bipolar patients to date), and given the reported efficacy of atypical drugs (e.g., olanzapine) in bipolar illness, the potential role of atypical antipsychotics in the long-term treatment of bipolar illness is being redefined. Indeed, these agents may prove beneficial not only for acute mania and prophylaxis against recurrent mania, but some clinicians have observed benefit for bipolar depressive symptoms as well.

Depression with Psychotic Features

Evidence from controlled studies suggests that depression with psychotic features is more effectively treated with the combination of an antidepressant and an antipsychotic drug (70%–80% response rate) than with either class of drug alone (30%–40% response rate). Electroconvulsive therapy appears to be the most effective treatment and is the treatment of choice if pharmacologic treatment fails or if the severity of symptoms demands extremely rapid treatment. In combined treatment as first studied, a high-potency typical antipsychotic drug was combined with a tricyclic antidepressant. The high-potency antipsychotic drug was used to minimize additive anticholinergic toxicity with tricyclic antidepressants. Combinations of atypical antipsychotic drugs with selective serotonin reuptake inhibitors (SSRIs) or other newer antidepressants are now standard practice, but some clinicians adhere to the older tricyclic antidepressants for the most severely depressed patients. Depression with psychotic features is more fully discussed in Chapter 3.

Schizoaffective Disorder

As defined in the *Diagnostic and Statistical Manual of Mental Disorders,* 4th edition (DSM-IV), schizoaffective disorder probably represents a heterogeneous group of patients rather than a single disease entity. The diagnosis is applied to patients who have periods of major manic or depressive symptoms or both, but who have prominent psychotic symptoms even at times when they are relatively free of affective symptoms. Clinically, affective symptoms often respond to lithium, antidepressants, or an anticonvulsant. Psychotic symptoms, especially those that occur between episodes of mood disorder, generally require treatment with antipsychotic medication. The dosages of antipsychotic medication for both acute florid symptoms and chronic maintenance are the same as for the analogous stages of schizophrenia. All atypical compounds are likely to be effective for schizoaffective disorder, although more study is warranted. Use of lithium and anticonvulsants in this disorder is discussed in Chapter 4.

Schizophreniform Disorder

As defined by the DSM-IV, schizophreniform disorder involves overt psychotic symptoms of less than 6 months' duration, with return to the premorbid level of functioning. The onset of symptoms tends to be rapid, rather than insidious, and patients may demonstrate confusion or perplexity at the height of their syndrome. Many, but not all, such patients lack the flat affect of typical schizophrenia.

Schizophreniform patients represent a heterogeneous group. Depending on the population studied, some investigators find predominantly mood disorders represented, whereas others find a heterogeneity, with perhaps half going on to manifest schizophrenia over time. The early stages of treatment for schizophreniform disorder are the same as for any acute psychosis (see later section on Therapeutic Usage). Given that the long-term prognosis for recovery of many of these patients is good, after the first episode an attempt can be made to taper and discontinue antipsychotic drugs entirely if symptoms fully remit and remain in remission for 6 months to a year. Many patients who meet criteria for schizophreniform disorder will also benefit from lithium or anticonvulsants (see Chapter 4) if symptoms of bipolar disorder emerge.

Delusional (Paranoid) Disorders

Patients with delusional (paranoid) disorder are often difficult to treat. They generally deny that they have a mental disorder, and their pervasive suspiciousness often extends to physicians and medical treatment. As a result, they are likely to be brought to treatment by others and are often noncompliant with treatment. If medication is introduced to the patient as a means of helping cope with anxiety, stress, or other complaints rather than explicitly confronting delusions, the initiation of treatment may be more acceptable. Nonetheless, over time it is best if the patient can be helped to develop insight into the distortions and misperceptions.

Antipsychotic drugs are effective in some patients with delusional disorder, especially in those whose symptoms are of recent onset. As with other psychotic disorders, the agents of choice are the atypical antipsychotics. For patients with chronic, systematized delusions, the response rate may be lower than for those with a more recent onset. Pending systematic studies of this clinical population, dosing guidelines should follow those for treating schizophrenia, while considering the possibility that lower doses may be adequate for some. If typical drugs are tried, low doses should be used initially (e.g., haloperidol 5 mg/day or the equivalent) to minimize side effects and enhance compliance. Consideration should be given to a trial of antidepressants or lithium if affective symptoms are apparent or if there is a family history of mood disorder.

Delirium and Acute Organic Psychoses

Delirium, acute confusional states, and *toxic/metabolic encephalopathy* are among the many terms that have been used to describe a clinical syndrome that consists of acute global depression of cerebral function generally accompanied by abnormalities in arousal. Delirium may result from a wide variety of medical causes, many of which are medical emergencies. The cornerstone of treatment for delirium is supportive care while specific therapy for the underlying disorder is provided. Because delirious patients are unpredictable and may either harm themselves by falling or by pulling out necessary lines and tubes in a hospital setting, or harm others, restraints or constant observation are generally indicated. Pending the results of specific therapy for an underlying disorder or while waiting for an offending drug to be metabolized and excreted, symptomatic use of psychotropics is often necessary, although use should be minimized if possible, especially when the diagnosis is unclear. The choice of agent will be dictated by the cause of the delirium and the patient's medical status.

Delirium due to ethanol, benzodiazepine, or barbiturate withdrawal is best treated with a cross-reactive agent, generally a benzodiazepine (see Chapter 5). Antipsychotic drugs are not effective treatments for ethanol withdrawal. When delirium is caused by anticholinergic drugs, it is also wise to avoid antipsychotics because of the risk of increasing anticholinergic toxicity. For many other causes of delirium, especially in medically fragile patients, an antipsychotic, but particularly the high-potency typical agent haloperidol, has long been the acute agent of choice because it has little effect on the cardiovascular system, little effect on respiratory drive, very low anticholinergic potency, and tablet, liquid, and rapidly acting parenteral formulations are available. Low-potency typical antipsychotic drugs lower the seizure threshold, increase the risk of postural hypotension, and may be strongly anticholinergic; thus, they should be avoided. In older patients, doses of haloperidol as low as 0.5 mg twice a day (b.i.d.) may be effective in symptomatic treatment of delirium. In younger patients, higher doses may be used at least initially (doses of 2–5 mg may be given parenterally every 30–60 min as needed). The major liability of haloperidol in older patients is the emergence of parkinsonian symptoms (although younger men are most at risk for acute dystonias). When elderly patients are given typical antipsychotics, however, they should be monitored frequently for cogwheel rigidity, changes in gait, and the development of masked facies. Late reemergence of agitation while a patient is on haloperidol should raise the suspicion of akathisia. If antipsychotic treatment beyond the acute intervention is required, the atypical agents are the treatments of choice. The availability of short-acting injectable atypical drugs (e.g., ziprasidone) should permit greater flexibility of administration of medication and increased use of atypical agents for this condition.

Dementia

In treating patients with dementing illnesses, antipsychotic drugs have two major roles: treating complicating psychotic symptoms that may occur (e.g., paranoid delusions) and treating severe agitation that cannot be helped by manipulation of the patient's environment. Because of greater vulnerability in the elderly to parkinsonism, low doses of atypical antipsychotic drugs are preferred. If D_2 antagonist typical agents are to be used, low doses of the higher potency agents (e.g., 0.5–5 mg of haloperidol or fluphenazine) are preferred. (The higher potency drugs have a lower risk of causing postural hypotension.)

Psychotic Symptoms with Parkinson's Disease

Patients with idiopathic Parkinson's disease may develop psychotic symptoms, associated with L-dopa therapy or in the context of dementia. Atypical antipsychotics are better tolerated than traditional compounds in this population; low doses are used initially. Quetiapine and clozapine would have the least detrimental effect on the underlying Parkinson's disease (D_2 binding is relatively lower with these drugs); sedation with both compounds and postural hypotension with clozapine must be monitored closely.

Tourette Syndrome

Tourette syndrome is characterized by multiple motor and phonic tics, which develop during childhood and are chronic in duration. The nature and severity of the symptoms vary markedly over time and among individuals. In addition to motor and phonic symptoms, patients may have difficulty with concentration, impulsiveness, obsessions, and compulsions.

When severe, this disorder is disabling and may require long-term drug treatment. Both haloperidol and pimozide have been used historically in the treatment of Tourette syndrome. Because of pimozide's cardiac side effects (increased QTc interval with risk of torsades de pointes ventricular tachycardia), the FDA has limited its dosage approval to 0.3 mg/kg or 20 mg/day, whichever is less. Both haloperidol and pimozide have been shown to be effective for Gilles de la Tourette syndrome at a mean dose of approximately 4 mg haloperidol and 11 mg pimozide. In the crossover portion of the study, haloperidol appeared to be slightly more effective than pimozide, without significantly worse side effects. Based on prior studies, however, it cannot be stated with certainty that haloperidol has advantages over pimozide; thus, the clinician should use the drug that is best tolerated by the patient. Haloperidol is usually begun at 1 mg/day in a single nightly dose, with slow dosage increases (e.g., 1 or 2 mg/wk) until adequate symptom control is attained. Dosages above 10 mg/day of haloperidol are rarely warranted. Because of the risk of cardiac toxicity, patients who are not optimally treated with 20 mg/day of pimozide should be switched to haloperidol. Long-term treatment studies with both of these agents and with newer atypical drugs are needed. For patients who cannot tolerate antipsychotic drugs, clonidine may prove to be a useful alternative (see Chapter 6).

Personality Disorders

Given their lack of proven effectiveness in treating personality disorders and the risk of TD, antipsychotic drugs should be rarely prescribed and only when other treatments (including nonpharmacologic therapies) have failed. The clinician should choose observable target symptoms that may be responsive to antipsychotic drugs. These symptoms should be monitored carefully, and the drug discontinued if there is no clear improvement. The antipsychotic drugs have been used in severe personality disorder (e.g., borderline) patients during periods of psychotic thinking and in treating and preventing episodes of impulsiveness, rage, and assaultiveness. When psychotic symptoms emerge, however, reconsider the diagnosis. Consider also the possibility of a mood disorder, complex partial seizures, drug abuse, or factitious symptoms. There are no established dosing guidelines for antipsychotics in personality disorders, but with the older agents, dosages greater than the equivalent of 10 mg/day of haloperidol did not appear to be warranted. The recommended duration of treatment, in the absence of long-term treatment data, is usually brief. The low risk of EPS with atypical compounds, however, favors their use should a trial of an antipsychotic drug seem appropriate.

THERAPEUTIC USAGE

Choosing an Antipsychotic Drug

For the first time in over 30 years, mental health care providers have available a group of drugs for the treatment of psychotic disorders that do not cause serious, sometimes life-threatening, neurologic or hematologic problems. The novel, atypical antipsychotics have a significantly lower incidence of such EPS symptoms as dystonia, tremor, stiffness and rigidity, akathisia, and altered affect, as well as greatly diminished risk of neuroleptic malignant syndrome (NMS) and TD. Risperidone and olanzapine are the most commonly used antipsychotics as the initial drug for a first episode. Standard of practice now dictate that the atypical compounds be used initially, with typical antipsychotics (i.e., haloperidol) reserved for nonresponders and partial responders.

Although clozapine heralded a new era in pharmacotherapy of psychosis, particularly with neuroleptic-resistant patients and other subpopulations (e.g., patients with Parkinson's disease), the risk of agranulocytosis complicated the use of this agent. The efficacy of clozapine for both positive and negative symptoms in acute and chronic schizophrenia is an additional feature of this compound and demonstrated that the effective treatment of psychoses was not inexorably linked with EPS. This observation prompted the search for similar compounds without the hematologic side effect.

All of the compounds approved as antipsychotic drugs in the United States are efficacious. Clozapine is more effective than the others in the treatment of schizophrenia; levels of efficacy of other atypicals is still a matter of investigation. The typical antipsychotic drugs differ only in their potency (the dosage needed to produce the desired effect) and side effects. Among the typical antipsychotics, drugs that are most potent tend to produce more EPS, and those that are less potent produce more sedation, postural hypotension, and anticholinergic effects

(Table 2.2). For example, 8 mg of haloperidol and 400 mg of chlorpromazine are equivalent with regard to antipsychotic efficacy; however, the patient receiving haloperidol would be more likely to develop extrapyramidal symptoms, and the patient on chlorpromazine would be more likely to feel sedated and to develop postural hypotension. The atypical compounds are much less likely to induce EPS than the typical compounds, but they all can cause sedation and postural hypotension, and, except possibly ziprasidone, can cause weight gain (particularly clozapine and olanzapine). Risperidone, among the atypicals, is especially likely to elevate plasma prolactin. With the exception of clozapine in treatment refractory schizophrenia, because there is no established difference in the therapeutic effectiveness of these drugs, side effect profiles are a central consideration when starting a patient on antipsychotic treatment.

A patient who has responded well to a particular psychotropic drug in the past is likely to do well on the same drug again. On the other hand, even if a patient has no history of severe EPS or other troublesome side effects with a particular typical antipsychotic, the physician should consider initiating therapy with an atypical compound that would have considerably less or no EPS or risk of TD over the long term. In considering the acute advantages offered by more sedating agents (e.g., for the young manic patient with severe insomnia), the clinician could also consider the acute use of a less sedating compound combined with temporary use of a benzodiazepine (e.g., clonazepam) to achieve sedation, so that when the acute episode passes, the sedation can be dissected from the treatment by stopping the hypnotic medication if desired.

For certain groups of patients, toxic effects determine drugs to avoid. Severely suicidal patients should not be given thioridazine, mesoridazine, or pimozide, because these antipsychotics can be cardiotoxic in overdose. Patients with glaucoma, prostatism, or other contraindications to anticholinergic drugs (e.g., patients taking other anticholinergic compounds such as tricyclic antidepressants) should not be given anticholinergic agents as with low-potency typical drugs, especially thioridazine. Clozapine should only be administered to patients who are adequately compliant so that they will comply with weekly blood drawing.

Use of Antipsychotic Drugs

Because antipsychotic drugs can produce striking changes in the thinking, language, and behavior (including motor behavior) of the patients who receive them, a thorough physical and mental status examination should be performed before initiating therapy. In psychotic disorders, the mental status may fluctuate markedly; thus, on occasion a brief initial period of drug-free observation may be helpful for the hospitalized patient when the diagnosis is unclear. A reliable history must always supplement the mental status examination. In all cases, but especially when the diagnosis is unclear, it is important to objectively rate target symptoms that can be monitored throughout treatment with antipsychotic drugs. The physician must have a clear notion of the symptoms that are likely to respond specifically to antipsychotic drugs and the symptoms (e.g., anxiety) that may be better treated by other classes of drugs.

The latency of response of psychotic symptoms such as delusions, hallucinations, and bizarre behavior is usually greater than 5 days, with nonspecific sedation occurring more rapidly. Full benefit in antipsychotic-responsive disorders usually takes at least 2 to 6 weeks. Unfortunately, physicians are often impatient in treating psychoses given the level of patient and family distress and the pressure of disruptive behavior on the inpatient unit. Thus, premature dosage increases occur, and when symptoms finally remit, the time course of improvement is often mistaken for a requirement for high doses of antipsychotic drugs. If dangerous behavior must be rapidly controlled, the physician may choose to increase the antipsychotic drug dosage temporarily to exploit its nonspecific sedative properties or perhaps more wisely choose to use an adjunctive benzodiazepine as needed. In either case, once the acute symptoms subside, extra dosages administered for sedation should be tapered and an optimal antipsychotic drug dosage established.

Switching from Older Antipsychotic Drugs to Atypical Compounds

The debate as to whether to switch stable patients on typical antipsychotics to newer agents is unfortunately not yet informed by data as to which populations will benefit most from changing their medication. (Patients initiating antipsychotic therapy should, in contrast, be started on an atypical compound without question.) In the cost-sensitive environment of managed health care, the significantly higher (sometimes 10-fold) cost of a regimen of atypical drugs versus traditional compounds raises questions about cost effectiveness of switching. Some fundamental points can be made presently regarding the question of switching a patient's regimen.

In the outpatient setting, the clinician should consider a switch if the patient is not doing well on an older typical antipsychotic medication, is able to comply with oral medication (accepts illness and can recognize symptomatic worsening), and there is family support for such a change. A switch should not be executed if compliance dictates use of a depot preparation, until a depot atypical compound is available. In the inpatient setting, a history of nonresponse or partial response on traditional antipsychotics and a clear history of compliance with oral medication are factors that should encourage a switch to an atypical compound. If the patient has a history of excellent response to a traditional drug, may not comply with an oral regimen, requires a depot preparation, or the side effect profile of the atypical drug is more challenging (e.g., an angina patient unable to tolerate hypotensive effects), a switch to atypical medication could be less advantageous. Generally, chronic schizophrenic patients who are doing well, without TD or EPS, and are stable on a traditional medication most probably can remain on their regimen. Patients who are not doing well on a traditional compound, are relatively unstable on traditional treatment, are having difficulty with EPS, and are able to comply with oral medicines should be given a trial course of atypical drugs.

Specific Clinical Situations

In the treatment of any psychotic disorder, certain paradigmatic situations arise, each requiring a distinct approach to the use of antipsychotic drugs. These include (a) acute psychoses in which the symptoms may constitute a medical emergency, (b) long-term treatment aimed at minimizing residual symptoms or prophylaxis of recurrent psychosis, and (c) use of antipsychotics on an as-needed basis.

Acute Psychosis

Acute psychosis is a clinical syndrome that may be caused by a wide variety of disorders (Table 2.5). Typically, patients present with rapid onset (days to weeks) of psychotic symptoms (e.g., hallucinations, delusions, ideas of reference), agitation, insomnia, and often hostility or combativeness. It is important to rule out acute medical illness by obtaining as much history as possible, monitoring vital signs, performing a physical examination, and ordering necessary laboratory work.

During an acute presentation (having excluded a medical disorder), it may still be difficult to make a definitive psychiatric diagnosis. Because a diagnosis cannot be made from mental status alone, and acutely psychotic patients often are poor historians, a definitive diagnosis may be difficult to establish immediately. To make a diagnosis, the following factors need to be considered:

1. Clinical presentation
2. Medical history, including any prescription or other drug use
3. Physical examination and any relevant laboratory tests
4. Past psychiatric history
5. Mental status examination
6. Baseline of premorbid functioning
7. Time course of onset of symptoms and overall duration of illness
8. History of prior treatment response, especially to traditional antipsychotics, antidepressants, lithium, or electroconvulsive therapy
9. Family history of psychiatric or neurologic disorders

When patients are extremely agitated, combative, or hyperactive, it may be necessary to begin treatment before a definitive diagnosis can be made. Fortunately, most acute primary psychotic disorders, and many psychoses secondary to medical and neurologic disorders, respond to antipsychotic drug treatment regardless of the specific disorder. Optimal long-term treatment requires that a correct diagnosis be made. In addition, it is important to identify conditions that might be worsened by some or all of the antipsychotic agents (e.g., low-potency antipsychotic drugs may worsen symptoms of phencyclidine toxicity or anticholinergic delirium; catatonic states may be caused by neuroleptic toxicity in some patients).

Table 2.5. Causes of acute psychotic syndromes

Major psychiatric disorders
  Acute exacerbation of schizophrenia
  Atypical psychoses (e.g., schizophreniform)
  Depression with psychotic features
  Mania

Drug abuse and withdrawal
  Alcohol withdrawal
  Amphetamines and cocaine
  Phencyclidine (PCP) and hallucinogens
  Sedative-hypnotic withdrawal

Prescription drugs
  Anticholinergic agents
  Digitalis toxicity
  Glucocorticoids and adrenocorticotropic hormone (ACTH)
  Isoniazid
  L-dopa and other dopamine agonists
  Nonsteroidal antiinflammatory agents
  Withdrawal from MAOIs

Other toxic agents
  Carbon disulfide
  Heavy metals

Neurologic causes
  AIDS encephalopathy
  Brain tumor
  Complex partial seizures
  Early Alzheimer's or Pick's disease
  Huntington's disease
  Hypoxic encephalopathy
  Infectious viral encephalitis
  Lupus cerebritis
  Neurosyphilis
  Stroke
  Wilson's disease

Metabolic causes
  Acute intermittent porphyria
  Cushing's syndrome
  Early hepatic encephalopathy
  Hypo- and hypercalcemia
  Hypoglycemia
  Hypo- and hyperthyroidism
  Paraneoplastic syndromes

Nutritional causes
  Niacin deficiency (pellagra)
  Thiamine deficiency (Wernicke-Korsakoff syndrome)
  Vitamin B_{12} deficiency

Because acutely psychotic patients are potentially dangerous to themselves and others, even if not immediately agitated or threatening, rapid treatment is an important goal. For the clinician, the question is: Which antipsychotic and what dose should be used?

The cornerstone of treatment for a wide variety of psychoses are the atypical antipsychotics, including risperidone, olanzapine, and quetiapine. An additional drug, ziprasidone, is likely to be approved by the FDA. Any one of the atypical antipsychotics are recommended as first-line treatment for new-onset psychosis, whether schizophrenia or as concomitant symptomatology of another illness (i.e., bipolar disorder, acute psychotic disorder). Their efficacy in well-controlled trials over 4 to 20 weeks is well established; the latency to full antipsychotic effect in the 75% of patients who respond remains approximately 2 to 4 week. If there is insufficient control of agitated behavior, it is recommended that additional dosing with a benzodiazepine (e.g., lorazepam, usually as needed 1–2 mg/4–6 h) be used over the course of the first week. The addition of a high-potency conventional antipsychotic should be reserved for patients not controlled with these two medications. They are often used as adjunctive treatment with the atypical drugs for patients who are particularly agitated or have a history of responding to a specific antipsychotic. Acute, sometimes life-threatening syndromes such as NMS or acute dystonic reactions, are far less likely with the newer compounds. Unfortunately, we do not have systematic data for the long-term use of these drugs, but evidence to date suggests a very low likelihood of TD. Following the acute phase of either a first episode of psychotic illness or exacerbation of a chronic disorder, the goal is eventual monotherapy with a single atypical drug.

Studies of acute mania suggest that the vast majority of patients improve on doses equivalent to less than 10 mg/day of haloperidol or 6 mg/day of risperidone. Because the occurrence and severity of EPS with the typical agents are dose-related, it is reasonable not to exceed the equivalent of 8 to 10 mg/day of haloperidol in the short-term treatment of acute mania. (Therapy with lithium or an anticonvulsant would likely be instituted concomitantly.)

Optimal dosing of the older agents in schizophrenia and schizoaffective disorder has been addressed in several studies. In one study (Van Putten et al., 1990), patients were treated with fixed doses of haloperidol (5, 10, or 20 mg/day) for 4 weeks. The 20-mg dose was superior to the 5-mg dose throughout the trial and was marginally superior to the 10-mg dose after the first 2 weeks of treatment. By the second week, however, the group given 20 mg/day experienced symptomatic worsening with respect to blunted affect, motor retardation, and emotional withdrawal. In addition, a significantly higher percentage of patients on the 20-mg dose left the hospital against medical advice than those on lower doses, suggesting that at high doses, toxicity of typical antipsychotics outweigh benefits. If a high-potency traditional antipsychotic drug is used, an anticholinergic drug often should be added as prophylaxis against dystonia; benztropine mesylate, 2 mg b.i.d., may be used. Evidence from various studies has demonstrated that such a regimen decreases the incidence of acute dystonia, which is a problem particularly in individuals younger than 40. If anticholinergic side effects become a problem, the dosage can be decreased to benztropine, 1 mg b.i.d.

Treatment studies with all atypical drugs have shown that their efficacy for acute psychosis is at least equivalent to that of traditional compounds, with 6 mg/day of risperidone, 20 mg/day of olanzapine, or 300 mg/day of quetiapine being reasonable doses to target.

It should be recognized that a substantial number of patients with schizophrenia will not benefit from first-line antipsychotic drugs. For these patients, very high doses are more likely to produce more side effects than therapeutic benefit. Schizophrenic patients who have been unresponsive to two or more adequate trials (8–12 weeks on therapeutic doses) of antipsychotic drugs should be considered for a trial of clozapine. Approaches to refractory mania are discussed in Chapter 4.

At the recommended doses of antipsychotic drugs, many patients will remain agitated in the short term. Therefore, in acute psychoses, in addition to effective doses of an antipsychotic drug, short-term use of benzodiazepines may be required. Lorazepam, which has a relatively short half-life, has no active metabolites, and is well absorbed intramuscularly, is a good choice. Other clinicians prefer the longer acting benzodiazepine clonazepam, which has the disadvantage of lacking a parenteral form. Lorazepam, 1 to 2 mg orally or i.m., or clonazepam, 0.5 to 1.0 mg orally, could be given every 2 hours as needed to calm an agitated patient. Benzodiazepines appear to be relatively free of dangerous side effects if used carefully in the short term, but avoided with clozapine. The physician should monitor the course of psychotic symptoms over the first 2 weeks of treatment, being alert to the fact that as the acute psychosis improves, the requirement of adjunctive benzodiazepine is likely to decrease. It is recommended that the sedative drug be tapered as agitation subsides.

Long-Term Use

Because most patients for whom antipsychotic drugs are effective have chronic or relapsing illnesses, long-term use of these drugs is usually indicated. When possible, the clinician should strive to use atypical antipsychotics for the long-term treatment of psychosis. Because with typical antipsychotic drugs the danger of producing TD is significant, the clinician should continually monitor their duration of treatment and consider alternative treatments whenever possible.

Although maintenance treatments are clearly efficacious, it is difficult to anticipate and recommend optimal maintenance dosages for individual patients based on the literature because of the variability of the studies. For example, one comprehensive review of typical antipsychotics (Baldessarini and Davis, 1980) found no correlation between dosage and effectiveness for long-term therapy. Throughout the course of long-term treatment, it is best to be flexible in adjusting the dosage with increases in the face of symptom worsening or episode prodromes, and seeking the lowest fully effective dosage over time.

LONG-ACTING PREPARATIONS. When patients with schizophrenia or other chronic psychoses relapse because of noncompliance, consideration should be given to the use of long-acting antipsychotic preparations. Of course, in some patients, noncompliance may respond to psychosocial measures, obviating the need for depot antipsychotic drugs.

The depot preparations available in the United States at the time of this writing are fluphenazine decanoate and haloperidol decanoate. Controlled studies of fluphenazine decanoate have covered a 100-fold range in dosage (1.25–125 mg every 2 weeks). High doses (25 mg every 2 weeks) appear to be associated with an inferior outcome. Although these studies may have been skewed by assignment of sicker patients to higher dosages, the general impression is that the dosages used in current clinical practice are often too high.

There are no ideal conversion ratios from oral dosages to depot preparations of fluphenazine. One reasonable estimate is that 0.5 mL of fluphenazine decanoate given every 2 weeks is equivalent to 10.0 mg/day of fluphenazine hydrochloride. For haloperidol decanoate, the ratio of decanoate to oral dose is about 10 to 15:1, so that 150 mg of the decanoate given every 4 weeks is equivalent to 10 mg/day of oral haloperidol. Because these conversions are only approximate, individual dosage adjustments will have to be made.

Because these are long-acting preparations, patients should be exposed to the oral form of the drug prior to their first injection to minimize the possibility of a long-lasting idiosyncratic reaction. It is safest to start long-acting agents at low dosages and then carefully adjust them to maximize the safety of therapy and minimize side effects. Because fluphenazine and haloperidol are high-potency typical antipsychotic drugs, extrapyramidal side effects are to be expected. Pending the availability of long acting atypical drugs, safe and effective use of these compounds can be achieved using the following recommendations:

1. Ensure that the patient has had a test of the drug orally to make certain that it is tolerated.
2. Start injections at low doses, for example, 5.0 to 12.5 mg (0.2–0.5 mL) of fluphenazine decanoate or 50 to 100 mg (1–2 mL) of haloperidol decanoate. Give fluphenazine decanoate every 2 weeks and haloperidol decanoate every 4 weeks.
3. With the initial low doses, oral supplementation may be necessary temporarily. Do not increase doses of the depot preparation too rapidly because steady state is only reached after four to five dosing intervals.
4. Average effective dosages are in the range of 12.5 mg (0.5 mL) every 2 weeks for fluphenazine and 150 mg (3 mL) every 4 weeks for haloperidol decanoate.
5. Observe patients for akinesia, depression-like symptoms, or increasing withdrawal. Because these symptoms may be drug induced, it may be necessary to lower the dosage. Parkinsonism and akathisia are also common and require treatment.
6. Recall that worsening of psychotic symptoms with dosage reduction may not become evident for several weeks;

hence, the clinician must monitor patients for an extended period of time before assuming that the reduction has been successful.

As-Needed Use

Antipsychotic drugs are often prescribed in the hospital on an as-needed basis for the acute treatment of psychotic symptoms or agitation. Although not an uncommon practice, the use of antipsychotics on an as-needed basis likely reflects absence of a clear diagnosis or treatment strategy. The time course of improvement for psychotic disorders in response to antipsychotic drugs is such that intermittent dosing is unlikely to help and may confuse the physician as to the amount of antipsychotic drug the patient is receiving daily. Patients receiving only intermittent antipsychotic drug doses for psychotic symptoms are more likely to do poorly; this would be much like using an antidepressant on an as-needed basis.

Frequent examinations by a physician are preferable to longstanding as-needed orders for antipsychotic drugs that may mask or exacerbate side effects or undiagnosed medical illness. For example, patients with akathisia on typical antipsychotics have been given extra (as-needed) doses of an antipsychotic drug because their symptoms were misinterpreted as agitation. If more medication is needed to provide sedation for an acutely disturbed patient, benzodiazepines (e.g., lorazepam) may be preferred to antipsychotic drugs because they are reliable and limit the side effects with higher doses of antipsychotics (e.g., >6 mg/day of risperidone) (see Chapter 5). It should be recalled that even hallucinations may worsen with anxiety, fear, and agitation and are likely to respond to adequate anxiolysis without additional antipsychotic drugs.

Clozapine

In well-designed clinical trials, albeit most of them short-term, and in clinical experience, clozapine has proved to be more effective in reducing symptoms of schizophrenia and in preventing relapses than traditional antipsychotic drugs. There is evidence that clozapine also may have advantages in schizoaffective disorders and in some treatment-refractory bipolar patients as well. Clozapine is also effective at lower doses in the treatment of L-dopa–induced psychotic symptoms in patients with Parkinson's disease, a patient group that cannot tolerate typical D_2 antagonist antipsychotic drugs. Clozapine has the significant advantage of being almost free of EPS and of not causing TD. Thus, it has not only produced improvement in previously refractory patients but has also been used effectively in some patients with severe EPS, including akathisia, who could not tolerate typical antipsychotic drugs. It has also been reported that clozapine may improve existing TD, but further data are needed to support this contention.

Unfortunately, clozapine has a rather severe side effect burden in its own right, which limits its general utility. Clozapine was first tested in the 1960s but was withdrawn from general use because of its association with high rates of agranulocytosis. It was initially introduced in the United States in 1990, bundled by its manufacturer with a mandatory program of weekly blood counts. Although the programs available for blood count determinations have since been broadened, weekly determination of granulocyte counts remains absolutely necessary with clozapine for the first 6 months of therapy, after which biweekly measures suffice. The rate of agranulocytosis with clozapine has been approximately 1%, although it has been greater in some trials. Despite appropriate monitoring, there have been fatalities due to agranulocytosis in the United States. More than 95% of cases of agranulocytosis occur within the first 6 months of treatment, with the period of highest risk between weeks 4 and 18. The risk also appears to increase with age and may be higher in women. The mechanism of agranulocytosis is not known.

As previously described, clozapine has a relatively low affinity for D_2 dopamine receptors compared with typical antipsychotic drugs and a higher ratio of affinity for D_4 versus D_2 dopamine receptors than older antipsychotic drugs. However, the role of D_4 dopamine receptors in treatment, if any, remains unclear. Its relatively low affinity for D_2 dopamine receptors and high affinity for $5\text{-}HT_{2A}$ serotonin receptors likely explains much of its low liability for causing EPS. It also interacts with D_1 and D_3 dopamine receptors, serotonin $5\text{-}HT_6$ and $5\text{-}HT_7$ receptors, α_1-adrenergic receptors, histamine H_1 receptors, and muscarinic cholinergic receptors. The mechanism of its unique efficacy remains unknown.

To minimize side effects, clozapine is begun with a single 12.5- or 25-mg daily dose, increased to 25 mg b.i.d., and then increased by no more than 25 mg/day to a dosage of 300 to 450 mg/day over a period of 2 to 3 weeks. Dosage should subsequently be increased no more rapidly than weekly in increments no greater than 100 mg. Careful monitoring for significant tachycardia and postural hypotension is important in the first month of treatment. Should these occur, the dosage may be temporarily decreased and then increased again more slowly. Most clozapine-responsive patients are effectively treated at dosages between 300 and 600 mg/day in divided doses. Some patients have been treated with dosages as high as 900 mg/day in divided doses, but at doses of 600 mg and above, the risk of seizures increases significantly (from 1%–2% to 3%–5%). The optimal duration of a trial to identify clozapine-responsive patients remains unknown. Patients should be treated for at least 12 weeks, and some clinicians would recommend considerably longer (e.g., 6-month) trials of clozapine before declaring the treatment ineffective.

In addition to agranulocytosis, seizures, and postural hypotension, other problematic side effects include sedation (which may be marked), siallorhea, tachycardia (which may be persistent), constipation, transient hyperthermia, and weight gain which can be substantial (20%–30% increase over baseline weight). Eosinophilia without serious consequences has also rarely been reported.

Some patients being discontinued from clozapine to start another antipsychotic drug, such as risperidone, have experienced marked agitation and even rebound psychotic symptoms.

The mechanism is unknown but likely represents a withdrawal syndrome. Slow tapering of clozapine rather than abrupt termination is recommended, even when switching to another antipsychotic drug.

Plasma concentrations of clozapine may be increased by drugs that inhibit P450 hepatic enzymes, such as cimetidine and SSRIs.

Risperidone

Risperidone combines high affinity for D_2 dopamine receptors with high affinity for $5-HT_{2A}$ receptors. The high D_2 affinity is similar to haloperidol (rather than clozapine), whereas the high $5-HT_{2A}$ affinity is similar to clozapine. Risperidone also has high affinity for α_1- and α_2-adrenergic receptors, but low affinity for muscarinic cholinergic receptors, making it devoid of anticholinergic effects. Based on the studies to date and early clinical experience, risperidone is as effective as haloperidol, and in some specific cases may be more effective. It is certainly better tolerated when used at the lower end of its dose range. It may still cause EPS, however, and regularly does so at higher doses. It also appears to lack the degree of enhanced efficacy exhibited by clozapine. Overall, given its efficacy and tolerability, it is justifiably a widely used first-line drug.

Since its introduction, the average doses of risperidone have decreased and the rate of titration has slowed. Patients may be started on 1 mg/day or b.i.d. (0.5 mg b.i.d. for the elderly or for those with impaired hepatic function). Although the dosage can be increased to 2 mg b.i.d. on day 2 and then 3 mg b.i.d. on day 3 if tolerated by the patient, recent practice has been to increase more slowly to the 4 to 6 mg/day range. The average dosage in use in the United States for schizophrenia is now just over 4 mg/day. Dosage increases should be slower in the elderly and in those who experience postural hypotension with initial dosing. Elderly schizophrenic patients benefit from doses ranging from 0.5 to 2 mg a day. Optimal antipsychotic effects for most schizophrenic patients are seen at 6 mg/day or less in divided doses. If response is poor, upward adjustments may be made, but dosages above 8 mg/day do not appear to offer added benefit, whereas EPS becomes more prominent. The incidence of EPS appears to be dose-related; at dosages of 10 mg/day or greater, the incidence of EPS is similar to that of haloperidol.

In addition to postural hypotension (and reflex tachycardia), risperidone may produce sedation, insomnia, and difficulty concentrating. Dizziness, galactorrhea, sexual dysfunction, and weight gain also have been reported. Like other D_2 receptor antagonists, risperidone may eventually reveal the potential to cause TD, and cases of NMS have been reported with this drug, although these risks at this point are decidedly less than those for the older agents. The combination of D_2 antagonism and high $5-HT_{2A}$ affinity likely explains risperidone's propensity to cause prolactin elevation, which accounts for the occasional report of galactorrhea and menstrual irregularities in women. The long-term implications of elevated prolactin levels, if any, particularly in the absence of side effects or menstrual irregularities is unclear.

Olanzapine

Olanzapine (2-methyl-4-(4-methyl-1-piperazinyl)-10H-thieno [2,3-b][1,5] benzodiazepine) is a thienobenzodiazepine compound related to clozapine. Like clozapine it has a complex pharmacology, interacting with D_1 and D_2 family dopamine receptors, multiple serotonin receptors (5-HT$_{2A}$, 5-HT$_{2C}$, and 5-HT$_6$), histamine H_1 receptors, and muscarinic cholinergic receptors (Table 2.2). In clinical trials olanzapine is at least as effective as haloperidol and far better tolerated. Some data indicate that it may be more effective than haloperidol for negative symptoms of schizophrenia, but this has been difficult to establish with certainty.

Olanzapine treatment of schizophrenia is typically begun with a single dose of 10 mg, although some patients who are particularly sensitive to sedation do best starting at 5 mg. The recommended maximum dose is 20 mg daily, but higher doses have been well tolerated. The average prescribed dosage is 10 to 20 mg/day. The drug reaches peak plasma levels in 5 to 8 hours and has a half-life of about 35 hours; drug–drug interactions are unlikely to influence olanzapine levels. Abnormalities of the QTc interval on electrocardiography (ECG) are unlikely to occur, so there is no need for a baseline ECG. With a typically benign side effect profile, the most common side effects are mild to moderate sedation, dizziness, and weight gain, but the latter, in a subgroup of patients, can be substantial. About 40% of patients in clinical trials gain weight, with reported anecdotes of significant weight gain associated with new onset of diabetes. EPS has not been observed at higher rates than placebo in dosages of up to 20 mg/day.

Quetiapine

Quetiapine (Seroquel) is a dibenzothiazepine compound with relatively low affinity for 5-HT$_{1A}$ and 5-HT$_{2A}$ receptors, moderate to high affinity for α_1, α_2, and H_1 receptors and weaker activity at D_1, D_2, D_3, D_4, and D_5 dopamine receptors. Some initial concerns among clinicians about the efficacy of quetiapine appear to have reflected inadequate dosing. Although the drug is more effective than placebo in the dosage range of 150 to 800 mg/day, 300 mg/day appears to be the initial target dosage for schizophrenia and 300 to 600 mg/day the expected range of dosing. It has a relatively mild side effect profile, especially with respect to EPS (no worse than placebo), with initial sedation being the main reason the drug should be started at low doses and titrated upward. Weight gain and orthostatic hypotension can occur, as can other effects such as insomnia, headache, and dry mouth. It does not elevate prolactin. Because it has a short half-life, b.i.d. or three times a day (t.i.d.) dosing has been recommended. For example, treatment may be initiated with 25 mg morning and night, and dosing increased as sedation diminishes. In actual practice, higher doses are typically given at bedtime. Weight gain has not been a major problem. The emergence of cataracts in toxicology studies of dogs has unclear, if any, implications for human use; although the current U.S. label advises baseline and subsequent slit-lamp examinations, there is no evidence that cataracts occur in relation to the drug in humans.

Ziprasidone

Ziprasidone is a 3-benzisothiazolyl-piperazine derivative with high 5-HT$_{2A}$ and moderate D$_2$ antagonism with antagonism at 5-HT$_{1D}$ and 5-HT$_{2C}$ receptors and antagonism at 5-HT$_{1A}$ and 5-HT$_{1C}$ receptors. Like other atypicals, it is a moderately potent α_1 and H$_1$ histamine receptor blocker. Its initial release was delayed by the FDA due to concerns about prolongation of the QTc interval. Following the accumulation of additional data bearing on this issue, the drug is expected to be approved for use in the year 2000. Thus, there is limited clinical experience with the agent at the time of this writing, but available clinical trial data indicate that it is efficacious, although not shown to be superior to other atypical drugs. Because it is expected to have a favorable profile with respect to weight gain and to exert minimal effects on prolactin, ziprasidone is expected to be a useful addition to the antipsychotic pharmacopoeia. Sedation may be the most common side effect but emerged in fewer than 20% of subjects in clinical trials. It is known to have a short half-life of 4 to 5 hours, and blood levels are increased with food; thus, dosing is expected to be b.i.d. with meals and although eventual dosing recommendations are not yet known, the range of efficacy is expected to be between 40 and 80 mg/day. Higher dosages have been studied. EPS was rare at the 40 mg dose but was reported in 9% of subjects on 80 mg/day with akathisia noted in 15%. A short-acting injectable preparation is expected for emergency use.

USE OF ANTIPSYCHOTIC DRUGS IN PREGNANCY AND NURSING

Antipsychotic medications, capable as they are of crossing the blood–brain barrier, are also generally able to cross the maternal placental barrier and to be present in the fetus and amniotic fluid. The effects of chlorpromazine have been the most carefully studied in pregnancy, although other agents also have been investigated with regard to teratogenicity. No clear patterns of teratogenicity have emerged. Given the relative paucity of safety data, it is best if possible to avoid antipsychotic agents in pregnancy, especially in the first trimester. Nonetheless, there are many situations in which failure to treat the mother creates a graver risk to the fetus than any established risk of antipsychotic drugs. Careful clinical judgment is required. Some recent reports and reviews suggest that pregnant women treated with traditional antipsychotics, clozapine, and atypical drugs have fared well, as have the newborn; in the face of a lack of systematic data, reasonable efforts should be made to avoid antipsychotic exposure during pregnancy, most particularly in the first trimester.

There are well-documented problems with the use of antipsychotics in late pregnancy. Chlorpromazine has been associated with an increased risk of neonatal jaundice. In addition, there are reports that mothers treated with antipsychotic drugs have given birth to infants with EPS. The washout time for these drugs in the fetus is at least 7 to 10 days. Therefore, to avoid EPS in the newborn, it has been recommended that the antipsychotic be discontinued 2 weeks before the due date. If the discontinuance predisposes the expectant mother to severe psychotic symptoms, the clinician must carefully weigh the risks of the psychotic disorder against the potential for neuroleptic toxicity in the child.

Antipsychotics are secreted in breast milk, although likely at very low levels. A nursing infant of a mother treated with antipsychotics is therefore at some risk for the development of EPS. Because the effect of antipsychotic drugs on development is unknown, mothers who must take antipsychotic agents should strongly consider alternatives to breast-feeding.

USE IN THE ELDERLY

The elderly have a slower hepatic metabolism of antipsychotic drugs (pharmacokinetic effects) and an increased sensitivity of the brain to dopamine antagonism and anticholinergic effects (pharmacodynamic effects). Thus, lower dosages should be used, and longer waiting periods should be respected before increasing doses. When typical antipsychotics are being used, recall that high-potency antipsychotic drugs are less likely than low-potency drugs to cause anticholinergic symptoms such as constipation, urinary retention, tachycardia, sedation, and confusion or to cause postural hypotension. Unfortunately, in the elderly, high-potency antipsychotic drugs have a higher likelihood of causing drug-induced parkinsonism and a higher risk of causing TD; with clozapine, there may be a higher risk of drug-induced agranulocytosis in elderly populations. Low dosages should therefore be the rule; dosages in the range of 0.5 to 2.0 mg/day of haloperidol are often adequate in the elderly. The atypical agents are of course the treatment of first choice for those not currently in treatment and doing well on older agents or who have not failed on atypical drugs.

SIDE EFFECTS AND TOXICITY

Neurologic Side Effects

Acute Dystonia

CLINICAL PRESENTATION. Acute dystonia is most likely to occur within the first week of treatment with typical antipsychotics. Despite the expected rarity of the event with the newer agents, the continued acute use of parenteral, high-potency typical neuroleptics in emergency settings indicates that clinicians need to be familiar with the recognition and treatment of acute dystonia. There is a higher incidence in patients under 40, in males, and in patients on high-potency typical antipsychotic drugs (haloperidol, fluphenazine). Patients may develop acute muscular rigidity and cramping, usually in the musculature of the neck, tongue, face, and back. Occasionally, patients report the subacute onset (3–6 hours) of tongue "thickness" or difficulty in swallowing. Opisthotonos and oculogyric crises also may occur. Acute dystonia can be very uncomfortable and frightening to patients, and occasionally it has serious sequelae; muscular cramps can be severe enough to cause joint dislocation, and, most dangerously, laryngeal dystonia can occur with compromise of the airway.

TREATMENT. Anticholinergic drugs (Table 2.6), such as benztropine, 2 mg i.m. or i.v., or diphenhydramine, 50 mg i.m. or i.v., usually bring rapid relief. Benztropine may be preferred because it lacks the antihistaminic effects of diphenhydramine. If there is no effect in 20 minutes, a repeat injection is indicated. If the dystonia is still unresponsive after two injections, a benzodiazepine, such as lorazepam 1 mg i.m. or i.v., may be tried. In cases of laryngeal dystonia with airway compromise, repeat dosing should occur at shorter intervals unless the dystonia resolves. The patient should receive 4 mg of benztropine i.v. within 10 minutes and then 1 to 2 mg of lorazepam i.v. slowly if needed.

With reversal of dystonia, if the antipsychotic medication is to be continued, standing doses of an anticholinergic drug (e.g., benztropine, 2 mg b.i.d.) should be prescribed for 2 weeks (Table 2.6). There is evidence that the prophylactic use of benztropine, 2 mg b.i.d., begun at the same time as the antipsychotic drug, significantly reduces the incidence of dystonia. Dystonias are much less likely with low-potency typical agents than with high-potency drugs.

Antipsychotic Drug-Induced Parkinsonism

CLINICAL PRESENTATION. Symptoms include bradykinesia, rigidity, cogwheeling, tremor, masked facies, stooped posture, festinating gait, and drooling. When these side effects are severe, akinesia, which can be indistinguishable from catatonia, may develop. Onset is usually after several weeks of therapy and is more common in the elderly and with high-potency drugs. These symptoms rarely limit therapy with the atypical drugs except for risperidone at doses of 8 mg and higher, and are rare to nonexistent with olanzapine or quetiapine. They are virtually absent with clozapine.

Switching treatment for a stable, psychotic patient from a typical agent to an atypical compound is certainly reasonable when that patient suffers drug-induced parkinsonism. If the clinician does choose to switch to an atypical antipsychotic, response must

Table 2.6. Commonly used antiparkinsonian drugs

Drug	Usual Dosage Range
Anticholinergic drugs	
Benztropine (Cogentin)	1–2 mg b.i.d.
Biperiden (Akineton)	1–3 mg b.i.d.
Trihexyphenidyl (Artane, Tremin)	1–3 mg t.i.d.
Anticholinergic antihistamine	
Diphenhydramine (Benadryl)	25 mg b.i.d. to q.i.d.
	50 mg b.i.d.
Dopamine-releasing agent	
Amantadine (Symmetrel)	100 mg b.i.d. to t.i.d.

be closely examined to assure comparable efficacy, in addition to reduced parkinsonian side effects.

TREATMENT. If the antipsychotic is to be unchanged, a fixed dose of an antiparkinson drug should be prescribed, and the antipsychotic drug dosage should be decreased to the lowest that is effective for the patient. In elderly patients, lower doses of antiparkinson drugs should be used (e.g., benztropine, 1 mg b.i.d.). A switch to a low-potency antipsychotic (especially thioridazine) may help in some cases, but a switch to an atypical is preferable. Because there is some evidence that long-term use of anticholinergics may increase the risk of TD, periodic attempts should be made to wean these drugs during maintenance therapy, assuming there remains a clinical rationale for use of the typical compound.

Akathisia

CLINICAL PRESENTATION. Akathisia is experienced subjectively as an intensely unpleasant sensation of restlessness and the need to move, especially the legs. Patients often appear restless, with symptoms of anxiety, agitation, or both. It can be difficult to distinguish akathisia from anxiety related to the psychotic disorder. Increased restlessness following the institution of typical antipsychotics should always raise the question of akathisia. Recent evidence suggests that akathisia may be more prevalent in patients treated with these drugs than previously thought. Akathisia is a leading cause of noncompliance and treatment refusal. The inescapable distress associated with akathisia may amplify the hopelessness of the patient and may be a factor in suicidal ideation. As with parkinsonism, akathisia is unlikely with risperidone at low doses, rare with olanzapine and quetiapine, and virtually absent with clozapine.

TREATMENT. Typical antipsychotic drugs should always be prescribed at the minimum effective dose. Low-potency typical antipsychotics, especially thioridazine, have a significantly lower incidence of akathisia than high-potency agents. A variety of compounds have been reported effective for the treatment of akathisia including β-adrenergic blockers as first-line remedies, anticholinergic drugs, and benzodiazepines. There have also been reports on the use of clonidine for akathisia, but the evidence in its favor is scant, and clonidine has the additional problem of causing hypotension.

In the treatment of akathisia, various situations, calling for differing approaches, can arise. We recommend the following:

A. When the patient is treated with a high-potency typical antipsychotic drug and does not have other EPS
    1. First choice: a β-adrenergic blocker, such as propranolol, 10 to 30 mg t.i.d. (nadolol also can be used) (see Chapter 6)
    2. Second choice: an anticholinergic, such as benztropine, 2 mg b.i.d.
    3. Third choice: a benzodiazepine, such as lorazepam, 1 mg t.i.d., or clonazepam, 0.5 mg b.i.d.

B. When the patient is treated with a low-potency typical antipsychotic drug (e.g., thioridazine) or an antipsychotic and a cyclic antidepressant and does not have other EPS
1. First choice: propranolol, 10 to 30 mg t.i.d.
2. Second choice: lorazepam, 1 mg t.i.d., or clonazepam, 0.5 mg b.i.d.
3. Third choice: benztropine, 1 mg b.i.d. (additive anticholinergic toxicity)

C. When the patient is treated with an antipsychotic and manifests other EPS (dystonias or parkinsonism)
1. First choice: benztropine, 2 mg b.i.d.
2. Second choice: benztropine with propranolol, 10 to 30 mg t.i.d.
3. Third choice: benztropine with lorazepam, 1 mg t.i.d., or clonazepam, 0.5 mg b.i.d.

D. When other EPS are present and akathisia is unresponsive to an anticholinergic alone
1. First choice: benztropine, 2 mg b.i.d., with propranolol, 10 to 30 mg t.i.d.
2. Second choice: benztropine, 2 mg b.i.d., with lorazepam, 1 mg t.i.d., or clonazepam, 0.5 mg b.i.d.

E. When EPS or akathisia are present, the clinician should review again the possibility of switching to an atypical antipsychotic, recognizing that when interchanging agents, comparable efficacy on a different drug is not certain.

Neuroleptic Malignant Syndrome

CLINICAL PRESENTATION. NMS is an extremely serious idiosyncratic reaction to neuroleptic drugs. The major symptoms of NMS are rigidity, fever, autonomic instability, and delirium. Symptoms usually develop over a period of several hours to several days, with rigidity typically preceding fever and autonomic instability. Fever may be high, with temperatures of 41°C or higher commonly reported. Lead pipe rigidity is typical, with increased muscle tone leading to myonecrosis in some cases. When patients are also dehydrated, the resulting myoglobinuria may be severe enough to cause renal failure. Autonomic symptoms include instability of blood pressure, often including both hyper- and hypotension, tachycardia, diaphoresis, and pallor. Cardiac arrhythmias may occur. In addition to rigidity, motor abnormalities including akinesia, tremor (which may fluctuate in severity), and involuntary movements have been reported. The patients are usually confused and often mute. There may be fluctuations in level of consciousness from agitation to stupor. Seizures or coma also may occur.

Neuroleptic malignant syndrome is a clinical diagnosis with a relatively wide continuum of severity. Because there are no clear criteria for making a diagnosis, especially in milder cases, it is difficult to state mortality rates. Although there are no specific laboratory findings, creatinine phosphokinase (CPK) is usually elevated. For unknown reasons, liver function test results also may be abnormal, including elevations of transaminases and lactic dehydrogenase. The white blood cell count also may be slightly elevated.

Risk factors for development of NMS include dehydration, poor nutrition, external heat load, and possible intercurrent medical illness. Although all typical neuroleptics have been associated with NMS, there is evidence to suggest that high doses of high-potency neuroleptics increase the risk. Although NMS is extremely rare with atypical drugs, a number of cases have been reported with risperidone, likely reflecting its potent dopamine-blocking activity and excessive doses that characterized its early use.

In severely psychotic patients, the following question often arises: Can the patient receive typical antipsychotics again after having had NMS? In fact, it appears that not all patients who have had NMS suffer a recurrence, even with the same drug that had previously caused the syndrome. Nonetheless, case reports accumulating in the literature suggest that a substantial percentage of patients who have developed NMS once have a recurrence. Given the serious morbidity and possible lethality of this syndrome, it is prudent to withhold typical antipsychotics from patients who have had NMS unless there are compelling indications to resume this treatment and no alternative can be found. We suggest that all patients with a high likelihood for a recurrence should receive a trial of an atypical compound. If for whatever reason this is not possible, the other alternative is to use the lowest possible doses of low-potency drugs, such as thioridazine. Ideally, treatment will not be resumed for at least 4 weeks after full resolution of NMS symptoms. The risks and benefits of such a decision should be fully discussed with the patient and, if appropriate, with his or her family.

TREATMENT. Meticulous supportive care is critical, including adequate hydration, use of cooling blankets for high fever, turning of patients to avoid decubitus ulcers, cardiac monitoring, and monitoring of urine output and renal function. Should renal failure occur, dialysis may be necessary, but dialysis cannot be expected to remove antipsychotics because they are highly bound to plasma proteins and peripheral tissues. Dantrolene, a direct-acting muscle relaxant, may decrease rigidity, secondary hyperthermia, and tachycardia. Response usually occurs quite rapidly. Dosages for this indication are not well established, but dosages in the range of 0.8 to 10.0 mg/kg/day have been advocated. In general, dosages of 1 to 3 mg/kg/day orally or i.v., divided into a four times a day regimen, seem to be effective. Dosages above 10 mg/kg/day have been associated with hepatotoxicity. The dopamine agonist bromocriptine is thought to act centrally to decrease some of the symptoms of NMS. There are conflicting opinions on whether bromocriptine speeds recovery. Full response is said to require several days of treatment. Treatment with bromocriptine usually begins at 2.5 mg orally t.i.d. and is increased as tolerated to 5 to 10 mg orally t.i.d.. Dantrolene and bromocriptine can be administered together. The duration of therapy with either drug is not well established, but it is prudent to continue the drugs for a week after symptoms of NMS have passed. In cases of rigidity and life-threatening hyperthermia, general anesthesia and paralysis may be life saving.

Tardive Dyskinesia

Tardive dyskinesia is a syndrome of long-standing or permanent abnormal involuntary movements that is most commonly caused by the long-term use of typical antipsychotic (neuroleptic) drugs. At least 20% of patients who are treated with neuroleptic drugs long-term develop TD. TD presents clinically as involuntary movements of the tongue, facial, and neck muscles, upper and lower extremities, truncal musculature, or occasionally muscle groups that subserve breathing and swallowing. Buccolingual–masticatory movements are usually seen early in the course of the disorder and are characterized by tongue thrusting (often visible to the observer as the tongue pushing against the cheeks or lips), tongue protrusions, lip smacking, puckering of the lips, chewing movements, and cheek puffing. Excessive unnecessary facial movements, including grimacing, blinking, and rapid ticlike movements of the face or periorbital musculature, also can be seen in the early phases of TD. Although the movements may occasionally be difficult to distinguish from stereotyped posturing that may occur spontaneously in chronically psychotic individuals, TD generally appears less voluntary and usually has a more choreoathetoid quality.

Tardive dyskinesia rarely develops in patients who have had less than 3 to 6 months of antipsychotic drug exposure. The only firmly established risk factor for TD besides typical antipsychotic drug exposure is being over age 50, although there is some evidence that women may be at greater risk than men. There is inconsistent evidence that patients with mood disorders may be at greater risk for developing TD and that intermittent dosing (particularly among patients with mood disorders) may increase the risk of TD. None of the typical antipsychotic drugs is known to be more or less likely to cause TD than another. There is no clear correlation between development of parkinsonism while on antipsychotic drugs and the risk for TD. There is some suggestion that chronic use of anticholinergic compounds may increase the risk of TD; thus, their use should be minimized if possible.

With the advent of the atypical antipsychotics, the clinician is compelled to consider a variety of factors in deciding the course of treatment for patients *on typical antipsychotics* at risk for TD. The choice may vary with the clinical situation, ranging from the patient doing very well on typical antipsychotics with no TD, to well-controlled psychotic patients with minimal TD, to well-controlled patients with moderate to severe TD, to poorly controlled patients with minimal TD, to poorly controlled patients with severe TD. Except for the well-controlled patient with no symptoms of TD, any evidence that TD is present compels the clinician to justify withholding a trial of atypical antipsychotics. Initial treatment of all patients, especially high-risk patients such as the elderly or those with a history of TD, should be with atypical antipsychotics. We believe that a very cogent argument could be made to switch from a typical to an atypical antipsychotic for a well-controlled psychotic patient *without TD*; certainly, with patients at risk for harm to self or others, clinical judgment must always be exercised before a change of regimen is contemplated.

Tardive dyskinesia often emerges while the patient is still on medication. However, antipsychotic drugs can mask the symptoms of TD, and the abnormal involuntary movements may only become apparent on discontinuation or lowering of the drug dosage. When TD-like movements occur after a decrease in drug dosage or discontinuation and then regress over several days or weeks, they are defined as withdrawal dyskinesia. If relatively permanent, they are defined as TD. Although there is no solid evidence to suggest that withdrawal dyskinesia portends TD if antipsychotics are resumed, it would be judicious to discontinue treatment with typical antipsychotic drugs if clinically possible. Treatment with an atypical antipsychotic should be considered in this situation.

There is some disagreement in the literature on the long-term prognosis for TD among patients with TD who continue to receive typical antipsychotic drugs. Some investigators find progression of TD, but other investigations have found that, once established, TD symptoms may plateau or, in some cases, improve. Pending additional research, the clinician must make a judgment for patients with serious psychotic disorders responsive to typical drugs who are unable to take clozapine or other atypical drugs. It currently appears that if the psychotic disorder has been serious, it may cause less morbidity to continue treatment, even with a typical antipsychotic drug, than to make TD the sole focus of the treatment. Clearly this clinical judgment requires a full discussion with the patient and family.

Tardive dystonia, a syndrome of late-onset refractory dystonias, has been reported uncommonly in schizophrenic patients treated chronically with typical antipsychotic drugs. There may be considerable overlap with TD. The natural history and risk factors are not well understood.

PREVENTION. There is no reliable treatment for TD. Thus, the optimal approach is to prevent it by limiting use of typical antipsychotics to situations in which they are truly indicated. In particular, patients with mood, anxiety, or personality disorders should not be treated with typical antipsychotic drugs for protracted periods of time unless there is some compelling clinical evidence to show that the benefits outweigh the potential risks of developing TD. It is also judicious to avoid long-term use of typical antipsychotics whenever possible in the treatment of mental retardation, organic brain syndromes, or in the elderly, because these patients may be at particular risk for TD.

The clinician should examine all patients prior to initiating antipsychotic drug treatment. Optimally, a standardized scale for abnormal movements should be used, such as the Abnormal Involuntary Movement Scale (AIMS), published by the National Institute of Mental Health. These examinations should be repeated no less than every 6 months while the patient is on antipsychotic drugs. If treatment with an antipsychotic is required for 1 year, the clinician should attempt to taper or discontinue the drug and perform the evaluation at a lowered dosage of antipsychotic or while the patient is off the drug. If evidence of TD is noted, the clinician should discuss the implications with the patient and family, so that an informed decision can be made with regard to continuing the antipsychotic drug or switching to an atypical antipsychotic.

DIFFERENTIAL DIAGNOSIS. A variety of primary neurologic disorders are similar to TD (Table 2.7).

TREATMENT. Although many treatments, including lithium, lecithin, physostigmine, and benzodiazepines have been tried, there is no consistently successful treatment for TD. Initial reports suggested that prophylaxis with the antioxidant vitamin E might prevent development or worsening of TD, but subsequent studies have been less encouraging.

Cardiac Toxicity

Pimozide and the low-potency antipsychotic drugs thioridazine and mesoridazine may slow cardiac conduction. Thus, they are mildly antiarrhythmic but can cause problems including heart block and prolongation of the QTc with risk of torsades de pointes ventricular tachycardia. Although the toxicity of these drugs is most likely to be evident in overdose, it may occur in therapeutic doses as well. Patients with known cardiac disease should therefore be treated with high-potency typical or newer atypical agents. One promising atypical agent, sertindole, was ultimately not marketed due to concerns about the potential for QT prolongation, risperidone has been associated with QT prolongation in some cases, and some initial uncertainties about the risk of prolonged QT with ziprasidone has delayed this agent's availability pending additional data. Available data did not appear to reveal significant ECG abnormalities. In patients with known elevated QTc, follow-up ECGs should be considered when these agents are used.

Clozapine is known to cause tachycardia independent of postural hypotension, which can be severe at times and may limit its use.

Table 2.7. Differential diagnosis of tardive dyskinesia

Neurologic disorders
  Wilson's disease
  Huntington's disease
  Brain neoplasms
  Fahr's syndrome
  Idiopathic dystonias (including blepharospasm, mandibular dystonia, facial tics)
  Meige's syndrome (spontaneous oral dyskinesias)
  Torsion dystonia (familial disorder without psychiatric symptoms)
  Postanoxic or postencephalitic extrapyramidal symptoms
Drugs and other toxicities
  Antidepressants
  Lithium
  Anticholinergics
  Phenytoin
  L-dopa and dopamine agonists
  Amphetamines and related stimulants
  Magnesium and other heavy metals

The ECG in patients on the older drugs, particularly the low-potency agents, may show an increase in the QT and PR intervals, ST segment depression, and increased heart rate, which may be of little clinical consequence, except in patients who have underlying cardiac disease or preexisting heart block. QT prolongation should prompt the physician to change to a high-potency neuroleptic (e.g., haloperidol) or an atypical drug.

Postural Hypotension

Postural hypotension most commonly develops with the use of the lower potency typical antipsychotic drugs, especially chlorpromazine, thioridazine, and clozapine. However, the high-potency atypical drug risperidone also produces postural hypotension, as can other atypical agents. This side effect is due to α-adrenergic receptor blockade by these compounds, and may be associated with reflex tachycardia. Postural hypotension may be severe enough to cause syncope. Hypotension almost always improves when the patient is supine; patients should be warned to get up from recumbency slowly.

Weight Gain

Both typical and atypical antipsychotic drugs may cause weight gain. The only antipsychotic drug that is convincingly free of this side effect is molindone. Of the atypical antipsychotic drugs, the greatest degree of weight gain has been associated with clozapine and the closely related compound olanzapine. Quetiapine and risperidone also have been associated with weight gain. Ziprasidone is expected to induce minimal weight gain. Given the long-term nature of antipsychotic drug use, this is more than a cosmetic issue. First, it may affect compliance. In addition, it puts patients at risk of obesity with associated risk of heart disease, hypertension, and diabetes. Cases of treatment-emergent diabetes have been observed with olanzapine. Because the clinician cannot readily predict in advance which patient on clozapine, olanzapine, or other agents will be among the subgroup (a minority, but up to 40% on olanzapine in some studies) to develop significant weight gain, patients should be informed of the risk, and exercise and diet counseling should be offered to minimize the likelihood of being surprised or overwhelmed by dramatic weight change. If weight gain occurs, a change to an agent less associated with increased weight can be instituted.

Ocular Side Effects

Blurred Vision

Because the low-potency agents such as chlorpromazine, thioridazine, mesoridazine, and clozapine are relatively anticholinergic, they may cause cycloplegia (the inability to accommodate). Patients may complain of blurred vision, usually with the greatest difficulty in reading. The medium-potency drugs (e.g., perphenazine) occasionally caused this effect as well. In addition, blurred vision can be caused by anticholinergic compounds given to treat EPS. Often, reading glasses can address the problem.

Glaucoma

Any anticholinergic drug may precipitate an attack of narrow-angle glaucoma; therefore, a history of glaucoma should prompt the use of a high-potency antipsychotic agent, avoidance of antiparkinson drugs, and an ophthalmologic follow-up. Narrow-angle glaucoma is a medical emergency. Patients with open-angle glaucoma can be managed on neuroleptics if their glaucoma is concomitantly treated by an ophthalmologist.

Ocular Pigmentation

This side effect can be divided into two categories. Pigmentation of the lens, cornea, conjunctiva, and retina (often associated with skin pigmentation) is one category. This occurs mostly with the use of low-potency antipsychotics and is unlikely to interfere with vision except in extremely severe cases. The second category is pigmentary retinopathy, which is associated with the use of thioridazine above dosages of 800 mg/day and which leads to irreversible degenerative changes with visual impairment. Thioridazine should never be used at dosages above 800 mg/day for this reason. Patients on thioridazine with visual complaints should be examined by an ophthalmologist.

Cutaneous Side Effects

As with any class of drugs in medicine, the antipsychotics can cause allergic rashes, usually within the first 2 months of treatment. These are most commonly maculopapular erythematous rashes that affect the upper trunk, face, neck, and extremities. Although rashes are usually mild, exfoliative dermatitis has been reported. Discontinuation of the drug is followed by a remission of these symptoms. The physician should choose a compound from another chemical class if antipsychotic treatment is to be resumed.

Low-potency typical antipsychotics can act as photosensitizers, leading to severe sunburn. In addition, there are rare reports of blue-gray discoloration of the patient's skin, usually associated with ocular pigmentary changes. Although cosmetically undesirable, this effect has not been shown to predispose patients to further cutaneous pathology.

Hypothalamic and Pituitary Side Effects

The major endocrinologic effect of risperidone, shared with the typical antipsychotic compounds, is hyperprolactinemia; the normal tonic dopaminergic inhibition of prolactin is blocked by these antipsychotics but not by clozapine and other atypical agents. In women this can result in galactorrhea (also seen rarely in men), amenorrhea, or both. In men, hyperprolactinemia may cause impotence. Because of its low affinity for D_2 dopamine receptors, clozapine has little or no effect on prolactin levels.

Although the effects are poorly understood, antipsychotics are known to predispose certain patients to **hyperthermia** or to marked **weight gain,** presumably by a hypothalamic mechanism. Severe neuroleptic-induced obesity may lead to drug refusal. There are several reports that molindone causes less obesity than the other typical antipsychotics, and some expectation that ziprasidone will have a favorable profile for weight gain when it becomes available.

Hepatic Side Effects

Antipsychotics, especially chlorpromazine, have been associated with cholestatic jaundice, probably secondary to a hypersensitivity reaction in certain predisposed individuals. This presents typically within the first 2 months of treatment and includes nausea, malaise, fever, pruritus, abdominal pain, and jaundice. Elevations of alkaline phosphatase and bilirubin accompanied by minor elevations of the transaminase are seen. Hepatitis should prompt discontinuation of the drug. The syndrome usually remits within 2 to 4 weeks after discontinuation. If further antipsychotic therapy is indicated, a different chemical class should be chosen.

Hematologic Side Effects

Agranulocytosis is a potentially life-threatening hematologic side effect seen most commonly with clozapine and very rarely with aliphatic and piperidine phenothiazine antipsychotics. The incidence with clozapine may be 1% to 3%. As emphasized previously, it is **imperative** to monitor white blood cell counts **weekly** for the entire treatment period with clozapine and for several weeks after discontinuation. A decrease of 50% or a white blood cell count of below 3,000 should lead to immediate discontinuation. Because the incidence of leukopenia in clozapine-treated patients has been lower than originally anticipated, the required weekly monitoring may be changed to biweekly after 6 months of treatment. Patients on other antipsychotics should be counseled to report signs of infection (e.g., sore throats) rather than to monitor blood counts. Symptomatic agranulocytosis requires immediate discontinuation of the medication. When agranulocytosis is associated with an antipsychotic drug in a particular patient, that drug should never be resumed.

OVERDOSAGE

Although the antipsychotic drugs have many toxicities that interfere with their therapeutic use, they have little potential for causing death if taken in overdose. Generally, the most serious complications of overdose are coma and hypotension, both of which should respond to volume expansion. Rarely, lethal cardiac arrhythmias may occur, probably most commonly with pimozide, thioridazine, and mesoridazine. These drugs may prolong the QT interval and precipitate heart block or torsades de pointes ventricular tachycardia.

The more common manifestations of overdose may differ between high- and low-potency antipsychotics. Low-potency drugs such as chlorpromazine and thioridazine generally produce CNS depression. Coma may result after 3 to 4 g of chlorpromazine. Low-potency drugs also may lower the seizure threshold markedly when taken in overdose, and thioridazine also has potent anticholinergic effects. In addition, these drugs have potent anti–α-adrenergic effects and may cause significant hypotension. Like all neuroleptics, these drugs may produce hypothermia or hyperthermia. Cardiac manifestations occur infrequently but may include QT prolongation and ventricular tachyarrhythmias, especially with thioridazine.

Higher potency antipsychotic drugs can produce either CNS depression or CNS excitation with agitation, delirium, and severe extrapyramidal effects, such as muscular rigidity, tremor, or catatonic symptoms. Thermoregulation also may be impaired. Cardiac arrhythmias are rare but have been reported.

With serious overdoses, the basis of treatment is meticulous supportive care. CNS excitation can be treated with low doses of lorazepam. Hypotension that does not respond to volume expansion will respond to vasopressors such as norepinephrine or phenylephrine. β-adrenergic agonists should be avoided because they may worsen vasodilatation. Hypothermia should be treated with slow warming. Hyperthermia should be treated with antipyretics and, if necessary, cooling blankets. Severe extrapyramidal effects should be treated with diphenhydramine, 50 mg i.m. or i.v., or benztropine, 2 mg i.m. or i.v. Because cardiac arrhythmias may occur, cardiac monitoring is necessary.

Ventricular tachyarrhythmias may be treated with lidocaine. Direct current (DC) cardioversion is the treatment for life-threatening tachyarrhythmias. Torsades de pointes ventricular tachycardia, which may occur with pimozide, thioridazine, or mesoridazine, is best managed with isoproterenol or overdrive pacing.

If an ingestion was recent, induction of emesis (which may be difficult because of the antiemetic properties of the drug) or evacuation of the gastric contents through a nasogastric tube is indicated. After emesis is complete, administration of activated charcoal with a cathartic is helpful in adsorbing any remaining drug. Forced diuresis or dialysis is not helpful in removing antipsychotic drugs.

BIBLIOGRAPHY

Mechanism of Action

Hyman SE, Nestler EJ. *Molecular foundations of psychiatry*. Washington, DC: American Psychiatric Press, 1993.

Kapur S, Zipursky RB, Remington G. Clinical and theoretical implications of 5-HT$_2$ and D$_2$ receptor occupancy of clozapine, risperidone, and olanzapine in schizophrenia. *Am J Psychiatry* 1999;156: 286.

Nyberg S, Eriksson B, Oxenstierna G, et al. Suggested minimal effective dose of risperidone based on PET-measured D$_2$ and 5-HT$_{2A}$ receptor occupany in schizophrenic patients. *Am J Psychiatry* 1999;156:869.

Tamminga CA. Principles of the pharmacotherapy of schizophrenia. In: Charney DS, Nestler EJ, Bunnery BS, eds. *Neurobiology of mental illness*. New York: Oxford University Press, 1999.

Schizophrenia and Other Schizoaffective Disorder

American Psychiatric Association. Practice guidelines for the treatment of patients with schizophrenia. *Am J Psychiatry* 1997;154 (4 suppl):1.

Breier A, Buchanan RW, Kirkpatrick B, et al. Effects of clozapine on positive and negative symptoms in outpatients with schizophrenia. *Am J Psychiatry* 1994;151:20.

Carlsson A, Waters N, Carlsson ML. Neurotransmitter interactions in schizophrenia-therapeutic implications. *Biol Psychiatry* 1999; 46:1388.

Kane J, Honigfeld G, Singer J, et al. Clozapine for the treatment-refractory schizophrenic: a double-blind comparison with chlorpromazine. *Arch Gen Psychiatry* 1988;45:789.

Kane JM. Pharmacologic treatment of schizophrenia. *Biol Psychiatry* 1999;46:1396.

Marder SR, Meibach RC. Risperidone in the treatment of schizophrenia. *Am J Psychiatry* 1994;151:825.

Robinson DG, Woerner MG, Alvir JMJ, et al. Predictors of treatment response from a first episode of schizophrenia or schizoaffective disorder. *Am J Psychiatry* 1999;156:544.

Small JG, Hirsch SR, Arvanitis LA, et al. Quetiapine in patients with schizophrenia: a high- and low-dose double-blind comparison with placebo. *Arch Gen Psychiatry* 1997;54:549.

Tollefson GD, Beasley CM, Tran PV, et al. Olanzapine versus haloperidol in the treatment of schizophrenia and schizoaffective and schizophreniform disorders: results of an international collaborative trial. *Am J Psychiatry* 1997;154:457.

Viguera AC, Baldessarini RJ, Hegarty JM, et al. Clinical risk following abrupt and gradual withdrawal of maintenance neuroleptic treatment. *Arch Gen Psychiatry* 1997;54:49.

Mood Disorders

Tohen M, Sanger TM, McElroy SL, et al. Olanzepine versus placebo in the treatment of acute mania. *Am J Psychiatry* 1999;156:702.

Zarate CA, Tohen M, Baldessarini RJ. Clozapine in severe mood disorders. *J Clin Psychiatry* 1995;56:411.

Other Psychiatric and Neurologic Disorders

Goldberg SC, Schulz C, Schulz PM, et al. Borderline and schizotypal personality disorders treated with low-dose thiothixene vs. placebo. *Arch Gen Psychiatry* 1986;43:680.

Pfeiffer RF, Kang J, Graber B, et al. Clozapine for psychosis in Parkinson's disease. *Mov Disord* 1990;5:239.

Shapiro E, Shapiro AK, Fulop G, et al. Controlled study of haloperidol, pimozide, and placebo for the treatment of Gilles de la Tourette syndrome. *Arch Gen Psychiatry* 1989;46:722.

Atypical Antipsychotic Drugs

Alvir JMJ, Lieberman JA, Safferman AZ, et al. Clozapine-induced agranulocytosis: incidence and risk factors in the United States. *N Engl J Med* 1993;329:162.

Brier AF, Malhotra AK, Su T-P, et al. Clozapine and risperidone in chronic schizophrenia: effects on symptoms, parkinsonian side effects, and neuroendocrine response. *Am J Psychiatry* 1999;156: 294.

Kane J, Honigfeld G, Singer J, et al. The Clozaril Collaborative Study Group: clozapine for the treatment-resistant schizophrenic. A double-blind comparison vs. chlorpromazine/benztropine. *Arch Gen Psychiatry* 1988;45:769.

Sanger TM, Lieberman JA, Tohen M, et al. Olanzapine versus haloperidol treatment in first-episode psychosis. *Am J Psychiatry* 1999;156:79.

Small JG, Hirsch SR, Arvantis LA, et al. Quetiapine in patients with schizophrenia. *Arch Gen Psychiatry* 1997;54:549.

Wahlbeck K, Cheine M, Essali A, et al. Evidence of clozapine's effectiveness in schizophrenia: a systematic review and meta-analysis of randomized trials. *Am J Psychiatry* 1999;156:990.

Wirshing DA, Marshall BD, Green MF, et al. Risperidone in treatment-refractory schizophrenia. *Am J Psychiatry* 1999;156:1374.

Depot Antipsychotic Drugs

Carpenter WT Jr, Buchanan RW, Kirkpatrick B, et al. Comparative effectiveness of fluphenazine decanoate injections every 2 weeks versus every 6 weeks. *Am J Psychiatry* 1999;156:412.

Side Effects and Toxicity

Allison DB, Mentore JL, Heo M, et al. Antipsychotic-induced weight gain: a comprehensive research synthesis. *Am J Psychiatry* 1999; 156:1686.

Arana GW, Goff D, Baldessarini RJ, et al. The effect of anticholinergic prophylaxis on neuroleptic-induced dystonia. *Am J Psychiatry* 1988;145:993.

Casey DE. Side effect profiles of new antipsychotic agents. *J Clin Psychiatry* 1996;57(suppl 11):40.

Chouinard G, Annable L, Ross-Choiunard A, et al. A 5-year prospective longitudinal study of tardive dyskinesia: factors predicting appearance of new cases. *J Clin Psychopharmacol* 1988;8(suppl): 21.

Fleischhacker WW, Roth SD, Kane JM. The pharmacologic treatment of neuroleptic-induced akathisia. *J Clin Psychopharmacol* 1990; 10:12.

Fulop G, Phillips RA, Shapiro AK, et al. ECG changes during haloperidol and pimozide treatment of Tourette's disorder. *Am J Psychiatry* 1987;144:673.

Gardos G, Casey DE, Cole JO, et al. Ten-year outcome of tardive dyskinesia. *Am J Psychiatry* 1994;151:836.

Rosebush P, Stewart T. A prospective analysis of 24 episodes of neuroleptic malignant syndrome. *Am J Psychiatry* 1989;146:717.

Rosenberg MR, Green M. Neuroleptic malignant syndrome: review of response to therapy. *Arch Intern Med* 1989;149:1927.

Drug Interactions

Ciraulo D, Shader RI, Greenblatt DJ, et al. *Drug interactions in psychiatry.* Baltimore: Williams & Wilkins, 1995.

Antipsychotic Drugs in the Elderly

Jeste DV, Lacro JP, Bailey A, et al. Lower incidence of tardive dyskinesia with risperidone compared with haloperidol in older patients. *J Am Geriatr Soc* 1999;47:716.

Antipsychotic Drugs in Pregnancy

Cohen LS, Altshuler LL. Pharmacologic management of psychiatric illness during pregnancy and the postpartum period. *Psychiatr Clin North Am* 1997;21:60.

Romeau-Rouguette C, Goujard J, Huel G. Possible teratogenic effect of phenothiazines in human beings. *Teratology* 1977;15:57.

Sloane D, Siskind V, Heinonen OP, et al. Antenatal exposure to the phenothiazines in relation to congenital malformations, perinatal mortality rate, birth weight, and intelligence quotient score. *Am J Obstet Gynecol* 1977;128:486.

Spielvogel A, Wile J. Treatment and outcomes of psychotic patients during pregnancy and childbirth. *Birth* 1992;19:3.

Viguera AC, Baldessarini RC. Neuroleptic withdrawal in schizophrenic patients. *Arch Gen Psychiatry* 1995;52:189.

3

Antidepressant Drugs

The antidepressant drugs are a heterogeneous group of compounds with major therapeutic effects in common, most importantly the treatment of major depressive illness. However, most of these drugs are also effective in the treatment of panic disorder and other anxiety disorders, and a subset are effective in the treatment of obsessive–compulsive disorder (OCD) and a variety of other conditions (Table 3.1). For consideration of therapeutic spectrum of action and patterns of side effects, antidepressants were traditionally subdivided into major groups: **(a) selective serotonin reuptake inhibitors (SSRIs), (b) tricyclic antidepressants (TCAs) and the related cyclic antidepressants (i.e., amoxapine and maprotiline), (c) monoamine oxidase inhibitors (MAOIs), and (d) other antidepressant compounds; the latter group has grown to include an array of newer agents with differing putative mechanisms of action and adverse event profiles (bupropion, mirtazapine, nefazodone, reboxetine, trazodone, and venlafaxine).** Because they overlap, the mechanisms of action and indications for use for the antidepressants are discussed

Table 3.1. Indications for antidepressants

Effective
  Major depression (unipolar)
  Bipolar depression
  Prophylaxis against recurrence of major depression (unipolar)
  Panic disorder
  Social phobia
  Depression with psychotic features in combination with an
    antipsychotic
  Bulimia
  Neuropathic pain (tricyclic drugs)
  Enuresis (imipramine best studied)
  Obsessive-compulsive disorder (clomipramine and SSRIs)
  Atypical depression (SSRIs or monoamine oxidase inhibitors)
Probably effective
  Attention-deficit/hyperactivity disorder
  Cataplexy due to narcolepsy
  Dysthymia (chronic depression)
  Generalized anxiety disorder
  Organic mood disorders
  Posttraumatic stress disorder
  Pseudobulbar affect (pathologic laughing and weeping)
Possibly effective
  School phobia and separation anxiety
  Personality disorders

53

together, but separate sections are provided for the method of administration and side effects.

MECHANISM OF ACTION

The precise mechanisms by which the antidepressant drugs exert their therapeutic effects remain unknown, although much is known about their acute actions within the nervous system. Their major interaction is with the monoamine neurotransmitter systems in the brain, particularly the norepinephrine and serotonin systems. Norepinephrine and serotonin are released throughout the brain by neurons originating in the locus ceruleus and brainstem raphe nuclei, respectively. Both of these neurotransmitters interact with multiple receptor types in the brain to regulate arousal, vigilance, attention, mood states, sensory processing, appetitive functions, and other global state functions. The importance of monoamine neurons in antidepressant action has been suggested by a number of observations. One of the classic animal models of depression uses the drug reserpine, which depletes neurons of monoamine neurotransmitters, including norepinephrine, serotonin, and dopamine. Similarly, reserpine has been shown to induce depression in some humans, which may be clinically indistinguishable from major depressive illness. In animal models, the cyclic antidepressants are partly able to reverse behavioral sedation induced by reserpine and other amine-depleting agents, such as tetrabenazine.

Norepinephrine, serotonin, and dopamine are removed from synapses after release by reuptake, mostly into presynaptic neurons. This mechanism of terminating neurotransmitter action is mediated by specific norepinephrine, serotonin, and dopamine reuptake transporter proteins. After reuptake, norepinephrine, serotonin, and dopamine are either reloaded into vesicles for subsequent release or broken down by the enzyme monoamine oxidase. The cyclic antidepressants and venlafaxine at higher doses block the reuptake of norepinephrine and serotonin in varying ratios, thus potentiating their action (Fig. 3.1). The SSRIs have not been shown at therapeutically relevant doses to have significant effects on norepinephrine reuptake in the human brain. Monoamine oxidase inhibitors may potentiate the action of biogenic amines by blocking their intracellular catabolism. Such observations initially suggested that antidepressants work by increasing noradrenergic or serotonergic neurotransmission, thus compensating for a postulated state of relative deficiency. However, this simple theory cannot fully explain the action of antidepressant drugs for a number of reasons. The most important of these include the lack of convincing evidence that depression is characterized by a state of inadequate noradrenergic or serotonergic neurotransmission. Indeed, many melancholic patients appear to have increased turnover of norepinephrine. Moreover, blockade of reuptake by the cyclic antidepressants and SSRIs and inhibition of monoamine oxidase by MAOIs occur rapidly (within hours) after drug administration, but antidepressants are rarely clinically effective prior to 3 weeks and may require 6 weeks or more.

These considerations have led to the idea that inhibition of monoamine reuptake or inhibition of monoamine oxidase by

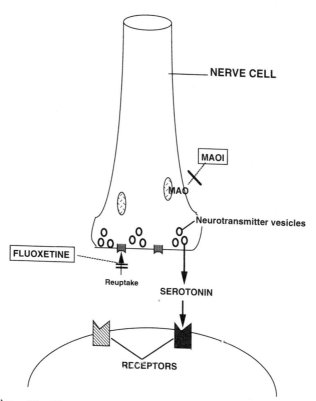

Figure 3.1. Fluoxetine blocks reuptake of serotonin into presynaptic serotonin neurons by blocking the reuptake transporter protein. The action of monoamine neurotransmitters in the synapse is terminated by reuptake via specific reuptake transporters. The selective serotonin reuptake inhibitors, such as fluoxetine, specifically block the serotonin transporter; the tricyclics and venlafaxine block both the norepinephrine and serotonin transporters. The resulting increases in synaptic neurotransmitters initiates slow adaptive responses that produce clinical improvement. *MAOI*, monoamine oxidase inhibitors.

antidepressants is an initiating event. The actual therapeutic actions of antidepressants, however, result from slower adaptive responses within neurons to these initial biochemical perturbations. Research investigating slow-onset changes in neurons that might better reflect the time course of antidepressant action is ongoing. It has been found, for example, that chronic (2 weeks) treatment of rats with cyclic antidepressants or MAOIs is associated with a reduction in number (downregulation) of β_1-adrenergic receptors, accompanied by a decreased activation of adenylyl cyclase by norepinephrine. Many antidepressants also downregulate α_2-adrenergic receptors and have variable effects on 5-HT$_2$ serotonin receptors. Changes in receptor number must currently be seen as correlates of long-term administration (established largely in normal rat brain), not a likely therapeutic mechanism. There is no convincing theory to explain how monoamine receptor regulation could have an effect on mood disorders. Slow-onset changes in the nervous system that may be related convincingly to the mechanism of action of antidepressants are actively being sought. Important candidates include antidepressant-induced changes in patterns of neuronal gene expression.

Although progress in understanding the mechanism of clinical action of antidepressants has been slow, receptor studies have been useful in understanding some of their side effects. For example, it has been found that the rank order of binding affinities of cyclic antidepressants at muscarinic cholinergic receptors generally parallels the potency of their clinical anticholinergic effects (e.g., amitriptyline, doxepin, imipramine, and desipramine). Similarly, doxepin and amitriptyline have high affinities for histamine H$_1$ receptors, partially explaining their strong sedative effects (sedation is also a function of muscarinic receptor blockade). Such information is very useful in the pharmaceutical industry for screening compounds for possible clinical use.

INDICATIONS

Given the roles of norepinephrine and serotonin neurons in regulating global brain states, it is not surprising that, by interacting with these systems, certain antidepressant drugs can treat not only mood disorders, but also anxiety disorders, eating disorders, OCD, and chronic pain syndromes. Additional uses are likely to be discovered. Indeed the term *antidepressant* is far too narrow and may raise issues in patient education when these drugs are prescribed for indications other than depression.

Since the introduction of fluoxetine, the SSRIs have become the most often prescribed initial treatment for major depression. The success of the SSRIs in displacing tricyclic drugs as first-choice agents is not based on established differences in efficacy, but rather on a generally more favorable side effect profile such as lack of anticholinergic and cardiac side effects, a high therapeutic index (ratio of lethal dose:therapeutic dose), combined with ease of administration. Furthermore, with certain comorbidities of depression to be discussed subsequently such as OCD, SSRIs offer advantages in efficacy over the tricyclics. Nonetheless, the tricyclic drugs remain useful alternative therapeutic options for the treatment of some patients with depression and anxiety disorders. Because of their toxicity and risk, MAOIs are a class of drug reserved for patients in whom other treatments have failed—MAOIs are frequently effective when other drugs have failed. As one would expect, the newer antidepressants all have safety and side effect advantages over the TCAs and MAOIs.

Suicide Risk

The tricyclic and related cyclic antidepressants (maprotiline and amoxapine) and the MAOIs have a narrow therapeutic index, making them potentially lethal in overdose, unlike the SSRIs and the other newer antidepressants. Thus, a careful evaluation of impulsiveness and suicide risk influences not only the decision as to the need for hospitalization but also the choice of an antidepressant, especially for those who will be treated as outpatients. For potentially suicidal or highly impulsive patients, the SSRIs and the newer agents would be a better initial choice than a cyclic compound or MAOI. Patients at elevated suicide risk who cannot tolerate these safer compounds or who do not respond to them should not receive large quantities or refillable prescriptions for tricyclics or MAOIs. Generally, patients who are new to treatment or those at more than minimal risk for suicide whose therapeutic relationship is unstable should receive a limited supply of any medication.

Evaluation for suicide risk must continue even after the initiation of treatment. Suicidal thoughts and intentions may be slow to respond to treatment, and patients may become demoralized before therapeutic efficacy is evident. Side effects and, most importantly, intercurrent life events may trigger suicidal thoughts prior to a full therapeutic response. Thus, rarely, for a variety of reasons, patients may temporarily become more suicidal following the initiation of treatment. Should such worsening occur, appropriate interventions may include management of side effects, more frequent monitoring, discontinuation of the initial treatment, or hospitalization.

Major Depression

For patients who meet the *Diagnostic and Statistical Manual of Mental Disorders,* 4th edition (DSM-IV) criteria for major depression, it can be expected that approximately 50% will fully recover with a single *adequate* trial (i.e., adequate dose for at least 6 weeks) of any effective antidepressant. Of the remainder, the majority will show some improvement, but 10% to 15% will not improve. For patients with comorbid psychiatric disorders, such as anxiety disorders, substance use disorders, personality disorders, or psychotic disorders, the response rates will be lower. For those who do not recover fully, combined treatments or selection of another antidepressant will benefit the majority.

Based on controlled trials, as many as 20% to 40% of patients who improve may be exhibiting a placebo response. An antidepressant response that emerges in the first 2 weeks of treatment and does not persist is more likely to reflect a placebo pattern than a true drug response. Therefore, loss of response early in the course may not represent loss of a true drug response and may indicate the need for more vigorous or prolonged treatment. Placebo response is less likely to occur with more severely depressed patients.

The most common reasons for failure of drug treatment are **inadequate drug dosage** and **inadequate length of drug trial.** For those who respond inadequately to initial treatment, there are literally dozens of alternatives when one considers the various permutations of switching agents, as well as augmenting and combining treatments. The majority of patients who fail adequate trials of drug therapy for moderate to severe depression could respond to electroconvulsive therapy (ECT), if the treatment were available and acceptable to the patient, although for most of these patients a continuation and maintenance treatment would still be required, a need that usually calls for continued efforts to find an effective pharmacologic regimen. Recent studies have suggested that some forms of short-term psychotherapy (cognitive and interpersonal therapies) may be as effective as pharmacotherapy in milder depressions and that the combination of an antidepressant with cognitive therapy can be more efficacious than either treatment alone. The more serious the depression, the clearer the advantage of drug therapy over psychotherapies in terms of efficacy. For residual depressive symptoms despite pharmacotherapy, cognitive therapy may prove to be particularly useful and the improvement in residual symptoms may remove one risk factor (negative cognitions) for recurrence of depression.

Subtypes of Depression

Even with the DSM-IV criteria, depression remains heterogeneous in its presentation and presumably in its etiology. Research addressing the question of valid subtypes of major depressive disorder continues, but it is already possible to identify groups of patients with specific features that differentiate them from other patients with major depression and that may predict differential treatment responses.

Depressed Phase of Bipolar Disorder

The classification of depression into unipolar and bipolar is well supported by longitudinal, family, and treatment studies. All classes of antidepressants are effective in treating episodes of depression in patients with bipolar disorder. Unfortunately, these drugs also have certain liabilities in bipolar patients:

1. As many as 30% to 50% of bipolar patients may develop a manic episode during treatment with an antidepressant. Concomitant therapy with lithium or anticonvulsants may only be partially protective against this switch into mania.
2. In some bipolar patients, antidepressants may initiate and maintain rapid cycling (a state with more than three episodes or two or more continuous complete cycles per year, often characterized by diminished response to lithium).

Given these concerns, it is clinically useful for each bipolar patient to make a chart graphically representing periods of depression, hypomania, mania, and mixed symptoms over time as deflections up or down from a euthymic baseline. The medications used should be recorded on this graphic time line as well. Such charting will help the clinician identify patterns of therapeutic efficacy and iatrogenically induced worsening should they occur.

If induction of mania occurs during antidepressant treatment, the antidepressant usually should be discontinued. If subsequent depressions occur, an antidepressant should be used for the shortest interval until symptoms improve and then treatment continued with mood stabilizers such as lithium or anticonvulsants. There is preliminary evidence to suggest that bupropion may be less likely than TCAs to precipitate mania in rapid-cycling bipolar type II patients (i.e., patients with depressions and antidepressant-induced hypomania), but like all antidepressants, it has been associated with the onset of mania in some patients. The switch into mania has been observed with all SSRIs, but suggestions from different studies raise the possibility that these and other newer agents may have lower risk of switch to mania than the TCAs. Low rates of manic switch, based on one or more clinical studies or case series, have raised the possibility of advantages over the older drugs for paroxetine, fluoxetine, nefazodone, and mirtazapine; however, adequately designed studies have not been accomplished to support these hypotheses. If a patient develops severe mania with antidepressants, despite lithium or anticonvulsant prophylaxis, it may prove necessary to attempt to ride out milder depressions without antidepressants and to use ECT for more severe episodes. However, even ECT may induce mania in a small number of patients. In general, chronic administration of antidepressants is best avoided, if possible, in bipolar patients. There has been interest in the possibility that the newer anticonvulsant lamotrigine might offer both antidepressant efficacy and mood stabilization.

Atypical Depression

Atypical depression historically has been used to refer to two different groups of depressed patients, generally classified as A or V type, the former referring to patients with prominent anxiety symptoms, including panic, and the latter referring to those with reversed vegetative signs, including hypersomnia and hyperphagia instead of insomnia and anorexia. As currently used, the term *atypical depression* refers to a group of patients with mood reactivity, who in addition report such symptoms as rejection sensitivity, hypersomnia, hyperphagia (e.g., carbohydrate craving), and prominent fatigue. These patients clearly respond better to MAOIs (phenelzine is best studied) than to tricyclics, although tricyclics are superior to placebo. Preliminary reports with fluoxetine suggested that the SSRIs might similarly offer efficacy advantages over the TCAs in individuals with atypical depression, but subsequent reports with other SSRIs failed to confirm superior efficacy but showed the expected side effect advantages. This form of depression tends to have onset at an early age and multiple recurrences; therefore, long-term treatment is likely to be necessary. Given their relative safety and ease of use, the SSRIs are preferred for an initial trial.

Hostile and Irritable Subtypes

Past attempts to discern subtypes of major depression yielded a possible hostile depressive subtype. Recent work indicates that a significant minority of outpatients with depressive illness are predominantly irritable while depressed and manifest intermittent outbursts of anger or rage, which may be termed *anger attacks*. Anger attacks emerge abruptly with minimal interpersonal provocation; they are associated with a paroxysm of autonomic arousal reminiscent of panic attacks but feature explosive verbal or physical anger, usually directed at close companions or family members. Both anecdotal and systematically ascertained data suggest an important therapeutic role for antidepressants, especially SSRIs and MAOIs, in these patients who appear to have decreased central serotonergic activity compared with patients without anger attacks. The depression in these irritable patients with anger attacks responds to antidepressants as well as it does in patients without anger attacks.

Grief, Bereavement, and Loss

Following bereavement, loss of a job, or a life event leading to significant loss of self esteem, individuals may experience symptoms of depression. It is important to distinguish depressive illness from normal grief or sadness. Although normally grieving individuals commonly sleep poorly and have decreased appetite, poor concentration, and other apparent neurovegetative symptoms immediately following the loss, these symptoms improve over several weeks' or months' time in the majority of cases. If depressive symptoms are particularly severe, persistent, or pervasive, are accompanied by serious suicidal thoughts or behavior, or are protracted beyond what might be expected for the precipitating stressor, specific treatment is indicated.

In many cases the preferred treatment modality is psychotherapy aimed at helping the patient appropriately mourn the loss or develop adequate coping skills to deal with problems that have arisen. However, if the depressive symptoms are severe and unremitting, antidepressant therapy should be considered. Indeed, patients may be better able to use psychotherapy if their depressive symptoms are alleviated. Dosages are the same as for the treatment of major depression, although the treatment duration may be shorter for a first episode, depending on the rapidity and completeness of the response.

Depression with Psychotic Features

Major depression accompanied by psychotic symptoms (e.g., delusions or hallucinations) responds poorly to treatment with antidepressants alone. Controlled studies demonstrate that depression with psychotic features is more effectively treated with the combination of an antidepressant and an antipsychotic drug (70%–80% exhibiting significant improvement) than if treated with either class of drugs alone (30%–50% response rate). ECT is at least as effective as the combined antidepressant–antipsychotic regimen and is the treatment of choice if this combination fails.

The recommended dosage of antipsychotic medication for depression with psychotic features has not been clearly established, but it appears that dosages slightly lower than those used in acute psychoses may be adequate, perhaps due to pharmacokinetic interactions with the antidepressant. Thus, patients might traditionally have been started on 4 to 6 mg of haloperidol or the equivalent in addition to **full doses of an antidepressant,** with individual dosage adjustments as needed. The combination of low-potency antipsychotics (e.g., thioridazine, mesoridazine, or chlorpromazine) with tricyclic or related cyclic antidepressants is to be avoided because of additive anticholinergic toxicity and postural hypotension. Combinations of antipsychotics with SSRIs are also effective. While diminishing the burden of anticholinergic, sedative, and hypotensive side effects, SSRIs may worsen the extrapyramidal side effects of typical antipsychotic drugs. Because of their relatively greater potential to inhibit the hepatic metabolism of drugs metabolized by the P450 2D6 isoenzyme, fluoxetine and paroxetine are more likely than sertraline or citalopram to produce increases in typical antipsychotic drug levels and thus side effects or toxicity. Fixed combinations (e.g., the old Triavil agent) do not allow the clinician to adjust medications individually and therefore are not recommended. For this reason we also did not recommend amoxapine, an antidepressant with metabolites possessing some neuroleptic effects, which has also been reported effective for depression with psychotic features.

The anticholinergic effects of many TCAs were often sufficient prophylaxis against extrapyramidal symptoms; thus, additional anticholinergics need not have been routinely prescribed when tricyclics were part of the combination. If multiple anticholinergic medication proved necessary for extrapyramidal symptoms, careful monitoring for anticholinergic toxicity was important.

A more subtle clinical point is that typical antipsychotic drugs may themselves cause masked facies, akinesia, and blunting of affect, which can be confused with depressive symptoms; thus, other target symptoms, such as sleep, guilt, or psychotic symptoms, may be better indicators of improvement when patients are on combined antipsychotic-antidepressant regimens.

Increasingly the atypical antipsychotics (e.g., olanzapine, risperidone) have replaced the typicals for use in mood-disordered patients given the relative lack of extrapyramidal adverse effects and the reduced risk for tardive dyskinesia for which mood-disordered patients appear to be more vulnerable. These drugs, particularly olanzapine and clozapine, also appear to offer some antidepressant potential. Whether they might be used alone, without antidepressants, for psychotic depression, remains to be demonstrated.

Given the serious morbidity and high suicide risk of depression with psychotic features, maintenance treatment must be considered. However, there are few data to guide the decision of whether to continue with combined treatment or either agent alone. For a patient who continues well, general clinical wisdom is to discontinue the antipsychotic drug first, while maintaining the antidepressant treatment longer term.

Depression Comorbid with Other Disorders

Depression with Anxiety

Anxiety symptoms (including panic attacks) commonly accompany major depression and generally respond to antidepressant treatment along with other symptoms of the depressive episode. Although pharmaceutical companies may market claims that one SSRI is superior in efficacy to another in depressed patients with prominent anxiety, the evidence is that the drugs of this class are equally efficacious in this population.

Many clinicians administer adjunctive benzodiazepines for symptomatic relief of anxiety in depressed patients. Adjunctive benzodiazepines offer initial relief of anxiety symptoms prior to onset of antidepressant efficacy. They also may be useful for residual symptoms that do not improve with the antidepressant (see Chapter 5). Because of its delayed onset of efficacy, buspirone is not used to provide initial relief. It is important to recognize that antidepressants are the essential therapeutic agents in these cases and that full antidepressant doses are needed whether or not a benzodiazepine produces initial improvements in such symptoms as anxiety and insomnia. Combining clonazepam with fluoxetine for initiation of antidepressant treatment has been reported to enhance treatment compliance and improve early response followed by tapering of the benzodiazepine as the antidepressant response emerges.

Depression Complicating Borderline Personality Disorder

Antidepressants, particularly the SSRIs, are used in patients with borderline personality disorder to (a) treat intercurrent major depression; (b) reduce chronic depressive symptoms that do not meet criteria for major depression; (c) modulate anger, hostility, and irritability; (d) diminish impulsivity; and (e) improve other comorbid conditions such as bulimia or panic attacks.

Both typical and atypical major depression frequently complicate the course of borderline personality disorder. In general, the presence of any personality disorder predicts a worse treatment outcome than expected for uncomplicated major depression; however, antidepressants are still superior to placebo, and in some studies, patients diagnosed with a personality disorder prior to treatment no longer meet criteria for that disorder after treatment. Because these patients are often impulsive, angry, and self-destructive, first-choice medications would be those with established efficacy for that profile and that are less dangerous in overdose, for example, the SSRIs.

Some patients with borderline personality disorder have pervasive depressive symptoms without meeting DSM-IV criteria for major depression or dysthymia. These patients may benefit from a trial of an antidepressant, particularly an SSRI or MAOI. Because of their difficulty of use, prescription of MAOIs in this population requires a strong alliance with the patient and great care.

Although SSRIs improve depressive symptoms, as well as anger and hostility, in one report the tricyclic compound amitriptyline produced worsening in a significant number of these patients in self-destructive episodes and global ratings.

Depression Comorbid with Substance Abuse

Secondary depression occurs in the context of alcohol abuse and abuse of other central nervous system (CNS) depressants (e.g., barbiturates). Often the depressive symptoms are presumed to be due to toxic effects of the alcohol; ideally, therefore, the primary treatment should be detoxification. Given the possibilities of drug interactions with alcohol or barbiturates (including altered pharmacokinetics and possible additive CNS depression), prescription of the older antidepressants to actively drinking alcoholics should be avoided if possible, and the newer antidepressants, although safer, are less likely to be efficacious. Generally, antidepressants are indicated only if depressive symptoms persist for 4 weeks or more after successful detoxification or if the history indicates that mood disorder may be primary and not secondary to substance abuse. There is some support for the potential of SSRIs to reduce drinking for some patients unrelated to an antidepressant effect, and for antidepressant treatment to increase the likelihood of abstinence in depressed alcoholics.

There also has been interest in the possibility that antidepressants may help maintain abstinence from cocaine based on early reports with desipramine and later anecdotes involving fluoxetine or other SSRIs, but the evidence for the usefulness of antidepressants in nondepressed cocaine abusers is not compelling.

Refractory Depression

A large number of patients respond partially or not at all to an initial antidepressant trial. It is important to ensure that the initial diagnosis was correct and that there is not an unsuspected comorbid condition (e.g., alcoholism or thyroid disease) impairing treatment response. There are three general strategies for treating refractory depression that can be used in an orderly fashion (these strategies are discussed in detail for each specific class of drug):

1. **Optimization**—ensuring adequate drug doses for the individual, which may be higher than initial doses (e.g., fluoxetine 40–80 mg, desipramine 200–300 mg), and adequate duration of treatment (6 weeks or longer). Also noncompliance, which is certainly more common than most practitioners appreciate, should be evaluated.
2. **Augmentation or combination**—addition to ongoing treatment of drugs that are not antidepressant agents themselves is termed *augmentation therapy*; well-studied augmentation strategies for TCAs included, for example, adjunctive lithium or L-triiodothyronine (T3). Combination treatment generally refers to the prescribing of more than one antidepressant. The array of putative augmentation strategies and the number of combinatory possibilities has dramatically increased with the newer antidepressant agents. Although there are many commonly used augmentations and combinations, few have been well studied and supported by clinical research.
3. **Substitution**—change in the primary drug, which is thought to have the greatest potential for efficacy when the switch is to an agent from a different drug class; for example, if the first drug were an SSRI, switch to bupropion, reboxetine, or venlafaxine. If, however, the first drug failed because of side effects, a drug within the initial class may be effective if it is tolerated. For reasons that are unclear but likely reflect the minor pharmacodynamic differences between SSRIs, switch within the class is clinically helpful for primary efficacy failures sufficiently often to warrant a second SSRI trial for some patients before switching out of class. If the patient remains seriously depressed despite additions or changes in medication, consideration should be given to the relative risks of additional trials (based on severity of symptoms and concern about time delay) versus the use of ECT.

Continuation and Maintenance Treatment

Originally based on studies with TCAs, patients with unipolar depression were observed to be at high risk for relapse when treatment was discontinued within the first 16 weeks of therapy. Therefore, in treatment responders, most experts favor a continuation of therapy for a minimum period of 6 months. The value of continuation therapy for several months to prevent relapse into the original episode also has been established for virtually all the newer agents. Risk of recurrence after this 6- to 8-month continuation period, that is, the development of a new episode after recovery from the index episode, is particularly elevated in patients with a chronic course before recovery, residual symptoms, multiple prior episodes (three or more), or a first episode in late life. For these individuals, the optimal duration of maintenance treatment is unknown but is measured in years. Based on research to date, prophylactic efficacy of an antidepressant has been observed for as long as 5 years with clear benefit. In contrast to the initial expectation that maintenance therapy would be effective at dosages lower than that required for acute treatment, the current consensus is that full-dose therapy is required for effective prophylaxis. In some cases, however, adequate maintenance control may actually require doses of antidepressants higher than those that were acutely effective.

In the past, maintenance treatment was difficult because some tricyclic side effects increased or emerged over time, such as weight gain, dental caries, and continuation of such unpleasant sensations and symptoms as dry mouth and constipation. With newer drugs, maintenance therapy is easier. The SSRIs and newer drugs have been found to remain effective for 6 months to 1 year. There have been patients, however, treated with each of the classes of antidepressants for whom the drug has lost efficacy over time. In such patients, the same considerations and strategies described for treating refractory depression are of potential value.

In a small number of patients on SSRIs, apathy has emerged as a side effect that can be mistaken for recurrent depression. Apathy in the absence of associated depressive symptoms should prompt a decrease rather than an increase in the dosage or the addition of a noradrenergic or dopaminergic agent.

Except for amoxapine, which possesses some neuroleptic properties and has been implicated in tardive dyskinesia, there are no known adverse effects specifically due to long-term antidepressant treatment except that the risk of a discontinuation syndrome with TCAs, MAOIs, SSRIs, and venlafaxine is more likely after abrupt interruption of chronic treatment especially with shorter half-life agents.

Dysthymia

Dysthymia is heterogeneous clinically and likely heterogeneous in etiology. Seventy percent of dysthymic patients have a comorbid medical or psychiatric disorder. This disorder may have profound consequences for quality of life and for effective functioning in multiple life roles; this morbidity is more reflective of the duration of dysthymia than of the number of symptoms. It was once thought that dysthymic patients would not respond to antidepressants, an opinion that may have reflected the mistaken idea that patients with milder symptoms should require only low doses of antidepressants, leading to inadequate dosing or duration of treatment for dysthymic patients. More recent studies of dysthymia treatment with SSRIs, nefazodone, and tricyclics indicate that this is a treatment-responsive condition; moreover, the benefit of treatment is maintained with continued therapy as in major depression. Inasmuch as one cannot predict ahead of time which dysthymic patients will respond to antidepressant treatment, and given the safety and efficacy of the SSRIs and nefazodone, a therapeutic trial should be considered for dysthymic patients. Because psychotherapies such as interpersonal therapy and cognitive therapy for depression have proven efficacious in patients with depressions of milder severity and in chronic depressions, these strategies should be considered as alternatives or adjuncts to antidepressant treatment.

Secondary Mood Disorders

Many medical illnesses and medications can produce secondary depressive syndromes (Table 3.2). When the depression is due to a treatable disorder or medication, it may remit with appropriate medical care or discontinuation of the offending drug. If, however, the depression is severe or does not remit after treatment of the medical condition, it would be reasonable to initiate antidepressant therapy.

Certain neurologic disorders (e.g., stroke, Parkinson's disease, Huntington's disease) commonly produce secondary depression. Stroke patients, in particular, develop secondary depression with an incidence greater than would be predicted by the degree of disability. Aggressive treatment of the depression may improve the patient's quality of life and his or her ability to participate in rehabilitation. For patients with depression secondary to an untreatable medical or neurologic illness, the duration of therapy is undetermined. Many patients with brain injuries or neurodegenerative disorders (e.g., Alzheimer's disease) manifest elevated susceptibility to the side effects of psychotropic medications.

Table 3.2.   Organic etiologies of depression

Drug induced: reserpine, β blockers, α-methyldopa, levodopa, estrogens, corticosteroids, cholinergic drugs, benzodiazepines, barbiturates and similarly acting drugs, ranitidine, calcium channel blockers

Related to drug abuse: alcohol abuse, sedative/hypnotic abuse, cocaine and other psychostimulant withdrawal

Metabolic disorders: hyperthyroidism (especially in the elderly), hypothyroidism, Cushing's syndrome, hypercalcemia, hyponatremia, diabetes mellitus

Neurologic disorders: stroke, subdural hematoma, multiple sclerosis, brain tumors (especially frontal), Parkinson's disease, Huntington's disease, uncontrolled epilepsy, syphilis, dementias, closed head injuries

Nutritional disorders: vitamin B_{12} deficiency, pellagra

Other: pancreatic carcinoma, viral infections (especially mononucleosis and influenza)

Panic Disorder

The core manifestation of panic disorder is recurrent unexpected panic attacks. In addition, a substantial proportion of patients with panic disorder develop anticipatory anxiety and phobic avoidance, which may prove more disabling than the panic attacks themselves. When severe, phobic avoidance in the form of agoraphobia (fear of situations in which it may be difficult to gain help or escape) may cause patients to become entirely housebound. TCAs, MAOIs, SSRIs, and high-potency benzodiazepines (alprazolam and clonazepam; see Chapter 5) have established efficacy in the treatment of panic attacks. Because of their side effect profile, the SSRIs are the first choice among the antidepressants for panic. As with the TCAs, increased jitteriness and anxiety may attend the initiation of treatment. Thus SSRIs or tricyclics should first be prescribed at the lowest doses possible (e.g., sertraline 25 mg, paroxetine 10 mg, fluoxetine 10 mg, imipramine 10 mg). Doses of fluoxetine under 10 mg can be accomplished with use of the liquid formulation or by dissolving the contents of a capsule in juice or water and aliquoting the juice. Among the TCAs, imipramine is the best studied, although it is likely that all of the tricyclics are effective. As with other disorders, MAOIs may be the most effective of all but are reserved for treatment-refractory patients because of their side effects and difficulty of use. The doses of antidepressants required for optimal treatment of this condition is higher than many clinicians appreciate, with full antidepressant dose levels yielding best response for some patients, as for example 40 to 60 mg of paroxetine.

The anticipatory anxiety and phobic avoidance observed in panic disorder may respond slowly following successful antidepressant monotherapy of panic attacks. Cognitive behavior therapy for panic disorder and agoraphobia is an alternative to pharmacotherapy but an especially useful adjunct as well to address the avoidant behavior, catastrophic thinking, and sensitivity to bodily sensations (anxiety sensitivity) that accounts for so much of the impairment, chronicity, and recurrence of this condition.

Comorbid depression is very common in panic disorder; its presence requires the selection of antidepressant treatment rather than a benzodiazepine as the primary treatment for both disorders. For panic disorder uncomplicated by depression or for residual anxiety symptoms, clinicians may choose a high-potency benzodiazepine. The major advantage of an antidepressant is low risk of dependence and less difficulty with discontinuation (see Chapter 5). The major disadvantages are delayed onset, more side effects, and perhaps less efficacy for anticipatory anxiety and less flexibility for as-needed use.

Obsessive–Compulsive Disorder

Obsessive–compulsive disorder involves recurrent intrusive thoughts that the patient recognizes as products of his or her own mind (obsessions) and/or repetitive, seemingly purposeful behavior designed to prevent or neutralize some dreaded consequence (compulsions). Of the drugs presently available in the United States, clomipramine and the SSRIs appear to have significant antiobsessional activity based on controlled studies and clinical experience.

Approximately 50% of patients receiving an adequate trial of one of these medications improve. It is striking that all of these drugs have potent and relatively selective effects on inhibition of serotonin reuptake (although the major metabolite of clomipramine has significant effects on norepinephrine reuptake as well).

There have been smaller studies and case reports of positive antiobsessional responses with many other drugs including TCAs (e.g., imipramine, desipramine, amitriptyline, and doxepin), MAOIs, and high-potency benzodiazepines, but these drugs have not proved reliably effective in large numbers of patients. Based on anecdotal evidence, MAOIs may be particularly effective for patients whose OCD is complicated by panic attacks, social phobia, or severe generalized anxiety. Although benzodiazepines are not generally effective in treating OCD, clonazepam did prove superior to placebo in one controlled trial. Because obsessions may be quite bizarre, patients are at risk for inappropriate diagnosis of psychosis and treatment with antipsychotic drugs. The use of antipsychotic drugs in the treatment of well-diagnosed obsessions should be restricted to nonresponders to standard treatment who have accompanying schizotypal features or clinically significant tics.

Psychopharmacologic treatment is most effective in treating obsessions. Patients presenting with predominantly compulsive rituals often respond better to behavior therapy, including exposure (e.g., getting the patient to handle a feared source of contamination) and response prevention (e.g., not allowing the patient to perform a ritual for a certain period of time). For many patients, a combination of pharmacotherapy and behavior therapy will prove optimal.

For OCD, clomipramine is typically used in dosages of 150 to 250 mg/day. Its use is limited by its anticholinergic effects. At dosages above 250 mg/day there is also a relatively high incidence of seizures. Treatment of OCD with SSRIs also at times requires higher doses than are typically recommended for depression. For fluoxetine, dosages of 60 to 80 mg/day are commonly required, and dosages as high as 120 mg/day have been used.

Symptoms of OCD respond more slowly than symptoms of major depression. Thus, trials of each medication should last for at least 12 weeks. Clomipramine at an average dosage of 180 mg/day (range 100–250 mg/day) also has been reported to be effective in the treatment of trichotillomania (hair pulling), a condition hypothesized to be related to OCD. In this same study, desipramine was not effective (Swedo et al., 1989).

Body Dysmorphic Disorder

Body dysmorphic disorder, previously referred to as dysmorphophobia or monosymptomatic hypochondriacal psychosis, involves preoccupation with an imagined physical defect. Antipsychotic drugs, most notably pimozide and haloperidol, have been used in the past and produced only modest benefit. More recently, SSRIs have been used successfully in high (OCD-like) doses.

Posttraumatic Stress Disorder

Following an extremely traumatic experience, such as rape, severe abuse, or combat, posttraumatic stress disorder (PTSD) may develop, which includes nightmares about the event, a heightened startle reflex, sudden feelings of reexperiencing the traumatic event (flashbacks), and avoidance of objects or situations that are reminders of the event. Such symptoms may be disabling in themselves and may lead to further impairment secondary to avoidant behaviors and depression. Fully effective treatments for the core symptoms of PTSD are lacking, but SSRIs (particularly fluoxetine) have been associated with substantial symptomatic improvement. These agents are best used in combination with psychosocial treatments. Some patients have had a partial or marked benefit from other antidepressants, including MAOIs or nefazodone.

Social Phobia (Social Anxiety Disorder)

Social phobia is defined as a persistent fear of social situations in which the individual feels open to scrutiny or humiliation. Several reports have identified MAOIs, specifically phenelzine and tranylcypromine, as potentially effective in reducing these fears and secondary avoidant behaviors (see also Chapter 5). Recent studies have also established the efficacy of SSRIs, with paroxetine the first SSRI agent to receive approval for social anxiety disorder from the U.S. Food and Drug Administration (FDA). Specific cognitive behavioral therapy protocols for social phobia are also efficacious alone or in combination with pharmacotherapy, but availability of well-trained practitioners is a limitation. The high-potency benzodiazepine clonazepam also has been demonstrated to be effective in social phobia and may be combined with SSRIs in difficult cases.

Bulimia

Several open and controlled trials support the use of SSRIs (fluoxetine is best studied), tricyclics, and MAOIs in the treatment of bulimia. Given the impulsiveness of these patients and the dangers of dietary indiscretions with MAOIs, this class of drugs is generally reserved for treatment-refractory patients who are nonetheless compliant with treatment. Bupropion also may be effective, but because of a high incidence of seizures in one study of bulimics, its use is not recommended in this disorder. Antidepressants produce improvement in binge frequency, vomiting and other purging, and attitude toward eating. In a multicenter placebo-controlled, double-blind trial of fluoxetine for bulimia, a dosage of 60 mg/day was superior to 20 mg/day, which was in turn superior to placebo. These data and clinical experience suggest that higher doses of SSRIs than are typically used for depression may be required to treat bulimia. Because higher doses of SSRIs are safer and better tolerated than higher doses of cyclic antidepressants, SSRIs have become the first-choice pharmacologic treatment for bulimia. Although some responsive patients who have been studied in antidepressant trials had depressive symptoms, many did not. Pharmacotherapy should generally be part of a comprehensive treatment program.

Antidepressants appear to be far less successful in treating anorexia nervosa than bulimia, although a prior history of anorexia nervosa does not seem to influence antidepressant response among current bulimics.

Attention-Deficit/Hyperactivity Disorder

Attention-deficit/hyperactivity disorder begins in childhood with symptoms of difficulty paying attention, impulsiveness, and hyperactivity. Although it is most frequently treated with psychostimulants (see Chapter 6), there is evidence for usefulness of bupropion in this condition. Some controlled trials have found the tricyclics imipramine and desipramine to be effective in treating the behavioral and cognitive disturbances associated with this disorder. Imipramine and desipramine have been used in dosages of 2 to 5 mg/kg/day. The advantage of antidepressants is a sustained effect and, for the tricyclics, once daily dosing; the disadvantage for tricyclics is that they have greater toxicity (e.g., anticholinergic and cardiac effects, with scattered reports of unexplained sudden death in children). Given the high rates of comorbid mood and anxiety disorders with ADHD, SSRIs have been helpful in the condition as well.

Chronic Pain Syndromes

Tricyclic antidepressants have been shown to be effective in a variety of chronic pain syndromes, even in the absence of diagnosable major depression, and often at lower doses than those used for depression. For example, in the treatment of neuropathic pain, analgesic effects of amitriptyline have been demonstrated at blood levels lower than those thought to be antidepressant and earlier (1–2 weeks after initiation of therapy) than an expected antidepressant effect. In animal studies, imipramine and amitriptyline both have been shown to potentiate morphine analgesia and to possess analgesic properties themselves.

Clinically, TCAs are used for treatment of chronic pain syndromes, especially neuropathic pain (e.g., diabetic neuropathy, postherpetic neuralgia, or trigeminal neuralgia). Empirical trials in patients with tension headaches, back pain, and other chronically painful conditions are occasionally successful. Imipramine and amitriptyline have been the most widely prescribed antidepressants for the treatment of chronic pain syndromes; however, one study demonstrated equivalent efficacy of desipramine to amitriptyline. In the same study, fluoxetine appeared to be ineffective. Because of its preferable side effect profile, patients might be started on desipramine, but nonresponders might be candidates for trials of imipramine, amitriptyline, or even clomipramine. Among the newer antidepressants, there is interest in the usefulness of mirtazapine and nefazodone for pain patients.

Tricyclics, especially amitriptyline, also have been studied in migraine prophylaxis, with mixed results. Although some trials have found amitriptyline to be superior to placebo, it appears to be less effective than propranolol for migraine prophylaxis. The effect of the SSRIs on headaches is variable, with some patients obtaining relief and others reporting worsened symptoms.

CHOICE OF ANTIDEPRESSANT

A large number of antidepressants are available (Table 3.3), including the SSRIs, tricyclic and related compounds, the MAOIs, and other compounds (bupropion, venlafaxine, nefazodone, mirtazapine, reboxetine, and trazodone). Successful use of antidepressants requires:

Table 3.3. Available preparations

Drug	Dosage Forms (mg)	Usual Daily Dose (mg/day)	Extreme Dosage (mg/day)	Therapeutic Plasma Levels (ng/mL)
Selective serotonin reuptake inhibitors				
Fluoxetine (Prozac)	C: 10, 20 LC: 20 mg/5 mL	20	5–80	
Fluvoxamine (Luvox)	T: 20, 30	150–200	50–300	
Paroxetine (Paxil)		20	10–50	
Sertraline (Zoloft)	T: 50, 100	100–150	50–200	
Cyclic compounds				
Imipramine (Tofranil and generics)	T: 10, 25, 50 C: 75, 100, 125, 150 INJ: 25 mg/2 mL	150–200	50–300	>225[a]
Desipramine (Norpramin and generics)	T: 10, 25, 50, 75, 100, 150 C: 25, 50	150–200	50–300	>125
Amitriptyline (Elavil and generics)	T: 10, 25, 50, 75, 100, 150 INJ: 10 mg/mL	150–200	50–300	>120 (?)[b]

Nortriptyline (Pamelor and generics)	C: 10, 25, 50, 75 LC: 10 mg/5 mL	75–100	25–150	50–150
Doxepin (Adapin, Sinequan, and generics)	C: 10, 25, 50, 75, 100, 150 LC: 10 mg/mL	150–200	25–300	100–250 (?)
Trimipramine (Surmontil)	C: 25, 50, 100	150–200	50–300	
Protriptyline (Vivactil)	T: 5, 10	15–40	10–60	
Maprotiline (Ludiomil)	T: 25, 50, 75	100–150	50–200	
Amoxapine (Asendin)	T: 25, 50, 100, 150	150–200	50–300	
Clomipramine (Anafranil)	C: 25, 50, 75	150–200	50–250	
Other compounds				
Bupropion (Wellbutrin)	T: 75, 100	200–300	100–450	
Venlafaxine (Effexor)		75–225	75–375	
Trazodone (Desyrel and generics)	T: 50, 100, 150, 300	200–300	100–600	
Nefazodone		200–300	100–600	
Monoamine oxidase inhibitors				
Phenelzine (Nardil)	T: 15	45–60	15–90	
Tranylcypromine (Parnate)	T: 10	30–50	10–90	

C, capsules; INJ, injectable form; LC, liquid concentrate or solution; T, tablets
[a]Sum of imipramine plus desipramine.
[b]Sum of amitriptyline plus nortriptyline.

1. Good patient selection as determined by a thorough diagnostic evaluation.
2. Choice of a drug with a tolerable side effect profile for the given patient.
3. Adequate dosage.
4. Drug trial of at least 4 weeks, preferably 6 weeks for depression or panic disorder, and at least 12 weeks for OCD.

Many patients with potentially treatable depression or panic disorder fail to improve because of inadequate dosing or duration of treatment or both.

As in the case of antipsychotic drugs, each physician need not be routinely familiar with prescribing every antidepressant on the market, but it is useful for the clinician to be comfortable prescribing several drugs that differ in mechanism and side effects. The most important considerations in choosing among these drugs are efficacy for the condition being treated and side effects. The efficacy of the available antidepressants for major depression, including various subtypes, and for other disorders is described under the section Indications. Although there are some differences in efficacy across the class of antidepressants for subtypes of depression and for OCD, the major clinically significant differences among the antidepressants are in their side effects. All of the TCAs and related compounds (maprotiline and amoxapine) cause some degree of anticholinergic side effects and postural hypotension, and all are potentially cardiotoxic in susceptible individuals or in overdose (Table 3.4). The consensus among experts in formulating depression treatment guidelines is that the first line of treatment should be a newer antidepressant (e.g., SSRI) in light of safety and tolerability concerns over the long-term. Although the SSRIs and venlafaxine may initially cause agitation, insomnia, nausea, and headache, and, over time, sexual dysfunction, among other side effects, they are generally more tolerable to patients than the older cyclic compounds. The MAOIs may cause significant side effects, including postural hypotension, and require dietary and drug interaction precautions.

At a minimum, general physicians should be comfortable prescribing at least two of the SSRIs, and at least one of the other newer agents. Because psychiatrists will often be called on to treat patients who have failed initial treatments, they should have broader experience, including experience with newer agents, tricyclics, and MAOIs. The following are general guidelines for choosing an antidepressant:

1. It is reasonable to prescribe a drug that was clearly effective in the past if it was well tolerated by the patient.
2. Avoid drugs (e.g., amitriptyline, protriptyline) with the highest levels of anticholinergic activity to maximize patient comfort and compliance. (Despite its high anticholinergic potency, clomipramine is useful because of its superior efficacy in treating OCD and possibly for severe depression.)
3. For patients with initial insomnia, some clinicians still select a sedating tricyclic compound (e.g., amitriptyline) given at bedtime. To avoid anticholinergic and cardiovascular side effects, however, the sleep-enhancing, newer agents mirtazapine or nefazodone would be preferred, with the expectation

that daytime sedation will abate over time with these medications. An alternative to prescribing a sedating antidepressant is the **temporary** use of a benzodiazepine or other hypnotic combined with an SSRI, with the expectation of tapering and discontinuing the hypnotic when the depression has improved. The sedating tricyclic drug amitriptyline has long been popular with physicians, but because it is among the most anticholinergic of the tricyclics, it should not be a first-choice agent. Trazodone, which lacks anticholinergic side effects, is very sedating, but its overall efficacy as monotherapy for depression is in question. Trazodone (50–300 mg at bedtime) has been used in place of a benzodiazepine to treat initial insomnia in patients treated for depression with an SSRI. For most depressed patients, if insomnia is related to depression, the sleep difficulties will improve with any effective antidepressant over time, even those without sedation as a side effect. With more sedating drugs, on the other hand, the side effect may persist after it is helpful and may interfere with daytime function and compliance.

4. The tricyclics are available generically and have the advantage of being the least costly treatments in terms of formulary cost. When one considers the other direct and indirect costs of treatment, however, the financial savings of the older agents disappears.

5. For patients who want to avoid sedation, the SSRIs are usually nonsedating, but bupropion, reboxetine, and venlafaxine are typically less so. Among the tricyclics, desipramine and nortriptyline are the least sedating.

6. In elderly patients, especially those with constipation or glaucoma, and in men with prostatic hypertrophy, the least anticholinergic drugs should be used, such as an SSRI or other newer agent. Among the tricyclics, desipramine and nortriptyline have lower but still significant anticholinergic potency.

7. The SSRIs bupropion, mirtazapine, reboxetine, and venlafaxine generally do not cause postural hypotension, whereas the older agents, tricyclics, and MAOIs have this risk. Some postural hypotension is associated with trazodone and less with nefazodone. Nortriptyline may have an advantage among the tricyclics in causing relatively less postural hypotension than the others (although this observation has been debated). The tricyclics have on rare occasion been associated with hypertension and at higher doses a small percentage of patients may have blood pressure elevation with venlafaxine.

8. In patients with cardiac disease or delay in intracardiac conduction, the tricyclics with their quinidine-like properties should be avoided.

9. Epileptic patients may develop a primary depressive disorder or secondary depression. Because all of the tricyclic and related cyclic antidepressants and bupropion may decrease the seizure threshold, the use of an SSRI or other newer agent is preferable. When combining any antidepressant with an anticonvulsant, the clinician must be alert for pharmacokinetic interactions.

Table 3.4. Antidepressants

Category and Drug	Sedative Potency	Anticholinergic Potency	Orthostatic Hypotensive Potency	Usual Adult Daily Dose (mg/day)	Dosage Rate (mg/day)
Selective serotonin reuptake inhibitors					
Citalopram	Low	Very low	Very low	20–40	20–80
Fluoxetine	Very low	Very low	Very low	20	10–80
Paroxetine	Low	Low	Very low	20	10–50
Sertraline	Very low	Very low	Very low	100–150	50–200
Other new-generation antidepressants					
Bupropion	None	Very low	Very low	300–450	200–450
Mirtazapine	High	Very low	Very low	30–45	15–45
Nefazodone	Moderate	Very low	Moderate	300–600	150–600
Reboxetine	Very low	Very low	Very low	8–10	4–12
Trazodone[a]	High	Very low	High	150–400	150–600
Venlafaxine	Low	Very low	[b]	75–225	75–375

Tricyclic and related cyclic compounds[c]

Amitriptyline	High	Very high	High	150–200	75–300
Amoxapine	Low	Moderate	Moderate	150–200	75–300
Clomipramine	High	High	High	150–200	75–250
Desipramine	Low	Moderate (lowest of the tricyclics)	Moderate	150–200	75–300
Doxepin	High	High	Moderate	150–200	75–300
Imipramine	Moderate	High	High	150–200	75–300
Maprotiline	Moderate	Low	Moderate	150–200	75–225
Nortriptyline	Moderate	Moderate	Lowest of the tricyclics	75–100	40–150
Protriptyline	Low	High	Low	30	15–60
Trimipramine	High	Moderate	Moderate	150–200	75–300
Monoamine oxidase inhibitors					
Isocarboxazid	—	Very low	High	30	20–60
Phenelzine	Low	Very low	High	60–75	30–90
Tranylcypromine	—	Very low	High	30	20–90

[a]Trazodone has been associated with cardiac arrhythmias and priapism.
[b]Venlafaxine causes dose-dependent increases in blood pressure in some individuals.
[c]All of the tricyclic and related cyclic compounds have well-established cardiac arrhythmogenic potential.

10. Most antidepressants may cause or worsen sexual dysfunction. The tricyclics have mainly been associated with erectile difficulties in men. The SSRIs, venlafaxine, and MAOIs are more likely to cause delayed orgasm or anorgasmia in men and women. (This side effect may prove a benefit in men with premature ejaculation.) Decreased libido also may occur. Trazodone has been associated with the serious, but uncommon, occurrence of priapism in males. Bupropion, nefazodone, reboxetine, and mirtazapine are the antidepressants least associated with sexual dysfunction.

11. Two cyclic compounds that we do not recommend are rarely used. Maprotiline has produced a high incidence of seizures at dosages above 200 mg/day (and occasionally at lower dosages), possibly limiting the prescription of adequate therapeutic doses. Amoxapine has neuroleptic effects, making it analogous to a combination drug containing both an antipsychotic and an antidepressant, but one in which the physician has no control over the ratio. In addition, the presence of neuroleptic side effects and risks with amoxapine, such as akathisia, can needlessly complicate therapy.

12. In general, fixed combination drugs, such as those older compounds that contained a tricyclic and an antipsychotic drug or a tricyclic and a benzodiazepine are not recommended because they do not allow optimal titration of the component drugs for any given patient.

13. The majority of patients seeking treatment for depression will have one or more comorbid conditions; the comorbid disorder should influence initial treatment selection in choosing an agent thought to be efficacious for the comorbid condition as well as the depression, as with SSRIs and OCD or bupropion and attention-deficit disorder.

SELECTIVE SEROTONIN REUPTAKE INHIBITORS

The recognition that specific neuronal uptake mechanisms for serotonin were present in the CNS suggested, as early as the late 1960s, a potential target for the development of antidepressants. By the early 1970s, the technology existed for the screening of molecules that could selectively inhibit serotonin uptake. In 1972, fluoxetine was shown to produce selective inhibition of serotonin uptake in rat synaptosomes. This drug, the first of a class that includes sertraline, paroxetine, citalopram, and fluvoxamine, was approved for release in the United States in December 1987. The impact of this class of drugs on the treatment of depression has been extraordinary, with, for example, more than 30 million people prescribed fluoxetine. The success of these drugs appeared to derive mainly from side effect advantages over older agents. The absence of anticholinergic, antihistaminergic, anti-α–adrenergic, weight gain, and cardiotoxic effects and potential for lethality in overdose generated wide patient and prescriber acceptance. This milder side effect profile made the delivery of adequate antidepressant doses available to patients for both acute and long-term treatment without the need for dose titration and the endurance of persisting unpleasant or dangerous side effects. The SSRIs are by no means free of side effects, but they appear to be more tolerable than those of the older drugs, and some patients are virtually free of any daily medication-related discomforts. The side effects of SSRIs include occasional initial anxiety or agitation, nausea and other gastrointestinal symptoms, and headaches in the short term and sexual dysfunction and occasionally apathy in the long term. Changes in libido or delayed ejaculation or anorgasmia may affect one third or more of patients on SSRIs. Although these side effects occasionally remit spontaneously, they frequently persist over time. As an alternative to switching drugs, anecdotal reports have touted an array of sexual dysfunction antidotes, including yohimbine (ranging from 2.7 mg as needed to 5.4 mg three times daily), amantadine (100–200 mg/day), cyproheptadine (4–8 mg/day, although this risks transient loss of antidepressant effect), adjunctive use of antidepressants that are not associated with sexual dysfunction such as bupropion, mirtazapine, or nefazodone, buspirone, sildenafil, gingko biloba, and cholinergics, and even stimulants. Although these are class-related side effects, some patients will tolerate one agent better than another or not suffer a particular adverse effect with a different SSRI. For example, the rates of sexual dysfunction appear to be higher on paroxetine than others. Although the SSRIs as a class tend to be weight neutral, especially over the short term, some weight gain may occur on occasion over the long-term. The average weight gain in the first months of treatment appears slightly higher with paroxetine than with sertraline or fluoxetine, and the likelihood of significant weight gain (>7% increase over baseline) over time is also higher on paroxetine than the other SSRIs. The majority of patients who report a history of treatment failure due to intolerance of one SSRI actually respond to treatment with a second SSRI.

Plasma levels of SSRIs have not been shown to correlate with efficacy and thus are not useful for therapeutic monitoring other than for compliance or to establish the safety of beginning an MAOI trial following treatment discontinuation of an SSRI.

Before Beginning SSRIs

A recent medical history, physical examination, and, if appropriate, laboratory work such as thyroid function tests should be accomplished for any patient newly diagnosed with depression. However, there are no medical tests specifically required before administering SSRIs. It is important to discuss fully with patients the common side effects that might occur, informing and reassuring the patient in this manner help the individual understand the physical symptoms that may be experienced and will enhance compliance. As with all antidepressants, it is important to stress to patients that onset of therapeutic benefit is most often delayed by several weeks and that the drugs are not effective if taken on an as-needed basis.

Drug Interactions with SSRIs

Given the similarities in efficacy across the SSRIs, the drug interaction profile has been marketed by some companies as a basis for discriminating the agent of first choice within the class. Concern about drug interactions, however, is pertinent to patients taking medications of narrow therapeutic margins that are metabolized by isoenzymes inhibited by the SSRI and if the prescriber is unfamiliar with or unable to determine the appropriate dose adjustment. Reports of clinically significant interactions with the SSRIs are remarkably rare, given their vast availability. Among the SSRIs, citalopram has the most favorable profile with respect to inhibition *in vitro* of CYP450 isoenzyme systems. Of the isoenzymes of most interest in predicting psychiatric drug–drug interactions (e.g., with tricyclics, antipsychotics, β blockers) the CYP450 2D6 isoenzyme is inhibited by fluoxetine and its metabolites, by paroxetine, and less so by sertraline. However, for all of the SSRIs, some vigilance is reasonable concerning the possibility of increased therapeutic or toxic effects of other coprescribed drugs metabolized by P450 2D6. In particular, if combining a tricyclic with an SSRI, the tricyclic should be initiated with low doses, and plasma levels should be monitored. Given the high capacity of the CYP450 3A3/3A4 system, inhibition of this isoenzyme is not a major concern for the SSRIs, although fluvoxamine and less so fluoxetine can inhibit it to some extent. Of little importance to drug interactions is the high rate of protein binding of the SSRIs because if other drugs are displaced from carrier proteins, the result is simply an increase in the rate and amount of free drug being metabolized.

Use in the Elderly

Elderly patients generally tolerate the side effects of the SSRIs (and other newer agents) better than they tolerate the anticholinergic and cardiovascular side effects of the tricyclic and related cyclic antidepressants. However, the elderly may have alterations in hepatic metabolic pathways, especially so-called phase I reactions, which include demethylation and hydroxylation, which are involved in the metabolism of both SSRIs and cyclic antidepressants. In addition, renal function may be decreased, and there may be increased end-organ sensitivity to the effects of antidepressant compounds. Because the elimination half-life of the SSRIs, cyclic antidepressants, and other antidepressants can be expected to be significantly greater than what it is in younger patients, accumulation of active drug will be greater and occur more slowly. Clinically this means that the elderly should be started on lower doses, that dosage increases should be slower, and that the ultimate therapeutic dose may be lower than in younger patients. However, given the wide margin of safety of the newer drugs, full-dose treatment in older patients, if tolerated, is required before considering treatment to have failed.

Use in Pregnancy

There is accumulating information about the use of SSRIs in pregnancy, although the bulk of available data is on fluoxetine. One prospective study of 128 pregnant women who took fluoxetine, 10 to 80 mg/day (mean 25.8 mg), during their first trimester did not find elevated rates of major malformations compared with matched groups of women taking tricyclics or drugs thought not to be teratogenic. There was a higher, albeit not statistically significant, rate of miscarriages in the fluoxetine (13.5%) and tricyclic (12.2%) groups compared with the women exposed to known nonteratogenic drugs (6.8%). Whether this increased rate of miscarriages is biologically significant and, if so, whether it relates to the drugs or to the depressive disorder could not be determined from this study. Decisions on continuing antidepressant drugs during pregnancy must be individualized, but it must be recalled that the effects of **severe** untreated depression on maternal and fetal health may be far worse than the unknown risks of fluoxetine or tricyclic drugs. A large registry of fluoxetine exposure during pregnancy is consistent with generally reassuring data from the tricyclic era that antidepressant agents are not evidently teratogens. Follow-up studies of children exposed *in utero* to fluoxetine were also reassuring, with an absence of any signal of interference with child development observed. That said, where possible, unnecessary exposure to any drug should be minimized, and thoughtful prepregnancy treatment planning and consideration of alternative interventions such as psychotherapies (e.g., cognitive behavior therapy [CBT]) are to be recommended. An alternative for severe depression that also appears to be safe is ECT.

Specific Drugs

Overall the SSRIs have similar side effect profiles and spectrum of efficacy. However, there are some differences meriting individual discussion.

Fluoxetine

Fluoxetine is clearly effective for major depression. There are anecdotal data that it may have particular advantages (as do MAOIs) over tricyclics in treating atypical depression (discussed previously). Questions remain as to whether SSRIs are as effective as tricyclics in the most serious melancholic depressions. Given the broad spectrum of mood and anxiety and other disorders for which SSRIs have proved useful, they might be considered psychopatholytics more than just antidepressants, with fluoxetine having a reported therapeutic role, in addition to depression and its subtypes, in OCD, PTSD, premenstrual syndrome and PMDD (premenstrual dysphoric disorder), panic disorder, social phobia, and bulimia. Fluoxetine is usually begun at a dosage of 20 mg/day given in a single daily dose. It is generally given in the morning because for some patients it may have an activating profile, although initial sedation is actually as likely as activation. Doses greater than 20 mg may be given in a single dose or divided. Although an initial antidepressant effect usually emerges within 2 to 4 weeks, remission will often require 6 to 12 weeks. For that reason and because of its half-life (2–4 days on average for fluoxetine and 7–9 days for its active metabolite norfluoxetine), it is reasonable to wait at least 4 weeks before increasing the dose.

Some patients may respond to doses as low as 5 mg/day. Therefore, patients with poorly tolerated side effects on 20 mg may use 10-mg capsules, mix their capsule contents in liquid, and take lower-dose aliquots or take fluoxetine every other day, which is possible because of its long half-life. Alternatively, patients may switch to another SSRI. Dosages of 60 to 80 mg/day may be required for OCD and bulimia, but 20 to 40 mg/day is usually adequate for depression. Use of the lowest effective dose will minimize side effects and therefore increase patient compliance. There is some evidence that maintenance treatment for some patients can be accomplished with a single weekly dose of 60 to 90 mg. Fluoxetine was the first antidepressant to demonstrate efficacy in the treatment of depression in children and adolescents.

The side effect of fluoxetine most likely to interfere with treatment acceptance initially is agitation, which may include neuromuscular restlessness (which resembles akathisia) and insomnia. If not mild, transient, and tolerated, this discomfort may respond to a dosage reduction or to temporary administration of a β-adrenergic blocker or benzodiazepine. Anecdotally, clonazepam, 0.25 to 0.5 mg twice daily, in particular has proven helpful for initial treatment with fluoxetine. Trazodone, 50 mg at bedtime, has proved superior to placebo for SSRI- or bupropion-induced insomnia. Clonazepam, 0.5 to 1.0 mg at bedtime, is an alternative. Some patients receiving both fluoxetine and trazodone complain of a loss of mental clarity. A minority of patients may develop daytime sedation from fluoxetine. Sexual dysfunction may occur in both men and women, most frequently delayed ejaculation or anorgasmia, which may lead to drug discontinuation by some patients. Unlike the cyclic antidepressants, fluoxetine does not appear to cause weight gain; some patients, especially those on higher doses, may lose weight. Fluoxetine may precipitate mania in bipolar patients. Other side effects include nausea, headache, and diarrhea.

The potential for drug–drug interactions should be recalled because it may remain a consideration for several weeks after treatment discontinuation given the drug's long half-life. Fluoxetine should not be used with MAOIs; because of its long half-life, fluoxetine should be discontinued 5 weeks before starting an MAOI. Its long half-life mitigates against symptoms induced by abrupt discontinuation, which have been reported with shorter acting SSRIs. These include dizziness, flulike symptoms, insomnia, nausea, or marked reemergence (rebound) of mood or anxiety symptoms. A major advantage of fluoxetine and other SSRIs and other newer agents is that these newer drugs are far less dangerous than cyclic antidepressants or MAOIs when taken in overdose.

Sertraline

Sertraline, like fluoxetine, is an SSRI effective for the treatment of major depression. Sertraline's spectrum of efficacy appears to be similar, with efficacy in panic disorder, OCD, social phobia, dysthymia, and atypical depressive disorders. Its efficacy and side effects in general clinical practice suggest a similar profile to other SSRIs. The half-life of sertraline is shorter than that of fluoxetine, approximately 25 hours; it has a less potently active metabolite with a half-life of 60 to 70 hours.

Sertraline is begun at 50 mg/day with a target dosage of at least 100 mg/day in healthy adults. The dosage range is 50 to 200 mg in single or divided daily doses. Compared with fluoxetine, it may have more gastrointestinal (nausea, diarrhea, and upper gastrointestinal symptoms) and less activating effects in some patients. Like fluoxetine, sertraline lacks the anticholinergic and cardiovascular side effects of cyclic antidepressants and is far less dangerous than cyclic antidepressants or MAOIs in overdose. Sertraline does not appear to cause weight gain. The most commonly reported side effects are nausea, diarrhea, agitation, and sexual dysfunction (delayed ejaculation in males or anorgasmia in males and females). Sertraline can precipitate mania. It should not be used with an MAOI. The recommended washout period before starting an MAOI is 14 days. For some prescribers, sertraline offers a reasonable choice because of its intermediate half-life and relatively favorable drug interaction profile. The optimum daily dose for treatment of depression tends to require titration to 100 mg or higher.

Paroxetine

Paroxetine was the third SSRI approved in the United States for major depression but the first to obtain approval by the FDA for use in the treatment of panic disorder. Consistent with this indication, its marketing tends to target the anxious depressed patient, although clinical trials do not demonstrate differential efficacy for this subtype across the SSRI class. As with other SSRIs, its relative efficacy, compared with the tricyclics, for the most serious cases of major depression with melancholia has been called into question (e.g., when clomipramine proved superior in one study of severely depressed inpatients). This finding more likely reflected the efficacy of clomipramine in this population, however, rather than that of tricyclics as a class. Paroxetine's spectrum of efficacy is similar to that of other SSRIs, and it has proved effective at higher doses in OCD and social phobia.

Paroxetine is begun at 20 mg in a single morning dose; elderly patients or those with serious hepatic or renal dysfunction should start at 10 mg daily. Patients who do not respond after 4 weeks can be increased to up to 50 mg/day or 40 mg/day in the elderly. For panic disorder, doses of up to 60 mg have proven efficacious.

Paroxetine has a side effect profile similar to that of other SSRIs in clinical trials but has been observed in some patients to be somewhat more sedating. Paroxetine also has been reported to cause more constipation than other SSRIs, presumed secondary to its anticholinergic potential. Other side effects are similar to those of other SSRIs, including insomnia or somnolence, nausea, asthenia, tremor, and delayed ejaculation or anorgasmia. The potential for weight gain and sexual dysfunction appears to be slightly greater with paroxetine than other drugs of the class. As an SSRI with a relatively shorter half-life and perhaps because it has nonlinear kinetics (it is a substrate and inhibitor of CYP450 2D6, thereby inhibiting its own metabolism at higher doses), paroxetine is the SSRI most associated with difficulties with abrupt discontinuation; therefore, taper upon termination after chronic treatment is essential to prevent patient distress. Paroxetine may enhance the effects of anticoagulants such as warfarin, suggesting the need for close monitoring of such patients. Paroxetine should not be given with an MAOI; the washout period before starting an MAOI is 14 days.

Citalopram

Citalopram was introduced to the U.S. market in late 1998, although it had been widely available for several years in the rest of the world. As the most selective of the SSRIs (lacking meaningful other pharmacodynamic effects besides uptake inhibition of the serotonin transporter), it has a favorable SSRI side effect profile, with low rates of anxiety or insomnia; nausea is the principal adverse effect to anticipate with the patient, and as with other SSRIs, it can be expected to resolve within days. Citalopram is used for the same spectrum of indications as the other SSRIs, including panic disorder and OCD. Its interaction with the CYP450 systems suggests that it is the least likely of the SSRIs to be associated with pharmacokinetic drug–drug interactions; its intermediate half-life of over 30 hours and linear kinetics predicts that discontinuation syndromes will be less than those with shorter half-lives. It does not appear likely to offer particular advantages with respect to sexual dysfunction.

The dose range for citalopram is 20 to 60 mg, with the higher dose used in the treatment of OCD. Dosing of citalopram usually begins with a single dose of 20 mg, but this can be reduced to 10 mg in the event of initial nausea. An adequate antidepressant dose for some will be 20 mg, but others will do better on or require 40 mg. Elderly patients with depressive illness appear to tolerate citalopram well, and the daily dosing range in this population is typically 20 to 40 mg.

Acceptance of citalopram was initially influenced by concerns about cardiac and overdose toxicity. The cardiac concern was based on observations of chronic high-dose toxicity studies in beagles that on investigation turned out to be a breed-specific issue of no relevance to humans, as evidenced by citalopram's FDA approval. The rare overdose deaths reported on very high dose ingestion, on review of all SSRIs, also did not implicate a citalopram-specific concern.

Fluvoxamine

Although fluvoxamine has been introduced into the United States with the labeled indication for OCD only, clinical trial data and clinical experience would predict a spectrum of efficacy similar to that of other SSRIs, including efficacy for depression. It is usually initiated in a single dose beginning with 50 mg, building up to a usual therapeutic range of 150 to 250 mg. It has a half-life of 15 hours. Its most common side effects are nausea, vomiting (apparently at a greater frequency than other SSRIs), headache, and insomnia or sedation. It is likely to cause sexual dysfunction but possibly less than the other SSRIs. Fluvoxamine may offer some drug drug interaction challenges because it inhibits CYP450 1A2, 2C9, and 3A4. As with all SSRIs, combination with MAOIs is to be avoided.

Augmentation and Combination Strategies with SSRIs

When one takes into consideration the number of patients who fail to achieve full remission with an initial adequate antidepressant trial, added to those who do not improve at all plus those who lose benefit in the continuation or maintenance phase of treatment, it is evident that the majority of depressed patients will require a next step in their treatment. Whereas for some patients higher doses or medication switches will be effective, many clinicians will use instead an augmentation or combination strategy. Although the usual goal of augmentation of combination treatment is to convert partial responders or nonresponders to full response or remission, some strategies also have been used to accelerate response, that is, to diminish the latency to response. Because augmentation and combination strategies appear to work quickly (in days rather than weeks), they have the potential to spare the patient the time and distress associated with washout or taper and start of a new treatment. Many of the strategies favored by clinicians are not supported by published clinical trials, but very large trials to examine these practices are underway in the United States. Some commonly used strategies are briefly reviewed below.

Lithium

Lithium is combined with antidepressants in two major instances: (a) treatment of acute bipolar depression as prophylaxis against a switch into mania and (b) augmentation of an antidepressant response. The latter is a very well studied and supported application with tricyclics. Patients who are poorly responsive to SSRIs, TCAs, or MAOIs may benefit from addition of lithium (usually at a plasma level of 0.4 mEq/L or higher). Approximately half of patients on tricyclics may improve with a time course of several days to several weeks. Lithium augmentation of SSRIs has not been as enthusiastically endorsed a strategy as with tricyclics, and some data suggest that the response is in fact more robust and enduring with tricyclics than with SSRIs. (See Chapter 4 for a more extensive discussion.)

L-Triiodothyronine

Another well-studied strategy with incomplete responders to tricyclics is use of T_3, 25 to 50 μg/day. The majority of responders are said to have had normal baseline thyroid function. In some reports, responders have more often been female with prominent fatigue or psychomotor retardation. When this treatment is successful, some improvement is usually seen within 2 weeks and maximal improvement within 4 weeks. Clinicians have been less impressed with this augmentation in SSRI-treated patients, favoring a number of other combination treatments.

Addition of a Second Antidepressant

The observation that some patients being transitioned from a TCA to an SSRI after a poor response to the former dramatically improved on the combination led to trials of adding low doses of secondary amine tricyclics such as desipramine or nortriptyline to partial responders or nonresponders on SSRIs. Beginning with doses as low as 10 mg of the tricyclic and ranging up to 75 mg, this combination was accepted in clinical practice as an intervention for treatment resistance or loss of benefit with SSRI therapy. Other work had suggested the possibility of a more rapid antidepressant response for some patients on a combination of fluoxetine and desipramine. Even though tricyclic doses used in this strategy are low, plasma level monitoring is recommended, because some patients will achieve substantial and possibly toxic tricyclic levels due to SSRI-induced inhibition of hepatic metabolism of the tricyclic. Surveys of practitioners indicate, however, that the early enthusiasm for this combination has waned, with greater current interest in SSRI combinations with other newer agents. For example, bupropion added to an SSRI, in some cases originally for management of sexual dysfunction, has been observed to offer an effective antidepressant regimen. The doses of bupropion used range from 100 mg a day up to full antidepressant doses. Reports of seizures with the combination are rare. The main limiting adverse effects are jitteriness and insomnia. The combination of an SSRI with bupropion also has been helpful for SSRI-induced apathy, comorbid attention-deficit disorder, and sexual dysfunction. Mirtazapine added to SSRIs also has been observed to increase response, occasionally benefit sexual dysfunction, and improve sleep. There is considerable interest in the potential of reboxetine, the selective norepinephrine reuptake inhibitor (NRI), to boost antidepressant response and to improve energy and motivation when combined with an SSRI. MAOIs should never be combined with SSRIs or with clomipramine because of the high risk of severe CNS toxicity (the so-called serotonin syndrome) and death.

Other Augmentation and Combination Strategies

Clinical practice, if not systematic study, has embraced a number of other potential pharmacologic additions to ongoing SSRI therapy for incomplete or poor responders, including psychostimulants, a dopamine agonist, and buspirone. Although psychostimulants may raise plasma levels of antidepressants somewhat, the improvement seen with stimulant addition is more likely due to enhancement of dopaminergic or noradrenergic neurotransmission. Effective stimulant doses are usually determined empirically but typically are in the range of 2.5 to 10.0 mg of dextroamphetamine twice daily or 10 mg twice daily to 20 mg three times daily for methylphenidate. Stimulant abuse has not been reported with this strategy, but circumspection is in order in treating those with past history of cocaine or stimulant abuse. Adequate long-term follow-up reports are not available; however, use of stimulants is not recommended in patients who have agitation or insomnia while receiving an SSRI. Other clinical strategies based on the potential benefit of enhancing dopaminergic mechanisms have been used by some clinicians, including limited success with bromocriptine, and pergolide, but some positive anecdotes with amantadine and especially pramipexole to augment antidepressant effects, but there are no systematic data demonstrating efficacy. Controlled trials of buspirone augmentation have been mixed, but the agent appears to have potential for accelerating or enhancing response to SSRIs. The atypical β blocker pindolol, in light of its antagonism of the 5-HT$_{1A}$ receptor, was hypothesized to enhance serotonergic activity and to serve as an augmentor of SSRIs. Studies and reports suggest that at doses of 2.5 to 5 mg three times daily the drug may accelerate initial response for some patients, but its efficacy in partial responders or nonresponders is doubtful. Of interest, a number of the antidepressant combinations have some potential to improve SSRI-induced sexual dysfunction such as bupropion, mirtazapine, dopaminergic agents, psychostimulants, and buspirone.

OTHER NEWER ANTIDEPRESSANTS

Bupropion

Bupropion is a phenelthylamine compound that is effective for the treatment of depression. Bupropion is structurally related to amphetamine and the sympathomimetic diethylpropion. Thus, it is not surprising that it has been reported to possess some stimulant-like effects when used for depression.

Patients are generally begun on 100 mg twice daily with an increase to 100 mg three times daily as tolerated. An initial antidepressant effect becomes apparent within 2 to 4 weeks. Although the agent is usually well tolerated, patients may develop agitation, restlessness, insomnia, and anxiety or gastrointestinal distress soon after initiation of treatment. Should agitation occur, the dosage can be temporarily decreased, or an adjunctive benzodiazepine may be administered. For insomnia due to bupropion, as for the SSRIs, clonazepam 0.5 mg or trazodone 50 to 150 mg orally at bedtime is usually effective. Patients who do not improve may have their bupropion dose increased to as high as 450 mg/day. Because of the risk of seizures, it is recommended that the total daily dose of bupropion be no higher than 450 mg and that no individual dose of the original bupropion formulation be higher than 150 mg; doses of 150 mg should be given no more frequently than every 4 hours. The incidence of seizures appears to be 0.4%, which is slightly higher than other marketed antidepressants. A sustained-release preparation of bupropion is available in 100- and 150-mg tablets that appears to reduce acute side effects and increase the safety of single doses up to 200 mg. Despite the absence of controlled trials, bupropion has become a popular combination treatment with SSRIs and venlafaxine.

Bupropion lacks anticholinergic properties and does not cause postural hypotension or alter cardiac conduction in a clinically significant manner. Although its CYP450 profile is not well characterized, bupropion appears to have CYP450 2D6 inhibition potential, which suggests that, when it is combined with fluoxetine or paroxetine, both 2D6 substrates, levels of the SSRI will increase. Compared with SSRIs, bupropion has the advantage of not being associated with sexual dysfunction; in fact, anecdotal reports impute libido-enhancing potential to this drug. Case reports and one small clinical trial also suggest that bupropion has lower risk than other antidepressants of precipitating mania for patients with bipolar depression and for rapid-cycling bipolar II patients, in particular. On the other hand, bupropion has been associated with switch into mania in some patients. Bupropion is not approved for use in patients with anorexia or bulimia because such patients were reported to have a very high incidence of seizures in prerelease studies. Its stimulant-like appetite-suppressing properties, however, may make it particularly useful for depressed patients who have hyperphagia or who have excessive weight gain when treated with standard TCAs. Under a different brand name, bupropion is marketed as a treatment to enhance smoking cessation, and it appears to be more efficacious for this indication than the nicotine patch.

Rare instances of ataxia, myoclonus, and dystonia have been reported. There are reports of bupropion causing psychotic symptoms and cognitive interference, but the incidence appears to be very low.

Venlafaxine   EFFEXOR

Introduced in the United States in 1994, venlafaxine at higher doses inhibits the uptake of both norepinephrine and serotonin. At lower doses (<150 mg) the drug acts essentially like an SSRI with a very short half-life. At higher doses, venlafaxine appears to recruit its noradrenergic mechanism. In this sense, it is like using an SSRI with a built-in combination treatment option accessed by increasing the dose if the first trial is ineffective. Venlafaxine lacks anticholinergic, antihistaminergic, and α_1-adrenergic blocking effects. Venlafaxine is metabolized by cytochrome P450 2D6, of which it is also a very weak inhibitor. Drugs that inhibit this enzyme may increase venlafaxine concentrations. Venlafaxine has a most favorable profile with respect to the CYP450 system in that it is not a meaningful inhibitor of the isoenzymes pertinent to drug metabolism. The half-lives of venlafaxine and its active metabolite o-desmethyl-venlafaxine are about 5 and 11 hours, respectively. The drug and this metabolite reach steady state in plasma within 3 days in healthy adults, and discontinuation must be accompanied by a very gradual taper to reduce the risk of intense discontinuation discomfort. Although many patients find that the recently introduced extended-release preparation reduced initial treatment-emergent adverse effects (e.g., nausea), the newer formulation would not be expected to extend the half-life or reduce the need for vigilance when discontinuing treatment.

The usual dosage range is 75 to 225 mg given in divided doses on a twice-daily schedule. Dosages as high as 450 mg/day have been used in seriously ill depressed inpatients. Although the extended-release form has only been labeled for use of up to 225 mg/day, there is no pharmacologic reason to limit treatment below the range of the immediate-release preparation (e.g., up to 375–450 mg/day if necessary).

The safety and side effect profile of venlafaxine is generally similar to that of the SSRIs. Anxiety or nervousness may emerge or worsen on initiation of treatment. Other side effects include nausea, insomnia, sedation, dizziness, and constipation. Unlike the SSRIs, but more like the tricyclics, venlafaxine may cause sweating. At the higher doses, 5% to 7% of patients may develop a modest but persisting increase in blood pressure. Thus, baseline blood pressure screening and periodic rechecks after upward titration of the dose should be performed. SSRI-like sexual side effects are observed with venlafaxine. Like other newer agents, venlafaxine is safer in overdose than older agents.

Some treatment-resistant depressed patients with well-documented treatment failures on prior antidepressant therapies have done well in one open study with venlafaxine treatment. Venlafaxine represents an alternative to tricyclics and is considered to have a similar efficacy profile but a more favorable acute and long-term side effect burden. Some clinical trial data suggest that the rate of remission with venlafaxine can be higher than for some of the SSRIs, but this claim remains controversial. Low doses (75 mg) of venlafaxine have been proven to be efficacious for generalized anxiety disorder, an indication for which FDA approval has been received in 1999. Its effects on blood pressure have not proven to be an obstacle to its use in clinical practice. For partial responders to venlafaxine, for those who lose benefit on it, or for very resistant cases, the same augmentation strategies as described for SSRIs can be considered (e.g., addition of mirtazapine to venlafaxine). Venlafaxine should be stopped 14 days prior to initiating therapy with an MAOI, and, again, stopping should always be done with a gradual taper.

Nefazodone

Nefazodone is a phenylpiperazine compound chemically similar to trazodone but with less α_1-adrenergic blocking properties and also less sedation and with no evident risk of priapism. Nefazodone weakly inhibits serotonin (and somewhat norepinephrine) uptake but is principally a blocker of postsynaptic 5-HT_2 serotonin receptors. The half-life of nefazodone is approximately 5 hours. Its most common side effects are headache, dry mouth, and nausea.

The usual starting dosage is 50 mg/day given at bedtime, titrated up in the absence of daytime sedation as rapidly as tolerated to achieve a usually effective antidepressant dosage in the 450 to 600 mg/day range. Slower dose titration is recommended in the elderly. Anxiety symptoms and insomnia often improve before the onset of an antidepressant effect. Its safety and side effect profile includes the potential for nausea, dry mouth, somnolence, dizziness, constipation, asthenia, and light-headedness. Sedation interferes most with rapid attainment of an effective antidepressant dose. Unusual but occasional adverse effects include visual disturbances (e.g., palinopsia) and irritability (possibly related to its mCPP [m-Chlorophenylpiperazine] metabolite, which may occur in higher levels in the presence of a CYP450 2D6 inhibitor). Nefazodone itself is an inhibitor of the CYP450 3A4 isoenzyme and thus may increase alprazolam or triazolam levels. The drug is helpful for depression-associated insomnia and does not cause sexual dysfunction or weight gain. In addition to treatment of major depression, there are preliminary data suggesting the drug can be useful for panic disorder, social phobia, PTSD, and dysthymia. Given its lack of weight gain and sexual dysfunction effects, and enhancement of the quality of sleep, nefazodone has a suitable profile for patients over the long-term, advantages that may offset the longer initial titration often necessary to accommodate to sedation.

Mirtazapine

Mirtazapine, a piperazino-azepine compound similar to an older agent in use in Europe, mianserin, is a tetracyclic agent with a unique pharmacologic mechanism of action profile. As an antagonist at 5-HT_{2A} and 5-HT_{2C} receptors and at α_2-adrenergic autoreceptors, the molecule influences both serotonergic and noradrenergic systems. It also blocks 5-HT_3 and histamine receptors, but does not inhibit serotonin or norepinephrine reuptake, muscarinic cholinergic receptors, or a_1-adrenergic receptors. It is an efficacious antidepressant with some data to assert a somewhat faster onset of action than SSRIs based on comparison trials. It has minimal anticholinergic effects, is not associated with adverse cardiac effects, and has been safe in overdose. It is quite sedating, and thus, generally administered at bedtime, but residual sedation is for some a limiting side effect, although typically diminishing with patient accommodation over days. Presumably due to its histamine-blocking effects, it is associated with increased appetite and weight gain especially in a subgroup of patients composed of younger women with previously normal weight. If weight gain is not observed in the first few months of therapy, it is unlikely to emerge later as a problem. Severe neutropenia has been rarely reported (1 in 1,000) with uncertain relationship to the drug, but as with other psychotropics, the onset of infection and fever should prompt the patient to contact their physician. The drug is most efficacious at doses of 30 to 45 mg (although 60 mg/day has been used in refractory cases) usually given in a single bedtime dose. Available in 15- and 30-mg scored tablets, the lower dose may be suboptimal, and compared with 15 mg, the 30-mg dose also may be less or at least not more sedating, possibly as a consequence of the noradrenergic effects being recruited at that dose. Mirtazapine has been successfully combined with SSRIs and venlafaxine for partial responders or nonresponders to the other drugs. In addition to enhanced efficacy with the combination, some SSRI side effects (e.g., sexual dysfunction, nausea) have been observed to improve as a likely consequence of the 5-HT$_2$– and 5-HT$_3$–blocking properties of mirtazapine. There is interest in the use of the drug in pain-depression syndromes as an alternative to tricyclics.

Reboxetine

The expected introduction of reboxetine, an NRI, is associated with renewed interest in the role of the neurotransmitter norepinephrine in depression after years of focus on serotonin. Like the SSRIs, an NRI offers one mechanism of action characteristic of the tricyclics but without the array of unwanted mechanisms that generated adverse effects or safety concerns. Whether initiating the antidepressant mechanism cascade via a noradrenergic as opposed to serotonergic input can predictably be associated with a different therapeutic profile is unknown at this time, but there is interest in the possibility that a noradrenergic agent might have advantages for the melancholic patient or the severely ill lethargic, elderly patient with a depressive illness. Early clinical studies comparing reboxetine to fluoxetine suggested that the noradrenergic agent might offer certain advantages in improving motivation, energy, and social interaction, without sexual dysfunction, despite comparable antidepressant effect. This observation requires further study.

Reboxetine, a morpholine compound, is chemically unrelated to the other antidepressants. It is highly protein bound and has a plasma half-life of about 13 hours. The drug does not appear to be a meaningful inhibitor of the CYP450 system and is metabolized itself by CYP450 3A4 isozyme with two inactive metabolites. Clinical data indicate that reboxetine has comparable efficacy to the TCAs and SSRIs but some different side effects, particularly increased heart rate, urinary hesitancy, constipation, sweating, and some insomnia. Increased blood pressure might be expected from the drug's mechanism in some patients but has not been reported to be a problem. The urinary hesitancy and constipation do not reflect anticholinergic but rather are noradrenergic effects. The usual dose range for reboxetine is 4 to 5 mg twice daily. Lower doses (2 to 3 mg twice daily) are recommended in those with hepatic or renal insufficiency and in the elderly. The possibility of combining this selective noradrenergic agent with selective serotonergic agents for treatment-resistant depression is intriguing. Other indications, such as attention-deficit/hyperactivity disorder are being explored, but preliminary studies reveal efficacy in panic disorder.

Trazodone

Trazodone, a triazolopyridine derivative, is chemically unrelated to the tricyclics or MAOI antidepressants. Trazodone very weakly inhibits serotonin reuptake and appears to act mainly postsynaptically as a 5-HT$_2$ antagonist. It also may have psychoactive properties through its major metabolite, m-chlorophenylpiperazine (m-CPP), a postsynaptic serotonin agonist. Trazodone is also an α blocker, which likely contributes to such side effects as sedation and postural hypotension.

Trazodone is rapidly absorbed following oral administration, achieving peak levels in 1 to 2 hours. It has a relatively short elimination half-life of 3 to 9 hours and is excreted mainly in urine (75%); m-CPP has a similar pharmacokinetic profile. Despite the short half-life, once-daily dosing appears reasonable because its effectiveness is likely to reflect long-term neurochemical changes in the brain.

The therapeutic range for trazodone is 200 to 600 mg/day, although this has not been clearly delineated. Therapeutic blood levels have not been established. Generally, a patient can be started on 100 to 150 mg/day either in divided doses or in a single bedtime dose and gradually increased to 200 to 300 mg/day. For optimal benefit, doses in the range of 400 to 600 mg may be needed. Most clinicians question whether trazodone is as effective as other antidepressants and see it mainly as an adjunctive agent for sleep. Trazodone does appear to be useful in the treatment of SSRI-, bupropion-, and MAOI-induced insomnia in a dose range from 50 to 300 mg. Patients combining SSRIs or MAOIs with trazodone occasionally complain of mental clouding. Common side effects of trazodone include sedation, orthostatic hypotension, and less commonly nausea, and vomiting. Side effects may be lessened if the drug is taken in divided doses and with meals. Trazodone is generally safe in overdose.

Trazodone lacks the quinidine-like properties of the cyclic antidepressants but has been associated in rare cases with cardiac arrhythmias. Thus, trazodone should be used with caution in patients with known cardiac disease. The most common cardiovascular toxicity of trazodone is postural hypotension.

Priapism may rarely occur with trazodone, most commonly early in therapy. Men given trazodone should be instructed to report abnormally prolonged erections to their physician or go to an emergency room. Should priapism occur, the drug should be permanently discontinued. Perhaps by a similar mechanism, trazodone may prove useful in the treatment of impotence.

TRICYCLIC AND RELATED CYCLIC ANTIDEPRESSANTS

Chemistry

The tricyclic compounds were first developed in the 1950s. The antidepressant properties of imipramine, a structural analog of chlorpromazine, were discovered fortuitously when it was being tested as a potential antipsychotic compound. A number of tricyclic and closely related tetracyclic compounds have been developed. Although the antidepressant market has grown enormously since the release of fluoxetine and despite the displacement of the older agents as first-line treatment by the newer agents, the actual volume prescribed, as opposed to market share, of the tricyclics has not decreased.

Pharmacology

Most of the antidepressants are available only as oral preparations, although amitriptyline, imipramine, and clomipramine are also available for parenteral use. The parenteral forms are not clearly established as more rapidly acting or more effective than oral preparations; their advantage lies in the possibility of administering them to patients who cannot or will not take oral medication. For such patients, they may provide an alternative to ECT.

Oral preparations of tricyclics and related drugs are rapidly and completely absorbed from the gastrointestinal tract; a high percentage of an oral dose is metabolized by the liver as it passes through the portal circulation (first-pass effect). The tricyclics are metabolized by the microsomal enzymes of the liver; the tertiary amines are first monodemethylated to yield compounds that are still active. Indeed, the desmethyl metabolites of amitriptyline and imipramine are nortriptyline and desipramine, respectively, and are marketed as antidepressants. Other major metabolic pathways include hydroxylation (which may yield partially active compounds) and conjugation with glucuronic acid to produce inactive compounds.

Tricyclic drugs are highly lipophilic, meaning the free fraction passes easily into the brain and other tissues. They are also largely bound to plasma proteins. Given their lipophilicity and protein binding, they are not removed effectively by hemodialysis in cases of overdose. The time course of metabolism and elimination is biphasic, with approximately half of a dose removed over 48 to 72 hours and the remainder, strongly bound to tissues and plasma proteins, slowly excreted over several weeks. There is considerable variation among individuals in their metabolic rate for cyclic antidepressants based on genetic factors, age, and concomitantly taken drugs. In fact, when metabolic differences are combined with variation in the degree of protein binding, as much as a 300-fold difference in effective drug levels may be found among individuals.

Method of Use

Before Beginning Cyclic Antidepressants

A medical history and examination are indicated before beginning cyclic antidepressants, particularly to determine whether the patient has cardiac conduction system disease, which is the major medical contraindication to tricyclic use. An electrocardiogram (ECG) should be obtained for any patient with a history of cardiac symptoms or known cardiac disease; it is also reasonable as a screening test for patients over age 40. Although it appears that minor conduction system disease, such as first-degree heart block, does not increase the risk of serious sequelae from cyclic antidepressants, the presence of conduction system abnormalities favors the use of an SSRI, or other newer agents, as the first-choice drug. Aside from the ECG, no other tests are generally indicated in healthy adults before starting a tricyclic.

As described for the SSRIs, it is important to discuss fully with patients both common side effects of cyclic antidepressants and the expected lag period before therapeutic effects can be anticipated. Informing and reassuring the patient in this manner helps the individual understand the physical symptoms that may be experienced and may enhance compliance. It should be stressed to patients that the drugs cannot be taken on an as-needed basis and are only effective if taken as prescribed. It is important for the physician to be available during the first weeks of an antidepressant trial, both to monitor the development of side effects and to help the patient differentiate effects that may be transient (e.g., dry mouth or sedation) from effects that may be more serious (e.g., postural hypotension). In this manner, both serious toxicity and noncompliance may be avoided.

Prescribing Cyclic Antidepressants

Tricyclics are started at a low dose with gradual increase until the therapeutic range is achieved. Finding the right tricyclic dose for a patient often involves a process of trial and error. The most common error leading to treatment failure is inadequate dosage. In healthy adults, the typical starting dose is 50 mg of imipramine or the equivalent. Nortriptyline is about twice as potent; thus, its starting dose is 25 mg. In some clinical situations, especially in the elderly and patients with panic disorder, it may be necessary to start with lower doses (as low as 10 mg of imipramine or the equivalent) because of intolerance to side effects.

Generally, tricyclics are administered once a day at bedtime to help with compliance and, when the sedating compounds are used, to help with sleep. Divided doses are used if patients have side effects due to high peak levels. The dosage can be increased by 50 mg every 3 to 4 days, as side effects allow, up to a dose of 150 to 200 mg of imipramine or its equivalent at bedtime (Table 3.3).

If there is no therapeutic response in 3 to 4 weeks, the dosage should be slowly increased, again as side effects allow. The maximum dosage of most tricyclics is the equivalent of 300 mg/day of imipramine, although rare patients who metabolize the drug rapidly may do well on higher dosages. The final dosage chosen is that at which the patient has a therapeutic response without severe side effects. Elderly patients should initiate treatment with one third to one half the usual adult dose with longer intervals between dosage changes. If the patient has been on a maximal dose for 4 to 6 weeks without response, the drug trial should be considered a failure. Discontinuation of treatment should be done with a taper to minimize the risk of discontinuation symptoms, including gastrointestinal distress and dizziness.

Blood Levels

There has been considerable interest in antidepressant blood levels because of the marked interindividual differences in steady-state blood levels produced by any given oral dose. Many investigators have hoped to demonstrate a correlation between blood levels and therapeutic response analogous to the correlations that exist for digoxin, aminophylline, and anticonvulsants. Blood levels of tricyclic and other cyclic antidepressants are difficult to measure because the drugs circulate in very low concentrations. In general, current methods of analysis use gas chromatography, high-performance liquid chromatography, and radioimmunoassay. The literature on the relationship between antidepressant blood levels and therapeutic response often has been inconclusive or conflicting.

Of the currently available cyclic and noncyclic antidepressants, only four drugs have been studied well enough to make generalizations about the value of their blood levels in treatment of depression: imipramine, desipramine, amitriptyline, and nortriptyline. Serum levels of the other cyclic and noncyclic antidepressants have not been well enough investigated to be clinically meaningful at present, except generally to confirm presence of the drug or to document extremely high serum levels.

The majority of studies of **imipramine** suggest a linear relationship between therapeutic response and blood levels of the parent compound and its desmethyl metabolite, desipramine; patients with a combined level of imipramine and desipramine greater than 225 ng/mL are believed to improve more than patients below that level. **Desipramine** given as a parent compound also appears to have a linear relationship to clinical improvement with a level greater than 125 ng/mL, producing a better response than lower levels.

Nortriptyline levels have been the best studied of the antidepressants. They reveal a more complex pattern than imipramine or desipramine—an inverted U shape correlation with clinical improvement, which is sometimes referred to as a therapeutic window. Clinical improvement correlates with levels of 50 to 150 ng/mL. The reason for poorer response above 150 ng/mL is not known, but it does not appear to relate to any measurable toxicity. On the other hand, the number of subjects in well-designed studies that indicate a window is small. Studies of **amitriptyline** levels have resulted in disagreement about the utility of levels, with linear, curvilinear, and lack of relationship reported by different investigators.

Reasons for the difficulty in unanimously establishing the utility of blood levels are unclear. It is possible that the studies reported in the literature have conflicting results because of the inclusion of mixed populations of individuals with depressive illness, some of whom were poor candidates for drug therapy, others of whom were appropriate for treatment, and some of whom spontaneously remitted despite subtherapeutic drug levels. In addition, the difficulty of performing tricyclic assays may have led to error in measurement of levels, especially in the early studies. On the other hand, plasma drug levels with the newer agents do not correlate with clinical response either.

Although clinical observation and judgment are still the best method to achieve maximal therapeutic benefit without producing intolerable side effects, blood levels for imipramine, desipramine, and nortriptyline might be useful in the following limited situations:

1. To assess compliance
2. To confirm rapid metabolism, resulting in lack of both therapeutic efficacy and side effects, often due to genetic differences or to induction of hepatic enzymes by anticonvulsants, cigarette smoking, or other agents
3. To discover slow metabolizers (i.e., patients with severe side effects at low oral doses as a result of high blood levels rather than somatization)
4. To document that a substantial level was obtained before terminating a drug trial

When used, blood levels should be drawn when the drug has achieved steady-state levels (at least 5 days after a dosage change in healthy adults; longer in the elderly) and 10 to 14 hours after the last oral dose. One final caveat regarding tricyclic blood levels is the variability that is evident among laboratories. It is worth establishing the reliability of local laboratories if tricyclic blood levels are to be used.

Discontinuation

As with all psychotropic drugs, it is good practice to taper cyclic antidepressants gradually rather than to discontinue them abruptly. The reasons for tapering are to prevent withdrawal symptoms and to catch reemergence of depressive symptoms so that effective doses for treatment can be rapidly restored if necessary. Withdrawal symptoms may in part represent cholinergic rebound, and include gastrointestinal distress, malaise, chills, coryza, and muscle aches. If depressive symptoms emerge during or after a drug taper, it would be reasonable to resume an effective antidepressant dosage for at least another 6 months.

Use in the Elderly

In general, the SSRIs are both safer and better tolerated than the tricyclics in the elderly. However, there have been some reports that the tricyclics may be more effective in severely ill, melancholic inpatients. Venlafaxine, with its tricyclic-like effect on both norepinephrine and serotonin at higher doses (e.g., >150 mg/day), but without tricyclic-like anticholinergic, hypotensive, and cardiac effects; mirtazapine, with impact on noradrenergic and serotonergic transmission; and the noradrenergic reboxetine may prove to be good alternatives for melancholic elderly patients.

As described previously, elderly patients may have slower metabolism of cyclic antidepressants, leading to greater drug accumulation and slower changes in steady-state levels with dosage changes. In addition, the elderly are more sensitive to the anticholinergic effects of the cyclic antidepressants. The clinical consequence is that if a cyclic antidepressant is to be used, a less anticholinergic compound, such as desipramine, should be chosen, and compounds with very long half-lives, especially protriptyline, should be avoided. Those drugs that are used should be administered at one third to one half the dosage given to young patients, and the interval between dosage changes should be longer (at least 5–7 days).

In addition to these pharmacokinetic effects, the elderly are more likely to have cardiac conduction system disease that would contraindicate the use of cyclic antidepressants, and they are at higher risk of injury if they fall because of postural hypotension. Thus, if a tricyclic is to be used in the elderly, careful medical supervision is prudent.

Use During Pregnancy

There are limited data on the use of cyclic antidepressants during pregnancy. There have been reports of congenital malformations in association with tricyclic use, but no convincing causal association. Overall, the tricyclics may be safe, but given the lack of proven safety, the drugs should be avoided during pregnancy, unless the indications are clearly compelling. Pregnant women who are at risk for serious depression might be maintained on tricyclic therapy. This decision should always be made very carefully and with extensive discussion of the risk–benefit factors. Due to more clinical experience, older agents, such as imipramine, may be preferred to newer drugs during pregnancy.

Tricyclics appear to be secreted in breast milk. Because their effects on normal growth and development are unknown, breast-feeding should be discouraged for mothers who are on tricyclics.

Augmentation of Tricyclics

As with the SSRIs, clinicians have used a number of augmentation or combination strategies for poor responders to a tricyclic.

Lithium

As with the SSRIs, lithium is combined with tricyclics in two major instances: (a) prophylaxis against a switch into mania in the treatment of bipolar depression and (b) augmentation of tricyclic effect in treatment nonresponders. For augmentation, lithium is generally added to an established tricyclic regimen at a dosage of 300 mg two to three times daily. Although initial reports found a high percentage of responders within 24 to 48 hours regardless of lithium level, later reports suggest a more variable response, with a delay of up to 2 weeks before improvement was evident. A small percentage of patients relapse despite initial improvement. (See also Chapter 4.)

L-Triiodothyronine

The strategy in using T_3 with tricyclics is similar to that described for its use with SSRIs. When patients have failed adequate trials of a cyclic antidepressant, 25 to 50 µg/day of T_3 may be added to their regimen. The mechanism of action does not appear to be an increase in tricyclic blood levels. Most responders are said to have had normal thyroid function at baseline. When this treatment is successful, some improvement is usually seen within 2 weeks and maximal improvement within 4 weeks.

Methylphenidate or Dextroamphetamine

The psychostimulants methylphenidate and dextroamphetamine have occasionally been used to augment a tricyclic regimen. For example, dosages of methylphenidate, 10 mg twice daily to 20 mg three times daily, have been used; although these dosages produce a small increase in tricyclic levels, this does not seem to be the mechanism by which patients improve. This combination is successful in a small number of patients and is usually well tolerated. Patients should be monitored for onset of insomnia or agitation. This strategy is not recommended for patients with a history of psychostimulant abuse (see also Chapter 6).

Monoamine Oxidase Inhibitors

Combined TCA–MAOI therapy has been used in occasional cases of refractory depression. This approach has not been well studied in a controlled fashion, but there are anecdotal reports of success in cases where conventional therapies failed. Severe reactions, including fatalities, also have been reported. The most severe reactions are more likely to involve hyperthermia, seizures, and delirium than hypertensive crisis. These reactions are most frequent when a tricyclic is added to an established MAOI regimen, although they may occur at any time. If this combination is to be used, patients should be fully informed of the risks. In general, an MAOI should be slowly added to an established tricyclic regimen, or the drugs can be started at low doses together. At present, this therapy is not recommended, except perhaps in carefully monitored inpatient settings, because the risks outweigh any established benefits. Indeed, clinical experience with responders to the combination typically reveals sustained benefit when the tricyclic is withdrawn and loss of benefit when the MAOI is discontinued, suggesting that the critical agent is the MAOI.

Side Effects and Toxicity of Cyclic Antidepressants

In general, the side effects of the tricyclics and related cyclic antidepressants are more difficult for patients to tolerate than the side effects of the newer drugs, such as the SSRIs, bupropion, or venlafaxine. It should be recognized, however, that many patients tolerate tricyclic drugs well, especially the less anticholinergic and less sedating compounds, such as desipramine and nortriptyline. In addition to side effects occurring with therapeutic use, another difficulty with the cyclic antidepressants (as well as the MAOIs) lies in their potential for lethality in overdose.

At therapeutic levels, tricyclics may produce postural hypotension, anticholinergic (antimuscarinic) effects, and quinidine-like effects on cardiac conduction and may decrease the seizure threshold. In addition, cyclic antidepressants cause weight gain that may be significant. Should this side effect interfere with treatment, an alternative is the use of an SSRI or bupropion, neither of which is associated with weight gain. Cyclic antidepressants may cause sexual dysfunction, most frequently erectile dysfunction in men. Also, patients may experience excessive sweating, which may interfere with quality of life; if severe enough, this side effect may prompt a switch to an SSRI or bupropion (venlafaxine also may cause sweating). Most side effects of cyclic antidepressants worsen with increased doses, although some may manifest even at lower doses (e.g., dry mouth, constipation, postural hypotension). Elderly patients are generally more susceptible to these side effects. The major medical contraindication to the use of cyclic antidepressants is serious cardiac conduction disturbances.

Complaints of side effects should be taken seriously; often, however, reassurance and symptomatic treatment (e.g., stool softeners for constipation, mouthwashes or sugar-free hard candies for dry mouth) are the best course. It is certainly better to help the patient tolerate side effects or to change to a different drug than to administer subtherapeutic doses. The use of subtherapeutic doses of these compounds exposes patients to side effects without providing a sufficient level of medication for treatment of the depression.

Orthostatic Hypotension

Orthostatic hypotension is the most serious common side effect of the TCAs and of trazodone. In the elderly, there is an increased risk of falls, with attendant increased risks of fractures and head injuries. Severe postural hypotension may limit therapy.

Postural hypotension is largely due to the α_1-adrenergic receptor antagonist properties of these drugs, although the exact mechanism is unclear. The side effect is not always dose related, as one would expect; it often occurs at low doses and may not always worsen with higher doses. In addition, patient factors are very important—depressed patients have a higher incidence of orthostatic symptoms than normal controls on an equivalent dose of drug.

None of the cyclic antidepressants is free of this hypotensive side effect. There are conflicting reports as to whether **nortriptyline** is less likely to cause hypotension. All patients beginning tricyclics should be warned to arise slowly from recumbency or sitting positions, especially on arising in the morning. Postural blood pressures should be obtained when a patient complains of dizziness, blackouts, or falling. The newer antidepressants, including SSRIs, bupropion, reboxetine, and venlafaxine, appear to be free of hypotensive properties.

Anticholinergic Effects

Mild anticholinergic effects are common with therapeutic doses of cyclic antidepressants. These effects include dry mouth, blurred near vision, constipation, and urinary hesitancy. More severe anticholinergic effects may occur in older patients even at therapeutic dosages. These include agitation, delirium, tachycardia, urinary retention, and ileus. A common reason for the appearance of a severe anticholinergic syndrome (Table 3.5) is the concomitant use of more than one anticholinergic drug. This often is seen in clinical situations when cyclic antidepressants

Table 3.5.   Symptoms and signs of anticholinergic toxicity

Systemic	Neuropsychiatric
Tachycardia	Agitation
Dilated, sluggishly reactive pupils	Motor restlessness
Blurred vision	Confusion
Warm dry skin	Disturbance of recent memory
Dry mucous membranes	Dysarthria
Fever	Myoclonus
Reduced or absent bowel sounds	Hallucinations (including
Urinary retention	visual)
	Delirium
	Seizures

are used in combination with low-potency antipsychotics (especially thioridazine), antiparkinsonian drugs, antihistamines, and over-the-counter sleep medications. It is important to be aware of the possibility of precipitating an attack of narrow-angle glaucoma. Patients with open-angle glaucoma can be treated with cyclic antidepressants so long as their intraocular pressures are checked by their ophthalmologist and their glaucoma medications are adjusted as needed.

If mild-to-moderate anticholinergic symptoms interfere with treatment, bethanechol chloride, a cholinergic agent that does not cross the blood brain barrier, may be prescribed. Effective doses range from 10 to 25 mg orally three times daily. For **acute urinary retention,** bethanechol chloride, 2.5 to 5.0 mg, may be given subcutaneously; rarely, a urinary catheter may be temporarily required. If an anticholinergic **delirium** or severe anticholinergic syndrome is suspected, the medication should be stopped. Although the use of physostigmine can be diagnostically useful in these situations, its short half-life and toxicity limit its therapeutic use.

Cardiac Toxicity

The cardiac toxicity of tricyclic and related cyclic antidepressants may limit their clinical use (Table 3.6). The toxicity is due to the quinidine-like effects of these drugs, slowing intracardiac

Table 3.6.   Cardiac toxicity of cyclic antidepressants

Sinus tachycardia
Supraventricular tachyarrhythmias
Ventricular tachycardia and fibrillation
Prolongation of PR, QRS, and QT intervals
Bundle branch block
First-, second-, and third-degree heart block
ST- and T-wave changes

conduction, and to a lesser extent to their anticholinergic effects. Patients at risk of serious cardiac toxicity are those with significant underlying conduction system disease. Except in overdose, major cardiac complications are extremely rare in patients with normal hearts (although benign ECG changes may occur).

In general, use of tricyclic and related cyclic antidepressants should be avoided in patients with bifascicular block, left bundle branch block, or a prolonged QT interval. Because the cyclic antidepressants slow intracardiac conduction, they are actually mildly antiarrhythmic, tending to decrease ventricular premature beats. Despite early reports to the contrary, cyclic antidepressants appear to have little, if any, clinically significant effects on cardiac contractility.

Sexual Dysfunction

It may be difficult to determine the true incidence of sexual dysfunction due to antidepressants because many depressed patients experience sexual dysfunction prior to initiation of treatment. Nonetheless, the incidence of sexual dysfunction with cyclic antidepressants, SSRIs, and MAOIs appears to be high in both men and women. Patients may be reticent about reporting sexual dysfunction; thus, the physician should inquire about this directly at follow-up. For cyclic antidepressants, sexual dysfunction appears to be dose related. Sexual arousal and orgasm may be impaired in both men and women. In men, erectile dysfunction is most common. The MAOIs and SSRIs also cause sexual dysfunction and therefore may not constitute a good alternative for many patients. Bupropion is the only antidepressant not associated with sexual dysfunction, and some reports indicate that it may increase libido. There are anecdotal reports that trazodone may improve sexual function in both men and women. However, it may rarely cause medically serious priapism in men. The clinician should warn male patients on trazodone to report abnormally prolonged or painful erections immediately.

Overdoses with TCAs

Acute doses of more than 1 g of TCAs are often toxic and may be fatal. Death may result from cardiac arrhythmias, hypotension, or uncontrollable seizures. Serum levels should be obtained when overdose is suspected both because of distorted information that may be given by patients or families and because oral bioavailability with very large doses of these compounds is poorly understood. Nonetheless, serum levels of the parent compound and its active metabolites provide less specific information about the severity of the overdose than one might hope. Serum levels of greater than 1,000 ng/mL are associated with serious overdose, as are increases in the QRS duration of the ECG to 0.10 second or greater. However, serious consequences of a TCA overdose may occur with serum levels under 1,000 ng/mL and with a QRS duration of less than 0.10 second.

In acute overdose, almost all symptoms develop within 12 hours. **Antimuscarinic effects** are prominent, including dry mucous membranes, warm dry skin, mydriasis, blurred vision, decreased bowel motility, and, often, urinary retention. Either **CNS depression** (ranging from drowsiness to coma) or an agitated delirium may occur. The CNS depressant effects of cyclic antidepressants are potentiated by concomitantly ingested alcohol, benzodiazepines, and other sedative-hypnotics. Seizures may occur, and in severe overdoses, respiratory arrest may occur. **Cardiovascular toxicity** presents a particular danger (Table 3.6). Hypotension often occurs, even with the patient supine. A variety of arrhythmias may develop, including supraventricular tachycardia, ventricular tachycardia or fibrillation, and varying degrees of heart block, including complete heart block.

Treatment of Overdose

Basic management of overdose includes induction of emesis if the patient is alert, and intubation and gastric lavage if the patient is not. Because bowel motility may have been slowed, it is worth giving 30 g of activated charcoal with a cathartic, such as 120 mL of magnesium citrate, to decrease the absorption of residual drug.

Basic cardiorespiratory supportive care should be administered if needed. Patients with depressed respiration will require ventilatory assistance. Hypotension will require the administration of fluid (however, this must be done cautiously if heart failure is present). In refractory hypotension, or if heart failure is present, pressors such as epinephrine or phenylephrine would be the agents of choice because they counteract the anti–α_1-adrenergic effects of the antidepressant.

Any patient with arrhythmias, a QRS duration of more than 0.10 second, or a serum tricyclic level of greater than 1,000 ng/mL requires continuous cardiac monitoring, preferably in an intensive care unit setting. It is sound practice to monitor levels serially and to discontinue cardiac monitoring until the QRS interval has normalized.

Sinus tachycardia usually requires no treatment. Supraventricular tachycardia contributing to myocardial ischemia or hypotension may be treated with direct-current (DC) cardioversion. Digoxin should be avoided because it might precipitate heart block, but propanolol appears to be safe in treating recurrent supraventricular tachycardia. Cardioversion is the treatment of choice for ventricular tachycardia or fibrillation. Administration of phenytoin may curtail ventricular arrhythmias. If lidocaine is administered, the likelihood of seizures may increase. If lidocaine fails to prevent further arrhythmias, propranolol and bretylium are the next agents of choice. Because quinidine, procainamide, and disopyramide may prolong the QRS interval and may precipitate heart block in tricyclic-overdosed patients, those agents should be avoided. Second- and third-degree heart block can be managed by insertion of a temporary pacemaker. Physostigmine is not generally effective in the treatment of most tricyclic-induced cardiac arrhythmias.

Central nervous system toxicity also can produce significant morbidity or death in tricyclic overdose. Generally, delirium is managed with a quiet environment and reassurance; severely agitated patients may need restraints. For patients with uncontrollable delirium that is threatening their medical condition, low doses of benzodiazepines may be effective. Because of its toxicity and short duration of action, physostigmine is not generally recommended as a therapeutic agent.

One of the most troublesome medical complications following overdose with cyclic antidepressants is seizures. First-line pharmacologic treatment for seizures induced by cyclic antidepressants is one of the benzodiazepines, diazepam or lorazepam. Diazepam is given intravenously in a dose of 5 to 10 mg at a rate of 2 mg/min. The dose may be repeated every 5 to 10 minutes until seizures are controlled. The risk of respiratory arrest can be minimized if intravenous benzodiazepines are given slowly, but resuscitation equipment should be available. Lorazepam is given intravenously in a dose of 1 to 2 mg over several minutes. The advantage of lorazepam is a longer biologic effect than diazepam in acute usage (hours as opposed to minutes) because of a smaller volume of distribution and perhaps a lesser tendency to respiratory depression (see Chapter 5). If a benzodiazepine fails, phenytoin should be given in a full loading dose of 15 mg/kg no more rapidly than 50 mg/min. Over-rapid administration of phenytoin causes severe hypotension.

Forced diuresis and dialysis are of no value because of protein and tissue binding of cyclic antidepressants and may exacerbate hemodynamic instability. Hemoperfusion may have a limited role in extremely severe cases, but its use must be considered experimental.

Drug Interactions

The cyclic antidepressants have a variety of important pharmacodynamic and pharmacokinetic drug–drug interactions that may worsen toxicity (Tables 3.7 and 3.8).

Table 3.7. Drug interactions with cyclic antidepressants

Worsen sedation
  Alcohol
  Antihistamines
  Antipsychotics
  Barbiturates, chloral hydrate, and other sedatives
Worsen hypotension
  α-methyldopa (Aldomet)
  β-adrenergic blockers (e.g., propranolol)
  Clonidine
  Diuretics
  Low-potency antipsychotics
Additive cardiotoxicity
  Quinidine and other type 1 antiarrhythmics
  Thioridazine, mesoridazine, pimozide
Additive anticholinergic toxicity
  Antihistamines (diphenhydramine and others)
  Antiparkinsonians (benztropine and others)
  Low-potency antipsychotics, especially thioridazine
  Over-the-counter sleeping medications
  Gastrointestinal antispasmodics and antidiarrheals (Lomotil and others)
Other
  Tricyclics may increase the effects of warfarin
  Tricyclics may block the effects of guanethidine

Table 3.8. Drugs that may affect levels of cyclic antidepressants

Increase Levels	Decrease Levels
Acetazolamide	Alcohol (chronic use)
Antipsychotics	Barbiturates and similarly acting
Disulfiram	sedative/hypnotics
Fluoxetine[a] and other SSRIs	Carbamazepine[a]
Glucocorticoids	Heavy cigarette smoking
Methylphenidate and	Phenobarbital[a]
amphetamines	Phenytoin[a]
Oral contraceptives	Primidone[a]
Salicylates	Rifampin[a]
Thiazides	
Thyroid hormone	

[a]Major effect.

MONOAMINE OXIDASE INHIBITORS

Iproniazid, the first of the MAOIs, was synthesized as an anti-tuberculous drug in the 1950s. It was noted clinically to have striking stimulant and antidepressant properties and was subsequently shown to be an inhibitor of the enzyme monoamine oxidase (MAO). Although its hepatotoxicity precluded its continued clinical use, other MAOIs were developed. The two MAOIs currently available in the United States for the treatment of psychiatric disorders are phenelzine and tranylcypromine.

Monoamine oxidase is found primarily on the outer membrane of mitochondria and is the enzyme primarily responsible for the intracellular catabolism of biogenic amines. In presynaptic nerve terminals, MAO metabolizes catecholamines that are found outside their storage vesicles. In the liver and gut, MAO metabolizes bioactive amines that are ingested in foods, thus serving an important protective function. It is known that MAO enzyme activity may vary markedly among individuals and appears to increase with age.

Two subtypes of MAO have been described (Table 3.9). Monoamine oxidase type A preferentially metabolizes norepinephrine and serotonin. Type B acts preferentially on phenylethylamine and benzylamine. Although selective MAOIs have been developed, the two approved for use in depression in the United States affect both the A and B types of the enzyme.

Chemistry

Phenelzine is a hydrazine derivative and an irreversible blocker of MAO, whereas tranylcypromine reversibly inhibits MAO. The other hydrazine agent, isocarboxazid, was recently delisted by the manufacturer but is now again commercially available. Tranylcypromine is the only available nonhydrazine MAOI antidepressant. It has structural characteristics similar

Table 3.9. Comparison of monoamine oxidase A and B

Type	Location	Preferred Substrates	Selective Inhibitors
A	Central nervous system, sympathetic terminals, liver, gut, skin	Norepinephrine, serotonin, dopamine, tyramine, octopamine, tryptamine	Clorgyline
B	Central nervous system, liver, platelets	Dopamine, tyramine, tryptamine, phenylethylamine, benzylamine, N-methylhistamine	Selegiline[a]

[a]Selectivity lost at higher doses (≥10 mg/day).

to amphetamine and has some stimulant properties (Fig. 3.1). An additional MAOI, selegiline, has been approved for the treatment of Parkinson's disease. In low doses (<10 mg/day), as used in Parkinson's disease, it is a selective inhibitor of MAO type B and therefore does not require a tyramine-free diet. At higher doses (e.g., 30 mg/day), it may have antidepressant effects but becomes a nonselective MAOI; therefore, dietary precautions must be observed.

Pharmacology

The MAOIs are well absorbed after oral administration. Parenteral forms are not available. As described, these compounds inhibit MAO in the CNS, peripheral sympathetic nervous system, and nonnervous tissues, such as liver and gut. They also partially inhibit other enzymes, but this effect probably is of little clinical consequence. With repeated dosing, maximal inhibition of MAO occurs in several days. Onset of action for antidepressant effect with MAOIs is 2 to 4 weeks, approximately equivalent to the latency of onset of other antidepressants. Because phenelzine irreversibly inhibits the enzyme, return of enzyme function after discontinuation may require 2 weeks (the time it takes for *de novo* synthesis of the enzyme). Although the bond with the MAO enzyme is not irreversible with tranylcypromine, restoration of enzyme activity may be similarly prolonged after discontinuation of the drug.

Metabolism

The metabolism of MAOIs is not well understood. There is controversy as to whether phenelzine is cleaved and acetylated in the liver. It is known that a sizable number of people are slow acetylators (a high percentage of Asians and about 50% of whites and blacks), but there is little evidence that the rate of acetylation is clinically significant for this class of drugs. Of clinical importance is the observation that metabolism of MAOIs does not seem to be affected by anticonvulsants.

MAO Levels

Although plasma levels of MAOIs are not well studied, the degree of enzyme inhibition produced by these drugs has been investigated. For phenelzine, inhibition of greater than 85% of baseline platelet MAO type B activity appears to correlate with therapeutic efficacy. Dosages greater than 45 mg/day are usually necessary to achieve this level of inhibition. This test is not useful for tranylcypromine because it maximally inhibits platelet MAO at subtherapeutic doses.

Interaction with Tyramine and Other Amines

Monoamine oxidase inhibitors inactivate intestinal and hepatic MAO (MAO type A). Thus, when patients taking MAOIs ingest vasoactive amines in foods, they are not catabolized but instead enter the bloodstream and are taken up by sympathetic nerve terminals. These exogenous amines may cause release of endogenous catecholamines, which can result in a hyperadrenergic crisis with severe hypertension, hyperpyrexia, and other symptoms of sympathetic hyperactivity including tachycardia, diaphoresis, tremulousness, and cardiac arrhythmias (the clinical syndrome is described below). A number of amines (especially tyramine, but also phenylethylamine, dopamine, and others) in foods may induce these sympathomimetic crises in MAOI-treated patients. For this reason, foods containing tyramine and other vasoactive amines and sympathomimetic drugs should not be ingested by patients on MAOIs.

Another potentially life-threatening drug interaction involves MAOIs and agents that are serotonergic, including certain tricyclics (e.g., clomipramine), SSRIs, and buspirone. The latter agents in combination with MAOIs may result in a serotonin syndrome, which if mild may feature tachycardia, hypertension, fever, ocular oscillations, and myoclonic jerks, but in its severe form may include severe hyperthermia, coma, convulsions, and death. There are similar life-threatening interactions with certain opioid derivatives, including meperidine and dextromethorphan.

Method of Use

Generally speaking, MAOIs are at least equally effective for major depressive illness and panic disorder compared with other agents if patient selection is appropriate and adequate doses are given. Older trials in which MAOIs appeared to be less effective than tricyclics suffered from poor patient selection and, more importantly, doses of MAOIs that would now be considered subtherapeutic. More recent controlled studies (e.g., using 45 mg/day of phenelzine) have shown equivalent or greater efficacy of MAOIs compared with tricyclics. In clinical practice, MAOIs are frequently effective when all other agents have failed, and they are particularly robust therapeutic options for atypical depressives.

Nonetheless, given the complexity of their use, including dietary restrictions, MAOIs are usually reserved for patients in whom non-MAOIs have failed or have not been tolerated. In the treatment of panic anxiety complicated by polyphobic behavior, at least one study has found phenelzine to be more effective than imipramine. An MAOI may be a first-choice agent in certain patients with atypical depression or depression with panic symptoms, although given their ease of use, SSRIs are now generally preferred.

Preparing Patients for Use of MAOIs

Before beginning therapy with MAOIs, it is important to educate the patient about the risks of interactions with amine-containing foods, beverages, and medications. Patients should clearly understand the need for dietary restrictions, and it is recommended that the physician fully describe these issues before medication is prescribed. Casual prescription of MAOIs must be avoided because the risks inherent in their use require a cautious approach and a cooperative patient.

It is most useful to have a prepared list of restrictions (Table 3.10) that can be given to the patient. It may be useful to enlist family support in planning meals that avoid proscribed foods. Symptoms of a hypertensive crisis should be discussed with the patient, with clear instructions to contact the treating physician immediately or proceed to an emergency room if symptoms occur. Patients should be questioned about compliance both with

**Table 3.10. Sample instructions for
patients taking monoamine oxidase inhibitors**

1. Certain foods and beverages must be avoided:
   All cheese except for fresh cottage cheese or cream cheese
   Meat
     Beef liver
     Chicken liver
     Fermented sausages
     Pepperoni
     Salami
     Bologna
     Other fermented sausages
     Other cured, unrefrigerated meats
   Fish
     Caviar
     Cured, unrefrigerated fish
     Herring (dried or pickled)
     Dried fish, shrimp paste
   Vegetables
     Overripe avocados
     Fava beans
     Sauerkraut
   Fruits
     Overripe fruits, canned figs
   Other foods
     Yeast extracts (e.g., Marmite, Bovril)
   Beverages
     Chianti wine
     Beers containing yeast (unfiltered)
   Some foods and beverages should be used only in moderation:
     Chocolate
     Coffee
     Beer
     Wine
2. If you visit other physicians or dentists, inform them that you are taking an MAOI. This precaution is especially important if other medications are to be prescribed or if you are to have dental work or surgery.
3. Take no medication without a doctor's approval.
   Avoid all over-the-counter pain medications except plain aspirin, acetaminophen (Tylenol), and ibuprofen.
   Avoid all cold or allergy medications except plain chlorpheniramine (Chlor-Trimeton) or brompheniramine (Dimetane).
   Avoid all nasal decongestants and inhalers.
   Avoid all cough medications except plain guaifenesin elixir (plain Robitussin).
   Avoid all stimulants and diet pills.
4. Report promptly any severe headache, nausea, vomiting, chest pain, or other unusual symptoms. If your doctor is not available, go directly to an emergency room.

medication dosage and dietary restrictions at follow-up visits. Any signs of noncompliance should be taken seriously and corrected. If patients report "safe" transgression of dietary rules, clarification should be given that certain foods may vary in tyramine content from portion to portion; thus, successful cheating on one occasion does not rule out the possibility of a hypertensive crisis on another occasion. Given the life-threatening nature of hypertensive crises, repeated or flagrant noncompliance with the prescribed dietary regimen should prompt the physician to consider discontinuation of the MAOI. Patients also should be made aware of proscribed medications and should be reminded to tell their other physicians and dentists that they are taking an MAOI.

In addition to dietary restriction, it is important to educate patients regarding common side effects, especially postural hypotension, insomnia, and possible sexual dysfunction. Informing patients about the latency of onset of therapeutic effects will minimize discouragement and noncompliance.

Choice of Drug

Although phenelzine has been better studied clinically, it has a greater incidence of side effects than tranylcypromine (most notably weight gain, drowsiness, anticholinergic-like effects such as dry mouth, and a greater incidence of impotence and anorgasmia). In addition, although hepatotoxicity is rare, phenelzine has a greater risk of causing serious or fatal hepatotoxicity than tranylcypromine. (It is believed that the hydrazine moiety is responsible for hepatotoxicity.)

Although tranylcypromine has a lower incidence of bothersome side effects, it does cause insomnia, which may be severe. Clonazepam 0.5 mg or trazodone 50 mg at bedtime may safely and effectively treat insomnia. Although there may be a slightly higher risk of hypertensive crisis with tranylcypromine, MAO enzyme function returns to normal more quickly when this drug is discontinued than when phenelzine is discontinued. Tranylcypromine might be the first-choice MAOI in patients who are intolerant of sedation.

Using MAOIs

Initially MAOIs are administered at low doses, with gradual increases as side effects allow. Some tolerance may develop to side effects, including postural hypotension. Phenelzine is usually started at 15 mg two to three times daily (7.5–15.0 mg/day in the elderly), isocarboxazid at 10 mg three times daily, and tranylcypromine at 10 mg two to three times daily (5–10 mg/day in the elderly). Dosages can be increased by 15 mg weekly for phenelzine and 10 mg weekly for isocarboxazid and tranylcypromine (as side effects allow) to 45 to 60 mg/day for phenelzine (30–60 mg/day in the elderly) and 30 to 40 mg/day for the others. Dosages as high as 90 mg/day of these drugs may be required, although these exceed the manufacturer's recommendations. Once depressive symptoms remit, full therapeutic doses are protective against relapse, although in managing patients on MAOIs, dose adjustments over time to manage side effects or clinical response are common.

Therapeutic effects often are not evident for 2 to 4 weeks. As with tricyclics, the aim is to achieve a therapeutic effect with the least possible toxicity. This is an empirical process that takes patience and careful dosage adjustment. Before abandoning a trial of phenelzine as a failure, some clinicians obtain a platelet MAO level. If there is inadequate suppression (85% of baseline if an initial measurement was made or 85% of normal otherwise), a higher dosage should be administered if clinically tolerated.

It is prudent to taper MAOIs over a week or more when discontinuing them; rarely, delirium has been reported with abrupt discontinuation. When MAOIs are stopped, MAO levels do not immediately return to normal. Thus, it is prudent to wait 2 or more weeks before discontinuing MAOI dietary and drug restrictions after discontinuing tranylcypromine and to wait 14 days after stopping phenelzine. During changes from an MAOI to a cyclic antidepressant, similar waiting periods should be observed. Severe and even fatal interactions have been reported when tricyclics have been added to MAOIs. It is generally recommended that tricyclics be stopped for 2 weeks, fluoxetine for 5 weeks, and other agents for 2 weeks before starting an MAOI.

Use in Pregnancy

There is little experience with the use of MAOIs in pregnancy. For this reason, their use should be avoided. If severe depression occurs, alternatives include SSRIs, tricyclics, and ECT.

Side Effects and Toxicity

Fear of MAOI toxicity has severely limited their use. Nonetheless, in compliant patients these drugs can be used safely and effectively.

Postural Hypotension

Postural hypotension is dose related and may limit therapy. This side effect may be worsened markedly if patients are also receiving diuretics or antihypertensives. Patients should be advised to arise slowly from sitting positions or recumbency, especially on awakening in the morning, and to lie down if they become dizzy. Except in overdose or combined treatment with antihypertensives, episodes of hypotension almost always respond to a supine position. In the rare event of severe and unremitting hypotension, intravenous fluids are required; pressor amines should be avoided if at all possible.

CNS Side Effects

Intractable insomnia and agitation can be troublesome with MAOIs. When this occurs, a trial on lower dosages should be considered, a benzodiazepine, or trazodone. Daytime somnolence may occur with MAOIs, especially phenelzine. Patients may develop tolerance to this side effect.

Hyperadrenergic Crises

Hyperadrenergic crises are caused by ingestion of sympathomimetic drugs or pressor amines, such as tyramine, which are found in some foods and beverages. These reactions are serious and may cause stroke or myocardial infarction. All sympathomimetic drugs can lead to crises, as can L-dopa and TCAs (Table 3.11). Symptoms include severe headache, diaphoresis, mydriasis, neuromuscular irritability, hypertension (which may be extreme), and cardiac arrhythmias.

Patients should be advised to contact their physician and to proceed to an emergency room if any such symptoms occur. For severe reactions, **treatment** consists of blockade of α-adrenergic receptors with phentolamine, 5 mg intravenously, repeated as necessary. Phentolamine can be administered over the next 12 to 36 hours (0.25–0.50 mg intramuscularly every 4–6 hours) as needed to control blood pressure. Sodium nitroprusside is extremely effective but requires continuous blood pressure monitoring for safe use. The most common strategy for mild to moderate reactions has been the use of the calcium channel blocker nifedipine, which in recent years has been considered controversial because of concerns over extreme decreases in pressure when used emergently for malignant hypertensive events. In the office or emergency room, the patient is instructed to bite a nifedipine capsule and swallow the contents. Doses of 10 or 20 mg are usu-

Table 3.11. **Interactions of monoamine oxidase inhibitors with other drugs**[a]

Drug	Effect
Sympathomimetics [e.g., amphetamines, dopamine, ephedrine, epinephrine (Adrenalin), isoproterenol (Isuprel), metaraminol, methylphenidate, oxymetazoline (Afrin), norepinephrine, phenylephrine (Neo-Synephrine), phenylpropanolamine, pseudoephedrine (Sudafed)]	Hypertensive crisis
Meperidine (Demerol and others)	Fever, delirium, hypertension, hypotension, neuromuscular excitability, death
Oral hypoglycemics	Further lowering of serum glucose
L-dopa	Hypertensive crisis
Tricyclic antidepressants,[b] venlafaxine[c]	Fever, seizures, delirium
SSRIs, clomipramine, tryptophan	Nausea, confusion, anxiety, shivering, hyperthermia, rigidity, diaphoresis, hyperreflexia, tachycardia, hypotension, coma, death
Bupropion	Hypertensive crisis

[a]This may include selegiline even at low doses.
[b]Tricyclics and MAOIs are occasionally used together.
[c]Likely effect.

ally initially effective and may be repeated over time to prevent or treat recurrence. Some clinicians have provided patients with capsules of nifedipine in case of emergency. β blockers should not be used because, as in the treatment of pheochromocytoma, a potential clinical effect would be to intensify vasoconstriction and thus worsen hypertension by leaving α-adrenergic effects unopposed. After acute treatment, it is important to identify the cause of the crisis; if the cause is deliberate dietary indiscretion, continuing therapy with MAOIs should be reconsidered. When a serotonergic agent is combined with an MAOI, a serotonin syndrome may occur (see later section on Overdose).

Sexual Function

Impotence or, more frequently, delayed ejaculation in men and anorgasmia in women occurs in a substantial minority of patients. It is worth inquiring about sexual function because some patients may be embarrassed about raising the issue themselves. Cyproheptadine has been used to treat MAOI-related sexual dysfunction, but its effectiveness is questionable and it has its own side effects. Anorgasmia occasionally resolves spontaneously.

Other Side Effects

Patients have reported weight gain on all MAOIs and occasionally weight loss more commonly on tranylcypromine. Anticholinergic-like side effects occur, although they are not due to muscarinic antagonism. These side effects are less severe than those seen with tricyclics, although patients on phenelzine may experience dry mouth. Elderly patients may develop constipation or urinary retention. Alternatively, nausea and diarrhea have been reported by some patients. Sweating, flushing, or chills also may occur. Rarely, hepatotoxicity may occur with phenelzine, which may be serious. Peripheral edema likely reflecting effects of the drug on small vessels may prove difficult to manage. Finally, some patients complain of muscle twitching or electric shock–like sensations. The latter may respond to clonazepam, although the emergence of neurologic or neuropathic symptoms may reflect interference with absorption of vitamin B_6 which should improve with dietary supplementation of pyridoxine (vitamin B_6) 50 to 100 mg/day.

Overdose

Monoamine oxidase inhibitors are extremely dangerous in overdose. Because they circulate at very low concentrations in serum and are difficult to assay, there are no good data on therapeutic or toxic serum levels. Manifestations of toxicity may appear slowly, often taking up to 12 hours to appear and 24 hours to reach their peak; thus, even if patients appear clinically well in the emergency room, they should be admitted for observation after any significant overdose. After an asymptomatic period, a serotonin syndrome may occur, including hyperpyrexia and autonomic excitation. Neuromuscular excitability may be severe enough to produce rhabdomyolysis, which may cause renal failure. This phase of excitation may be followed by CNS depression and cardiovascular collapse. Death may occur early due to seizures or arrhythmias, or later due to asystole, arrhythmias, hypotension, or renal failure. Hemolysis and a coagulopathy also may occur and contribute to morbidity and mortality.

Treatment should include gastric emptying followed by oral administration of a charcoal slurry. With the emergence of symptoms such as delirium, hyperpyrexia, and hypertension or hypotension, meticulous supportive care is required. CNS excitation can be treated with lorazepam or diazepam intravenously. These agents should not be used excessively, however, because they may potentiate CNS depression later. If multiple doses are to be used, lorazepam is preferred because of its shorter elimination half-life. Neuroleptics, especially low-potency agents, such as chlorpromazine, should be avoided because they can produce or worsen hypotension. Seizures may be treated with lorazepam 1 to 2 mg or diazepam 5 to 10 mg, given slowly intravenously and repeated every 10 to 15 minutes as needed. Severe neuromuscular irritability or rigidity may occur and may be so severe as to impair respiration because of decreased chest wall compliance. Muscular irritability and rigidity may contribute to fever, a hypermetabolic state, and rhabdomyolysis. There are several case reports of successful use of dantrolene sodium, a directly acting muscle relaxant, to treat these problems. A dosage of 2.5 mg/kg intravenously every 6 hours for 24 hours was used successfully in one patient; it is prudent to continue therapy with lower doses for several days afterward. A severe serotonin syndrome with hyperpyrexia and muscular rigidity may be best treated with anesthesia and muscle paralysis. Severe hypertension may be treated with phentolamine 5 mg intravenously, repeated as necessary, or with sodium nitroprusside (which requires continuous blood pressure monitoring). Ventricular arrhythmias can be safely treated with lidocaine, but bretylium should be avoided because of its adrenergic effects.

The serotonin syndrome produced by the interaction of MAOIs with meperidine, dextromethorphan, clomipramine, and SSRIs, and occasionally with cyclic antidepressants, may be similar clinically to overdose, with similar principles of management applying.

Drug Interactions

Important drug interactions are listed in Table 3.11.

BIBLIOGRAPHY

Antidepressant Mechanism of Action

Hyman SE, Nestler EJ. *The molecular foundations of psychiatry.* Washington, DC: American Psychiatric Association, 1993.

Hyman SE, Nestler EJ. Initiation and adaptation: a paradigm for understanding psychotropic drug action. *Am J Psychiatry* 1996; 153:15.

Indications for Antidepressants

Fluoxetine Bulimia Nervosa Collaborative Study Group. Fluoxetine in the treatment of bulimia nervosa. *Arch Gen Psychiatry* 1992;49:139.

Goldbloom DS, Olmstead MP. Pharmacotherapy of bulimia nervosa with fluoxetine: assessment of clinically significant attitudinal change. *Am J Psychiatry* 1993;150:770.

Golden RN, Rudarfer MV, Sherer MA, et al. Bupropion in depression: I. Biochemical effects and clinical response. *Arch Gen Psychiatry* 1988;45:139.

Greist JH, Jefferson JW, Kobak KA, et al. Efficacy and tolerability of serotonin transport inhibitors in obsessive compulsive disorder: a meta-analysis. *Arch Gen Psychiatry* 1995;52:53.

Hellerstein DJ, Yanowitch P, Rosenthal J, et al. A randomized double-blind study of fluoxetine versus placebo in the treatment of dysthymia. *Am J Psychiatry* 1993;150:1169.

Katzelnick DJ, Kobak KA, Greist JH, et al. Sertraline for social phobia: a double-blind placebo controlled crossover study. *Am J Psychiatry* 1995;152:1368.

Max MB, Lynch SA, Muir J, et al. Effects of desipramine, amitriptyline, and fluoxetine on pain in diabetic neuropathy. *N Engl J Med* 1992;326:1250.

Oehrberg S, Christiansen PE, Behnke K, et al. Paroxetine in the treatment of panic disorder: a randomized, double-blind placebo-controlled study. *Br J Psychiatry* 1995;167:374.

Quitkin FM, Stewart JW, McGrath PJ, et al. Phenelzine versus imipramine in treatment of probable atypical depression: defining syndrome boundaries of selective MAOI responders. *Am J Psychiatry* 1988;145:306.

Robinson RG, Kubos KL, Starr LB, et al. Mood disorders in stroke patients. *Brain* 1984;107:81.

Robinson RG, Parikh RM, Lipsey JR, et al. Pathological laughing and crying following stroke: validation of a measurement scale and a double-blind treatment study. *Am J Psychiatry* 1993;150:286.

Roose SP, Glassman AH, Attia E, et al. Comparative efficacy of selective serotonin reuptake inhibitors and tricyclics in the treatment of melancholia. *Am J Psychiatry* 1994;151:1735.

Sachs GS, Lafer B, Stoll AL, et al. A double-blind trial of bupropion versus desipramine for bipolar depression. *J Clin Psychiatry* 1994;55:391.

Salzman C, Wolfson AN, Schatzberg A, et al. Effect of fluoxetine on anger in symptomatic volunteers with borderline personality disorders. *J Clin Psychopharmacol* 1995;15:23.

Spiker DG, Weiss JC, Dealy RS, et al. The pharmacological treatment of delusional depression. *Am J Psychiatry* 1985;142:430.

Steiner M. Fluoxetine in the treatment of premenstrual dysphoria. *N Engl J Med* 1995;332:1529.

Swedo SE, Leonard HL, Rapoport JL, et al. A double-blind comparison of clomipramine and desipramine in the treatment of trichotillomania (hair pulling). *N Engl J Med* 1989;321:497.

Walsh BT, Stewart JW, Roose SP, et al. Treatment of bulimia with phenelzine. *Arch Gen Psychiatry* 1984;41:1105.

Yonkers KA, Halbreich U, Freeman E, et al. Symptomatic improvement of premenstrual dysphoric disorder with sertraline. *JAMA* 1997;278:983.

Zisook S, Braff DL, Click MA. Monoamine oxidase inhibitors in the treatment of atypical depression. *J Clin Psychopharmacol* 1985;5:131.

Therapeutic Usage of Antidepressants

Fontaine R, Ontiveros H, Elie R, et al. A double-blind comparison of nefazodone, imipramine, and placebo in major depression. *J Clin Psychiatry* 1994;55:234.

Joffe RT, Singer W, Levitt AJ, et al. A placebo-controlled comparison of lithium and triiodothyronine augmentation of tricyclic antidepressants in unipolar refractory depression. *Arch Gen Psychiatry* 1993;50:387.

Kupfer DJ, Frank E, Perel JM, et al. Five-year outcome for maintenance therapies in recurrent depression. *Arch Gen Psychiatry* 1992;49:769.

Quitkin FM, Rabkin JG, Ross D, et al. Identification of true drug response to antidepressants. *Arch Gen Psychiatry* 1984;41:782.

Quitkin FM, Stewart JW, McGrath PJ, et al. Loss of drug effects during continuation therapy. *Am J Psychiatry* 1993;150:562.

Renaud J, Axelson D, Birmaher B. A risk-benefit assessment of pharmacotherapies for clinical depression in children and adolescents. *Drug Safety* 1999;20:59.

Task Force on the Use of Laboratory Tests in Psychiatry, American Psychiatric Association. Tricyclic antidepressants: blood level measurements and clinical outcome. *Am J Psychiatry* 1985;142:155.

Antidepressant Side Effects and Their Management

Garland EJ, Remick RA, Zis AP. Weight gain with antidepressants and lithium. *J Clin Psychopharmacol* 1988;8:323.

Gitlin MJ. Psychotropic medications and their effects on sexual dysfunction: diagnosis, biology, and treatment approaches. *J Clin Psychiatry* 1994;55:406.

Johnston AJ, Lineberry CG, Ascher JA. A 102-center prospective study of seizure in association with bupropion. *J Clin Psychiatry* 1991;52:450.

Marshall JB, Forker AD. Cardiovascular effects of tricyclic antidepressant drugs: therapeutic usage, overdose, and management of complications. *Am Heart J* 1982;163:401.

Nelson JC, Jatlow PI, Brock J, et al. Major adverse reactions during desipramine treatment. *Arch Gen Psychiatry* 1982;39:1055.

Nierenberg AA, Adler LA, Peselow E, et al. Trazodone for antidepressant-associated insomnia. *Am J Psychiatry* 1994;151:1069.

Rabkin J, Quitkin F, Harrison W, et al. Adverse reactions to monoamine oxidase inhibitors. Part I: A comparative study. *J Clin Psychopharmacol* 1984;4:270.

Rabkin J, Quitkin F, McGrath P, et al. Adverse reactions to monoamine oxidase inhibitors. Part I: Treatment correlates and clinical management. *J Clin Psychopharmacol* 1985;5:2.

Rosenstein DL, Nelson C, Jacobs SC. Seizures associated with antidepressants: a review. *J Clin Psychiatry* 1993;54:289.

Shulman KI, Walter SE, MacKenzie S, et al. Dietary restriction, tyramine, and the use of monoamine oxidase inhibitors. *J Clin Psychopharmacol* 1989;9:397.

Sternbach H. The serotonin syndrome. *Am J Psychiatry* 1991;148:705.

Walker PW, Cole JO, Gardner EA, et al. Improvement in fluoxetine-associated sexual dysfunction in patients switched to bupropion. *J Clin Psychiatry* 1993;54:459.

Antidepressant Overdose

Barbey JT, Roose SP. SSRI safety in overdose. *J Clin Psychiatry* 1998;59(suppl 15):45.

Boehnert MT, Lovejoy FH. Value of the QRS duration versus the serum drug level in predicting seizures and ventricular arrhythmias after an acute overdose of tricyclic antidepressants. *N Engl J Med* 1985;313:474.

Linden CH, Rumack BH, Strehlke C. Monoamine oxidase inhibitor overdose. *Ann Emerg Med* 1984;13:1137.

Antidepressants in Pregnancy

Cohen LS, Altshuler LL. Pharmacological management of psychiatric illness during pregnancy and the postpartum period. *Psychiatr Clin North Am* 1997;4:21.

Pastuszak A, Schick-Boschetto B, Zuber C, et al. Pregnancy outcome following first-trimester exposure to fluoxetine (Prozac). *JAMA* 1993;269:2246.

4

Mood Stabilizers

The mood stabilizers are a diverse group of drugs used primarily in the treatment of manic–depressive illness; as a class these drugs are effective in acute mania, generally less effective in acute depression, and act to dampen mood swings over time. The established mood stabilizers are lithium and the anticonvulsants, valproate and carbamazepine. Newer anticonvulsants and the atypical antipsychotic drug, clozapine, have also shown promise as mood stabilizers in small clinical trials. Other drugs that have shown mixed success as mood stabilizers are the calcium channel blocker verapamil, as well as the high-potency benzodiazepine clonazepam. Clinical trial data are greatest for lithium and, despite its wide acceptance, more modest for valproate.

GENERAL COMMENTS ON THE USE OF MOOD STABILIZERS

Bipolar disorder is a serious mental disorder in which recurrences of both mania and depression are the rule, and for a minority of patients symptoms become chronic. A great weight of evidence favors long-term prophylaxis against recurrences after effective treatment of acute episodes. The mainstay of treatment for bipolar disorder for the past three decades has been lithium. Given its long use, lithium's efficacy, limitations, and side effects are extremely well documented. Despite far less documentation of the benefits and risks of therapy with valproate, many experienced clinicians find that it has efficacy equivalent to that of lithium, but greater acceptability to many patients based on side effects and ease of use. As a result, it is becoming a first-line treatment. No existing treatment for bipolar disorder is fully satisfactory, however, and it is good news that several new anticonvulsants are now in clinical trials for use as mood stabilizers.

From the distance of the classroom, we often teach our trainees to avoid polypharmacy because of the risk of cumulative side effects and drug interactions. Although a bipolar patient may require only one agent such as valproic acid as the mainstay of the treatment, over time, given the nature of bipolar illness, interventions are likely to include the addition of antidepressants, antipsychotics, benzodiazepines, and other compounds. For example, approximately two thirds of patients in contemporary studies fail to achieve complete remission or long-term stability on lithium monotherapy.

If possible, one drug should ideally be used as the anchor medication for the disease; for example, a fully unsatisfactory response to valproic acid should lead the clinician to consider the use of lithium or carbamazepine alone. In actual practice, however, the clinician does not have the luxury of sequential pure trials of the many drugs available. Therefore, usual practice is to add either lithium or another anticonvulsant to the ongoing treatment with the first agent while watching for possible interactions. When the goal is monotherapy and moving from one compound to another, this can be done by cross-tapering treatment: tapering the first drug and gradually increasing the second.

Bipolar illness is often a severe and life-altering, if not life-threatening, disease, and as with other serious medical conditions (cancer, hypertension, etc.), the clinician should not shrink from combination therapies. The combined use of valproic acid, or whichever compound is the anchor medication (lithium, carbamazepine, gabapentin), and an additional mood stabilizer is recommended when a partial response is achieved with one mood stabilizer. The clinician may combine, for example, from an array of choices including lithium, carbamazepine, gabapentin, or lamotrigine and topiramate, while acknowledging that controlled studies of each of these combinatorial possibilities have not yet been accomplished. Combination therapy always must be administered with caution, watching for combined toxicities. Some combined regimens are best managed when the clinician monitors blood levels of both compounds. One common error of polypharmacy in bipolar patients is leaving a patient on an antidepressant for too long, risking induction or even maintenance of a manic state.

Over time, the clinician, in partnership with the patient, should be encouraged to vary doses and regimens, always searching for the optimal combination of compounds and doses. Daily mood charting of longitudinal treatment by bipolar patients, with careful documentation of the effect of specific regimens on the various phases of the affective illness, is critical to optimize outcomes.

Lithium

Lithium is the lightest solid element in the periodic table; it is active as a psychopharmacologic agent in the form of its singly charged cation. The therapeutic value of lithium was discovered serendipitously by Cade in 1949 when he noted its calming effect on animals. He then tried it on 10 manic patients and found dramatic improvement. The therapeutic usage of lithium was thereafter rapidly explored in Australia and Europe. Its approval for use in the United States, however, was delayed until 1970 because of severe and sometimes fatal cases of lithium poisoning in the 1940s in patients who had unrestricted use of it as a salt substitute. By the time it was approved in the United States, its efficacy as a treatment for mania had been demonstrated beyond question by research in Europe.

PHARMACOLOGY

Absorption

Lithium tablets and capsules (Table 4.1) are available as the carbonate salt, which is less irritating to the gastrointestinal tract than the chloride. Each 300-mg tablet contains 8 mmol of lithium. Because lithium is a monovalent ion, 8 mmol is equal to 8 mEq. Lithium is also available as lithium citrate syrup, containing 8 mmol of lithium per 5 mL. Lithium is well absorbed after oral administration. Standard preparations produce peak serum levels in 1.5 to 2.0 hours; slow-release preparations that

Table 4.1.   Available preparations of lithium

Form	Brand Name	How Supplied
Lithium carbonate	Eskalith	300-mg capsules, tablets
	Lithium carbonate	300-mg capsules, tablets
	Lithonate	300-mg capsules
	Lithotabs	300-mg tablets
Lithium carbonate, slow release	Lithobid	300-mg tablets
	Eskalith CR	450-mg tablets
Lithium citrate syrup	Cibalith-S	8 mEq/5 mL[a]
	Lithium citrate syrup	8 mEq/5 mL[a]

[a]8 mEq of lithium is equivalent to 300 mg of lithium carbonate.

achieve peak levels in 4.0 to 4.5 hours also are available. No parenteral forms are available.

Blood Levels

Lithium therapy must be guided by measurement of serum levels. Serum level, not oral dose, is highly correlated with both therapeutic and toxic effects. Levels may be reported either as milliequivalents per liter (mEq/L) or millimoles per liter, or millimolar (mM), which are equivalent because lithium ion is monovalent. Lithium levels are accurately measured by flame-photometry or atomic absorption methods that are identical to those used for sodium and potassium. Standards for interpreting serum lithium levels are based on measurement 12 hours after the last oral dose (generally prior to the first morning dose). Regimens in which the entire dose is given at bedtime will produce morning levels 10% to 20% higher than regimens with divided dosing.

Distribution

Lithium distributes throughout total body water, although neuronal levels may be slightly lower than serum levels. There is some lag in penetration into the cerebrospinal fluid, but equilibration between blood and brain occurs within 24 hours. Like sodium, lithium circulates unbound to plasma proteins. In the elderly, there is a reduction in lean body mass (and thus total body water) of 10% to 15%; thus, lithium has a smaller volume of distribution in elderly patients than in younger patients. This reduction, along with age-related decreases in glomerular filtration rate (GFR), contributes to the need for lower oral doses in the elderly.

Excretion

Lithium is excreted almost entirely (95%) by the kidney. It is filtered by the glomerulus, and like sodium, it is 70% to 80% reabsorbed in the proximal renal tubules; lithium is also reabsorbed to a lesser extent in the loop of Henle, but unlike sodium it is not further reabsorbed in the distal tubules. Thus, its excretion is not facilitated by diuretics (such as thiazides), which act at the distal tubules. In fact, because proximal reabsorption of lithium and sodium is competitive, a deficiency of sodium, as may be produced by thiazide diuretics, dehydration, or sodium restriction, increases retention of lithium by the proximal nephron and thus increases serum lithium levels. Typically, thiazides increase lithium levels by about 30% to 50%, thus requiring dosage reductions in lithium if they are coadministered. On the other hand, the diuretic furosemide, which acts proximally to thiazides in the nephron (at the loop of Henle), apparently blocks lithium reabsorption to an adequate degree that it does not generally elevate serum lithium levels. Nonetheless, lithium levels must be monitored closely in any patient initiating diuretic therapy.

The renal excretion of lithium is maximal in the first few hours after peak levels are achieved and then proceeds more slowly over several days. In healthy adults, the **elimination half-life** of lithium is approximately 24 ± 8 hours. Lithium excretion is directly related to GFR. In the elderly, who have a diminished GFR, the elimination half-life may be significantly prolonged; it also may be increased with renal dysfunction. Conversely, conditions that increase GFR, such as pregnancy, increase lithium clearance.

MECHANISM OF ACTION

Mechanism of Action of Lithium and Other Mood-Stabilizing Drugs

Lithium has many known actions in the nervous system at concentrations that approximate the therapeutic serum concentration of 1 mM. Lithium has acute and chronic effects on the release of serotonin and norepinephrine from nerve terminals; at higher concentrations, it has effects on transmembrane ion pumps. Chronic lithium administration has been shown to alter the coupling of a number of neurotransmitter receptors to their signal-transducing G proteins. These interesting effects notwithstanding, the leading candidate mechanisms of lithium action currently are the inositol depletion hypothesis and the action of lithium on the wnt signaling pathway. For neither of these hypotheses, though, has a direct link to the treatment of manic–depressive illness been established.

Inositol Depletion Hypothesis

Many neurotransmitter receptors (e.g., α_1-adrenergic, 5-HT$_2$–serotonergic, and muscarinic cholinergic receptors) are linked via the G protein, Gq, to the enzyme phospholipase C, which hydrolyzes the membrane phospholipid phosphatidylinositol bisphosphate (PIP$_2$), to yield two second messengers, diacylglycerol and inositol triphosphate (IP$_3$) (Fig. 4.1). Diacylglycerol activates protein kinase C, and IP$_3$ binds its receptor on the endoplasmic reticulum to release intracellular Ca^{2+}, itself a critical second messenger. Phosphatidylinositol is synthesized from free inositol and a lipid moiety. Most cells can obtain free inositol directly from the plasma, but neurons cannot, because

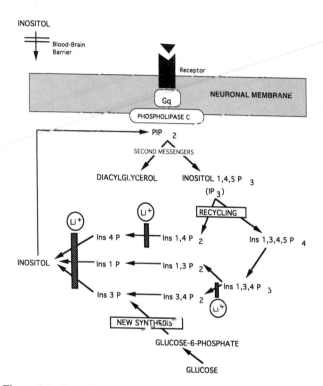

Figure 4.1. The effects of lithium (Li+) on the phosphatidylinositol cycle. Lithium blocks the recycling of inositol phosphates and new synthesis of inositol from glucose, thus inhibiting the ability of neurons to generate the second messengers diacylglycerol and inositol 1,4,5-triphosphate (IP_3). Gq is the signal-transducing G protein that activates this system. PIP_2, phosphatidylinositol 4,5-bisphosphate. (Adapted from Hyman SE, Nestler EJ. *The molecular foundations of psychiatry.* Washington, DC: American Psychiatric Association, 1993:141.)

inositol does not cross the blood–brain barrier. As a result, neurons must either recycle inositol by dephosphorylating inositol phosphates after they are generated from hydrolysis of phosphatidylinositols, or synthesize it *de novo* from glucose-6-phosphate, a product of glycolysis. Lithium, at therapeutically used concentrations, inhibits inositol monophosphatase (IMPase). This blocks the ability of neurons to generate free inositol from recycled inositol phosphates or glucose-6-phosphate. Lithium-exposed neurons, therefore, have a diminished ability to resynthesize PIP_2 after it is hydrolyzed in response to neurotransmitter receptor activation. It has been hypothesized that, when firing rates of neurons are abnormally high, lithium-treated neurons will become depleted of PIP_2, and neurotransmission dependent on this second messenger system will be dampened.

However, even if this hypothesis is correct, it remains incomplete. The critical cells in the brain that are targets of lithium's therapeutic action remain unknown, and it is unclear which of the many phosphatidylinositol-dependent neurotransmitter systems must be dampened for lithium to have its therapeutic effects.

Regulation of the wnt Pathway and Glycogen Synthase Kinase 3β

In addition to its antimanic effects, lithium has teratogenic effects on embryos of the African clawed toad, *Xenopus laevis*. Inhibition of IMPase was thought not only to be a candidate mechanism for mood stabilization (as stated above), but also to explain the dramatic effects of lithium on early development in some model organisms. The teratogenic effects of lithium have now been found to be due not to inhibition of IMPase, but to its ability to inhibit the activity of glycogen synthase kinase 3β (GSK-3β). The GSK-3β pathway is a negative regulator of the cellular signaling pathway in which the key intercellular signaling molecule is a peptide called wnt. Inhibition of wnt by molecular means reproduces the teratogenic effects of lithium in several species. The possibility that a pathway involved in brain development might also be involved in brain remodeling in response to pharmacologic agents is an intriguing one. Given the continuing difficulty, after more than a decade, of pinpointing a mechanism by which inhibition of IMPase can produce antimanic effects, the implication of GSK-3β has given new impetus to this field. The generation of selective inhibitors of GSK-3β will be needed to test this hypothesis in humans.

Lithium Regulation of Adenylyl Cyclase

As mentioned above, lithium acutely inhibits adenylyl cyclase in most tissues, including brain. Although the concentrations required to exert this effect in the brain appear to be higher than clinically relevant levels, this effect of lithium may account for some of its peripheral side effects. Lithium inhibits the normal activation of adenylyl cyclase by thyroid-stimulating hormone (TSH) and antidiuretic hormone (vasopressin), which may partly explain its antithyroid effects and its tendency to cause defects in the ability to concentrate urine.

INDICATIONS

Lithium has been shown to be effective in bipolar disorder, both for the treatment of acute mania and for prophylaxis against recurrences. Its usefulness in other psychiatric disorders is less well established (Table 4.2).

Bipolar Disorder

Lithium is the best studied and a broadly effective treatment for bipolar disorder. Approximately 70% of bipolar patients gain at least moderate benefit from lithium during some stage of their treatment. For most patients, however, lithium is not, by

Table 4.2.   Indications for lithium treatment

Effective agent of choice
  Acute mania
  Bipolar prophylaxis
  Augmentation of TCAs
Effective, other agents preferable
  Acute bipolar depression, primary treatment
Possibly effective
  Cyclothymia
  Schizophreniform disorder
  Schizoaffective disorder
  Unipolar prophylaxis (most recent episode mild)
Conflicting or preliminary evidence for effectiveness
  Aggressive behavior
  Affectively unstable personality disorders
Unproven or ineffective
  Alcohol abuse
  Anxiety
  Bulimia
  Schizophrenia

itself, a fully adequate treatment for all phases of their illness. Lithium is most effective in the treatment of acute mania and the prophylaxis of manic recurrences, moderately effective in the prophylaxis of depressive recurrences, and generally inadequate as a sole acute treatment for depressive episodes. In each of these situations, lithium may be supplemented by other drugs. During acute manias, supplementation with antipsychotic drugs and benzodiazepines is often beneficial. During acute depressive episodes, supplemental use of antidepressants is most often indicated. Because of such complexities, the clinical phases of bipolar disorder are treated separately below.

Acute Mania

Many controlled studies have demonstrated that at a serum level of approximately 1 mM, lithium is effective treatment for manic episodes in approximately 70% to 80% of cases. Lithium also has been shown to be more effective overall than antipsychotic drugs used as single agents in treating acute mania. Onset of improvement with lithium usually takes at least 10 to 14 days, and full improvement may take 4 weeks or more. When manic symptoms are not so severe as to require immediate control of abnormal behavior, lithium may be used alone. However, when mania is severe, especially in settings where hospitalization time is limited, the onset of the therapeutic response to lithium is impractically slow. Thus, early in the treatment of acute mania, antipsychotic drugs are often used as adjuncts to lithium therapy. They are effective when administered at full antipsychotic doses (e.g., 8–10 mg of haloperidol). In contrast to the benzodiazepines, which provide only sedation, the antipsychotic drugs possess true antimanic properties. With the introduction of relatively less toxic third-generation antipsychotic medications, the clinician can more easily add these drugs without the prospect of extrapyramidal symptoms (EPS), danger of neuroleptic malignant syndrome (NMS), or incidence of dystonia that attended the use of typical antipsychotics. Nonetheless, to minimize undesirable side effects at higher doses of antipsychotic drugs (see Chapter 2), benzodiazepines are often used if temporary additional sedation is required during the early treatment of acute mania (e.g., lorazepam 1–2 mg or clonazepam 0.5 mg every 2 hours as needed), either in addition to lithium alone or with an antipsychotic drug. A modest series of uncontrolled and controlled reports have suggested that verapamil, a calcium channel blocker commonly used to treat hypertension, may be effective in acute mania. Verapamil can be used as the single agent, combined with lithium or an antipsychotic, and in combination with benzodiazepines (see Chapter 5). Similarly, lithium can be used in conjunction with antiseizure medications such as valproate, carbamazepine, gabapentin, or lamotrigine for refractory manic episodes (see later section on Treatment-Refractory Mania). Milder cases of mania can be treated with lithium alone. However, even mild episodes that occur in the context of lithium prophylaxis generally require the temporary addition of **other compounds.** If, at the time of a hypomanic or manic breakthrough, the patient's lithium level has been maintained at 0.8 mM or less, the lithium dosage can be increased to achieve a level of 1.0 mM (as side effects allow) and an antipsychotic drug added until the symptoms are well controlled. The treating physician must then weigh the frequency of relapses against side effects experienced by the individual patient and decide whether to attempt future prophylaxis with a higher serum level of lithium.

In treating any acutely manic patient, a low-stimulation environment should be provided. Limits should be set clearly and firmly, and provocative interactions avoided. If hospitalized patients attempt to feign compliance with medication, mouth checks and use of liquid preparations, such as lithium citrate, may be necessary. When patients refuse treatment because their judgment is impaired by mental illness, a mechanism of substituted judgment is required. Most states require evidence that there is a high risk of serious harm if the patient remains untreated leading to a judicial process for establishing substituted judgment.

Treatment-Refractory Mania

Predictors of poor response to lithium in acute mania include a prior history of poor response, rapid cycling, dysphoric symptoms, mixed symptoms of depression and mania, psychiatric comorbidity (including personality disorders), and medical comorbidity. Medical illnesses may complicate attempts to achieve adequate lithium levels. For example, the presence of renal disease alters lithium excretion and therefore requires careful monitoring of both lithium levels and salt balance. The presence of sinoatrial node dysfunction raises the question of whether it is safe to use lithium in the absence of a cardiac pacemaker. The presence of even mild dementia complicates the use of lithium (as well as all other psychotropic drugs) by increasing the risk of drug-induced encephalopathy. Comorbidity of mania with either a medical disorder or a nonaffective psychiatric disorder decreases the likelihood that patients will receive adequate lithium doses or respond well if they do.

For patients who have not shown significant response to their initial mood stabilization treatment after 2–3 weeks at therapeutic levels, reconsider the possibility of an undetected complicating medical, psychiatric, or drug abuse disorder. Patients who do not respond to the combination of lithium and an antipsychotic drug may respond to treatment with one of the anticonvulsants, valproate or carbamazepine. Indeed many clinicians now use valproate as their initial treatment for bipolar disorder.

There is reasonable evidence to suggest that some patients who do not respond to lithium alone or an anticonvulsant alone respond to combination therapy. There are literally dozens of ways to mix and match seizure medications, valproate, carbamazepine, gabapentin, lamotrigine, and clonazepam with or without lithium and antipsychotics to reduce symptomatology in treatment-resistant patients. However, combined therapy does increase the risk of central nervous system side effects, especially in elderly patients. There have been reports of success with a valproate–carbamazepine combination in lithium-refractory or lithium-intolerant patients. Because of pharmacokinetic interactions, the dose of valproate will usually have to be increased and the dose of carbamazepine decreased if this combination is used. Carbamazepine also may speed the metabolism of concomitantly administered antipsychotic and benzodiazepine drugs that are metabolized by CYP450 3A4 (see later section on Psychiatric Uses of Anticonvulsants). Very severe episodes of mania that do not respond satisfactorily to first-line treatments may respond to electroconvulsive therapy (ECT). ECT has the advantage of rapidity, with remission often occurring after six treatments (with treatments given three times weekly). ECT is not a first-line treatment, in part because the treatment of bipolar disorder requires long-term prophylaxis, which is not provided by ECT. Thus, even after successful ECT treatment, it is still necessary to find an effective prophylactic regimen. ECT is safe and effective in patients receiving lithium or antipsychotic drugs; use of valproate or carbamazepine will elevate the seizure threshold, requiring some adjustments in treatment.

Acute Bipolar Depression

In the long-term course of bipolar disorder, antidepressant therapy will clearly prove necessary at times. However, it is now widely accepted that antidepressant treatment in bipolar patients poses a risk of triggering a switch into mania or hypomania, or inducing rapid cycling. Switch into mania has been observed with virtually every antidepressant treatment and ECT. Thus, the central rule in treatment of bipolar depression is that when antidepressants are used, they should be used together with a mood stabilizer, and that antidepressants should be used for the briefest time possible, quite a different approach than in unipolar patients (see Chapter 3). Over the long term, some patients who are chronically suicidal may actually do better with lithium alone (the impact of other mood stabilizers on suicidality is less well documented) than with chronic antidepressant administration. If psychosis is present during a depressive episode, an antipsychotic drug should be added or ECT considered.

All antidepressants in current use are effective in bipolar depression; bupropion appears to have a somewhat lower likelihood of initiating a switch into mania than other antidepressants, but is not free of risk. Despite claims in the older literature, lithium is not broadly effective as a sole treatment for acute bipolar depression, although it may be efficacious in a selected minority. Of the other mood stabilizers, valproate is more effective as an antimanic agent than as an antidepressant. Preliminary data indicate that lamotrigine has antidepressant potential, but the selection of patients who might be candidates for lamotrigine monotherapy for bipolar depression is unclear.

Electroconvulsive therapy is effective in all phases of bipolar disorder, including depression, and should be considered where medications are unsuccessful or in the presence of psychosis, catatonia, active suicidal plans, and pregnancy.

In summary, if a depression occurs in a bipolar patient who is not currently on lithium or another mood stabilizer, treatment should be started with lithium or valproate plus an antidepressant, appropriate psychotherapy, or both. The choice will depend on the patient's prior history of responsiveness and the severity of the episode. More severe episodes favor initiation of combination therapy with an antidepressant. When depression occurs in bipolar patients on long-term lithium therapy, the clinician is cautioned that lithium may cause hypothyroidism, which may masquerade as or exacerbate depressions.

Should manic symptoms emerge, the antidepressant should be discontinued and therapy continued with a mood-stabilizing agent (lithium, valproate, or an alternative). Antidepressant-precipitated mania often continues, however, after the antidepressant is stopped, requiring institution of full antimanic treatment, which may include adjunctive use of antipsychotic or benzodiazepine drugs as well as the mood stabilizer. It is prudent to withdraw the antidepressant, if possible, in bipolar patients after acute depressive episodes have passed and then to maintain the patients on a mood stabilizer alone (see Chapter 3).

Mixed Episodes

When an episode is characterized by mixed symptoms of mania and depression, the episode is best treated like acute mania, that is, with a mood-stabilizing drug (lithium, valproate, carbamazepine, gabapentin, or lamotrigine) or a combination. As in acute mania, ECT is generally reserved for patients who are refractory to initial drug treatments and who are so severely ill that rapid treatment is required. Patients who respond to ECT will still need subsequent pharmacologic prophylaxis. In mixed episodes, as in acute mania, adjunctive antipsychotic drugs may be indicated. Benzodiazepines are the drugs of choice for adjunctive sedation. Antidepressants are to be avoided because they are likely to worsen the overall course of the episode. Some investigators have recommended use of thyroid hormone [thyroxine (T_4) or L-triiodothyroxine (T_3)] for refractory mixed episodes, with the goal of bringing thyroid hormone levels into the upper range of normal. This approach requires additional study.

Prophylaxis in Bipolar Disorder

Bipolar disorder must be treated with a longitudinal view of the illness because essentially all patients will suffer recurrences. Many open and double-blind placebo-controlled studies have confirmed that lithium decreases the frequency and severity of both manic and depressive recurrences. Lithium does not, however, eliminate recurrences. Lithium also may improve minor, but troublesome, subsyndromal mood swings that occur in untreated bipolar patients. Overall experience suggests that lithium is somewhat more effective in preventing manic than depressive recurrences. Episodes of mild depression are reported by many patients. Lithium appears to be less effective for patients with a history of frequent recurrences, especially if they are rapid cyclers (more than three cycles per year). Rapid withdrawal of lithium from previously stable patients appears to predispose them to early manic relapses, suggestive of a rebound phenomenon (see later section on Discontinuation of Lithium Therapy).

If the most recent episode was a mania, prophylaxis should generally be undertaken with a continuation of the mood-stabilizing drug or drugs (lithium, valproate, carbamazepine, gabapentin, or lamotrigine) that were effective for that episode. Any adjunctive antipsychotic drugs used during the acute episode should generally be tapered and discontinued. (The exception is the patient on mood stabilizers known to relapse without an antipsychotic.) Whenever possible, atypical antipsychotics are preferred to minimize the risk of side effects, including tardive dyskinesia. For some treatment-refractory patients, clozapine has proven particularly efficacious.

If the most recent episode was depressive, recently added antidepressants should be tapered and discontinued, if possible, and prophylaxis continued with mood stabilizers alone. There are conflicting data on optimal lithium serum levels for prophylaxis. Although effective prophylaxis has been reported with serum levels of lithium as low as 0.4 mM, a randomized double-blind prospective study of 94 patients found levels of 0.8 to 1.0 mM clearly superior to levels of 0.4 to 0.6 mM (Gelenberg et al., 1989). Patients assigned to the lower range had a threefold higher risk of serious recurrence, predominantly mania, than those assigned to the higher range. Moreover, patients with levels in the lower range had higher rates of cycling within episodes (mania and depression within a single relapse). The main cost of higher levels is worsened side effects, which affect quality of life. However, long-term treatment with standard levels is most unlikely to result in renal failure or other life-threatening complications. It is prudent to start prophylaxis with a target level of 0.8 to 1.0 mM and to educate and reassure patients about side effects. For patients who cannot tolerate these levels, alternative mood stabilizers should be considered.

For patients who fail lithium prophylaxis after a 6- to 12-month trial, an alternative therapy should be instituted, generally valproate alone or in combination with lithium. Additionally, there is an early but encouraging body of literature on the use of gabapentin and lamotrigine as adjunctive treatment for refractory bipolar disorder. Although most available reports represent small trials without rigorous design, several groups have found that the addition of either of these two newer anticonvulsants to ongoing monotherapy or combined therapy has offered an approximately 50% improvement of symptoms in these treatment-resistant patients (see below). Carbamazepine use in long-term prophylaxis is less well supported by the existing data. Intermittent addition of an antipsychotic drug is a commonly used strategy, and is far more acceptable now with the availability of newer atypical compounds that incur fewer short-term and long-term side effects than the typical antipsychotics. Given the risk of tardive dyskinesia, which may be elevated in patients with mood disorders, the total lifetime use of typical antipsychotics should be minimized.

Despite the burden of side effects of prophylaxis, given morbidity and life disruption caused by manic and depressive recurrences, prophylaxis is the rule. Some patients are resistant to the idea of long-term prophylaxis (this is particularly true in adolescent populations) and insist on a trial of cessation of medication. It is critical that the patient be well stabilized prior to a trial off medication (i.e., without substantial residual symptoms), that medications be discontinued very slowly to avoid a rapid relapse, and that there a plan for close observation be in place that ideally involves family members.

Prophylaxis for Rapid-Cycling Bipolar Disorder

A minority of bipolar patients have more than three recurrences per year. These patients, defined as rapid cyclers, have a diminished response to lithium treatment, although lithium remains superior to placebo. There is evidence that valproate may be preferable as a first-line treatment in this population.

Rapid cycling is more common in women. It occurs in pedigrees along with classic bipolar disorder, suggesting that it does not have a different genetic basis. A high percentage of patients have onset of rapid cycling while being treated with antidepressants. All classes of antidepressants and even ECT have been implicated in initiating rapid cycling in some cases. It also has been reported that thyroid abnormalities may predispose to rapid cycling, although this finding has not always been replicated.

In managing rapidly cycling patients, it is useful to have the patient graphically chart mood state and medications. Thyroid abnormalities should be vigorously sought and treated. Many clinicians would advocate administration of T_4 for TSH elevations even in the absence of abnormalities in free T_4 levels, although this has not been systematically studied. Trials of lithium or valproate should not be terminated too quickly because some rapid cyclers will only begin to show improvement after a year of treatment, especially if antidepressants can be avoided. Antipsychotic drug use, although common in difficult to stabilize bipolars, was recommended to be used sparingly because of the long-term risk of tardive dyskinesia. It is widely assumed that there will be less risk of tardive dyskinesia with the newer atypical antipsychotic drugs, especially, although more evidence is needed, with use of the least D_2-blocking members of the atypical group: olanzapine, quetiapine, or ziprasidone [when approved by the U.S. Food and Drug Administration (FDA)]. Clozapine, which is relatively free of EPS, has shown promise in the treatment of rapidly cycling individuals. Antidepressant drugs should be avoided if possible in rapid cyclers; however, patients who do not respond to mood stabilizers alone should not be left untreated during serious depressive episodes. When needed, antidepressants should be used for the shortest time possible. If one antidepressant clearly shortens cycle length, an antidepressant from another chemical class should be tried. Bupropion, mirtazapine, nefazodone, and perhaps the selective serotonin reuptake inhibitors (SSRIs) have all had reason to claim advantage over other tricyclic antidepressants (TCAs) at risk for manic switch, but this is not well established. Selective inhibitors of monoamine oxidase A are also said to be advantageous in this population, but none is currently available in the United States. ECT may be the best antidepressant modality in some rapidly cycling patients, although it too may precipitate switches into mania.

Acute Unipolar Depression

Most studies concur that although lithium as a single agent exhibits some antidepressant properties in selected bipolar patients, it is not a generally effective treatment for unipolar depression. Its major use in unipolar depression is in augmentation regimens (see also Chapter 3).

Lithium Augmentation of Antidepressants

Approximately 30% of patients with major depression do not improve substantially with their initial antidepressant treatment, and another 30% do not respond fully. Because it may take many weeks to observe improvement when changing from one antidepressant to another, a number of strategies, which include adding a second drug to the initial antidepressant, have been developed to convert refractory patients or partial responders to responders. The effectiveness of adding lithium to an unsuccessful antidepressant trial has been confirmed in placebo-controlled double-blind studies, case reports, and clinical practice. Lithium augmentation can be successful with a wide range of antidepressants, including SSRIs, TCAs, and monoamine oxidase inhibitors, although there is evidence that the rate and duration of response is superior with TCA than SSRI augmentation. Negative studies also have been reported. In addition, lithium augmentation has been reported to induce mania in a few cases. No correlation of clinical response with serum lithium level has been found.

Lithium augmentation may benefit approximately 50% of patients who receive it. Patients who are nonresponders on a fully adequate antidepressant regimen are generally started on lithium, 300 mg two to three times daily. A blood level should be checked after 5 to 7 days or if there are severe side effects to ensure that the drug level is not in the toxic range. Patients who respond generally do so within 2 to 3 weeks of augmentation therapy, although some patients respond more rapidly. Although some patients respond with low doses, a lithium level of 0.4 mEq/L is considered a minimum effective level.

Atypical Psychoses: Schizoaffective and Schizophreniform Disorders

As defined by the *Diagnostic and Statistical Manual of Mental Disorders,* 4th edition (DSM-IV), schizoaffective patients have prominent psychotic symptoms at times when they do not meet syndromal definitions for mania or depression, and they also have periods during which they do meet criteria for major depression or mania.

As defined by DSM-IV, schizophreniform disorder involves symptoms of schizophrenia, but of less than 6 months' duration. The onset of symptoms tends to be rapid rather than insidious, and patients may demonstrate confusion or perplexity at the height of their syndrome. Many, but not all, such patients lack the flat affect typical of schizophrenia.

Patients with schizoaffective and schizophreniform presentations are clearly heterogeneous, with diverse long-term outcomes. However, the clinician must still decide which patients, in addition to antipsychotic drugs, should receive a trial of treatments for possible mood disorders (i.e., lithium, valproate, or other anticonvulsants, antidepressants, or ECT).

From the current state of knowledge, the following guidelines for the use of lithium or valproate in schizoaffective, schizophreniform, and other atypical psychotic disorders can be tentatively suggested:

1. Clearly, acute onset from good baseline functioning is more suggestive of a mood disorder than schizophrenia. A family history of mood disorder helps corroborate this diagnosis. Dysphoric mania with psychosis may be confused with schizophreniform disorder.
2. When patients have moderate to severe mood disturbance with neurovegetative signs during the course of a schizoaffective illness, lithium, valproate or other anticonvulsants, or antidepressants should be tried as appropriate. Lithium, valproate, and possibly the atypical antipsychotics are the initial drugs of choice for schizomanic presentations. Antidepressants are the drug of choice for schizodepressed presentations. These treatments may help with abnormalities of mood, sleep, and appetite, even if hallucinations, delusions, or thought disorder prove resistant.
3. The presence of paranoia as the sole or predominant psychotic symptom should raise the possibility of atypical mania or depression, especially if there is a family history of mood disorders or if there are neurovegetative signs.

Cyclothymia

Cyclothymia is defined as a chronic mood disturbance with periods of hypomania and depressed mood or loss of interest or pleasure; however, episodes are not severe enough to meet criteria for mania or major depression. There is often a positive family history for mood disorders in such patients. Personality disorders and drug abuse may masquerade as cyclothymia, so caution is required in making the diagnosis. Lithium is often helpful, although less clearly so than in bipolar disorder. As with rapid-cycling bipolar patients, it may be necessary to employ an extended trial of lithium for a year or more to see improvement. Lithium in these patients is used in the same blood level range as in long-term treatment of bipolar patients.

Eating Disorders

There are scant data to suggest that lithium may be effective in bulimia. Given the dangers of lithium toxicity in individuals who abuse laxatives and diuretics, and the now well-established utility of the SSRIs and other antidepressant drugs as components of treatment for bulimia, lithium should be reserved only for bulimic patients who are also bipolar who do not do well on valproate or another anticonvulsant.

Alcohol Abuse

Lithium is not effective for the primary treatment of alcoholism. Alternatives such as naltrexone have far greater promise. Lithium or valproate are indicated, however, if after detoxification it becomes apparent that a patient's alcohol abuse is secondary to or coexists with bipolar disorder. Because active alcohol abuse may complicate the safe use of lithium, the drug ideally should not be prescribed prior to detoxification.

Personality Disorders

The literature is quite divided on the utility of lithium or other mood stabilizers in treating affective lability, emotional instability, and dyscontrol in patients with borderline and other personality disorders. A potential confounding variable in the study of personality disorders is the possibility that those individuals who responded to lithium (or antidepressants) had a comorbid mood disorder or a primary mood disorder that manifested itself as a personality disorder, or at least exacerbated a personality disorder.

Serum lithium levels in positive responders have usually been reported to be in the range of 0.6 to 1.2 mM. Although further research is needed to define lithium's usefulness, if any, in these emotionally unstable patients, lithium, carbamazepine, or valproate might be tried in those patients in whom mood swings and affective lability are prominent and disabling symptoms, so long as the mood stabilizer is not portrayed as a panacea, it is discontinued if it proves ineffective after an adequate trial (e.g., 12 weeks), and other treatment modalities continue.

Explosive and Violent Behavior

Some investigators have reported that lithium is effective in controlling episodic violence, both in adults with antisocial personality histories and in nonpsychotic, aggressive children with conduct disorders. Serum lithium levels between 0.6 and 1.3 mM have reportedly been used. Although lithium's efficacy for this indication needs further research, it might be tried in violent individuals if there is a family history of mood disorders or if the patient has symptoms suggesting that violent behavior might be a manifestation of a mood disorder. Lithium's use should be presented to the patient and family as an empirical trial rather than a proven treatment.

THERAPEUTIC USE

Before Starting Lithium

Some consensus has developed on the minimum workup of patients prior to starting lithium therapy (Table 4.3). Many clinicians also obtain a pretreatment complete blood count (CBC) because lithium may cause a benign elevation of the white blood cell count. Because lithium may depress sinoatrial node function, patients with sick sinus syndrome probably should be treated only if they have a cardiac pacemaker. There is no need to withhold lithium while waiting for the results of thyroid function tests, because there is no danger to the patient. If the patient proves to have a thyroid abnormality, it can be treated after lithium therapy has commenced. A pretreatment 24-hour creatinine clearance is not needed prior to beginning lithium unless the patient has known renal disease. If a lithium test dose is used for dosage prediction and low lithium clearance is discovered, or if the patient develops very high lithium levels on low doses when therapy begins, a creatinine clearance should then be performed. Measurement of creatinine clearance is also indicated if during the course of therapy there is a significant increase in the serum creatinine or a significant unexplained increase in lithium levels.

Methods have been developed to predict individual dosage requirements using a test dose of lithium. In healthy adults, 600 mg can be given and a blood level drawn 24 hours later. The expected daily dose requirement can be read from a nomogram.

Table 4.3. Summary: method of lithium use

Before beginning lithium
   Medical history
   Physical examination
   Blood urea nitrogen, creatinine
   T_4, T_3 resin uptake, TSH
   Electrocardiogram (ECG) with rhythm strip recommended if
      patient is over age 50 or has history of cardiac disease
   CBC (optional)
   Human chorionic gonadotropin (pregnancy test), if appropriate
Initial dosing
   Usually 300 mg t.i.d.
   Lower doses in elderly or with renal disease (150–300 b.i.d.)
Blood vessels
   Draw approximately 12 h after the last oral dose
   At start of therapy, every 5 days to adjust dose
   Draw less frequently as levels stabilize
   For stable long-term patients, draw every 3–6 mo
   Draw immediately if toxicity suspected
Follow-up monitoring (stable patients)
   Creatinine, TSH every 6 mo
   For patients over age 40 or with cardiac disease, follow-up ECGs
      as indicated

Table 4.4.   Prediction of lithium dose

Level	Predicted Total Daily Dosage
<0.05	3,600 mg
0.05–0.09	2,700 mg
0.10–0.14	1,800 mg
0.15–0.19	1,200 mg
0.20–0.23	900 mg
0.24–0.30	600 mg
>0.30	Use with extreme caution

Dosages required to achieve a serum lithium level of 0.9 ± 0.3 mEq/L predicted
from a lithium level drawn 24 hours after a single dose of 600 mg.
Adapted from Cooper TB, et al. *Am J Psychiatry* 1976;133:440.

Lower test doses should be used in the elderly (Table 4.4). This
test can be useful in identifying patients who are at the extremes
of the dosage range, including some patients with unsuspected
renal failure. However, because optimal care requires slow dosage
increases as side effects allow, dosage prediction from a nomogram
is no substitute for careful monitoring of side effects and levels.

Prior to starting lithium, patients should be told not to be discouraged if the onset of efficacy is slow and that extra doses are
not helpful and may be dangerous. They should also be
instructed not to alter their sodium intake, embark on a weight
reduction diet, or take diuretics or nonsteroidal antiinflammatory agents (NSAIDS) without medical supervision. This last
warning is particularly important now that NSAIDS such as
ibuprofen and naproxyn are available over the counter.

Blood Levels

Safe and effective lithium therapy is monitored by serum levels; oral dosage is not an adequate guideline. Because lithium
levels vary widely from peak to trough with most dosing schedules, it is best to draw blood levels as close to 12 hours after the
last oral dose as possible, usually in the morning prior to the
first daily dose. This must be emphasized to patients because a
misunderstanding will result in confusing or uninterpretable
levels. Regimens in which the entire dose is given at bedtime are
being used increasingly. These will produce morning levels 10%
to 20% higher than regimens using divided dosing.

Because the half-life of lithium is approximately 24 hours and
the time to steady state for any drug is four to five half-lives, levels should be drawn no sooner than 5 days after a change in
dosage unless toxicity is suspected. Levels drawn before equilibration is complete can be misleading because they may still be
on the rise. In the elderly and in patients with renal disease, the
elimination half-life and hence the time to equilibration is prolonged (often 7 days or more). If toxicity is suspected, lithium
should be withheld and a level determined immediately. Interpretation of the level requires that the time since the last dose
be taken into account.

Using Lithium

In healthy adults, the usual starting dosage is 300 mg three times daily, but smaller dosages (e.g., 150 mg twice daily) should be used if the patient is elderly or has renal disease. At the beginning of therapy, it is useful to draw levels after 5 days and to use results to adjust the dosage upward to the therapeutic range even if a dosage prediction nomogram has been used.

Many side effects that occur early in therapy, such as nausea and tremor, are due to absolute levels but also may occur at lower levels of lithium if the levels are rising too rapidly. It is best to increase the dosage slowly to avoid such side effects and to maximize patient comfort and eventual compliance. If troublesome side effects emerge at the beginning of therapy, the oral dosage should be temporarily decreased and then slowly increased again after several days as side effects allow. If there is pressure to obtain rapid symptom control, temporary use of antipsychotics or benzodiazepines may be more expedient.

Dosage Forms and Dosing Intervals

One of the major problems with long-term lithium therapy is patient compliance. Compliance is clearly improved when dosing regimens are simplified. Most patients tolerate lithium well on a twice-daily regimen, allowing omission of the often forgotten midday dose. Indeed there is evidence that lithium may be best tolerated by the kidney in a single nightly dose. Patients on a single daily dose have less polyuria and fewer renal structural abnormalities than patients on multiple daily doses (see later section on Renal Effects). The data suggest that the kidney is able to tolerate higher peak levels reached with single daily dosing but benefits from lower troughs. From the current evidence, it would appear appropriate to treat patients with single daily doses, especially if they have compliance problems or severe polyuria. In any case, there appears to be no reason to give lithium more frequently than twice daily unless the patient has serious peak level side effects. Slow-release lithium may help patients who have side effects at peak levels such as severe tremor or nausea, but a minority of patients will only tolerate lithium on a regimen of smaller, more frequent daily doses. The slow-release preparations available in the United States have excellent bioavailability and result in less dose fluctuation during the day than standard lithium. Because their absorption is delayed, however, these preparations have a greater tendency to cause diarrhea than regular lithium preparations.

Target Plasma Levels

As described previously, regimens in which the entire dose is given at bedtime will produce morning levels 10% to 20% higher than regimens with divided dosing. The target levels described in this section are based on divided dosing regimens. For **acute mania,** a therapeutic response is usually achieved at serum levels of 1.0 to 1.2 mM. There is no convincing justification for higher levels; levels greater than 1.5 mM are likely to be toxic. The oral dose that produces therapeutic levels varies with the size of the patient and his or her GFR. In healthy adults, the typical oral dose to produce a level of 1.0 mM is in the range of 1,500 ± 300 mg, but extreme doses range from 300 to 3,000 mg. Some clinicians report that early in the treatment of acute mania the oral doses needed to produce a given level may be higher than later in treatment. The reasons for this clinical observation are unknown.

For **prophylaxis,** levels of 0.8 to 1.0 mM have been shown to be more effective than lower blood levels, although they result in more side effects. If side effects are severe and may compromise therapy, the lowest effective serum level for that patient should be determined empirically. If a patient cannot tolerate lithium in the therapeutic range, substitution of valproate or carbamazepine should be considered.

Monitoring Long-Term Therapy

Following initiation of lithium therapy, patients should have a follow-up serum creatinine drawn after reaching a therapeutic blood level. Follow-up electrocardiograms (ECGs) should be performed as clinically indicated. Lithium can be expected to cause a variety of benign changes in the ECG, including a pattern similar to that of hypokalemia. (It is important to make sure that the patient is not, in fact, hypokalemic.) Therapy should only be interrupted if a potentially dangerous arrhythmia emerges.

During long-term lithium use, serum levels for stable patients can be obtained every 3–6 months as indicated (more frequently if toxicity is suspected, if noncompliance is a problem, or if mood symptoms emerge). Serum creatinine and TSH should be drawn every 6 months or if signs of renal or thyroid toxicity emerge. An unexplained increase in serum lithium levels requires an investigation of renal function.

Discontinuation of Lithium Therapy

Both open and controlled trials have documented that there is a substantial risk of new episodes of mania or depression following discontinuation of lithium even after years of stability on lithium. A review of existing studies found a high early risk of recurrent manias in bipolar patients following relatively abrupt lithium discontinuation, with over half of the recurrences occurring within the first 3 months after discontinuation. Depressive recurrences tended to come later. More striking, the survival time to 50% recurrence was 5 months, far shorter than during lithium treatment and even shorter than in previous untreated cycles (11.6 months) (Suppes et al., 1991). These data suggest a rebound effect with rapid discontinuation. In a prospective study, this group found that gradual (2–4 weeks) discontinuation of lithium diminished the risk of early recurrence (Faedda et al., 1993). Given these data, it would be prudent to taper lithium no more rapidly than 300 mg per month, unless side effects demand a more rapid taper. Concern also has been raised that discontinuation of lithium may cause later unresponsiveness to lithium. However, no evidence of such lithium resistance has emerged in recent follow-up analyses. Controlled longitudinal studies in bipolar disorder are required.

USE IN PREGNANCY

Women with bipolar disorder may experience significant affective symptoms during pregnancy and are at elevated risk of developing postpartum manias or depressions. However, use of lithium, valproate, or carbamazepine during the first trimester of pregnancy is associated with increased risk of major birth defects. All women with bipolar disorder considering pregnancy or who become pregnant should receive counseling on the relative risks of pharmacologic treatment versus no treatment in their particular case. A contingency plan should be made (and discussed with the family) concerning a course of action should a severe episode occur, especially during the first trimester of pregnancy.

First-trimester use of lithium has been associated with risk of Ebstein's anomaly (right ventricular hypoplasia and tricuspid valve insufficiency). Recent epidemiologic and case control studies suggest that the rates in the original Lithium Register were likely overestimates due to an over-reporting bias. Although there does appear to be an association (with a risk in the general population estimated at 1 in 20,000 births) between first trimester lithium exposure and risk of Ebstein's anomaly, the revised estimate is about 1 in 2,000 for exposure, a 10-fold increase over the general population. Thus, the absolute risk is low and certainly does not itself justify a recommendation of termination of pregnancy. Further modern sensitive fetal ultrasound technology can detect the presence or absence of Ebstein's anomaly by week 16 of gestation. Because of the risks posed by all mood stabilizers, ECT is the treatment of choice for severe manic or depressed episodes. Alternatives that appear to be safer than lithium, valproate, or carbamazepine include high-potency antipsychotic drugs, benzodiazepines, and, for depression, imipramine or fluoxetine.

Lithium use later in pregnancy may pose potential complications for the mother. Regulation of the lithium level may be complicated by changes in maternal blood volume, which increases during pregnancy by 50%, and GFR, which increases by 30% to 50%. At parturition, diuresis may lead to shifts in plasma lithium levels, which must be monitored to avoid lithium toxicity.

Lithium is secreted in breast milk at about half the serum levels in the mother. The effects of lithium on growth and development are unknown. Therefore, breast-feeding is typically discouraged among mothers who take lithium to reduce the risk of postpartum illness.

USE IN THE ELDERLY

Given the decrease in GFR and the decreased ratio of water to fat that occurs with increasing age, several precautions should be taken when using lithium in the elderly. Elderly patients should be started at lower dosages (e.g., 150–300 mg twice daily) depending on age and presence of renal dysfunction. Level drawing and dose changing should be slower to reflect the increased time to steady state (>7 days). In addition, the physician must be aware of any underlying cardiac disease. Elderly patients are often on drugs, such as diuretics and NSAIDs that may predispose to lithium toxicity. Finally, elderly patients are more sensitive to the neurologic toxicity of lithium. The physician should carefully document the patient's cognitive function before beginning lithium and then monitor the patient for the emergence of subtle confusional states. Risks of producing confusional states are greater if the patient is on combined therapy with other drugs such as antidepressants, antipsychotics, anticonvulsants, or anticholinergics.

SIDE EFFECTS

Use of lithium is complicated by its **low therapeutic index.** At serum levels not much higher than therapeutic, significant toxicity may occur. Even at therapeutic levels, perhaps 80% of patients experience some side effects, although only 30% would be characterized as moderate or severe. Mild to moderate side effects can be bothersome enough to patients to limit therapy. The most common side effects include thirst, increased urination, tremor, and weight gain. Side effects are often a particular problem at the initiation of therapy when levels are rising or several hours after dosing when peak levels are achieved. Patients who develop bothersome side effects within several hours of a dose may do better on a slow-release preparation; alternatively, the dosage schedule can be altered so that the medication is administered in more frequent smaller doses, but multiple daily dosing makes compliance more difficult.

As serum levels increase, more serious toxic symptoms can be expected, but because patients have varying susceptibility, lithium toxicity is primarily a clinical diagnosis for which serum levels provide confirmation. In general, some toxicity is to be expected at levels above 1.5 mM. Severe toxicity may manifest at levels as low as 2.0 mM and is almost always evident at levels above 3.0 mM. In addition to its dose-related toxicities, lithium may produce several idiosyncratic reactions, such as dermatologic reactions, which may occur at any level.

Gastrointestinal Side Effects

Patients treated with lithium may experience nausea, vomiting, anorexia, diarrhea, or abdominal pain. These symptoms are dose related, emerging at higher serum levels or with rapidly increasing serum levels at the initiation of treatment even if the actual level is not high. Thus, these symptoms are common at the start of treatment and are usually transient. If they occur with rising levels at the start of treatment, the dosage can be temporarily decreased and then increased again more slowly when the symptoms abate. Nausea may be minimized if lithium is given with meals or if slow-release preparations are used. However, slow-release preparations may result in a higher incidence of diarrhea than regular lithium. Patients who do not tolerate either preparation of the carbonate salt may have less gastrointestinal distress with lithium citrate syrup. Gastrointestinal symptoms that emerge late in treatment suggest the presence of toxic levels.

Renal Effects

Although lithium commonly causes defects in urine concentration ability, it rarely causes renal failure in patients whose lithium levels are maintained in the therapeutic range. An early report of serious abnormalities, including glomerulosclerosis and interstitial fibrosis on renal biopsies of patients on long-term lithium therapy, however, raised the concern that long-term lithium therapy might lead to renal failure. Longitudinal studies have failed to confirm this fear, and have not offered comparable reassurance for patients who have had periods of significant lithium toxicity. In a naturalistic study, 46 patients who had taken lithium for a mean of 8 years were compared with 16 patients undergoing renal biopsies for other reasons. The number of sclerotic tubules and atrophic glomeruli in the lithium-treated patients were slightly higher than those in controls, but the differences did not achieve statistical significance; changes in glomerular function were not clinically significant. However, the proportion of sclerotic glomeruli and atrophic tubules among lithium-treated patients was higher in patients who received lithium in divided daily doses than in those patients on once-daily dosing.

Polyuria

The most common renal problem due to lithium therapy is polyuria. This may be partly due to the antagonistic effect of lithium on the renal actions of ADH (antidiuretic hormone), leading to an inability to produce appropriately concentrated urine. However, other renal processes may contribute. Polyuria may occur in 50% to 70% of patients on long-term therapeutic doses of lithium; about 10% have a urine output of greater than 3 L/day, thus qualifying as having nephrogenic diabetes insipidus. Currently, lithium therapy is the most common cause of nephrogenic diabetes insipidus. Whether polyuria progresses with duration of therapy is unclear. One study of 32 patients on lithium for an average of 10 years found no interval change in polyuria in the most recent 2-year period of follow-up (Hetmar et al., 1987).

Polyuria, nocturia, and thirst can be very troublesome to patients. When severe, these symptoms may interfere with normal living habits and sleep. These symptoms may improve with dosage reduction and usually abate entirely when lithium is discontinued. A small number of patients, however, seem to have long-term (many months) or permanent urine-concentrating defects that suggest structural damage to the kidney.

MANAGEMENT OF POLYURIA. Patients who are symptomatic from polyuria should first be established at the minimum effective lithium levels for them. Second, lithium can be administered as a single bedtime dose. Third, diuretics can be administered, because diuretics paradoxically decrease urine outputs in lithium-induced polyuria.

The potassium-sparing diuretic amiloride markedly decreases urine volumes without a major effect on lithium or potassium serum levels, so long as the patient has normal renal function. Amiloride is started at 5 mg twice daily and can be increased to as much as 10 mg twice daily if the effect is inadequate. Total dosages above 20 mg/day do not have an added benefit. With amiloride, patients can remain on normal diets with unrestricted sodium. Nonetheless, it is prudent to monitor weekly lithium and potassium levels for several weeks after beginning amiloride to be sure that there are no changes.

Should amiloride not be tolerated, hydrochlorthiazide, 50 mg/day, can be substituted; should amiloride be tolerated but prove inadequately effective, hydrochlorthiazide, 50 mg/day, can be added. However, it must be recalled that thiazides alone or in combination with amiloride may increase lithium levels substantially. Thiazide diuretics reduce extracellular volume, leading to a compensatory increase in sodium reabsorption, thereby producing increased lithium reabsorption and elevation of lithium levels. Typically, thiazides used alone increase lithium levels by 30% to 50%. Thus if thiazides are used with or without amiloride, the lithium dosage should initially be halved and lithium levels monitored weekly; the needed oral dose to achieve the patient's therapeutic blood level can then be established. Thiazides have the additional problem of causing potassium depletion; even if the patient is also on amiloride, potassium levels should be monitored, initially on a weekly basis, until it is determined whether the patient is wasting potassium and needs potassium supplementation. When patients are on diuretics, it is prudent to obtain potassium levels when lithium levels are drawn.

Other Renal Problems

Rarely, patients have an **acute increase in serum creatinine** with the institution of lithium therapy, usually with a benign urinalysis (i.e., no cells or casts). Such cases are more common than is reported in the literature. These patients generally do not require a diagnostic renal biopsy. The majority have interstitial nephritis (tubulointerstitial nephropathy). In general, when the creatinine increases significantly in the context of lithium therapy, lithium should be discontinued and a 24-hour creatinine clearance performed. Of course, the physician should be sure that the problem is not due to an episode of lithium toxicity, dehydration, obstruction, or the addition of another medication. Patients who have acute interstitial nephritis will have markedly decreased creatinine clearance. Fortunately, when these changes are detected early, they are reversible with permanent discontinuation of lithium.

A small number of patients have been reported to develop **nephrotic syndrome** in association with lithium therapy (Wood et al., 1989). Nephrotic syndrome is usually reversed by discontinuation of lithium, but occasionally corticosteroids have proved necessary. Renal biopsies have revealed fusion of renal epithelial foot processes (minimal change disease). These patients should not be treated with lithium again.

Edema

A minority of patients develop intermittent **edema** of the lower extremities or face, unrelated to any changes in renal function. The edema often resolves spontaneously. If a medical etiology has been ruled out and the edema poses a problem for the individual, lithium-related edema can be treated with the diuretic spironolactone. If spironolactone is administered, lithium levels and electrolytes should be monitored (lithium levels may increase with the use of this drug).

Neurologic Side Effects

Mild neurologic side effects may occur with increasing lithium levels at the start of therapy or with stable therapy, especially at times of peak levels. These complaints include lethargy, fatigue, weakness, and action tremor. The **tremor** is a 7- to 16-Hz action tremor similar to physiologic or essential tremor and unlike the pill-rolling tremor of parkinsonism. It is aggravated by anxiety and performance of fine motor movements. It also may be aggravated in some patients by concomitant administration of antidepressants. Tremor may be embarrassing for some patients and may impair normal daily activities involving delicate motor movements. Tremor can often be controlled by decreasing the lithium dosage, if possible, and decreasing or stopping caffeine intake and, if these maneuvers fail, by adding a β-adrenergic blocker, such as propranolol. Propranolol, 10 to 20 mg, can be taken 30 minutes prior to an activity in which tremor will be a serious problem. For patients who require suppression of tremor all day, propranolol may be started at 10 to 20 mg twice daily with the dose titrated upward as needed. Patients who develop central nervous system side effects from propranolol may do better on the less lipophilic drug atenolol, 50 mg/day in a single daily dose. Coarsening of the tremor may be a sign of lithium toxicity.

Lithium may independently cause EPS in a minority of patients and may worsen neuroleptic-induced EPS in some patients. The balance of the evidence suggests that lithium neither prevents nor predisposes to tardive dyskinesia. There have been case reports of lithium causing recurrence of NMS when used in place of antipsychotic drugs in patients recovering from NMS. This may be due to the same mechanisms by which lithium causes EPS. Given the rarity of such reports, lithium may be used safely in patients who have recovered from NMS, but the possibility of recurrence should be kept in mind.

Several cases of **benign intracranial hypertension** (pseudotumor cerebri) occurring in association with lithium therapy have been reported. Patients presented with headache, blurred vision, and papilledema. If lithium is causally related to pseudotumor at all (perhaps by inhibiting cerebrospinal fluid reabsorption), the problem appears to be extremely rare. Therefore, screening fundoscopic examinations appear to be unnecessary. However, it would be prudent to perform a fundoscopic examination and to consider this diagnosis in patients who complain of severe headaches or new visual abnormalities while on lithium.

Lithium may produce **electroencephalographic changes** in a large proportion of patients, but only variable and minor effects on seizure threshold have been reported. Although worsening has been reported in some patients with complex partial (temporolimbic) epilepsy, many other such patients have improved behaviorally without a worsening pattern of seizures. In an open study of bipolar patients with seizure disorders (primary generalized seizures or complex partial seizures), lithium was effective in treating the mood disorder and did not increase the seizure frequency in patients with active seizures or induce seizures in patients whose seizures had remitted (Shukla et al., 1988). Pending new data, lithium should not be withheld from patients who have both mood and seizure disorders, but careful clinical monitoring is needed. Lithium does not affect serum levels of anticonvulsants.

The appearance of new neurologic symptoms during the course of therapy, even if mild, should raise the suspicion of lithium toxicity. A lithium level should be drawn and subsequent doses withheld until the question of toxicity is resolved. Patients may develop **moderately severe neurologic symptoms** at lithium levels not much higher than therapeutic ones. Some elderly patients or patients with brain lesions or dementia may develop such toxic symptoms even in the conventional therapeutic range. Moderate neurologic toxicity includes neuromuscular irritability, including twitching and fasciculations, EPS, ataxia, coarsening of tremor, dysarthria, incoordination, difficulty in concentrating, confusion, visual disturbance, and altered levels of consciousness. Symptoms of encephalopathy due to lithium, such as confusion or hallucinations, may be difficult to distinguish from the underlying illness, especially in patients who have a concomitant dementia. Lithium combinations with typical antipsychotics (commonly used in mania) are more likely to produce EPS and encephalopathy than either drug alone.

Severe neurologic toxicity can cause ataxia, seizures, hallucinations, delirium, coma, and death. With lithium poisoning, permanent memory impairment, nystagmus and cerebellar ataxia may occur.

Cognitive and Psychological Side Effects

Patients on lithium may complain of dull affect, a sense of depersonalization, a general "graying" of their mental life, or loss of creativity. Patients also may complain of memory disturbance and cognitive slowing. It has been difficult to quantify these complaints, some of which may reflect loss of valued hypomanias or mild depression. Schou (1984) followed artists on lithium and found that creativity increased, decreased, or was unchanged on lithium, depending on the individual. Several investigators have found that subjective complaints of memory disturbance in their study population were partly explained as effects of aging and depression, although lithium could not be completely exonerated from impairing certain cognitive tasks. Joffe and associates (1988) tested attention, concentration, visuomotor function, and memory in 12 normal controls and 18 patients on lithium (serum levels 0.7–0.9 mM) and on carbamazepine. The lithium and carbamazepine patients did not differ from controls. Further study with larger sample sizes is necessary to decide this issue. For the present, when patients complain of such side effects it makes sense to attempt prophylaxis with the lowest possible lithium level that affords the patient effective treatment. When patients complain of cognitive difficulty, a mental status examination should be performed and symptoms of depression should be elicited to rule out a treatable condition. In some cases, alternative therapies, such as an anticonvulsant, will be necessary.

Thyroid Side Effects

Lithium interferes with the production of thyroid hormones at multiple steps, including iodine uptake, tyrosine iodination, and release of T_3 and T_4. Inhibition of the TSH-responsive adenylyl cyclase in thyroid cells may be responsible. Clinically, patients may develop goiter with or without some degree of hypothyroidism. Overall, approximately 5% of patients on long-term lithium develop hypothyroidism (compared with 0.3%–1.3% in the general population, predominantly women). Perhaps 3% of patients on lithium will develop goiter. On the other hand, a much larger percentage develop increased levels of TSH. The clinical importance of this latter finding is not clear; treatment of TSH abnormalities in the absence of abnormalities in T_3 or T_4 is controversial. Patients with antithyroid antibodies prior to onset of lithium therapy appear to be at higher risk for development of hypothyroidism. The timing of onset of thyroid problems during lithium therapy is extremely variable.

Because of lithium's thyroid toxicities, it is important to perform baseline thyroid studies (TSH, T_4, and T_3 resin uptake). In follow-up, patients should be observed for development of goiter, and thyroid function tests (at least a TSH, which is the most sensitive for hypothyroidism) should be drawn every 6 months. Development of thyroid abnormalities does not necessitate a change in lithium therapy but rather treatment of the thyroid problem, usually in consultation with an endocrinologist or general internist. Should hypothyroidism or goiter develop, they can generally be treated by addition of thyroid hormone (e.g., synthetic T_4). Because hypothyroidism, including lithium-induced hypothyroidism, can present refractory depression (Yassa et al., 1988), it is important to check thyroid function if the patient's pattern of depressive episodes changes in character or becomes treatment resistant.

Cardiac Toxicity

It is reasonable to question patients about cardiac symptoms or history of cardiac disease before initiating lithium therapy. Patients over age 50 or those who have a cardiac history should have a baseline ECG with follow-up ECGs as clinically indicated. If there is any question about cardiac disease, a consultation with an internist should be obtained. During follow-up visits, patients should be asked about dizziness, palpitations, or irregular heartbeats when they are asked about other possible side effects of lithium.

Many patients treated with lithium develop **ECG changes** such as T-wave flattening or inversion. These changes correlate poorly with serum levels, are reversible with discontinuation of lithium, and are almost always benign. It is important, however, that other possible causes of T-wave abnormalities, such as hypokalemia, are not ignored because the patient is on lithium.

Arrhythmias due to lithium have been described, almost always in patients with preexisting cardiac disease. Sinoatrial node dysfunction, including sinoatrial block and tachycardia, have been reported. These may present with dizziness, syncope, or palpitations or may be asymptomatic. They are reversible with discontinuation of lithium. Patients with preexisting sinoatrial node dysfunction (sick sinus syndrome) can only be safely treated if they have a cardiac pacemaker. Because the calcium channel blocker verapamil is occasionally used as a treatment of bipolar disorder, there is a possibility that it will be used together with lithium. Cases of serious bradycardia with this combination have been reported.

Ventricular arrhythmias also have been reported, although rarely. In several case reports, patients were also receiving antipsychotic drugs. Now that it is known that some antipsychotics (e.g., thioridazine and trifluoperazine) are calcium antagonists, it is possible that the cause for the arrhythmias should be reassigned to the antipsychotic or to combined toxicity.

Dermatologic Reactions

Dermatologic reactions appear to be idiosyncratic rather than dose related. They include acne and psoriasis (which are the most frequent), maculopapular eruptions, folliculitis, and extremely rare cases of exfoliative dermatitis. This last, a presumed hypersensitivity reaction, may be life threatening; patients who recover should not receive lithium again.

Acne

Acneiform eruptions are probably the most common dermatologic reaction to lithium. They may prove to be a major stumbling block to acceptance of lithium by adolescents and young adults unless vigorously treated. The acne usually begins as a monomorphic eruption (all lesions in the same stage) and may occur on the face, neck, shoulders, and back. The eruptions may be new or an exacerbation of preexisting acne. The acne usually responds to vigorous treatment with standard anti-acne regimens. If the acne does not respond, a dermatologic consultation might be useful, especially if lithium refusal could result from the patient's cosmetic concerns.

Psoriasis

Lithium may cause exacerbations of preexisting psoriasis or onset of new psoriasis. Psoriasis due to lithium tends to be treatment resistant but usually regresses with discontinuation of the drug. The decision to stop lithium must obviously be balanced with the risks to the patient from affective illness. The anticonvulsants do not appear to have any effects on this skin disorder. Some patients with preexisting psoriasis do not worsen on lithium; thus, a history of psoriasis is not an absolute contraindication to lithium therapy, although patients with severe disease or psoriatic arthritis might be more safely treated with anticonvulsants, including valproate, carbamazepine, gabapentin, or lamotrigine.

Other Dermatologic Reactions

Maculopapular rashes (usually pruritic) have been reported to occur occasionally early in treatment. These often regress by themselves. Asymptomatic folliculitis, which may occur as hyperkeratotic erythematous follicular papules on extensor surfaces, the abdomen, and the buttocks, also has been reported. It appears to pose little problem for patients and should not require changes in lithium therapy.

Hair loss is a rare side effect of lithium therapy. When hair loss occurs, it is important to check for hypothyroidism and other possible causes of alopecia.

Hematologic Effects

Lithium produces a benign, relative leukocytosis, increasing neutrophil mass without impairing function. There is no known adverse effect; in fact, leukocytosis induced by lithium has been exploited in the treatment of leukopenic patients. It is important to be aware of this effect of lithium to avoid unnecessary medical workups for elevated white blood cell counts. The total white blood cell count rarely exceeds 15,000 as a result of lithium therapy alone.

Weight Gain

A side effect that can be extremely troublesome and lead to noncompliance or lithium refusal is weight gain (Garland et al., 1988). In some studies, lithium has been associated with weight gain of more than 10 kg in 20% of patients on long-term therapy. Lithium has been reported to have insulin-like effects on carbohydrate metabolism. Antipsychotic drugs and cyclic antidepressants also may cause obesity (a hypothalamic mechanism has been the hypothesized cause for this). Patients who are polyuric should be advised not to replace their fluid losses with high-calorie beverages such as beer or sugary sodas. Some will benefit from dietary consultation. For some patients who have developed severe obesity, substitution of another drug for lithium might be considered.

Calcium Metabolism

Anecdotal reports and several small studies have associated lithium therapy with mild elevations in calcium and parathyroid hormone. These elevations appear to be rarely, if ever, clinically significant. However, because alterations in calcium level are associated with neuropsychiatric symptoms, serum calcium levels might be obtained if there is a change in a patient's pattern of symptoms, especially depressive symptoms.

EVALUATION AND TREATMENT OF LITHIUM TOXICITY DUE TO ELEVATED LEVELS

For **mild toxicity,** lithium should be withheld until levels return to the patient's usual therapeutic range. If an obvious cause for the change in level cannot be found, a renal workup should be undertaken, including urinalysis and creatinine clearance.

For **moderate to severe lithium toxicity,** the patient is best admitted to a hospital. Adequate sodium should be given, and lithium levels should be checked several times a day to make sure that they are decreasing. If the patient does not have congestive heart failure or renal failure, intravenous administration of normal saline at a rate of 150 to 200 mL/h is often effective in reducing lithium levels rapidly; this is safe as long as urine output is adequate.

Acute Lithium Intoxication

Acute lithium intoxication, manifested by a severe clinical syndrome or levels above 3.0 mM, is a medical emergency. Because the severity and reversibility of toxic symptoms are related both to the serum level and to the duration of high levels, rapid aggressive treatment is necessary even if the patient appears clinically well. Indeed, early in lithium poisoning the patient's symptoms may be relatively mild despite high levels, giving the physician a false sense of security. Symptoms of serious intoxication include both systemic and neurologic symptoms, including nausea, vomiting, diarrhea, renal failure, neuromuscular irritability or flaccid-

ity, ataxia, dysarthria, coarse tremor, confusion, delirium, hallucinations, seizures, and stupor. Protracted coma and glucose intolerance have been reported. Lithium poisoning also may cause
death. Survivors of serious toxicity may suffer permanent cerebellar ataxia and severe permanent anterograde amnesia.

In treating acute lithium intoxication, the therapeutic goal is
to remove lithium from the body as rapidly as possible. It is
important to obtain a toxic screen to know what other agents the
patient has ingested, especially if the case appears to be an
intentional overdose. If the patient is stuporous or comatose, protection of the airway, with intubation if necessary, and cardiorespiratory support should be the first priority. In overdose
cases in which the drug was taken less than 4 hours prior to
treatment, induction of vomiting in alert patients or gastric
lavage in comatose patients will help diminish the risk of worsening toxicity. Because lithium levels are often high in gastric
secretions, continuous gastric aspiration can be helpful.

Despite the fact that most reports of lithium intoxication are
either anecdotal or retrospective, there seems to be strong evidence that management should be aggressive. If lithium levels
are less than 3 mM and signs of intoxication are mild, fluid and
electrolyte abnormalities should be corrected and normal saline
may be administered at a rate of 150 to 200 mL/h, as long as
urine output is adequate. If the lithium level is greater than 3
mM and signs of toxicity are severe, or if there is poor urine output or renal failure, prompt institution of dialysis is indicated. If
the lithium level is above 4 mM and does not respond within a
few hours to saline diuresis at a rate of 250 mL/h, dialysis is
indicated regardless of the patient's clinical appearance.
Hemodialysis is most effective, but where unavailable, peritoneal dialysis may be used. Lithium will reequilibrate from the
tissues after a dialysis treatment, so frequent monitoring of the
lithium level is important. A reasonable end point is a lithium
level of 1.0 mM or less 6 hours after a dialysis treatment.

Causes of Intoxication

Although overdosage is an important cause of toxic serum levels, the most common cause of toxicity among compliant patients
is an **alteration in sodium balance.** Any condition that leads to
sodium depletion will elevate lithium levels; thus, dehydration,
changes in dietary habits (either with sodium restriction or overall weight reduction diets), or administration of sodium-wasting
diuretics will cause elevations in lithium levels. There has been
concern that heavy exercise or fever, both of which produce sweating, could result in lithium toxicity. However, it appears that
sweat contains enough lithium that heavy perspiration does not
elevate lithium levels. Other renal causes of lithium retention
include many NSAIDS (not aspirin, however) in susceptible individuals, intrinsic renal disease, and systemic diseases (e.g., congestive heart failure or cirrhosis) that decrease renal blood flow.

DRUG INTERACTIONS

Alcohol and other central nervous system depressants, including prescribed psychotropic drugs and antihypertensive agents,
may interact with lithium to produce sedation or confusional

Table 4.5. Pharmacokinetic interactions with lithium

Interactions that Increase Lithium Levels	Interactions that Decrease Lithium Levels
Diuretics	Acetazolamide
Thiazides	Theophylline, aminophylline
Ethacrynic acid	Caffeine (mild effect)
Spironolactone	Osmotic diuretics
Triamterene	
Nonsteroidal antiinflammatory agents	
Antibiotics	
Metronidazole (Flagyl)	
Tetracyclines	
Angiotensin-converting enzyme inhibitors	

states. NSAIDS and thiazide diuretics may increase lithium levels with resultant intoxication (Table 4.5). Metronidazole has been reported to cause serious renal toxicity when used in combination with lithium.

PSYCHIATRIC USES OF ANTICONVULSANTS

This section focuses on the psychiatric uses of anticonvulsants. Epilepsy and other neurologic disorders are mentioned only briefly because a full discussion would occupy an entire volume. Two anticonvulsants have proved particularly useful in the treatment of bipolar disorder, several others currently are being studied for both affective disorders and other psychiatric illnesses such as substance abuse. Carbamazepine was the first anticonvulsant used to treat mania, but clinicians now favor valproic acid. Valproic acid is a widely accepted agent in the treatment of bipolar disorder. Carbamazepine is also a useful treatment for bipolar disorder and has been tried in several other conditions. Like lithium, both valproic acid and carbamazepine are more effective in treating and preventing manic episodes than depressive episodes. Phenytoin and the barbiturates do not appear to possess mood-stabilizing properties that would make them useful in the treatment of bipolar disorder. Several recently approved anticonvulsants require further study for psychiatric applications. Clonazepam, a benzodiazepine with high enough potency and a long enough half-life to be used as an anticonvulsant, is effective in panic disorder and is a useful adjunct in the treatment of some patients with bipolar disorder or other psychotic conditions who require greater anxiolysis or sedation than is provided by their primary therapeutic agents. Clonazepam is fully discussed in Chapter 5.

Lithium had been the first-choice treatment for bipolar disorder; nonetheless, more than 30% of bipolar patients either have a poor response to lithium or cannot tolerate it. Given the side effects of the typical antipsychotic drugs and their long-term risk of tardive dyskinesia (which may be elevated in patients with mood disorders), the use of the older antipsychotics in bipolar disorder should be minimized if possible. Clozapine is not likely to cause tardive dyskinesia but has many side effects that adversely affect quality of life. Other atypicals have not been well studied as to their long-term safety and efficacy in the maintenance treatment of bipolar disorder. ECT is effective in the treatment of acute mania and depression; however, it does not appear to be a viable long-term treatment. Thus, the development of additional anticonvulsants as alternatives to lithium is desirable.

VALPROATE

A number of well-designed studies suggest that valproate is as effective as lithium for bipolar disorder. Valproate was initially approved as an anticonvulsant and is effective in the control of absence (petit mal), myoclonic, and generalized tonic–clonic seizures. It is less effective in partial seizures with or without complex symptomatology. Approved by the FDA in 1995 for the treatment of acute mania, valproate appeared superior to lithium in rapid cycling and dysphoric mania. Moreover, in contrast to lithium, the antimanic effect of valproate is not diminished by a history of a large number of prior episodes. Based on the existing efficacy data and side effects, many clinicians now use valproate as the first choice therapy in the treatment of mania, particularly in mixed states or when mania cooccurs with other disorders.

Pharmacology

Valproic acid is available in several different preparations and dosage forms (Table 4.6). Valproic acid is available in capsule or syrup form. Divalproex sodium is an enteric-coated form that contains equal parts valproic acid and sodium valproate. Both valproic acid and valproex circulate in their ionized form, valproate. Valproic acid is rapidly absorbed after oral administration, achieving peak levels in 1 to 2 hours if taken on an empty stomach and in 4 to 5 hours if taken with food. Divalproex

Table 4.6. Available preparations of valproic acid and carbamazepine

Form	Brand Name	How Supplied
Valproic acid	Depakene	250-mg capsules
	Depakene	250 mg/5 mL syrup
	Valproic acid	250-mg capsules
Divalproex sodium	Depakote	125-, 250-, 500-mg tablets
	Depakote	125-mg sprinkle capsules
Carbamazepine	Atretol	200-mg tablet
	Tegretol	100-, 200-mg tablets
	Tegretol	100 mg/5 mL suspension
	Carbamazepine	200-mg tablets
	Carbamazepine	100-mg chewable tablets

sodium is more slowly absorbed, reaching peak serum concentrations in 3 to 8 hours.

In plasma, valproic acid is 80% to 95% protein bound. It is rapidly metabolized by the liver; it has no known active metabolites. Interactions with other protein-bound or hepatically metabolized drugs occur. Valproic acid has a short elimination half-life of approximately 8 hours; thus, three times daily dosing is usually recommended for epilepsy. The need for divided dosing in bipolar disorder has not been established.

There is a poor correlation between serum levels and antimanic effects, but levels in the range of 50 to 150 µg/mL are generally required. Blood levels are measured by immunoassay or gas chromatography.

The precise **mechanism of action** in both bipolar disorder and epilepsy is unknown, but valproic acid is known to increase synaptic levels of gamma-aminobutyric acid (GABA), the principal inhibitory neurotransmitter in the brain. Experimentally, it blocks the convulsive effects of the $GABA_A$ receptor antagonists picrotoxin and bicuculline. Whether it also shares mechanisms with lithium (e.g., in the GSK-3β/wnt pathway) is currently a matter of investigation.

Psychiatric Indications

Bipolar Disorder

As described above, there is now enough evidence for many clinicians to use valproate as the first-choice therapy for bipolar disorder. When valproate fails as monotherapy, it may be combined with lithium, carbamazepine, or other agents. Valproic acid is generally better tolerated than lithium, and unlike carbamazepine, tolerance to valproate is rare. Valproate is now used by many clinicians for long-term prophylaxis, despite the lack of adequate evidence from well-designed studies. Based on open studies, it appears that when used for prophylaxis, valproate is more effective in preventing manic than depressive recurrences. Open studies and anecdotal clinical data do not currently support the use of valproate as an antidepressant. However, it may decrease the risk of mania in bipolar patients being treated with an antidepressant.

Schizoaffective Disorder

Open trials and case reports suggest that valproate may be substituted for lithium in mood stabilization or during maniclike episodes in schizoaffective disorder. Valproate does not appear to be effective for well-diagnosed schizophrenic patients or schizoaffective patients whose episodes of mood disorder are exclusively depressive.

Other Psychiatric Indications

Valproate is an alternative to benzodiazepines (see Chapter 5) in the treatment of alcohol withdrawal, a state that is not uncommonly associated with hospitalization for mania.

Therapeutic Use

There is no standardized workup prior to initiation of valproic acid therapy, but it is optimal to obtain a general medical history and examination, with particular attention to other drugs used by the patient and any history of liver disease or bleeding disorder. Ideally, baseline liver function tests (LFTs) and a CBC with platelets also should be obtained. Valproic acid should not be administered to patients with known liver disease.

Valproic acid therapy should be initiated slowly to minimize side effects. A first test dose of 250 mg is best given with a meal. Gradually the dosage can be increased to 250 mg three times daily over several days as gastrointestinal symptoms and sedation allow. Further dosage increases, probably up to 1,800 mg/day, can be made as needed to control symptoms. Optimal blood levels for both seizure disorders and mania are debated but appear to be in the range of 50 to 150 µg/mL. Blood levels may be obtained weekly until the patient is stable. Many clinicians also obtain LFTs and a CBC at the same time. Antimanic effects are generally seen within 1 to 2 weeks of achieving target levels.

An alternative approach to initiating valproic acid treatment for inpatients is an oral loading strategy using 20 to 30 mg/kg body weight. The onset of reduction in manic symptoms occurs more quickly, within a few days of starting treatment, diminishing the need for antipsychotics early in the course of therapy. The prophylactic effect of valproic acid over the long-term is roughly comparable with that of lithium.

In stable, asymptomatic patients, blood levels, LFTs, and a CBC may be obtained every 6 months. However, new onset of side effects after stable therapy has been achieved should prompt measurement of drug levels and additional appropriate workup. For example, late onset of nausea, anorexia, or fatigue is an indication for obtaining levels and LFTs, including ammonia levels.

Use in Pregnancy

Valproic acid has not been well studied in pregnancy, but it has been associated with major congenital malformations, including spina bifida. Given reports of neural tube defects as high as 5% in offspring of women treated with valproate in the first trimester, the drug is not a preferred choice over lithium; however, if a woman does remain on treatment, there is a suggestion that supplemental folate may reduce the risk. Alterations in clotting function also may pose risks to mother and fetus later in pregnancy and at parturition. Alternative treatments for mania that appear to be safer include ECT and high-potency antipsychotic drugs (see earlier section regarding lithium in Use in Pregnancy). Valproic acid is secreted in breast milk at concentrations 1% to 10% of serum concentration. The effect on the developing child is unknown.

Side Effects and Toxicity

Minor side effects are common at the start of treatment with valproic acid and are often transient. These include gastrointestinal effects (including nausea, vomiting, anorexia, heartburn, and diarrhea), sedation, tremor, and ataxia (Table 4.7). Administration with food or use of enteric-coated preparations, such as divalproex, may help diminish gastrointestinal effects. Histamine H_2 receptor blockers such as ranitidine also may decrease upper gastrointestinal distress but risk possible drug interactions. Approx-

Table 4.7. Side effects and toxicity of valproic acid

Common side effects
  Gastrointestinal: nausea, vomiting, anorexia, heartburn, diarrhea
  Hematologic: thrombocytopenia, platelet dysfunction
  Hepatic: benign elevation of transaminases
  Neurologic: sedation, tremor, ataxia
  Other: alopecia, weight gain
Less common side effects
  Hematologic: bleeding tendency
  Metabolic: hyperammonemia
  Neurologic: incoordination, asterixis, stupor, coma, behavioral
    automatisms
Serious idiosyncratic side effects
  Hepatitis/hepatic failure
  Pancreatitis
  Drug rashes, including erythema multiforme

imately half of those treated initially experience some degree of sedation. This tends to diminish with chronic use. Sedation may become a severe problem when valproic acid is coadministered with other anticonvulsants, especially phenobarbital (which is not used for bipolar disorder). Valproic acid appears to cause mild impairment of cognitive function with chronic use; in this regard it is slightly inferior to carbamazepine, but superior to phenytoin or barbiturates. The other common side effects of valproic acid are alopecia and weight gain.

Hepatotoxicity

Valproic acid may cause transient dose-dependent asymptomatic increases in aspartate and alanine transaminases in 15% to 30% of patients, which are an indication for monitoring but not for stopping treatment. These laboratory abnormalities are generally maximal during the first 3 months of treatment. Isolated hyperammonemia, which may be accompanied by confusion or lethargy, has been reported rarely. These hepatic effects usually improve with decreased dosage. Rare cases of fatal hepatotoxicity associated with valproate have been reported. Between 1978 and 1984, 37 cases were discovered. All but one patient had medical conditions in addition to the seizure disorder for which valproate was being prescribed, such as mental retardation, developmental delay, congenital abnormalities, or other neurologic disorders. Between 1985 and 1986, the rate of fatal hepatotoxicity was 2.5 in 100,000 patients. For patients receiving valproate as their only anticonvulsant drug, the rate of fatal hepatotoxicity was 0.85 in 100,000 patients. No hepatic fatalities have been reported in patients above age 10 receiving valproate as their only anticonvulsant. Given the experience with valproate–lithium combinations in populations with psychiatric rather than seizure disorders, the risk of hepatic toxicity in psychiatric use appears to be very low, and certainly far lower than the risk to life from undertreated bipolar disorder. Minor elevations in hepatic transaminases are commonly seen with the use of this medication and should not be viewed as a warning that liver function studies will continue to worsen. Should significant liver function abnormalities or symptoms of hepatitis occur (e.g., malaise, anorexia, jaundice, abdominal pain, or edema), the drug should be immediately discontinued and the patient carefully monitored.

Neurotoxicity

As noted previously, sedation is the most serious problem, and hand tremor is the most common long-term neurologic side effect. If troublesome, these side effects generally diminish if the dosage is decreased. There are anecdotal reports of tremor responding to β-adrenergic blockers, such as propranolol (as in the case of lithium tremor; see Chapter 6), but β blockers have been associated with their own central nervous system side effects, including depression-like symptoms. Ataxia may occur at higher doses of valproic acid. Rarely, asterixis, stupor, coma, and behavioral automatisms have been reported.

Hematologic Toxicity

Valproic acid can cause thrombocytopenia or platelet dysfunction, but only rarely is it associated with bleeding complications. This effect is usually only observed in patients on high doses. Patients on valproate should have their platelet count and bleeding time checked before any surgery.

Other Serious Idiosyncratic Toxicities

Rarely, hemorrhagic pancreatitis may occur, usually in the first 6 months of treatment, and may be fatal. Agranulocytosis is also a rare idiosyncratic side effect. Drug rashes, including erythema multiforme, also have been reported. There is concern that the rates of polycystic ovary disease may be increased in women treated with valproic acid; pending further study, it is not clear whether the association with valproate is causal or related to other factors such as obesity or epilepsy.

Serious Dose-Related Toxicities and Overdoses

Excessive serum levels may occur in the context of drug–drug interactions or intentional overdose. The symptoms of overdose include severe neurologic symptoms. Overdose with valproic acid can be treated with hemodialysis. Only rare fatalities have been reported.

Drug Interactions

Valproic acid may have pharmacodynamic interactions with other psychotropic drugs, including carbamazepine, lithium, and antipsychotic drugs, producing combined central nervous system toxicity. Whenever multiple psychotropic drugs are coadministered, patients must be monitored for deterioration of mental status.

Valproic acid also produces pharmacokinetic interactions with many drugs. It inhibits the metabolism of drugs that are oxidized by the liver; thus, it may increase levels of cyclic antidepressants and possibly SSRIs, phenytoin, phenobarbital, and other drugs. Valproic acid also may increase the effective levels of other protein-bound drugs, or conversely, it may be displaced from protein binding by drugs such as aspirin, precipitating valproic acid toxicity. Thus, patients who must take other protein-bound drugs, such as warfarin, must be monitored closely at the initiation of combined therapy.

Valproic acid concentrations may be decreased by drugs, such as carbamazepine, that induce hepatic microsomal enzymes. Its concentrations may be increased by drugs, such as SSRIs, that inhibit hepatic microsomal enzymes.

It should also be noted that valproic acid is partially eliminated in the urine as a ketometabolite, which may lead to false interpretations of urine ketone tests.

CARBAMAZEPINE

Carbamazepine is an iminostilbene anticonvulsant that is structurally similar to the tricyclic antidepressant imipramine. It is generally considered to be the drug of first choice in the treatment of partial epilepsy with or without complex symptomatology; it is also effective for primary generalized seizures. Carbamazepine is also the treatment of choice in trigeminal neuralgia and is used in other neuropathic pain syndromes that have a lancinating component.

Several reports in the neurologic literature suggested that carbamazepine improved mood symptoms in patients treated for epilepsy. It was first reported as a primary treatment for manic–depressive illness in Japan in the early 1970s. Since that time, many studies of carbamazepine for acute mania have been performed, although few have been well designed. Carbamazepine is more effective than placebo for acute mania. It remains unclear whether it is as effective as lithium. It appears to be useful for some patients in long-term bipolar prophylaxis, but its general utility for this indication has not been established, and some reports have suggested diminishing effectiveness over time. On the basis of small studies and case reports, some investigators have suggested that carbamazepine may be particularly effective for patients with forms of bipolar disorder that are often relatively refractory to lithium [i.e., patients with mixed bipolar symptoms (both manic and depressed symptoms present), dysphoric mania, and rapid-cycling bipolar disorder]. Carbamazepine is now under study for a variety of psychiatric disorders other than bipolar disorder.

Pharmacology

Carbamazepine is available for oral administration as 100-mg and 200-mg tablets and as a suspension (Table 4.6). No parenteral forms are available. Its absorption is slow and erratic, with peak levels usually achieved in 4 to 8 hours, but occasionally later. Slow-release forms appear to produce more stable serum concentrations than regular tablets. Carbamazepine is poorly soluble in gastrointestinal fluids; after oral administration, 15% to 25% is excreted unchanged in the feces. The effect of food on absorption does not appear to be clinically significant. In the blood it is 65% to 80% protein bound.

Blood levels can be measured by gas–liquid chromatography, high-pressure liquid chromatography, and immunoassays. Therapeutic levels for epilepsy are in the range of 4 to 12 µg/mL (core range 6–10 μg/mL), with the lower end of the range typically effective for tonic–clonic seizures and the higher end effective for partial seizures with or without tonic–clonic seizures. For bipolar disorder, initial studies suggested that blood levels in the range of 8 to 12 μg/mL corresponded to therapeutic efficacy. More recently this correlation has appeared less certain. A therapeutic effect is unlikely with a level of less than 4 μg/mL; however, many clinicians no longer recommend use of blood levels to titrate efficacy in bipolar disorder.

Carbamazepine is metabolized by the liver. Its 10-, 11-epoxide metabolite (which may reach levels 20% as high as the parent compound) is an effective anticonvulsant; it is unknown whether it is also an active antimanic agent. The elimination half-life of carbamazepine in a single dose in healthy volunteers is 18 to 55 hours; however, with repeat dosing the half-life decreases to 5 to 20 hours (longer in the elderly). This reduction in half-life with repeat dosing is due to the drug inducing its own metabolism by hepatic P450 enzymes. This induction may be clinically significant. An oral dose, which is effective early in therapy, may become ineffective due to decreasing levels after several weeks. This autoinduction effect generally plateaus within 3 to 5 weeks. Carbamazepine metabolism also can be induced by other drugs, especially the anticonvulsants phenytoin, phenobarbital, and primidone, resulting in lower serum levels.

Mechanism of Action

Carbamazepine has two known mechanisms that may be relevant to its antiepileptic effect. Opening of voltage-sensitive sodium channels is central to the mechanism of neuronal action potentials. These channels become temporarily inactive after use. Carbamazepine binds to an inactivated state of sodium channels, resulting in use-dependent and voltage-dependent block. Thus, carbamazepine inhibits repetitive firing of action potentials. This effect of carbamazepine seems particularly to affect sodium channels localized on neuronal cell bodies. Carbamazepine also appears to block presynaptic sodium channels, thus inhibiting depolarization of presynaptic terminals in response to action potentials propagated down the axon. Because the depolarizing effect of the sodium action potential is blocked, voltage-gated calcium channels are secondarily inhibited. The result is decreased calcium entry into the presynaptic terminal and a decrement in neurotransmitter release. Mechanisms of this type could have widespread effects on neural function in addition to treating epilepsy. Their relevance to mood disorder is not known.

There are a variety of animal models in epilepsy. Carbamazepine appears to be the most active anticonvulsant in blocking the development of seizures in the kindling model. Kindling involves the repetitive application of subthreshold electrical or chemical stimuli to produce an autonomous epileptic focus. The effectiveness of carbamazepine in this model has led to a great deal of theorizing that mood disorders and other psychiatric disorders may represent a kindling process. Although no convincing mechanistic models of kindling in mood disorders have emerged to date, speculation about kindling has produced valuable reexaminations concerning the course of psychiatric disorders, focusing attention on the observation that episodes may become more frequent and more autonomous (less related to environmental precipitants) over time in a subset of patients.

Indications

Acute Mania

In both published studies and clinical practice, carbamazepine appears to be effective in the treatment of acute mania; however, the number of patients studied in placebo-controlled double-blind fashion remains small, and many study populations are atypical. Thus, carbamazepine appears to be effective for acute mania, but it is not clear whether it is as effective as lithium or valproate.

At present, the effective oral dose for each patient must be determined empirically by upward dosage titration, using the attainment of therapeutic effects and the emergence of side effects to guide dosing. For acute mania, an average effective dosage is approximately 1,000 mg/day (range 200–1,800 mg/day). After a therapeutic dosage is established, patients must be carefully observed because after several weeks carbamazepine may induce its own metabolism, requiring a dosage increase. Therapeutic dosage levels for bipolar disorder have not been established; many clinicians use the levels that have been established for epilepsy as a general guide.

If an episode of mania is mild, carbamazepine alone may be adequate treatment. For severe manic episodes, however, carbamazepine is usually begun along with an antipsychotic drug or a benzodiazepine to gain more rapid control of manic behavior. Neuroleptic dosages equivalent to those of haloperidol, 8 to 10 mg/day, are usually effective. Higher doses carry a risk of worsened side effects without strong evidence of added benefit. If possible, the antipsychotic medication should be tapered and discontinued after the acute symptoms have resolved, and the patient should be maintained on carbamazepine alone. Some patients who do not respond to lithium or carbamazepine as single agents respond to the combination at full therapeutic doses. The most compelling evidence for this synergy comes from longitudinal "on-off-on" trials, but only small numbers of patients have been studied, generally in an unblinded fashion. Similarly, combined therapy with carbamazepine and valproic acid has been reported effective in some refractory patients with acute mania.

Bipolar Prophylaxis

Several studies have suggested that carbamazepine may be effective for prophylaxis against recurrences in bipolar disorder, but there is a paucity of placebo-controlled or double-blind studies. Taken together, the published studies and clinical experience underscore the point that long-term prophylactic use of carbamazepine in bipolar disorder is less well established than its use in acute mania. For example, while one unblinded prospective study of lithium-refractory patients found carbamazepine to be effective in bipolar prophylaxis as a single agent in some patients and in combination with lithium in others over a mean of 20.2 months (Stuppaeck et al., 1990), a retrospective study found carbamazepine to be relatively ineffective after 3 to 4 years in lithium-refractory patients (Frankenburg et al., 1988). Interpretation of these contrasting studies is made difficult by serious methodologic problems in each report. Clearly more research is necessary, but for the present, it is reasonable to use carbamazepine for long-term prophylaxis either singly or with lithium in patients who have been treated with that regimen for their acute mania. The effectiveness of carbamazepine or any other prophylactic agent can only be judged after a sufficiently long period of time to compare the patient's rate of cycling on carbamazepine with the patient's prior rate of cycling. This will vary depending on the patient's base rate. Dosage for prophylaxis is not established; it is reasonable to use the same dosage that is effective for the patient during acute manic episodes and to decrease the dosage only if side effects may limit therapy. The current evidence suggests that carbamazepine may be more effective in prophylaxis against manic than against depressive recurrences.

Rapid-Cycling Bipolar Disorder

Lithium is less effective for rapidly cycling patients (i.e., those with more than three cycles per year) than for patients with more typical bipolar disorder. Despite the lack of clear proof that carbamazepine is effective for long-term bipolar prophylaxis, there is some evidence that it may be more effective than lithium for rapid cyclers. In a small, partially blinded longitudinal trial, Post and associates (1983) compared the course of illness of seven rapidly cycling, lithium-resistant bipolar patients before and after administration of carbamazepine. The patients were followed for an average of 1.7 years on carbamazepine, with a decrease in total (manic and depressive) recurrences from 16.4 to 5.6 per year. It is important to note that although carbamazepine improved the course of rapid-cycling illness, it did not suppress all affective recurrences. It may take 6 months to a year to judge the efficacy of carbamazepine for this population.

Acute Depression

Despite a few case reports to the contrary, carbamazepine does not appear to be effective as an antidepressant. Like lithium and valproate, it may prevent induction of mania in bipolar depressed patients being treated with an antidepressant.

Atypical Psychoses: Schizoaffective and Schizophreniform Disorders

Use of mood stabilizers in schizoaffective and schizophreniform disorders are more fully discussed earlier in this chapter. Based on clinical reports, mood stabilizers, including lithium, valproate, and carbamazepine, may be indicated for schizoaffective patients, especially those with manic symptoms, or for schizophreniform patients. On this basis, a trial of carbamazepine might be indicated in selected schizoaffective or schizophreniform patients who are unresponsive to or intolerant of lithium.

Neuropathic Pain

Pain may develop in response to an injury to peripheral or central sensory afferents. Because of damage to the nociceptive pathways, there is generally some loss of normal pain sensation (hypalgesia), but severe neuropathic pain may follow after a delay. Such pain may be produced by processes such as amputation, nerve avulsion, cordotomy, or peripheral neuropathy. Phantom limb pain, causalgia, postherpetic neuralgia, and thalamic pain are all forms of neuropathic pain.

The symptoms of neuropathic pain may include persistent burning or unprovoked paroxysms of lancinating pain referred to the deafferented region. Patients also may describe dysesthesias (e.g., pins and needles, numbness or tingling, or formication, a feeling of insects crawling on the skin). In addition, mildly noxious stimuli may provoke severe pain in the region (hyperpathia), and even innocuous stimuli applied to this region may produce perverted sensations or severe pain (allodynia).

Carbamazepine is the drug of choice in the treatment of trigeminal neuralgia (tic douloureux) and a related syndrome that occurs in the distribution of the glossopharyngeal nerve. It appears to be somewhat more effective in these conditions than phenytoin, although the latter is also effective. The high-potency benzodiazepine clonazepam also may have some role in these conditions. Carbamazepine also may be effective for neuropathic pain due to diabetic neuropathy, multiple sclerosis, postherpetic neuralgia, and other conditions, especially if there is a paroxysmal, lancinating component. In these latter conditions, however, most clinicians begin with a tricyclic antidepressant (see Chapter 3). Carbamazepine is begun at low doses (e.g., 100 mg twice daily) and slowly increased until relief occurs (usually in the range of 400–800 mg/day).

Carbamazapine as a Detoxification Agent

Several open and controlled trials have suggested that carbamazepine is effective in the treatment of alcohol withdrawal. One randomized double-blind study of 86 men with severe alcohol withdrawal found carbamazepine, 800 mg/day, as effective as oxazepam, 120 mg/day, with no difference in side effects (Malcolm et al., 1989). Given the long track record of safety and efficacy for benzodiazepines, more study would be required before carbamazepine could be recommended as a detoxification agent for ethanol.

A small number of reports also have suggested that carbamazepine, 200 to 800 mg/day, may be a useful adjunct for withdrawal from alprazolam and other benzodiazepines. Although this strategy may aid individual patients, a large controlled study failed to show evidence of efficacy. Should this approach be attempted, there are few data to guide the clinician on the appropriate duration of carbamazepine treatment to maintain patients benzodiazepine free. In one trial, patients were placed on carbamazepine, 400 mg, for 1 to 2 weeks prior to detoxification at a rate of 25% per week. Carbamazepine was maintained for 14 days after the benzodiazepine taper ended (Schweizer et al., 1991).

Seizures

The use of carbamazepine as an anticonvulsant (Table 4.8) is fully reviewed in other sources. The method of administration and side effect monitoring is the same for epilepsy as is described below for psychiatric disorders.

Table 4.8.   Use of carbamazepine for seizure disorders

Effective	Ineffective
Simple partial	Generalized absence
Complex partial	
Generalized tonic–clonic	
Mixed seizure patterns that include complex partial, tonic–clonic, or other partial or generalized seizures	

Therapeutic Use

Preliminary Workup

Patients who are candidates for carbamazepine treatment should have a medical history and physical examination with emphasis on prior history of blood dyscrasias or liver disease. Laboratory tests should include a CBC with platelets and liver and renal function tests. Patients with hematologic abnormalities should be considered at high risk for serious blood dyscrasias if treated with carbamazepine; they therefore deserve closer follow-up than usual. Patients with significant hepatic disease should not receive this drug unless there are no better alternatives; they should be started on one third to one half the normal starting dosage, with longer than usual time (5–7 days) between dosage adjustments.

Beginning Carbamazepine

In patients over the age of 12, carbamazepine is begun at 200 mg once or twice a day. The dosage is increased by no more than 200 mg every 2 to 4 days until therapeutic levels or effects are achieved. The clinical situation determines how aggressively the dosage may be increased. In hospitalized patients with acute mania, the dosage might be increased daily in 200-mg increments up to 800 to 1,000 mg unless side effects develop, with slower increases thereafter as indicated. In less acutely ill outpatients, dosage adjustments should be slower. Rapid dosage increases may cause patients to develop nausea and vomiting or mild neurologic toxicity such as drowsiness, dizziness, ataxia, clumsiness, or diplopia. Should such side effects occur, the dosage can be decreased temporarily and then increased again more slowly once they have passed. As noted previously, therapeutic blood levels for bipolar disorder have not been established. Some clinicians use the core range for epilepsy, 6 to 10 µg/mL, as a guide. Blood levels are typically observed to decrease after 2 to 4 weeks of treatment, resulting from carbamazepine's autoinduction of CYP450 3A4 isoenzymes; carbamazepine induces its own metabolism and, when this occurs, an upward adjustment of dose is required. Should blood levels be obtained to document a therapeutic trial or to establish an effective level for a given patient, trough levels are most meaningful and are conveniently drawn prior to the first morning dose. Given its elimination half-life, carbamazepine levels should be drawn no more frequently than 5 days after a dosage change. **Maintenance dosages** both for bipolar and epileptic patients average about 1,000 mg/day, but the dosage range in routine clinical practice is large (200–1,800 mg/day). The manufacturer recommends dosages no higher than 1,600 mg/day.

Combinations with Lithium

Carbamazepine is used most often for bipolar patients who prove **resistant to treatment with lithium or valproic acid.** In many situations, therefore, the patient will already have a pharmacologic treatment for bipolar disorder that has been judged to be inadequate. In acute mania, carbamazepine can be either substituted for lithium or valproic acid or added to the initial drug. The primary danger of adding carbamazepine to lithium or valproic acid (and, in these situations, often a neuroleptic and perhaps an antiparkinsonian or benzodiazepine) is risk of an acute combined central nervous system toxicity, for example, producing a confusional state. However, if the manic symptoms are severe enough to create pressure for rapid treatment, the physician may choose to add carbamazepine to the existing regimen because some patients respond only to combined therapy. If the patient improves, an attempt should be made to taper the lithium (or valproic acid) once the patient has stabilized. Some patients will worsen and require resumption of combined treatment. When such a combined regimen is undertaken, it is also essential to minimize the dose of any typical antipsychotic drug (e.g., in the range of 8–10 mg of haloperidol or the equivalent). Unneeded anticholinergics and sedatives should also be decreased or omitted. In addition, it is important to have a clear idea of the patient's mental status and to consider the possibility of drug toxicity if the mental status worsens.

In the elderly and in patients whose mania is not so severe, it is preferable to substitute carbamazepine for lithium or valproic acid rather than add it. If the patient remains unresponsive, lithium or valproic acid can be added later. Whether a patient responds to carbamazepine alone or in combination with another mood stabilizer, it is good practice to taper and discontinue antipsychotic drugs once the acute episode has abated to minimize the risk of tardive dyskinesia.

Use in Pregnancy

Carbamazepine and other anticonvulsants cross the placenta. Fetal malformations caused by phenytoin (fetal hydantoin syndrome) have been well documented, and carbamazepine had been thought to be safer. However, carbamazepine is also teratogenic. A prospective study of 35 children exposed to carbamazepine alone *in utero* found that 11% had craniofacial defects, 26% had fingernail hypoplasia, and 20% had developmental delay, similar to the abnormalities found with phenytoin. Pending further clarification, carbamazepine should be avoided if possible during pregnancy. Carbamazepine is secreted in breast milk at about 60% the level found in the mother. Nursing children have been reported to become excessively drowsy. All anticonvulsants, including carbamazepine, are cleared more rapidly in pregnant women, leading to a decrease in serum levels.

Side Effects and Toxicity

Although carbamazepine is associated with several serious toxicities (e.g., hepatitis, severe blood dyscrasias, and exfoliative dermatitis), these are fortunately extremely rare. In general, this drug is well tolerated, with fewer than 5% of patients discontinuing the medication because of side effects. This compares favorably with the older anticonvulsant phenytoin. Most of carbamazepine's side effects (Table 4.9) are neurologic or gastrointestinal symptoms due to too rapid a dosage increase or excessively high serum levels. These side effects can usually be avoided by increasing dosages slowly and using the minimum effective dosage.

Neurologic Side Effects

Neurologic side effects are relatively common and may limit the dosage that patients can tolerate. The most common are drowsiness, vertigo, ataxia, diplopia, and blurred vision. When such side effects occur, a decrease in dosage is indicated, but these side effects do not represent a reason to stop therapy. When such side effects occur at the initiation of therapy, a temporary dosage decrease with a slower subsequent increase is often successful in permitting achievement of a therapeutic dosage. Carbamazepine also can produce confusion, the risk of which is higher when it is combined with antipsychotic drugs or lithium. Risk factors for confusional states include old age or

Table 4.9.   Side effects and toxicity of carbamazepine

Common dosage-related side effects
  Dizziness
  Ataxia
  Clumsiness
  Sedation
  Dysarthria
  Diplopia
  Nausea and gastrointestinal upset
  Reversible mild leukopenia
  Reversible mild increases in liver function tests
Less common dosage-related side effects
  Tremor
  Memory disturbance
  Confusional states (more common in elderly and in combination
    treatments with lithium or neuroleptics)
  Cardiac conduction delay
  Syndrome of inappropriate antidiuretic hormone secretion
Idiosyncratic toxicities
  Rash (including cases of exfoliation)
  Lenticular opacities
  Hepatitis
  Blood dyscrasias
    Aplastic anemia
    Leukopenia
    Thrombocytopenia

underlying organic brain disease. In the absence of frank confusional states, carbamazepine appears to have little effect on memory or other cognitive functions and is better than phenytoin in this regard.

Hematologic Toxicity

Carbamazepine has both benign and severe hematologic toxicities. It frequently is associated with clinically unimportant decreases in white blood cell counts and rarely is associated with serious or irreversible depression of red blood cells, white blood cells, or platelets, or a combination of these. Estimates of the rate of severe blood dyscrasias in the literature suggest an incidence of about 1 in 20,000 patients treated. As of 1982, there were 22 case reports of aplastic anemias (6 in the first month of treatment) and 17 cases of agranulocytosis.

Because carbamazepine often produces minor hematologic effects, it is important to have guidelines for identification of severe reactions, requiring discontinuation of the drug and close medical attention. Although there are no prospectively derived guidelines for psychiatric patients, Hart and Easton (1982) have made the following recommendations based on a review of the literature and clinical experience in neurologic patients:

1. Perform CBC and LFTs prior to treatment.
2. Consider patients with baseline abnormalities to be at high risk with closer follow-up monitoring.
3. During the first 2 months, check blood counts and LFTs every 2 weeks.
4. If no laboratory abnormalities appear and no symptoms of bone marrow suppression or hepatitis occur, obtain counts and LFTs every 3 months.
5. Stop the drug if white blood cell count drops below 3,000/μL or neutrophil count drops below 1,500/mL, or in case of a threefold increase in LFTs.

More recent practice by neurologists and psychiatrists is not as conservative as these recommendations, with less frequent blood monitoring generally acceptable over time, although recognizing the increased risk of blood dyscrasia in the first weeks and months of therapy. Of special importance, however, is the recommendation that patients should be instructed to report fever, sore throat, pallor, unaccustomed weakness, petechiae, easy bruising, or bleeding. Concomitant use of lithium could potentially mask (but not reverse) carbamazepine-induced leukopenia. Thus, lithium should not be added to carbamazepine at times when a potentially serious decrease in the white blood cell count has occurred.

Cardiovascular Effects

Carbamazepine slows intracardiac conduction and may worsen preexisting cardiac conduction disease. Both sinus bradycardia and varying degrees of atrioventricular block have been reported. Carbamazepine is less dangerous in this regard than tricyclic antidepressants, but the existence of a high degree of heart block is a relative contraindication to its use. Other cardiovascular side effects listed by the manufacturer (e.g., congestive heart failure) are rare and may not be causally related to the drug.

Gastrointestinal Effects

Nausea and vomiting are relatively common dose-related side effects that do not necessitate termination of therapy. They are common at the start of therapy and, like dose-related neurologic side effects, can be minimized by increasing the dosage slowly. Mild, nonprogressive elevations of LFTs are also relatively common and require follow-up. The decision to continue the medication in the presence of mild LFT abnormalities must be individualized and should involve consultation with an internist or gastroenterologist.

Rarely, idiosyncratic, non–dose-related hepatitis may occur, usually in the first month of treatment. Patients generally manifest other signs of a hypersensitivity reaction, including fever and rash. Twenty cases were reported by 1985, of which about five were fatal. In the presence of such a reaction, carbamazepine should be permanently discontinued.

Dermatologic Effects

Rashes may develop in up to 3% of patients taking carbamazepine. Patients with urticaria and pruritic erythematous drug rashes should have the medication discontinued. Rarely, patients have developed Stevens-Johnson syndrome, which may be fatal.

Effects on Electrolytes

Carbamazepine has antidiuretic properties that can lead to **decreases in serum sodium.** These are usually clinically unimportant, but on rare occasions more severe hyponatremia may occur. Risk is highest in the elderly and in patients with a low serum sodium level at baseline. Appearance of new mental symptoms during carbamazepine treatment merits a check of serum electrolytes. Carbamazepine does not appear to be helpful in reversing lithium-induced polyuria.

Effects on Thyroid

Although long-term studies of patients on carbamazepine show decreases in free T_3 and T_4, reports of clinical hypothyroidism are anecdotal and rare. Carbamazepine is much less likely to produce significant effects on the thyroid than lithium, but hypothyroidism should be considered if a patient develops refractory depression.

Drug Interactions

Carbamazepine, like most anticonvulsants, may induce hepatic microsomal enzymes, CYP450 3A3 and 3A4 in particular, resulting in increased metabolism of compounds that undergo hydroxylation or demethylation in the course of elimination. Significant drug interactions are listed in Table 4.10.

Overdose

Because of carbamazepine's slow absorption, peak levels in overdose may not be reached until the second or third day after

Table 4.10. Drug interactions with carbamazepine

Diminishes Effects of	Unpredictable Effects on	May Augment Effects of	Carbamazepine Levels Decreased by	Carbamazepine Levels Increased by
Warfarin	Phenytoin	Digitalis (may induce or exacerbate bradycardia)	Phenobarbital	Erythromycin (marked increase)
Ethosuximide			Primidone	Isoniazid (marked increase)
Valproic acid			Phenytoin	Propoxyphene
Tetracycline				Cimetidine
Haloperidol (probably)				SSRIs
Cyclic antidepressants (probably)				
Benzodiazepines, including clonazepam				

the ingestion. Although it has a tricyclic structure, carbamazepine appears to be less dangerous in overdose than the tricyclic antidepressants. The major concerns in carbamazepine overdose are the development of high degrees of atrioventricular block (meriting cardiac monitoring) and stupor and coma, with risk of aspiration pneumonia. At higher doses, depression of respiration may occur, but it is usually relatively mild. Other symptoms and signs of overdose that have been reported include nystagmus, tremor, ballistic movements, mydriasis, ophthalmoplegia, orofacial dyskinesias, myoclonus, hypo- or hyperreflexia, rigidity, and seizures.

Management of carbamazepine overdoses is supportive. Because the drug is highly protein bound, hemodialysis is of no benefit. Hemoperfusion confers uncertain benefit and does not appear to be indicated.

Lamotrigine

Lamotrigine, a phenyltriazine originally approved for adjunctive use in the treatment of partial seizures, has in small studies and case series been shown to have efficacy in the treatment of mania, both as a single agent and in combination with lithium or valproate. Early observations suggested that lamotrigine may be particularly effective in the treatment of rapid cycling and in the depressed phase of bipolar disorder. The mechanism of action of lamotrigine in bipolar disorder is not known. At the cellular level, lamotrigine inhibits the release of the excitatory amino acid glutamate, thus diminishing central nervous system excitation, and *in vitro* it also inhibits low-voltage sodium channels.

Method of Use

Lamotrigine is begun at a low dose, 25 mg/day. The daily dose may be increased by 25 mg every 1 to 2 weeks in order to minimize side effects. It is usually administered on a twice-daily schedule. Although case reports have noted daily doses of up to 500 mg, the typical maintenance range is 100 to 200 mg/day. The dose is generally higher when combined with carbamazepine, because the latter induces enzymes that metabolize lamotrigine, and lower with valproic acid, which can inhibit lamotrigine metabolism. Lamotrigine does not affect P450 hepatic enzymes itself.

Side Effects

Although side effects are generally mild, rash may occur in 10% of individuals. Although generally benign, Stevens-Johnson syndrome, which may be fatal, has been reported. Rashes appear to depend at least partly on starting dose and rate of increase; therefore, slow dosage increments are recommended ("no rush, no rash"), particularly when the drug is used in combination with valproate, which inhibits the metabolism of lamotrigine. The risk of severe or fatal rashes is much higher in the pediatric than adult age group; therefore, the drug is contraindicated in patients under 16 years of age. Other side effects of lamotrigine include headache, central nervous system symptoms (diplopia, ataxia, blurred vision), and nausea and vomiting. No adverse cognitive effects of up to 4 weeks' dosing with lamotrigine were seen in young adult healthy volunteers. The safety of lamotrigine or the other newer anticonvulsants in pregnancy is not yet known.

Gabapentin

Gabapentin (Neurontin), an antiepileptic drug indicated as adjunctive therapy for partial seizures, has a structure similar to GABA although it does not appear to bind to GABA receptors. It is thought, however, to be GABAergic by increasing brain GABA levels, but it has influences on other neurotransmitter systems as well. There is mainly anecdotal evidence to suggest that gabapentin may be efficacious in bipolar disorder for acute mania and mood stabilization, including rapid cycling. It also has been reported to be efficacious in anxiety disorders, including panic disorder and social phobia. Although a substantial number of patients have been described, controlled trial data are still lacking.

Method of Use

Gabapentin is typically started at a dose of 300 mg at night, and titrated up to daily doses of 900 to 2,400 mg. It has a short half-life of 5 hours, which, coupled with reduced absorption at high doses, requires a multiple daily dose schedule. It is unusual among the anticonvulsants in that it is excreted unchanged by the kidney; dosing therefore should be reduced in the presence of kidney disease. Gabapentin does not appear to alter single-dose lithium pharmacokinetics.

Side Effects

Gabapentin is a benign and well-tolerated compound and has not been associated with serious adverse effects, the most common treatment-emergent complaints being sedation, fatigue, dizziness, and ataxia. Overactivation and weight gain are occasionally reported. No hepatic or hematologic abnormalities have been described. No significant drug–drug interactions have been reported. Tolerability may in fact be the main feature to recommend it in bipolar disorder, given the weakness of evidence for its efficacy. Clinicians do observe, however, that some patients benefit from its adjunctive use; whether that reflects true mood stabilization or its more evident anxiolytic potential is unclear.

Topiramate

Topiramate a fructopyranose compound, is approved for adjunctive treatment of refractory partial seizures in adults. Currently the published literature in bipolar disorder consists of uncontrolled case reports and series, mostly describing add-on therapy in mixed patient samples with refractory mood disorders. Unlike other anticonvulsants, topiramate is more generally associated with weight loss than weight gain. Topiramate enhances GABAergic transmission, blocks glutamate receptors, inhibits carbonic anhydrase, and modulates sodium conductance.

Method of Use

Topiramate has generally been started at 25 mg twice a day when added to ongoing treatments. The dose is than increased every few days or once a week, in 25- to 50-mg increments. Most clinical trials have used daily doses of 200 to 500 mg. Topiramate is not extensively metabolized, with 70% of a dose excreted unchanged in urine. The half-life is 21 hours. Topiramate does interact pharmacokinetically with other anticonvulsants such as carbamazepine and valproate, making it imperative to check levels when topiramate is added.

Side Effects

Common side effects of topiramate include somnolence (which may not appear until 1 or 2 weeks after initiation of treatment), fatigue, nervousness, dizziness, ataxia, and anxiety. Dose-related weight loss can be clinically significant, and some patients describe a loss of appetite and mild nausea. The potential for use as a weight-loss treatment, particularly to offset the weight gain caused by other psychotropics, has been reported anecdotally. Concentration or attention difficulties have been reported both in patients and healthy volunteers. These have limited the acceptability of treatment for some patients who report "feeling stupid." Other adverse effects, which probably relate to the carbonic anhydrase inhibition properties of topiramate, are paresthesias and increased risk of kidney stones.

CLONAZEPAM

Clonazepam, a potent benzodiazepine recently FDA approved for the treatment of panic disorder, has been used primarily as an anxiolytic, but was originally labeled as an anticonvulsant drug, especially in the treatment of some childhood epilepsies. Uses of clonazepam in seizure disorders include:

Absence (petit mal) seizures (ethosuximide preferred)
Atypical absence seizures
Infantile spasms
Myoclonic seizures
Complex partial seizures (carbamazepine, phenytoin, and phenobarbital preferred)

Its use as an anticonvulsant has required high doses, with a correspondingly high incidence of sedative side effects, development of tolerance, reports of paradoxical excitement, and, rarely, induction of psychotic-like symptoms. It has been shown to be effective at lower dosages (1–3 mg/day) in the treatment of panic disorder with few side effects. Like all benzodiazepines, it is a safe and effective sedative when used as an adjunct to lithium and antipsychotic drugs in treating acute mania or other acute psychoses. A number of case reports and small studies have suggested that clonazepam has specific antimanic (as opposed to general sedative) properties, but the evidence is not strong and there also have been negative studies. Clonazepam is fully discussed in Chapter 5.

TIAGABINE

Tiagabine, a nipecotic acid derivative, was recently introduced as an adjunctive antiepileptic for the treatment of partial seizures. Its mechanism of action is uncertain, but *in vitro* it has inhibited glial reuptake of GABA. Although there is interest in whether it offers potential for psychotropic or mood-stabilizing effects, there is minimal evidence to date. In epilepsy, dosing begins with 4 mg/day and is increased each week by 4 mg/day to a maximum dosage of 56 mg/day. Side effects include dizziness, somnolence, nervousness, and tremor. Although dosing in bipolar disorder is unknown, case reports describe dosages in the 8 to 12 mg/day range. Use with carbamazepine increases tiagabine metabolism, whereas combined therapy with valproate yields increased free tiagabine levels.

Nutritional Supplements

Omega-3 fatty acids are hypothesized to dampen signal transduction pathways in a manner similar to the more established mood stabilizers. In a preliminary trial, Stoll and associates (1999) found a combination of the two main omega-3 fatty acids in high doses (9.6 g/day) to be superior to placebo in preventing an acute illness episode and on a variety of symptom rating scale measures during 4 months of maintenance treatment of 30 patients with bipolar disorder. With a range of initial mood states, the continuation of previous medications during the trial in most subjects, and the apparently unsuccessful effort at blinding the fishy aftertaste of the active fatty acid capsules, these findings must be accepted with caution (Stoll et al., 1999; More definitive research is required.

BIBLIOGRAPHY

Pharmacology

Hardy BG, Shulman KI, Mackenzie SE, et al. Pharmacokinetics of lithium in the elderly. *J Clin Psychopharmacol* 1987;7:153.

Vitiello B, Behar D, Malone R, et al. Pharmacokinetics of lithium carbonate in children. *J Clin Psychopharmacol* 1988;8:355.

Mechanism of Action

Berridge MJ, Downes CP, Hanley MR. Neural and developmental actions of lithium: a unifying hypothesis. *Cell* 1989;59:411.

Klein PS, Melton DA. A molecular mechanism for the effect of lithium on development. *Proc Natl Acad Sci U S A* 1996;93:8455.

Manji HK, Lenox RH. Lithium: a molecular transducer of mood-stabilization in the treatment of bipolar disorder. *Neuropsychopharmacology* 1998;19:161.

Indications

Mood Disorders

Black DW, Winokur G, Bell S, et al. Complicated mania. *Arch Gen Psychiatry* 1988;45:232.

Bowden CL, Brugger AM, Swann AC, et al. Efficacy of divalproex vs. lithium and placebo in the treatment of mania. *JAMA* 1994; 271:918.

Faedda GL, Tondo L, Baldessarini RJ, et al. Outcome after rapid vs. gradual discontinuation of lithium treatment in bipolar patients. *Arch Gen Psychiatry* 1993;50:448.

Gelenberg AJ, Kane JM, Keller MB, et al. Comparison of standard and low serum levels of lithium for maintenance treatment of bipolar disorder. *N Engl J Med* 1989;321:1489.

Price LH, Heninger GR. Lithium in the treatment of mood disorders. *N Engl J Med* 1994;331:591.

Prien RF, Kupfer DJ, Mansky PA, et al. Drug therapy in the prevention of recurrences in unipolar and bipolar affective disorders. *Arch Gen Psychiatry* 1984;41:1096.

Shapiro DR, Quitkin FM, Fleiss JL. Response to maintenance therapy in bipolar illness: effect of an index episode. *Arch Gen Psychiatry* 1989;46:401.

Small JG, Klapper MH, Kellams JJ, et al. Electroconvulsive treatment compared with lithium in the management of manic states. *Arch Gen Psychiatry* 1988;45:727.

Suppes T, Baldessarini RJ, Faedda GL, et al. Risk of recurrence following discontinuation of lithium treatment in bipolar disorder. *Arch Gen Psychiatry* 1991;48:1082.

Varanka TM, Weller RA, Weller EB, et al. Lithium treatment of manic episodes with psychotic features in prepubertal children. *Am J Psychiatry* 1988;145:1557.

Lithium Augmentation of Antidepressants

Bauman P, Nil R, Souche A, et al. A double-blind, placebo-controlled study of citalopram with and without lithium in the treatment of therapy-resistant depressive patients: a clinical, pharmacokinetic, and pharmacogenetic investigation. *J Clin Psychopharmacol* 1996;16:307.

de Montigny C, Cournoyer G, Morisette R, et al. Lithium carbonate addition in tricyclic antidepressant-resistant depression: correlations with the neurobiological actions of tricyclic antidepressant drugs and lithium ion on the serotonin system. *Arch Gen Psychiatry* 1983;40:1327.

Garbutt JC, Mayo JP Jr, Gillette CM, et al. Lithium potentiation of tricyclic antidepressants following lack of T$_3$ potentiation. *Am J Psychiatry* 1986;143:1038.

Heiligenstein MH, Tollefson GD, Faries DE. A double-blind trial of fluoxetine 20 mg and placebo in outpatients with DSM-III-R major depression and melancholia. *Int Clin Psychopharmacol* 1993;8:247.

Pope HG, McElroy SL, Nixon RA. Possible synergism between fluoxetine and lithium in refractory depression. *Am J Psychiatry* 1988;145:1292.

Price LH, Charney DS, Heninger GR. Variability of response to lithium augmentation in refractory depression. *Am J Psychiatry* 1986;143:1387.

Alcoholism

de la Fuente JR, Morse RM, Niven RG, et al. A controlled study of lithium carbonate in the treatment of alcoholism. *Mayo Clin Proc* 1989;64:177.

Dorus W, Ostrow DG, Anton R, et al. Lithium treatment of depressed and nondepressed alcoholics. *JAMA* 1989;262:1646.

Fawcett J, Clark DC, Aagesen CA, et al. A double-blind, placebo-controlled trial of lithium carbonate therapy for alcoholism. *Arch Gen Psychiatry* 1987;44:248.

Other Indications for Lithium

Schiff HB, Sabin TD, Geller A, et al. Lithium in aggressive behavior. *Am J Psychiatry* 1982;139:1346.

Other Issues in Management of Bipolar Patients

Faedda GL, Tondo L, Baldessarini RJ, et al. Outcome after rapid vs. gradual discontinuation of lithium treatment in bipolar disorder. *Arch Gen Psychiatry* 1993;50:448.

Kane JM. The role of neuroleptics in manic–depressive illness. *J Clin Psychiatry* 1988;49(suppl):12.

Post RM, Roy-Byrne PP, Uhde TW. Graphic representation of the life course of illness in patients with affective disorder. *Am J Psychiatry* 1988;145:844.

Shukla S, Mukherjee S, Decina P. Lithium in the treatment of bipolar disorders associated with epilepsy: an open study. *J Clin Psychopharmacol* 1988;8:201.

Wehr TA, Goodwin FK. Rapid cycling in manic–depressives induced by tricyclic antidepressants. *Arch Gen Psychiatry* 1979;37:555.

Wehr TA, Goodwin FK. Can antidepressants cause mania and worsen the course of affective illness? *Am J Psychiatry* 1987;144:1403.

Wehr TA, Sack DA, Rosenthal NE, et al. Rapid cycling affective disorder: contributing factors and treatment responses in 51 patients. *Am J Psychiatry* 1988;145:179.

Method of Use

Cooper TB, Simpson GM. The 24-hour lithium level as a prognosticator of dosage requirements: a two-year follow-up study. *Am J Psychiatry* 1976;133:440.

Jefferson JW, Greist JH, Clagnaz PJ, et al. Effect of strenuous exercise on serum lithium level in man. *Am J Psychiatry* 1982;139:1593.

Perry PJ, Dunner FJ, Hahn RL, et al. Lithium kinetics in single daily dosing. *Acta Psychiatr Scand* 1981;64:281.

Post RM, Roy-Byrne PP, Uhde TW. Graphic representation of the life course of illness in patients with affective disorder. *Am J Psychiatry* 1988;145:844.

Side Effects and Toxicity

Acute Lithium Intoxication

Schou M. The recognition and management of lithium intoxication. In: Johnson FN, ed. *Handbook of lithium therapy.* Lancaster, England: MTP Press, 1980.

Simard M, Gumbiner B, Lee A, et al. Lithium carbonate intoxication: a case report and review of the literature. *Arch Intern Med* 1989; 149:36.

Lithium and the Kidney

Battle DC, von Riotte AB, Gavira M, et al. Amelioration of polyuria by amiloride in patients receiving long-term lithium therapy. *N Engl J Med* 1985;312:408.

Bendz H, Aurell M, Balldin J, et al. Kidney damage in long-term lithium patients: a cross-sectional study of patients with 15 years or more on lithium. *Nephrol Dialysis Transplant* 1994;9:1250.

Bowen RC, Grof P, Grof E. Less frequent lithium administration and lower urine volume. *Am J Psychiatry* 1991;148:189.

De Paulo JR Jr, Correa EI, Sapir DG. Renal function and lithium: a longitudinal study. *Am J Psychiatry* 1986;143:892.

Hetmar O, Brun C, Clemmsen L, et al. Lithium: long-term effects on the kidney: II. Structural changes. *J Psychiatr Res* 1987;21:279.

Hetmar O, Clemmsen L, Ladefoged J, et al. Lithium: long-term effects on the kidney: III. Prospective study. *Acta Psychiatr Scand* 1987;75: 251.

Kosten TR, Forrest JN. Treatment of severe lithium-induced polyuria with amiloride. *Am J Psychiatry* 1986;143:1563.

Plenge P, Raaelson OJ. Lithium treatment: Does the kidney prefer one daily dose instead of two? *Acta Psychiatr Scand* 1982;66:121.

Wood IK, Parmelee DX, Foreman JW. Lithium-induced nephrotic syndrome. *Am J Psychiatry* 1989;146:84.

Neurologic Toxicities

Apte SN, Langston JW. Permanent neurological deficits due to lithium toxicity. *Ann Neurol* 1983;13:452.

Engelsmann F, Katz J, Ghadirian AM, et al. Lithium and memory: a long-term follow-up study. *J Clin Psychopharmacol* 1988;8:207.

Joffe RT, MacDonald C, Kutcher SP. Lack of differential cognitive effects of lithium and carbamazepine in bipolar affective disorder. *J Clin Psychopharmacol* 1988;8:425.

Saul RF, Hamberger HA, Selhorst JB. Pseudotumor cerebri secondary to lithium carbonate. *JAMA* 1985;253:2869.

Schou M. Long-lasting neurological sequelae after lithium intoxication. *Acta Psychiatr Scand* 1984;70:594.

Other Toxicities

Deandrea D, Walker N, Mehlmauer M, et al. Dermatological reactions to lithium: a critical review of the literature. *J Clin Psychopharmacol* 1982;2:199.

Franks RD, Dubovsky SL, Lifshitz M, et al. Long-term lithium carbonate therapy causes hyperparathyroidism. *Arch Gen Psychiatry* 1982;39:1074.

Garland EJ, Remick RA, Zis AP. Weight gain with antidepressants and lithium. *J Clin Psychopharmacol* 1988;8:323.

Lyman GH, Williams CC, Dinwoodie WR, et al. Sudden death in cancer patients receiving lithium. *J Clin Oncol* 1984;2:1270.

Mitchell JE, Mackenzie TB. Cardiac effects of lithium therapy in man: a review. *J Clin Psychiatry* 1982;43:47.

Susman VL, Adonizio G. Reintroduction of neuroleptic malignant syndrome by lithium. *J Clin Psychopharmacol* 1987;7:339.

Yassa R, Saunders A, Nastase C, et al. Lithium-induced thyroid disorders: a prevalence study. *J Clin Psychiatry* 1988;48:14.

Drug Interactions

Miller F, Meninger J. Lithium-neuroleptic neurotoxicity is dose dependent. *J Clin Psychopharmacol* 1987;7:89.

Ragheb M. The clinical significance of lithium-nonsteroidal anti-inflammatory drug interactions. *J Clin Psychopharmacol* 1990; 10:350.

Use in Pregnancy

Cohen LS, Friedman JM, Jefferson JW, et al. A reevaluation of risk of *in utero* exposure to lithium. *JAMA* 1994;271:146.

Zalstein E, Koren G, Einarson T, Freedom RM. A case control study on the association between 1st trimester exposure to lithium and Ebstein's anomaly. *Am J Cardiol* 190;65:817.

Valproic Acid

Use in Bipolar Disorder

Bowden CL, Brugger AM, Swann AC, et al. Efficacy of divalproex vs lithum and placebo in the treatment of mania. *JAMA* 1994;271: 918.

Bowden CL, Brugger AM, Swann AC, et al. Efficacy of divalproex vs lithium and placebo in the treatment of mania. The Depakote Mania Study Group. *JAMA* 1994;271:918.

Calabrese JR, Markovitz P, Kimmel SE, et al. Spectrum of efficacy of valproate in 78 rapid-cycling bipolar patients. *J Clin Psychopharmacol* 1992;12(suppl):53.

Swann AC, Bowden CL, Calabrese JR, et al. Differential effect of number of previous episodes of affective disorder on response to lithium or divalproex in acute mania. *Am J Psychiatry* 1999; 156:1264.

Swann AC, Bowden CL, Morris D, et al. Depression during mania. Treatment response to lithium or divalproex. *Arch Gen Psychiatry* 1997;54:37.

Side Effects and Toxicity

Dreifuss FE. Valproic acid hepatic fatalities: revised table. *Neurology* 1989;39:1558.

Dreifuss FE, Langer DH, Moline KA, et al. Valproic acid hepatic fatalities. II: U.S. experience since 1984. *Neurology* 1989;39:201.

Smith MC, Black TP. Convulsive disorders: toxicity of anti-convulsants. *Clin Pharmacol* 1991;14:97.

Wisner KL, Perel JM. Serum levels of valproate and carbamazepine in breastfeeding mother-infant pairs. *J Clin Psychopharmacol* 1998;18:167.

Carbamazepine

Use in Bipolar Disorder

Lusznat RM, Murphy DP, Nunn CMH. Carbamazepine vs. lithium in the treatment and prophylaxis of mania. *Br J Psychiatry* 1986; 153:198.

Placidi GF, Lenzi A, Lazzerini F, et al. The comparative efficacy and safety of carbamazepine versus lithium: a randomized, double-blind three-year trial in 83 patients. *J Clin Psychiatry* 1986;47: 490.

Small JG, Klapper MH, Milstein V, et al. Carbamazepine compared with lithium in the treatment of mania. *Arch Gen Psychiatry* 1991; 48:915.

Stuppaeck C, Barnas C, Miller C, et al. Carbamazepine in the prophylaxis of mood disorders. *J Clin Psychopharmacol* 1990;10:39.

Use in Other Psychiatric Disorders

Malcolm R, Ballenger JC, Sturgis ET, et al. Double-blind controlled trial comparing carbamazepine to oxazepam treatment of alcohol withdrawal. *Am J Psychiatry* 1989;146:617.

Schweizer E, Rickels K, Case WG, et al. Carbamazepine treatment in patients discontinuing long-term benzodiazepine therapy. *Arch Gen Psychiatry* 1991;48:448.

Sramek J, Herrera J, Costa J, et al. A carbamazepine trial in chronic, treatment-refractory schizophrenia. *Am J Psychiatry* 1988;145: 748.

Uhde TW, Stein MB, Post RM. Lack of efficacy of carbamazepine in the treatment of panic disorder. *Am J Psychiatry* 1988;145:1104.

Side Effects and Toxicity

Hart RG, Easton JD. Carbamazepine and hematological monitoring. *Ann Neurol* 1982;11:309.

Heh CWC, Sramek J, Herrera J, et al. Exacerbation of psychosis after discontinuation of carbamazepine treatment. *Am J Psychiatry* 1988;145:878.

Joffe RT, MacDonald C, Kutcher SP. Lack of differential cognitive effects of lithium and carbamazepine in bipolar affective disorder. *J Clin Psychopharmacol* 1988;8:425.

Joffe RT, Post RM, Roy-Byrne PP, et al. Hematological effects of carbamazepine in patients with affective illness. *Am J Psychiatry* 1985;142:1196.

Roy-Byrne PP, Joffe RT, Uhde TW, et al. Carbamazepine and thyroid function in affectively ill patients. *Arch Gen Psychiatry* 1984; 41:1150.

Trimble MR, Thompson PJ. Anticonvulsant drugs, cognitive function, and behavior. *Epilepsia* 1983;24(suppl 1):55.

Drug Interactions

Arana GW, Goff D, Friedman H, et al. Does carbamazepine-induced lowering of haloperidol levels worsen psychotic symptoms? *Am J Psychiatry* 1986;143:650.

Ketter TA, Post RM, Worthington K. Principles of clinically important drug interactions with carbamazepine: Parts I and II. *J Clin Psychopharmacol* 1991;11:198.

Use in Pregnancy

Altshuler LL, Cohen L, Szuba MP, et al. Pharmacologic management of psychiatric illness during pregnancy: dilemmas and guidelines. *Am J Psychiatry* 1996;152:592.

Jones KL, Johnson KA, Adams J. Pattern of malformations in children of women treated with carbamazepine during pregnancy. *N Engl J Med* 1989;320:1661.

Rosa FW. Spina bifida in infants of women treated with carbamazepine during pregnancy. *N Engl J Med* 1991;324:674.

Other Anticonvulsants

Calabrese JR, Bowden CL, McElroy SL, et al. Spectrum of activity of lamotrigine in treatment-refractory bipolar disorder. *Am J Psychiatry* 1999;156:1019.

Calabrese JR, Bowden CL, Sachs GS, et al. A double-blind placebo-controlled study of lamotrigine monotherapy in outpatients with bipolar I depression. Lamictal 602 Study Group. *J Clin Psychiatry* 1999;60:79.

Marcotte D. Use of topiramate, a new anti-epileptic as a mood stabilizer. *Affect Disord* 1998;50:245.

Young LT, Robb JC, Hasey GM, et al. Gabapentin as an adjunctive treatment in bipolar disorder. *J Affect Disord* 1999;55:73.

Other Agents

Ghaemi SN, Goodwin FK. Use of atypical agents in bipolar and schizoaffective disorders: review of the empirical literature. *J Clin Psychopharmacol* 1999;12(suppl):57.

Marcotte D. Use of topiramate, a new anti-epileptic as a mood stabilizer. *J Affect Disord* 1998;50:245.

Suppes T, Webb A, Paul B, et al. Clinical outcome in a randomized 1-year trial of clozapine versus treatment as usual for patients with treatment-resistant illness and a history of mania. *Am J Psychiatry* 1999;156:1164.

Stoll AL, Severus WE, Freeman MP, et al. Omega 3 fatty acids in bipolar disorder: a preliminary double-blind, placebo-controlled trial. *Arch Gen Psychiatry* 1999;56:407.

Tohen M, Sanger TM, McElroy SL, et al. Olanzapine versus placebo in the treatment of acute mania. *Am J Psychiatry* 1999;156:702.

Benzodiazepines and Other Anxiolytic Drugs

The benzodiazepine drugs have anxiolytic, sedative, anticonvulsant, and muscle relaxant properties, all of which are useful in clinical practice. A large number of benzodiazepines (Table 5.1) are currently available; drugs chemically unrelated to the benzodiazepines but with some similar receptor action (zolpidem and zaleplon) have been introduced in the United States. Prior to the introduction of the benzodiazepines in 1960, a variety of other compounds were used to treat anxiety and insomnia. These included bromides early in the century, ethanol and structural analogs such as paraldehyde and chloral hydrate in the 1940s, followed by the barbiturates and propanediol drugs, including meprobamate, in the 1950s.

Benzodiazepines, like the older sedative-hypnotics, are central nervous system (CNS) depressants, with anxiolytic properties at relatively low doses and sedative-hypnotic effects (i.e., induction of drowsiness or sleep) at higher doses. The benzodiazepines have several clear advantages over the older drugs. Compared with barbiturates and similarly acting drugs, benzodiazepines have (a) a greater dose margin between anxiolysis and sedation, (b) less tendency to produce tolerance and dependence, (c) less abuse potential, and (d) a higher ratio of the median dose producing lethality to median effective dose ($LD_{50}:ED_{50}$). Indeed, the barbiturates and similarly acting drugs are quite dangerous in overdose, potentially causing coma, respiratory depression, and death, whereas the benzodiazepines are rarely associated with death from overdose alone. Since the introduction of benzodiazepines, the number of sleeping pill–related suicides and accidental deaths has decreased markedly. Given the advantages of benzodiazepines, the use of most of the older compounds (e.g., secobarbital, pentobarbital, meprobamate, glutethimide, or ethchlorvynol) for anxiolysis or sedation is irrational. Nonbenzodiazepines, with relatively selective affinity for the type 1 benzodiazepine receptor, are now also available that appear to offer some clinical advantages over benzodiazepines for the treatment of insomnia.

BENZODIAZEPINES

The effectiveness and relative safety of the benzodiazepines combined with the high frequency of complaints of anxiety and insomnia in medical practice have led to their extensive use. Despite a sharp decline in prescriptions for benzodiazepines over the past 20 years because of concerns about addiction and abuse, they are still widely prescribed. It is true that dependence and discontinuation difficulties on benzodiazepines can occur even at therapeutic doses in the course of long-term use (6 months), and more rapidly with high-potency, short-acting benzodiazepines.

Nonetheless it appears the risks of serious problems with dependence in the course of proper therapeutic use have been exaggerated; many patients continue to benefit from benzodiazepines with long-term use without obvious deleterious effects. Indeed, it is likely that, at present, excessive fears of addicting patients may be contributing to withholding potentially effective therapy from many anxious patients. On the other hand, the potential for inducing dependence, especially with some of the more potent short-acting drugs such as alprazolam and lorazepam, must be considered by physicians when making therapeutic choices. In general, benzodiazepines should neither be withheld because of prejudice nor prescribed indiscriminately without a careful diagnostic evaluation. Rational use of benzodiazepines is based on:

1. Presence of a benzodiazepine-responsive syndrome.
2. Use of appropriate nonpharmacologic therapies when indicated.
3. Assessment of the approximate duration of treatment (e.g., avoiding open-ended treatment of insomnia, but recognizing that many anxiety disorders may require long-term therapy).
4. Consideration of the risk–benefit factors associated with benzodiazepine treatment for individual patients (e.g., benzodiazepines should be avoided in patients with a history of alcohol or drug abuse unless there is a compelling indication, no good alternative, and close follow-up).
5. Adjustment of dosage to optimize therapeutic effects and minimize side effects (e.g., drowsiness).
6. Monitoring for abuse (unsupervised dose acceleration or diversion to other individuals).
7. Slowly tapering the drug after an appropriate trial to determine the need for any further treatment.
8. Reconsideration of diagnosis and treatment choice if the patient is poorly responsive, if medication is needed longer, or if higher doses than originally estimated are needed.

Chemistry

The benzodiazepines are a group of closely related compounds. The name *benzodiazepine* is derived from the fact that the structures are composed of a benzene ring fused to a seven-member diazepine ring.

Pharmacology

Dependence

Clinically, the major pharmacologic problem with benzodiazepines is their tendency to cause dependence, that is, a risk of significant discontinuation symptoms, especially with long-term use. Long-term benzodiazepine use occurs in medical settings because both panic disorder and generalized anxiety disorder (GAD) often run chronic courses. Discontinuation symptoms may pose a serious clinical problem in some patients, causing distress or inability to discontinue treatment. However, it is the widespread confusion of **pharmacologic dependence with drug addiction** that has most complicated the clinical use of benzodiazepines.

Table 5.1.   Available anxiolytic and hypnotic preparations

Available Preparations	Regular Oral Dosage Forms (mg)	Slow-Release Forms (mg)	Parenteral Forms (mg)
Alprazolam (Xanax)[a]	0.25, 0.5, 1.0, 2.0 (tablet)		
Buspirone (BuSpar)[b]	5, 10 (tablet)		
Chlordiazepoxide[c] Librium and others	5, 10, 25 (tablet) 5, 10, 25 (capsule)		100 mg/2 mL (ampule)
Clonazepam (Klonopin)	0.5, 1.0, 2.0 (tablet)		
Clorazepate (Tranxene) and generics	3.75, 7.5, 15.0 (tablet) 3.75, 7.5 (capsule)	11.25, 22.5	
Diazepam (Valium and generics)	2, 5, 10 (tablet)	15	10 mg/2 mL (ampule or syringe) 50 mg/10 mL (vial)
Estazolam (ProSom)	1, 2 (tablet)		

Flurazepam (Dalmane) and generics	15, 30 (capsule)
X Lorazepam (Ativan)[a] and generics	0.5, 1.0, 2.0 (tablet)
Midazolam (Versed)	20 mg/10 mL, 40 mg/10 mL (vial) 2 mg/mL, 4 mg/mL (syringe)
Oxazepam (Serax and generics)	1 mg/mL 5 mg/mL (vial) 15 (tablet) 10, 15, 30 (capsule)
Quazepam (Doral)	7.5, 15.0 (tablet)
Temazepam (Restoril) and generics	7.5, 15.0, 30 (capsule)
Triazolam (Halcion)	0.125, 0.25 (tablet)
Zolpidem (Ambien)[b]	5, 10 (tablet)

[a]Tablets can be taken sublingually for use requiring more rapid onset of action.
[b]Nonbenzodiazepines.
[c]Available with clidinium bromide (Librax, Clipoxide) and amitriptyline (Limbitrol).

Dependence means that on drug cessation, an individual experiences pathologic symptoms and signs. In the past, it was often taught that physical dependence, as manifested by physical withdrawal symptoms (e.g., tremor or elevated blood pressure) appearing with drug cessation, was the key indicator of drug addiction. This concept has now appropriately been abandoned. Some highly addictive drugs, such as cocaine, do not produce a physical withdrawal syndrome. Moreover, many medically useful drugs, such as the antihypertensive drugs clonidine and propranolol, may produce physical dependence (e.g., rebound hypertension or angina on cessation) without producing addictive behaviors. Rather than basing the concept of addiction on physical dependence, addiction is now understood as a cluster of cognitive, affective, behavioral, and physiologic signs that indicate compulsive use of a substance and inability to control intake despite negative consequences such as medical illness, failure in life roles, and marked interpersonal difficulties.

The *Diagnostic and Statistical Manual of Mental Disorders,* 4th edition (DSM-IV) does not use the term *addiction* because it has collected a variety of imprecise and pejorative meanings. However, the DSM-III and DSM-IV use of drug dependence to signify addiction raises the specter of serious misunderstandings among both physicians and patients for the medical use of benzodiazepines (and of narcotic analgesics). The terminal cancer patient with severe pain is likely to become both physically and psychologically dependent on prescribed opiate analgesics but is not an addict; that is, the person has not lost control over the drug and is not engaged in maladaptive compulsive drug-seeking behaviors. Moreover, were the pain to stop, the individual would not experience drug craving. Similarly, the patient with panic disorder also may become dependent on prescribed benzodiazepines; that is, the patient might have rebound anxiety and even withdrawal symptoms (e.g., tachycardia) with discontinuation but is not an addict. The confusion of dependence and addiction can lead to unnecessary shame for patients and, more importantly, to undermedication even when the drug is indicated. Although it is true that polydrug abusers may misuse benzodiazepines and become addicted to them in the true sense of the term, benzodiazepines are intrinsically far less addictive than opiates, cocaine, alcohol, barbiturates, or nicotine. Restrictive prescribing laws (e.g., as in New York) effectively decrease benzodiazepine prescriptions but may lead to increased prescription of more dangerous and less effective drugs such as meprobamate, methyprylon, and barbiturates. Such laws also put stigma and other obstacles in the way of appropriate anxiolytic therapies.

Choosing a Benzodiazepine

All benzodiazepines have similar mechanisms of action and side effects. Of all of the drugs used in psychiatry, benzodiazepines are the class in which pharmacokinetic considerations play the greatest role in selecting a drug for a particular situation. The dosage forms, rate of onset of action, duration of action, and tendency to accumulate in the body vary considerably and can influence both side effects and the overall success of the treatment. The other major consideration in choosing a benzodiazepine drug is potency; for example, the most potent agents have demonstrated utility in the treatment of panic disorder and certain epilepsies.

Route of Administration

ORAL USE. Most benzodiazepines are well absorbed when given orally on an empty stomach; many achieve peak plasma levels within 1 to 3 hours, although there is a wide range among the benzodiazepine drugs (Table 5.2). Antacids seriously interfere with benzodiazepine absorption; thus, benzodiazepines should be taken well ahead of any antacid dose.

The rate of onset of action after an orally administered benzodiazepine (Table 5.2) may be an important variable in choosing a drug. For example, rapid onset is important when emergency sedation is required or for the individual who has trouble falling asleep. On the other hand, a more slowly acting drug might be prescribed when insomnia occurs later in the night. Drugs with a rapid onset achieve higher peak levels than equivalent doses of drugs with slow onset, whose peaks are spread over time (Fig. 5.1). The psychotropic effects of drugs with rapid onset, such as diazepam or clorazepate, are often distinctly felt by patients both because of the rapid change in drug level and because the peak level is high. Patients may experience rapidly acting drugs as positively or negatively reinforcing; some patients expect to feel the onset of action of a dose, interpreting this as therapeutic. Others have a dysphoric response, complaining of sedation or loss of control. This latter group of patients often do better on a drug with a slow onset of action. It is worth asking about such reactions in follow-up. Patients who are drug abusers may interpret peak effects as a desirable high; thus, patients with drug abuse histories might be given an agent with slow onset (e.g., oxazepam), if given a benzodiazepine at all.

The available benzodiazepines differ markedly in the rate of onset of their therapeutic effect (Table 5.2), offering a wide choice of drugs to fit the patient's needs. Diazepam, a rapidly absorbed compound, usually achieves peak levels within 1 hour after an oral dose.

SUBLINGUAL USE. Several benzodiazepines (nongeneric forms of lorazepam, alprazolam, and triazolam) are compounded to permit either sublingual or oral administration. The time to peak levels appears to be only slightly faster by the sublingual route and may not represent a clinically significant difference from the oral route. However, the sublingual route may be a useful alternative for patients who cannot swallow pills or for patients who have a full stomach, which would delay oral absorption. Furthermore, the placebo effect of the expectation of rapid onset may be considerable. When used sublingually, tablets should be placed under the tongue and allowed to dissolve passively. Dry mouth may lead to a lack of dissolution of the tablet. Depending on how they are compounded, generic forms may not be absorbed sublingually.

INTRAMUSCULAR USE. Absorption of benzodiazepines after intramuscular administration varies according to drug and site of administration. Drugs are better absorbed from better per-

Table 5.2. Data on available benzodiazepines

Available Preparations	Oral Dosage Equivalency (mg)	Onset After Oral Dose	Distribution Half-life	Elimination Half-life (h)[a]
Alprazolam (Xanax)	0.5	Intermediate	Intermediate	6–20
Chlordiazepoxide (Librium and generics)	10.0	Intermediate	Slow	30–100
Clonazepam (Klonopin)	0.25	Intermediate	Intermediate	18–50
Clorazepate[b] (Tranxene)	7.5	Rapid	Rapid	30–100
Diazepam (Valium and generics)	5.0	Rapid	Rapid	30–100
Estazolam (ProSom)	2.0	Intermediate	Intermediate	10–24
Flurazepam (Dalmane)	30.0	Rapid–intermediate	Rapid	50–160
Lorazepam (Ativan and generics)	1.0	Intermediate	Intermediate	10–20
Midazolam (Versed)	—	Intermediate	Rapid	2–3
Oxazepam (Serax)	15.0	Intermediate–slow	Intermediate	8–12
Quazepam (Doral)	15.0	Rapid–intermediate	Intermediate	50–160
Temazepam (Restoril)	30.0	Intermediate	Rapid	8–20
Triazolam (Halcion)	0.25	Intermediate	Rapid	1.5–5

[a]The elimination half-life represents the total for all active metabolites; the elderly tend to have the longer half-lives in the range reported. Chlordiazepoxide, clorazepate, and diazepam have desmethyldiazepam as a long-lived active metabolite. Flurazepam and quazepam share N-desalkylflurazepam as a long-lived active metabolite. With chronic dosing, these active metabolites represent most of the pharmacodynamic effect of these drugs.

[b]Clorazepate is an inactive prodrug for desmethyldiazepam, which is the active compound in the blood.

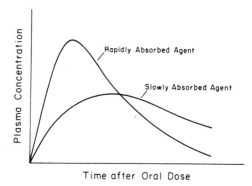

Figure 5.1. Comparison of peak levels achieved related to
rate of absorption. The curves could represent a comparison of
levels for a single drug given rapidly versus slowly intravenously.
The curves also could represent peak levels for equivalent
doses of two similar drugs with different rates of absorption.
The more rapidly absorbed drug achieves a higher peak level.

fused muscle groups. Specifically, it appears that lorazepam,
midazolam, and perhaps diazepam are well absorbed if given in
the deltoid muscle, a site that is preferable to the vastus lateralis
or gluteus maximus. Chlordiazepoxide is not reliably absorbed
when administered intramuscularly, regardless of site; therefore,
chlordiazepoxide should not be administered by this route.

INTRAVENOUS USE. Benzodiazepines are commonly administered intravenously for preoperative sedation and in treating
seizures. In psychiatric practice, benzodiazepines are used intravenously only in emergency situations. Intravenous diazepam,
lorazepam, or midazolam is useful for the control of antipsychotic-induced laryngeal dystonia if anticholinergics fail (see
Chapter 2) and for emergency sedation in extremely agitated or
delirious states. Of these three drugs, lorazepam has the longest
lasting effects after a single intravenous dose because it is less
quickly and extensively distributed into lipid stores than
diazepam, which is a critical parameter after a single emergency
dose (see section on Duration of Effect). Midazolam has an
extremely short elimination half-life.

Whenever benzodiazepines are given intravenously, they should
be given slowly (over a minute or two) instead of by rapid push;
too rapid administration can produce very high blood levels,
resulting in excessive risk of respiratory arrest (Fig. 5.1). Benzodiazepines should only be given intravenously if personnel are
trained and equipped to deal with possible respiratory arrest.

Duration of Effect

For benzodiazepines, simple half-life data are potentially misleading, regarding duration of clinical effect. Clinical efficacy
depends on the presence of at least a minimum effective concentration in the blood, which is reflected by levels in well-perfused
tissues such as those in the brain. After a single dose, the levels

may decrease to ineffective concentrations, either (a) by being distributed into peripheral tissues, such as fat (referred to as α phase, with a time course described by the distribution half-life), or (b) by metabolic inactivation or elimination from the body altogether (referred to as β phase, with a time course described by the elimination half-life).

The volume of distribution represents the size of the pool of tissues into which the drug may be drawn; this is determined by the drug's lipid solubility and tissue-binding properties. With repeated drug dosing, its volume of distribution becomes saturated, and the elimination half-life becomes the more important parameter in describing its behavior. Benzodiazepines differ markedly in their half-lives of distribution and elimination, producing varying clinical effects.

These pharmacokinetic considerations have clear clinical relevance in the use of benzodiazepines (Table 5.3). When acute doses of benzodiazepines are to be used (e.g., in emergency situations), the rates of absorption and distribution are critical (the latter because benzodiazepines lose their biologic effect by redistribution into the tissues much more rapidly than by elimination from the body). With repeated dosing, on the other hand, distribution is complete, and the elimination half-life, which determines the steady-state levels of the drug, becomes the important factor.

These points can be demonstrated in the clinical use of two commonly used drugs, diazepam and lorazepam. The distribution half-life (α phase) for oral diazepam is 2.5 hours, whereas the elimination half-life (β phase) is more than 30 hours. Desmethyldiazepam, diazepam's major active metabolite, extends the overall elimination half-life to 60 to 100 hours (up to 200 hours in the elderly). This means that a single dose of diazepam will be active for a relatively short period of time based on the rapid distribution of the drug, whereas with repeated administration, elimination half-life becomes the important parameter to consider, making diazepam a very long-acting drug (i.e., one that will accumulate in the body to high levels). Conversely, despite the relatively short elimination half-life

Table 5.3.   Clinical relevance of pharmacokinetics of benzodiazepines

Situations in which single-dose kinetics are important
 Treatment of insomnia (one night)
 Sleep during travel across time zones
 Emergency treatment of acute anxiety or agitation
 Emergency sedation of patients with acute psychosis
 Status epilepticus
 Preoperative sedation
 Induction of anesthesia
Situations in which multiple-dose kinetics are important
 Long-term treatment of anxiety
 Nightly treatment of insomnia (consecutive nights)
 Intermediate-term adjunctive use with antidepressants
 Long-term treatment of neuroleptic-induced akathisia

of lorazepam (10 hours) and its lack of active metabolites, it has a smaller volume of distribution than diazepam and therefore a longer action when given as a single dose. Thus, for a single emergency dose (e.g., for acute sedation or an intravenous dose for status epilepticus), lorazepam would have a significantly longer lasting clinical effect than diazepam and might therefore be preferable. With repeated dosing, however, lorazepam is shorter acting than diazepam and is therefore unlikely to build up to high levels, as diazepam does (Table 5.4).

Another important clinical issue related to duration of effect applies to the use of the high-potency, short-acting benzodiazepines, alprazolam, triazolam, and midazolam, and to a lesser extent lorazepam. Such drugs pose a potential clinical problem because their high potency may make them more liable to cause dependence and their rapid termination of effect unmasks any dependence that develops. Patients may therefore experience rebound symptoms between scheduled doses. For example, some patients treated with alprazolam for panic disorder develop rebound anxiety between doses, unless their dose frequency is increased to four to five doses per day. Patients treated with triazolam for insomnia may develop rebound symptoms, as manifested by early morning awakening or anxiety. Such problems can be addressed by switching to longer acting drugs when indicated (e.g., replacing alprazolam with clonazepam for panic anxiety; method described in the section Tolerance and Discontinuation Symptoms) or by replacing triazolam with temazepam or flurazepam for insomnia.

Metabolism

Except for lorazepam, oxazepam, and temazepam, the commonly used benzodiazepines are metabolized by hepatic microsomal enzymes to form demethylated, hydroxylated, and other oxidized products that are pharmacologically active. These active metabolites are, in turn, conjugated with glucuronic acid; the resulting glucuronides are inactive, and because they are more water soluble than the parent compounds, they are readily excreted in the urine. Major metabolic pathways for benzodiazepines are shown in Fig. 5.2.

Some of the active metabolites of benzodiazepines, such as desmethyldiazepam and desalkylflurazepam, have extremely long half-lives and with repeat dosing may come to represent most of the pharmacologically active compound in serum. In contrast, under normal circumstances (e.g., excluding cirrhosis) the active metabolic products of alprazolam, triazolam, and midazolam are of little clinical importance.

Lorazepam, oxazepam, and temazepam are metabolized only by conjugation with glucuronic acid with no intermediate steps, and they have no active metabolites. Unlike the pathways involved in the initial metabolism of other benzodiazepines, glucuronidation is less affected by aging and liver disease; thus, if benzodiazepines are to be used in elderly patients or those with cirrhosis, lorazepam and oxazepam are the drugs of choice. In cirrhosis, the elimination of benzodiazepines metabolized by oxidation and demethylation may be reduced by as much as fivefold; thus, routine doses could lead to toxicity. In cirrhosis, even

Table 5.4. Clinical importance of long versus short half-life of elimination with repeat dosing

	Long Half-life		Short Half-life	
	Advantages	Disadvantages	Advantages	Disadvantages
	Less frequent dosing	Accumulation (problem in the elderly)	No accumulation	More frequent dosing
	Lack of interdose rebound anxiety or insomnia	Greater risk of next-day sedation after use for insomnia	Less daytime drowsiness after repeated nightly use as hypnotic	Rebound insomnia (especially after use of high-potency compounds on several consecutive nights)
	Withdrawal problems less severe			Interdose rebound anxiety and early morning anxiety (with high-potency compounds)

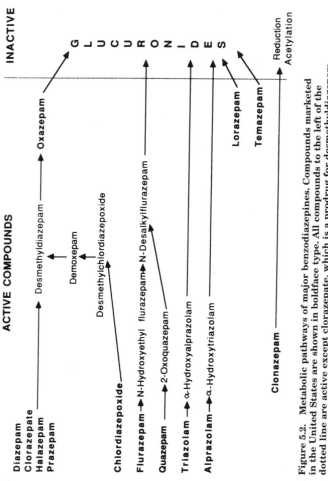

Figure 5.2. Metabolic pathways of major benzodiazepines. Compounds marketed in the United States are shown in boldface type. All compounds to the left of the dotted line are active except clorazepate, which is a prodrug for desmethyldiazepam.

alprazolam, triazolam, and midazolam may accumulate to dangerous levels.

Mechanism of Action

Acting through its gamma-aminobutyric acid A ($GABA_A$) receptor, the amino acid neurotransmitter GABA is the major inhibitory neurotransmitter in the brain. $GABA_A$ receptors are ligand-gated channels, meaning that the neurotransmitter-binding site and an effector ion channel are part of the same macromolecular complex. Because $GABA_A$ receptor channels selectively admit the anion chloride into neurons, activation of $GABA_A$ receptors hyperpolarizes neurons and thus is inhibitory on neuronal firing. Benzodiazepines produce their effects by binding to a specific site on the $GABA_A$ receptor.

The pharmacology of $GABA_A$ receptors is complex; $GABA_A$ receptors are the primary site of action not only of benzodiazepines but also of barbiturates and of some of the intoxicating effects of ethanol. The multiple drug and neurotransmitter-binding sites associated with the $GABA_A$ receptor are schematized in Fig. 5.3. Benzodiazepines and barbiturates act at separate binding sites on the receptor to potentiate the inhibitory action of GABA. They do so by allosterically regulating the receptor (changing its conformation) so that it has a greater affinity for GABA. In addition, each drug increases the affinity of the receptor for the other. Ethanol also allosterically modifies the receptor so that it has increased affinity for GABA and the other drugs. It does so not by binding to the receptor itself, but by altering the membrane environment of the receptor. At higher doses, barbi-

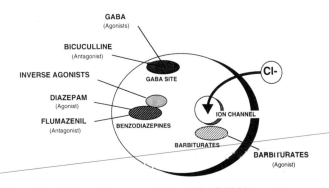

Figure 5.3. Schematic representation of the GABAA receptor. This diagram illustrates three of the major binding sites on the GABAA receptor and the chloride channel, but does not represent the actual subunit structure of the receptor. The chloride channel opens when two molecules of GABA bind to their site on the receptor. The proconvulsant compound bicuculline blocks the binding of GABA to its site. The benzodiazepine and barbiturate binding sites are physically separate from the GABA site and from each other. Compounds such as flumazenil, with no intrinsic activity, compete with benzodiazepines such as diazepam for binding and thus serve as benzodiazepine antagonists.

turates and ethanol, but not benzodiazepines, also can open the chloride channel within the receptor independent of GABA. The fact that benzodiazepines, barbiturates, and ethanol all have related actions on a common receptor explains their pharmacologic synergy (and therefore the dangers of combined overdose) and their cross-tolerance. Their cross-tolerance is exploited in detoxification of alcoholics with benzodiazepines.

It has recently become clear that $GABA_A$ receptors are constructed of multiple subunits. Active $GABA_A$ receptors appear to contain two α subunits, two β subunits, and a γ or δ subunit. Only those $GABA_A$ receptors that contain γ subunits can interact with benzodiazepines. Multiple different α, β, and γ subunits have been discovered. The actual diversity of $GABA_A$ receptors in the brain (i.e., how the different types of subunits are mixed and matched) is being exploited for new drug development. The diversity of $GABA_A$ receptors underlies the emergence of more selective benzodiazepine-like drugs in the future, drugs with the potential to be anxiolytic with less sedative effects or even with less tendency to produce dependence.

Although it is known that benzodiazepines and zolpidem produce their primary actions by allosterically regulating $GABA_A$ receptors, it is not entirely clear how they function as anxiolytics. Specifically, given the ubiquity of $GABA_A$ receptors in the brain, it is not clear how benzodiazepines achieve specificity as anxiolytics when used at therapeutic doses. It must be asked which of the many GABAergic synapses in the brain are actually relevant to benzodiazepine-induced anxiolysis and what are their normal functions. Based on animal models, it is believed that the anxiolytic properties of benzodiazepines reflect their inhibitory actions on neurons within the limbic system, including the amygdala, and on serotonergic (5-HT) and noradrenergic neurons within the brainstem. In contrast, the anticonvulsant actions of benzodiazepines may represent action on cortical neurons.

ZOLPIDEM AND ZALEPLON

Zolpidem, a nonbenzodiazepine hypnotic of the imadazopyridine class, and zaleplon, a pyrazolopyramidine, are designed to interact with a smaller subset of $GABA_A$ receptors than the benzodiazepines, that is, the type 1 benzodiazepine receptors. They are therefore pharmacologically cross-reactive with the benzodiazepines to a degree but offer reduced muscle relaxant and anxiolytic potential. Both are effective for short-term treatment of insomnia and, relative to the benzodiazepines, lack significant anxiolytic, muscle relaxant, or anticonvulsant effects. They are rapidly and completely absorbed from the gastrointestinal tract, reaching peak serum levels in 1 to 2 hours. Absorption is delayed by food, so for optimal hypnotic effect, they should be ingested on an empty stomach. Both are metabolized by the liver, with short elimination half-lives of 2.5 hours for zolpidem and 1 hour for zaleplon. Thus, there is very little carryover of daytime sedation. The half-life is prolonged in the elderly and in patients with liver disease. The recommended doses are 5 or 10 mg for both zolpidem and zaleplon. The lower doses are recommended for the elderly or possibly for initiation of treatment, especially in the patient naive to hypnotics. Given its rapid clearance, zaleplon in doses up to 20 mg has been observed to be safe and effective without residual daytime impairment. There are data that these drugs are associated with less rebound insomnia on discontinuation of treatment than the benzodiazepines, but subjective reports of increased sleep latency on discontinuation of treatment are common. Because zaleplon is relatively recently approved, there is relatively less experience with the agent, but studies suggest that rapid tolerance does not occur, interaction with alcohol is less than the benzodiazepines, and amnestic and residual effects at therapeutic doses are minimal to nonexistent. For example, 10- to 20-mg doses 5 or 10 hours beforehand did not interfere with driving. The safety profile of these agents with respect to risk for dependence and withdrawal appears to be greatly improved over the benzodiazepines, but vigilance is still indicated, especially if patients are taking high dosages. These agents may be safely coprescribed with the selective serotonin reuptake inhibitors (SSRIs) or other nonsedating antidepressants for short-term management of insomnia. Possible side effects of these drugs, besides drowsiness, are nausea, vomiting, diarrhea, headache, and dizziness. Like benzodiazepines, zolpidem may at higher doses produce some next day anterograde amnesia. Their safety in overdose appears to be high while liability for abuse appears to be low.

BUSPIRONE

Buspirone is a nonbenzodiazepine anxiolytic that has been approved for treatment of GAD. It is a member of a chemical group called the azaspirodecanediones. Buspirone has no direct effects on $GABA_A$ receptors; it has no pharmacologic cross-reactivity with benzodiazepines or barbiturates, and it lacks the sedative, anticonvulsant, and muscle relaxant effects of benzodiazepines. A major advantage of buspirone is that it does not produce dependence, and it has no abuse potential.

Buspirone is believed to exert its anxiolytic effect by acting as a partial agonist at $5\text{-}HT_{1a}$ receptors. Serotonin is thought to act as an anxiogenic neurotransmitter in limbic structures. Because $5\text{-}HT_{1a}$ receptors are autoreceptors, their activation by buspirone decreases serotonin turnover, so according to the theory, buspirone is anxiolytic. However, investigations of the role of serotonin in anxiety suggest that there is a complex relationship between the neurotransmitter and anxiety symptoms and behaviors. Of interest, buspirone has an active metabolite, 1-phenyl-piperazine (1-PP), that acts via α_2-adrenergic receptors initially to increase the rate of firing of locus ceruleus neurons. Because the ratio of the plasma level of this metabolite to the parent compound increases with treatment over time, this stimulation of adrenergic systems may play a key role in the agent's therapeutic as well as adverse effects. Indeed, the noradrenergic properties of the buspirone metabolite 1-PP may account for the drug's potential usefulness as an SSRI augmentation strategy and for its putative role in improving SSRI-associated sexual dysfunction and as a second-line therapy for attention-deficit/hyperactivity disorder.

Buspirone is 100% absorbed from the human gastrointestinal tract but undergoes extensive first-pass metabolism by the liver so that only 4% may be bioavailable. Buspirone is metabolized by the liver; the half-life of the parent compound is 2 to 11 hours.

When used to treat GAD, buspirone has been found to be as effective as standard benzodiazepine treatments in some but not all studies. Buspirone is most often ineffective as a sole treatment for panic disorder. It appears that patients with GAD who have taken benzodiazepines within 4 weeks prior to taking buspirone may be less likely to benefit from buspirone. Unlike benzodiazepines, buspirone is effective only when taken regularly. It takes 1 to 2 weeks to show its initial effects, and maximal effectiveness may be reached only after 4 to 6 weeks. This must be clearly explained to patients who are accustomed to using benzodiazepines. Because of this time course of effectiveness, buspirone is not useful in emergencies or when rapid onset of anxiolysis is required. The initial dosage of buspirone is 5 mg three times daily; in most trials, 20 to 30 mg/day in three divided doses has been effective, but a total dosage of up to 60 mg/day may be required for an optimal response.

Due to its lack of cross-reactivity with benzodiazepines, buspirone cannot prevent benzodiazepine withdrawal symptoms. Therefore, when switching patients from a benzodiazepine to buspirone, the benzodiazepine must be slowly tapered as if no new drug were being introduced. If buspirone is started before the taper has concluded (which should be safe), it is important not to confuse benzodiazepine withdrawal or rebound symptoms with buspirone side effects.

Buspirone does not cause sedation; it may occasionally produce restlessness. It does not appear to impair psychomotor performance. Headache, gastrointestinal distress, dizziness, and paresthesia have been reported but are infrequent. Buspirone does not appear to be highly toxic in overdose.

Buspirone has been somewhat disappointing in general clinical use in that a smaller percentage of anxious patients benefit from buspirone than from benzodiazepines. Whether this reflects inappropriate expectations and inadequate dose and duration of treatment on the part of both physicians and patients who are accustomed to the rapid effects of benzodiazepines is unclear. For patients who respond to buspirone, it has the marked advantages of being free of sedation, lacking any prominent discontinuation symptomatology, and at higher doses having some antidepressant potential. Buspirone has been more recently used as an antidepressant augmentation agent with SSRIs (typically in 30 to 45-mg daily doses) and as an antidote for SSRI-induced sexual function for which there are some positive reports.

INDICATIONS FOR BENZODIAZEPINES, ZOLPIDEM, ZALEPLON, AND BUSPIRONE

Although benzodiazepines are marketed for different indications, such as flurazepam, temazepam, and triazolam for insomnia, or diazepam for anxiety, muscle relaxation, and preoperative sedation, it is likely that all of the drugs in this class share most of their therapeutic properties. The differences in approved indications largely reflect selective research and marketing decisions rather than rational therapeutics. In other words, diazepam works well for insomnia, and flurazepam would serve as an anxiolytic. In most cases, drug choice is best made on the basis of pharmacokinetic differences and potency (as discussed previously). Potency is particularly important in the treatment of panic attacks, in which high-potency benzodiazepines (e.g., alprazolam and clonazepam) have clear therapeutic advantages. The high-potency and long half-life of clonazepam make it uniquely valuable in the treatment of certain epilepsies. The nonbenzodiazepine buspirone may be effective for some patients with generalized anxiety, but not for panic disorder. Its major disadvantages are slow onset of effect and inconsistent efficacy.

Anxiety

Anxiety is a ubiquitous human emotion. Most instances of anxiety do not call for medical treatment. However, anxiety can become severe enough that it impairs the ability of the individual to act adaptively; in such circumstances, treatment should be considered. Anxiety may be (a) a normal response to stressful life events, (b) a symptom of an anxiety disorder, (c) a symptom of another psychiatric disorder such as depression, or (d) a symptom of a medical illness, such as thyrotoxicosis.

Situational or Stress-Related Anxiety

This is usually self-limited and rarely calls for medical treatment. When patients complain of anxiety due to a specific life stress, the questions to address include the following:

1. Is the anxiety harmful to the individual? In many situations anxiety may be helpful in terms of motivation to respond, cope, or adapt, but in other situations anxiety can lead to maladaptive behavior or extreme dysphoria. In such situations, treatment is indicated.
2. Would psychosocial treatment be effective and acceptable to the patient?
3. What are the risks of short-term benzodiazepine treatment? Specifically, the physician must consider side effects, the acceptability of pharmacologic treatment to the individual, possible dependency, and possible interactions with other medications or medical disorders.

If drug treatment is indicated, a low-potency, long-acting benzodiazepine might be prescribed. Such compounds have the lowest risk of causing dependence and subsequent withdrawal symptoms. A typical regimen might be diazepam, 5 mg three times daily or the equivalent. Doses may be increased as needed, but the equivalent of 30 mg of diazepam or less should suffice for almost all cases of situational anxiety. The duration of treatment should be limited, guided by the time course of the stressor that precipitated the anxiety.

Benzodiazepines also can be useful for the symptomatic treatment of transient anxiety, fear, or tension associated with medical illnesses (e.g., postmyocardial infarction) and surgical illnesses (e.g., for pre- or postoperative anxiety). The dosage is similar to that for other situational anxieties, usually less than the equivalent of 30 mg/day of diazepam. In the elderly or in patients with compromised hepatic function, lorazepam or oxazepam is a better choice because it will not accumulate; in such patients, lower doses are prudent.

Social Phobia and Performance Anxiety

Social phobia, or social anxiety disorder, as defined by DSM-IV, represents persistent fears of one or more social situations in which the person is exposed to possible scrutiny by others and fears humiliation. Perhaps the best known example is public speaking anxiety, in which an individual is unable to speak before an audience. Other specific social phobias include being unable to eat in front of others, write or sign one's name under scrutiny, use public urinals, or speak on the telephone; in the generalized form of the condition, the sufferer avoids or experiences intense distress in any social situation where the potential exists for observation by others. Social phobia, like panic disorder, is associated with marked impairment in social and work function and is often comorbid with other anxiety disorders.

In **stage fright** or performance anxiety, the major troublesome symptoms are autonomic, such as pounding heart, dry mouth, and tremor. Because benzodiazepines may adversely affect mental acuity, the treatment of choice is usually a β-adrenergic blocker, such as propranolol, which is likely to have fewer cognitive side effects (see Chapter 6). Clinical reports also have suggested efficacy of the longer acting β-adrenergic blocker atenolol for discrete social phobias, but not for the generalized form of the disorder. Cognitive and behavior therapies, whether offered in individual or group settings, are a treatment of choice for diminishing distress and avoidance and also may be combined with pharmacotherapies.

For other types of social phobia, there is evidence that benzodiazepines may be efficacious. If the phobic situation is encountered rarely, as-needed use of a benzodiazepine (e.g., diazepam 5 mg) may be helpful. For individuals whose social phobia causes pervasive avoidance of interpersonal interactions, prescription of a regular dose of a benzodiazepine may be indicated, especially if combined with cognitive/behavioral therapies. Anecdotal reports support the use of alprazolam, and a randomized clinical trial established clonazepam for treatment of social phobia. There is also controlled trial evidence for efficacy of the monoamine oxidase inhibitors (MAOIs) phenelzine and tranylcypromine in social phobia (see Chapter 3). Weighing issues of safety, efficacy, and tolerability, however, the consensus drugs of first choice for social phobia are the SSRIs.

Generalized Anxiety Disorder

Generalized anxiety disorder is characterized by unrealistic and excessive ongoing worry (6 months) accompanied by specific anxiety symptoms such as motor tension, autonomic hyperactivity, or excessive vigilance. Whether GAD represents a valid diagnostic entity or a heterogeneous group of patients remains to be seen, but the diagnosis may be clinically useful because it provides criteria for identifying a group of patients who have similar treatment needs and whose management poses similar difficulties. Family/genetic studies, course of illness, and even treatment responsiveness suggest that GAD is more closely related to major depressive disorder than to other anxiety disorders.

It is important to be careful about the diagnosis of GAD because generalized anxiety symptoms are often features of other major psychiatric disorders, medical disorders, or medications or drugs (secondary anxiety). Anxiety symptoms often accompany depression, psychoses, obsessive–compulsive disorder, and other psychiatric disorders. They also may be the manifestation of medical illnesses such as angina, congestive heart failure, arrhythmias, asthma, and other obstructive pulmonary diseases, and hyperthyroidism, or they may result from overuse of aminophylline, thyroid supplements, caffeine, or over-the-counter decongestants or appetite suppressants. Secondary anxiety also may be the result of withdrawal from alcohol or other CNS depressants. Secondary anxiety is best approached by treatment of the underlying disorder, although in many situations, short-term or intermittent use of adjunctive benzodiazepines may be helpful. In some cases (e.g., in certain respiratory disorders), however, a benzodiazepine may prove harmful.

The treatment research on GAD has proven difficult because of the high placebo response in acute studies of the disorder, a feature of the condition that has limited new drug development. When antidepressants have been used at adequate dose and duration of therapy, they are typically efficacious, at least comparably so to the benzodiazepines, as seen, for example, in the studies leading to the GAD indication for venlafaxine. Benzodiazepines are reliably helpful for symptom reduction but are best combined with a nonpharmacologic treatment (e.g., cognitive or behavior therapy) for an optimal long-term improvement. Generally, low-potency, long-acting benzodiazepines are safe and effective. High-potency, short-acting compounds, such as alprazolam, carry a higher risk of dependence and interdose rebound symptoms. Typically, dosages of 15 to 30 mg/day of diazepam or the equivalent are effective, but occasional patients have required the equivalent of 40–60 mg/day of diazepam. Some patients with generalized anxiety improve with short-term (2–6 weeks) treatment, but the majority will have recurrences if treatment is stopped at that time. Long-term treatment (6 months) appears to be safe and effective for many patients; nonetheless, it is worth trying to taper the medication slowly and periodically to see if the underlying symptoms have improved. When tapering medication, it is important to distinguish recurrence of the original symptoms from transient rebound or withdrawal symptoms.

An alternative to benzodiazepines for GAD is buspirone. Buspirone is typically started at 5 mg three times daily. Average effective dosages are 30 mg/day in three divided doses, although total doses of up to 60 mg/day have been used. Buspirone is a good initial choice in detoxified alcoholic patients who may be at increased risk for benzodiazepine abuse.

The approval of venlafaxine for GAD underscores the usefulness of antidepressants for GAD; when studied in the past, even tricyclics were comparably efficacious to the benzodiazepines. Venlafaxine is superior to placebo in doses ranging from 75 mg, but some patients will do best on 150 mg or more. Antidepressants are also useful in addressing the frequent comorbidity of GAD with depression and other anxiety disorders such as panic disorder and social phobia.

Panic Attacks and Panic Disorder

The core manifestation of panic disorder is recurrent unexpected panic attacks. In addition, a substantial proportion of patients with panic disorder develop anticipatory anxiety and phobic avoidance, which may prove more disabling than the panic attacks themselves. When severe, phobic avoidance in the form of agoraphobia (fear of situations in which it may be difficult to gain help or escape) may cause patients to become entirely housebound.

Optimal therapy involves prevention of panic attacks, combined with treatment of anticipatory anxiety, phobic avoidance, and depression if present. Antidepressants, particularly the SSRIs are considered first-line treatments for the disorder because of their potential efficacy across these several domains of symptoms. Besides the SSRIs, tricyclic antidepressants including clomipramine, MAOIs (see Chapter 3), and probably venlafaxine, reboxetine, and nefazodone are efficacious. In the United States, paroxetine and sertraline were the first antidepressants to receive U.S. Food and Drug Administration (FDA) approval for a panic disorder indication. The high-potency benzodiazepines alprazolam and clonazepam are non-antidepressants with FDA approval for panic disorder, and they have demonstrated comparable efficacy to the antidepressants for the reduction of panic attacks, anticipatory anxiety, and phobic avoidance. Nonpharmacologic treatments, especially packaged interventions of cognitive and behavior therapy techniques (e.g., panic control therapy), are also first-line interventions, demonstrating comparable efficacy and superior durability after treatment is discontinued versus a drug therapy. Given the high rates of chronic and recurrent distress, many patients require multimodal treatment or more than one drug. Some patients with severe agoraphobia may be unable to leave their homes to attend treatment without short-term benzodiazepine therapy or may benefit from temporary use of a benzodiazepine to mitigate early activating side effects of an antidepressant.

If they could be given in adequate doses, it is possible that all benzodiazepines might prove effective in preventing panic attacks; however, the required doses of lower potency compounds, such as diazepam, would be so high as to produce oversedation. Therefore, the high-potency compounds are the ones most clinically useful for this indication. There is some evidence to support the clinical utility of lorazepam as well.

Alprazolam is generally administered in dosages of 2 to 6 mg/day, although dosages as high as 10 mg/day have been studied. Because it has a short duration of action, it is usually given in three to four divided doses a day. Clonazepam is generally used in dosages of 1 to 4 mg/day, usually divided into two daily doses, although total daily doses as low as 0.5 and as high as 6.0 mg/day have been used. Clonazepam has some advantages and disadvantages with respect to alprazolam. The major problem with alprazolam is twofold:

1. It has a tendency to produce greater dependence with more rebound and withdrawal symptoms. Thus, it may be more

difficult to stop treatment with alprazolam after a therapeutic trial or successful course of treatment.
2. Because of its short half-life, a substantial minority of patients develop interdose rebound anxiety. Despite frequent doses throughout the day, such patients may endure more distress as the effects of the last dose wear off, leading to clock watching and, potentially, dosage acceleration.

It is generally easier to taper treatment with clonazepam than with alprazolam, principally because of its longer half-life, although the ultimate success of full discontinuation of therapy with panic disorder patients may not differ between the two drugs. The long half-life of clonazepam makes interdose rebound uncommon. Patients unable to wean themselves from alprazolam or patients with severe interdose rebound anxiety on alprazolam might do well to switch to clonazepam. A possible disadvantage of clonazepam is that it may be more commonly associated with the emergence of depression than alprazolam. This observation remains anecdotal, and the emergence of depression has also been reported during treatment with alprazolam. The anticonvulsants valproic acid and gabapentin have been reported as useful for some patients as well.

The availability of multiple drug therapies for panic disorder permits the clinician to tailor treatment individually. An antidepressant would be preferred for a patient with a history of drug or alcohol abuse or of recurrent depression. A benzodiazepine might be chosen for patients extremely intolerant of medication side effects or when a more rapid clinical response is needed. In many situations, however, the clinician will have a wide range of choices. The advantage of benzodiazepines is the ease of starting therapy (i.e., rapid effect and few side effects beyond temporary sedation). The disadvantages become clearer later in therapy, when many patients find it difficult to discontinue benzodiazepines. The optimal duration of therapy for panic disorder with benzodiazepines or antidepressants is unknown, but it makes sense to try to taper pharmacologic therapy after 6 months of being symptom free. Many patients with panic disorder, however, have a history of vulnerability to anxiety symptoms across the life cycle, beginning with anxiety difficulties in early childhood, including separation anxiety and school avoidance, followed by social anxiety in adolescence, and panic attacks in early adulthood; these individuals also have family histories of anxiety disorders and more comorbidity with anxiety disorders. It is unrealistic to expect these patients to continue to feel and function well over time without treatment in contrast to those with a more defined, acute syndrome, which may more often remit with treatment.

Simple Phobias

Benzodiazepines are generally not the treatment of choice for simple object phobias, such as of bees, dogs, snakes, spiders, or heights. Behavior therapies that emphasize exposure appear to be successful with few contraindications. Nonetheless, if a patient with a simple phobia of a situation that can be anticipated or is likely to endure (e.g., storms, airplanes) must confront the phobic stimulus on particular occasions (e.g., an airplane flight), as-needed use of a benzodiazepine (1–2 mg of lorazepam or 5–10 mg of diazepam) may be helpful.

Obsessive–Compulsive Disorder

Benzodiazepines are not generally effective as sole treatments in obsessive–compulsive disorder, although case series and one clinical trial indicated efficacy of clonazepam compared with placebo. This disorder is best treated with clomipramine or an SSRI in combination with behavior therapy (see Chapter 3). Clonazepam also has been used adjunctively with these agents for incomplete responders. Buspirone may have some use as an adjunct to fluoxetine in the treatment of obsessive–compulsive disorder, but the support for this recommendation is inconsistent.

Depression

Benzodiazepines are not effective as primary treatments for major depressive illness, even when anxiety is a prominent symptom. When first introduced, alprazolam was thought to have antidepressant potential, but the consensus based on subsequent studies and clinical experience has not supported those early claims. Given the evident evolution of depression from anxiety symptoms early in life or in some cases early in the course of an episode, however, anxiolytics may yet prove to have a role in the prevention and treatment of depression (or buffering against stress that might worsen or precipitate depression), but for those with a depressive syndrome, anxiolytics are at best adjunctive. Coadministration of clonazepam with fluoxetine, for example, has been observed to improve the early response to fluoxetine.

Depression with Anxiety

When anxiety is a prominent symptom of depressive illness, temporary adjunctive use of a benzodiazepine (1–4 weeks) may be helpful while waiting for the onset of action of the antidepressant. It should be emphasized that benzodiazepines are not a substitute for effective antidepressant treatment and that patients should be prepared for the short-term use of benzodiazepine therapy (see Chapter 3). Depression with a comorbid anxiety disorder, such as panic disorder or social phobia, may be more resistant to treatment and thus be more likely to be treated with more than one class of drug.

Depression with Insomnia

Patients with major depressive illness often have trouble sleeping. However, many of the antidepressants with the most favorable side effect profiles (e.g., the SSRIs, venlafaxine, desipramine, nortriptyline, and bupropion) are relatively nonsedating or may even cause insomnia as a side effect in some patients (e.g., SSRIs, bupropion, or tranylcypromine). The clinician may approach depression with insomnia in one of two ways: (a) by relying on a more sedating antidepressant compound, such as nefazodone or mirtazapine (with the entire dose given at bedtime), or sedating tricyclic antidepressants, such as doxepin or amitriptyline at the expense of anticholinergic, and possible cardiovascular, side effects; or (b) with temporary use of a sedative-hypnotic at bedtime in addition to the antidepressant. Zolpidem, zaleplon, benzodiazepines, and trazodone (50 mg at bedtime; see Chapter 3) are the most widely used sedatives for this purpose. In general, the duration of their use is limited (e.g., 1–3 weeks) pending the therapeutic response to the antidepressant. Longer term use of a hypnotic or adjunctive trazodone is advised when the patient is having a good response to the primary antidepressant (e.g., fluoxetine) but is having continued insomnia as a side effect of that antidepressant.

Insomnia

Insomnia is a common symptom that can result from a wide variety of causes. Insomnia should be thoroughly investigated prior to prescribing a drug for symptomatic treatment. It is important to determine the onset, duration, and nature of the sleep disturbance; to review the medical and psychiatric histories, with special attention to medication, caffeine, alcohol, or other drug use; and to perform a physical and mental status examination. Although insomnia often proves to be idiopathic or due to an identifiable transient stressor, difficulty in sleeping is not infrequently a symptom of serious medical or psychiatric disorder, such as depression or alcoholism, or of a specific sleep disorder (Table 5.5). Clinically, insomnia of only a few days' duration is most often the result of pain, situational anxiety, stress, or drug or medication use. Insomnia lasting more than 3 weeks is more likely to be secondary to a medical or psychiatric disorder.

For short-term insomnia, zolpidem, zaleplon, benzodiazepines, and trazodone are effective symptomatic treatments, but should follow the use of nonpharmacologic interventions:

1. Patients should be advised to stop using alcohol or stimulants such as caffeine near bedtime.
2. Excessive and inappropriate medications should be withdrawn.
3. Patients should avoid daytime naps.
4. The patient's bedroom should be sufficiently dark and quiet.
5. Important life stressors should be ascertained and addressed.
6. Any obsessional overconcern with sleep that might contribute to insomnia must be addressed.

If prescribing a benzodiazepine, a small amount should be given, usually no more than a 2-week supply. For long-term insomnia for which no primary medical or psychiatric cause can be found, long-term use of benzodiazepines also may be helpful, but the ratio of benefit (long-term efficacy) to risk (dependence, impairment of psychomotor performance, subtle changes in mood) must be considered.

The greatest benefit of hypnotic medications appears to be reduced sleep fragmentation during the night. Benzodiazepines have many effects of unknown clinical significance: they suppress rapid eye movement (REM) sleep, prolong REM latency, increase stage 2 sleep, and decrease stages 1, 3, and 4 sleep. Flurazepam, temazepam, triazolam, quazepam, estazolam, and the nonbenzodiazepine zolpidem are specifically marketed for insomnia, although, as noted, the benzodiazepine hypnotics have no special features to distinguish them from other benzodi-

Table 5.5.   Causes of insomnia

Common medically related
  Pain
  Respiratory problems such as chronic cough or paroxysmal
    nocturnal dyspnea
  Nocturnal angina
  Hyperthyroidism
  Esophageal reflux, diarrhea, and other gastrointestinal
    complaints
  Nocturia

Drug and alcohol related
  Chronic alcoholism
  Alcohol use prior to retiring
  Caffeine and other psychostimulant use
  Withdrawal from alcohol, sedative-hypnotics, or narcotics
  Discontinuation of hypnotic drugs
  Neuroleptic-induced akathisia
  SSRIs, bupropion tranylcypromine

Psychiatric disorder related
  Depression
  Mania
  Anxiety disorders (including posttraumatic stress disorder)
  Dementing disorders, especially with superimposed delirium

Specific sleep disorder related
  Sleep apnea (obstructive or central)
  Nocturnal myoclonus
  Restless legs syndrome

Environmental and behavioral related
  Change in sleeping environment
  Current life stress
  Preoccupation with falling asleep
  Air travel across time zones

Idiopathic

---

azepines such as diazepam. Outside the United States, a variety of other benzodiazepines are marketed as hypnotics, including brotizolam, loprazolam, lormetazepam, and nitrazepam. The nonbenzodiazepine zolpidem has little effect on stages of sleep perhaps because of its binding profile for a subset of benzodiazepine receptors. Whether this offers unique clinical benefits is unknown but is potentially an advantage.

In healthy adults, the standard hypnotic dose of flurazepam and temazepam is 30 mg, although 15 mg is effective for some individuals. Quazepam is given at 15 mg; 7.5 mg may be adequate for some individuals and is the manufacturer's recommended dose for the elderly. Because of the risk of accumulation, flurazepam and quazepam should not be used in the elderly if more than a few days' use is contemplated, in which case temazepam, 15 mg, would be a better choice. Triazolam is given at 0.125 to 0.25 mg nightly (0.125 mg in the elderly). Zolpidem is available as a 10-mg tablet for usual adult dosing, but the 5-mg strength should be selected for the elderly and is often adequate for other adults with insomnia. Zaleplon is available in 5- and 10-mg capsules.

The two major considerations in choosing a benzodiazepine hypnotic are rapidity of onset and half-life. For patients who report difficulty in falling asleep, the rapidity of onset of the drug is particularly important. After oral administration, diazepam and flurazepam act rapidly, achieving peak plasma concentrations in 0.5 to 1.0 hour. Triazolam (1.3 hours to peak) and quazepam (1.5 hours to peak) have intermediate rates of absorption. Temazepam has a slower rate of onset, with peak levels achieved after only 3 hours, making it less helpful for sleep-latency insomnia unless taken 1 hour prior to bedtime. To improve absorption, all benzodiazepines should be administered on an empty stomach.

The other important consideration in choosing a hypnotic is half-life. Flurazepam has a long-lived metabolite, N-desalkylflurazepam (Fig. 5.2), which reaches its peak plasma concentration approximately 10 hours after an oral dose. After 2 weeks of nightly administration, this metabolite [which has a half-life of 50–160 hours (200 hours or more in the elderly)] accumulates to levels seven to eight times its peak level on the first night. Although only 3.5% of N-desalkylflurazepam is free (not protein bound), after 2 weeks this represents a great deal of pharmaco-dynamic activity; indeed, with repeat dosing, this metabolite may represent most of the active compound in plasma. Quazepam is metabolized to oxoquazepam and then to N-desalkylflurazepam, which, as in the case of flurazepam, represents most of the drug's pharmacodynamic activity with chronic dosing. With repetitive administration, this drug is not likely to differ significantly from flurazepam in its effects.

Two advantages of long-acting drugs are that they may decrease early morning awakening and treat daytime anxiety. However, the trade-off may be residual daytime drowsiness, possible cognitive impairment, and possible interactions with other CNS depressants, such as ethanol, that might be consumed during the day (although most patients develop tolerance to daytime effects and experience no hangover and little impairment). In the elderly, the level of accumulation may be greater and thus more likely to produce intoxication or delirium; therefore, in the elderly, repetitive dosing with long-acting compounds, such as flurazepam, quazepam, or diazepam, is not recommended.

Short-acting benzodiazepines do not accumulate but may be more associated with rebound insomnia after treatment discon-tinuation. Rebound insomnia may occur when short-acting ben-zodiazepines (e.g., triazolam, alprazolam, or lorazepam) are used on several consecutive nights. The shortest period necessary to produce rebound is unclear, but it may be only several days. Rebound is common when triazolam is used at dosages of 0.5 mg nightly; it is less of a problem at a dosage of 0.25 mg nightly but is still reported by many patients. On the first or second night after discontinuation of short-acting benzodiazepines, patients may complain of increased sleep latency and increased total wake time. After discontinuing triazolam 0.5 mg, there may be a 25% reduction in total sleep time on the first night after discontinuation. Especially if misinterpreted as reemergence of underlying chronic insomnia, rebound may reinforce chronic benzodiazepine use and risk of dependence. In addition to rebound after discontinuation, triazolam, which has a very short half-life, may occasionally cause rebound symptoms within the same night, manifested by early morning awakening and morning anxiety symptoms. Rebound side effects from triazolam may occur even if it was ineffective for the original complaint of insomnia. Rebound insomnia appears to be uncommon with temazepam and with very long-acting drugs such as flurazepam. If rebound insomnia occurs with flurazepam, it might not be expected until 4 to 10 nights after discontinuation. Because of their short half-lives, rebound would have been expected with zolpidem and zaleplon, but their more selective mechanism of action may be responsible for less than expected observation of rebound insomnia.

Barbiturates, such as secobarbital, pentobarbital, and amobarbital, and related drugs, glutethimide and ethchlorvynol, essentially have no place in the treatment of insomnia because of their high risk of causing tolerance and dependence and their danger in overdose. Of the barbiturate-like drugs, chloral hydrate appears to be the least problematic, with relatively low abuse potential. Thus, it is still used as an alternative to benzodiazepines by some physicians. For patients with a history of adverse reactions to benzodiazepines or a history of alcohol or sedative-hypnotic abuse, sedating antihistamines are sometimes used, but they are less effective in reducing sleep latency than benzodiazepines and are associated with residual daytime sedation and anticholinergic effects. Diphenhydramine is most commonly used, often at a dose of 50 mg (range 25–100 mg). Its half-life is 3.4 to 9.3 hours. Hydroxyzine, with a half-life of 7 to 20 hours, and doxylamine, with a half-life of 4 to 12 hours, are also sometimes used as hypnotics. All sedating antihistamines are strongly anticholinergic, and caution should be used in prescribing them in combination with other anticholinergic compounds. It is important to monitor elderly patients for emergence of anticholinergic toxicity. The sedating tricyclic antidepressants amitriptyline and doxepin, and the nontricyclic trazodone have often been used in dosages lower than necessary to treat depression for primary insomnia. Compared with the benzodiazepines, they have not been well studied for primary insomnia with respect to efficacy and the development of tachyphylaxis, but they appear to be safe in sleep apnea. The disadvantages, at least of the tricyclics amitriptyline and doxepin, are that they are strongly anticholinergic, are dangerous in overdose, and have cardiac side effects (see Chapter 3). Trazodone has been shown to be better than placebo in treatment of insomnia induced by SSRIs or bupropion. The sedating antidepressants mirtazapine and nefazodone are useful in insomnia associated with major depression.

Alcohol Withdrawal

Because of their effectiveness and safety, benzodiazepines are the agents of choice for the treatment of withdrawal from ethanol. The effectiveness of benzodiazepines is based on their pharmacologic cross-tolerance with ethanol.

Mechanism of Action

Benzodiazepines and ethanol increase activation of GABA$_A$ receptors. With chronic high-dose ethanol (or barbiturate or benzodiazepine) use, there is an apparent decrease in efficacy of GABA$_A$ receptors (a mechanism of tolerance and dependence). When high-dose ethanol is discontinued, this downregulated state of GABAergic transmission is unmasked. GABA is the most important inhibitory neurotransmitter in the brain; therefore, this state is manifested by anxiety, insomnia, agitated delirium, and a tendency to have seizures. By augmenting the effectiveness of GABA at its GABA$_A$ receptors, benzodiazepines restore adequate CNS inhibition. Slow withdrawal of the benzodiazepine detoxification agent presumably permits recovery of GABAergic systems to normal levels of activity.

Clinical Indications

Benzodiazepine treatment of alcohol withdrawal helps with anxiety, agitation, insomnia, and autonomic symptoms, and it may prevent seizures. Additionally, benzodiazepines make patients more comfortable and therefore more likely to complete detoxification. Adequate benzodiazepine therapy also may prevent progression to the life-threatening syndrome of delirium tremens. Benzodiazepines are therefore especially important for patients at high risk for delirium tremens, including those with a complicating medical illness, malnutrition, dehydration, or a prior history of delirium tremens. Should delirium emerge, benzodiazepines are effective sedatives.

Once a diagnosis of alcohol withdrawal has been established, aggressive treatment is indicated for hypertension, tachycardia, tremulousness, agitation, and other objective signs of withdrawal. Ideally, a calm state should be produced as swiftly as possible without making the patient excessively drowsy. All benzodiazepines are probably effective in the treatment of alcohol withdrawal, provided that an adequate dosage is used. Patients with hepatic dysfunction should be treated with either oxazepam or lorazepam; these short-acting benzodiazepines are metabolized by glucuronidation (a metabolic pathway that is relatively preserved in liver disease), and they have no active metabolites. Other patients are probably best served by using a long-acting benzodiazepine, such as chlordiazepoxide or diazepam, because these drugs minimize the chance that symptoms will emerge between doses and because long-acting drugs are usually easier to taper than short-acting ones.

Dosing

Whenever possible, benzodiazepine dosages should be adjusted to control symptoms rather than keeping to an arbitrary dosage schedule because the dosages required to achieve adequate sedation vary markedly. For example, some patients may require 2,000 mg of chlordiazepoxide on the first day, whereas others may be oversedated by a dose of 200 mg. Oral doses in the range of 25 to 100 mg of chlordiazepoxide, or 5 to 20 mg of diazepam every 4 hours as needed, are usually effective in the treatment of withdrawal symptoms.

Other Drugs for Withdrawal

The β-adrenergic blocker atenolol has been reported to be an effective adjunct to benzodiazepines in the treatment of alcohol withdrawal (see Chapter 6). Because it does not produce cross-tolerance with alcohol, β-adrenergic blockers cannot replace benzodiazepines as sole agents of detoxification. Preliminary studies also suggested a possible role for carbamazepine in alcohol withdrawal (see Chapter 4). Antipsychotic drugs cannot substitute for benzodiazepines. High-potency antipsychotic drugs (e.g., haloperidol 5 mg) may be useful in the emergency treatment of intoxicated belligerent alcoholics. High-potency antipsychotics also may be useful in the treatment of alcoholic hallucinosis (i.e., auditory, visual, or tactile hallucinations caused by alcohol withdrawal); however, benzodiazepines will still be required for the remainder of the withdrawal symptomatology. Low-potency antipsychotic drugs, such as chlorpromazine and thioridazine, should be avoided during alcohol withdrawal because of their adverse effect on the seizure threshold and their tendency to precipitate postural hypotension.

Delirium Tremens

Once a patient develops full-blown delirium tremens, with hypertension, fever, and delirium, symptoms may be very difficult to control. The development of this syndrome constitutes a medical emergency because it carries a substantial risk of mortality. Preferably, patients should be treated in an intensive care setting. In addition to supportive care and workup for other medical illnesses (e.g., pneumonia or subdural hematoma), aggressive use of benzodiazepines is indicated. Benzodiazepines should be given intravenously if possible to ensure absorption. Lorazepam, 2 mg every 2 hours, or diazepam, 5 to 10 mg every 2 hours, can be used as starting dosages. The final dosages used should be a function of the patient's symptoms and not based on any arbitrary maximum dosage. Risk of oversedation is greatest if repeated dosing is given before the prior dosage has reached peak effect.

Use in Mania and Psychotic Disorders

Acute Mania and Other Agitated Psychoses

Small studies and case reports have suggested that clonazepam may be effective for acute mania either as a sole agent or in combination with lithium; there also have been negative reports. To date there is no convincing evidence that clonazepam has a specific antimanic action. Clonazepam and other benzodiazepines do have a role as adjunctive sedatives in the treatment of mania, as described below.

Many patients with mania and other psychoses require sedation, especially early in the course of illness. Benzodiazepines are safe and reliable sedatives that are relatively free of unwanted acute side effects. Benzodiazepines should not be permitted to interfere with the primary treatment, which will consist of a mood stabilizer or an antipsychotic drug depending on the diagnosis. However, benzodiazepines have some advantages over as-needed use of the older antipsychotic drugs for acute control of dangerous or hyperactive behavior. Although as-needed doses of antipsychotic drugs have frequently been used for control of disruptive behavior and hyperactivity, the typical neuroleptic drugs have side effects, including akathisia, which may worsen the patient's agitation. The atypical antipsychotics such as olanzapine and risperidone appear to be quite effective in managing mania. A sample regimen for severe acute mania could well include using a benzodiazepine such as clonazepam or lorazepam along with an atypical or typical antipsychotic on an as-needed basis until a calming effect is achieved. The interval between doses can then be extended. Benzodiazepines can generally be tapered within 2 to 3 weeks, thus making dependence unlikely.

Bipolar Prophylaxis

For bipolar prophylaxis, the data about clonazepam's potential for prophylaxis are mixed. In one retrospective study of patients requiring both lithium and antipsychotics, clonazepam, 0.5 to 3.0 mg/day, successfully replaced the antipsychotic drugs in 6 of 17 bipolar patients (lithium therapy was continued unchanged). A less satisfactory outcome was found in a prospective study (Aronson et al., 1989) in which antipsychotics were replaced by clonazepam, 2 to 5 mg/day, in severely ill refractory patients while lithium was continued. The trial was terminated after only five patients were enrolled because all patients relapsed rapidly, one within 2 weeks and four within 10 to 15 weeks. The impetus to replace maintenance neuroleptic treatment of nonpsychotic bipolars with clonazepam is considerably diminished by the availability of the atypical antipsychotics, which greatly reduce the risk to the bipolar patient of extrapyramidal symptoms (EPS) and tardive dyskinesia. Recent data, however, indicate that bipolar patients on mood stabilizers were in fact less likely to relapse when clonazepam was included in the regimen as compared with placebo.

At present, the efficacy of clonazepam as an adjunct for bipolar prophylaxis is unclear, but for nonpsychotic stable bipolar patients who experience the onset of insomnia, a potential precursor or trigger of manic relapse, an acute intervention with clonazepam at bedtime may offer benefit by restoring sleep, reducing anxiety, and perhaps having some specific antimanic effect.

Catatonic Symptoms

Parenteral lorazepam has been reported to reverse both neuroleptic-induced and psychogenic catatonia. Doses of 1 to 2 mg intravenously or 2 mg intramuscularly have been reported to produce rapid and dramatic reversal of catatonic states. Although the percentage of catatonic patients who actually respond to lorazepam is unknown, it is reasonable to try lorazepam in catatonia because it is relatively safe when given intramuscularly or slowly intravenously (safer than amobarbital). This may be an especially useful option for patients in whom it is unclear whether the catatonic syndrome is the result of typical neuroleptics and from whom neuroleptics should therefore be withheld. Because lorazepam has multiple effects on the nervous system, its effectiveness does not clarify the diagnosis. For example, lorazepam also might be effective if apparent catatonia was due to complex partial status epilepticus.

Long-Term Use in Chronic Nonaffective Psychoses

Benzodiazepines are commonly administered as long-term adjuncts to antipsychotic drugs during the chronic phase of schizophrenia and other psychotic disorders. Although this indication has not been well studied in a controlled fashion, it appears from case reports and clinical practice that judicious use of benzodiazepines may improve anxiety related to the psychotic disorder and also may decrease neuroleptic-induced akathisia. Although some clinicians have found the high-potency compound alprazolam partially effective for ameliorating negative (deficit) symptoms of schizophrenia, use of long-acting low-potency benzodiazepines, such as diazepam, may be advantageous because of their lower risk of producing dependence.

Symptomatic Treatment of Agitated Delirium

The key to treating delirium is supportive care while specific therapy for the underlying disorder is given. However, symptomatic treatment with sedatives is often necessary when no cause for the delirium can be found or while awaiting the effect of specific therapy. Because delirious patients are unpredictable, restraints are generally indicated. When used, sedatives should be given at the lowest effective dosage. Delirium due to ethanol withdrawal is best managed with a benzodiazepine. Delirium due to withdrawal from barbiturate-like drugs is best managed with phenobarbital, although long acting benzodiazepines also may be used. In other types of delirium, especially in the eldorly, the high-potency antipsychotic drug haloperidol may be preferable because it is less likely than benzodiazepines to produce inattention, thereby worsening confusion. Haloperidol also has little effect on cardiorespiratory status (see Chapter 2).

If haloperidol is ineffective or not tolerated, a benzodiazepine could be used; lorazepam and oxazepam are good choices because they have short half-lives, have no active metabolites, and are metabolized by glucuronidation, which is relatively preserved in the elderly and in cirrhosis. Lorazepam has the advantage of a parenteral form and more rapid absorption when given orally. Lorazepam can be given intramuscularly with reliable absorption or intravenously. The very short-acting benzodiazepine midazolam is also sometimes used for sedation, but if repeat administration is contemplated, a longer acting compound would be preferable.

Depending on the patient's age and degree of agitation, lorazepam, 0.5 to 2.0 mg, can be given slowly intravenously; slow administration reduces the risk of respiratory arrest. Nonetheless, intravenous benzodiazepines should only be given if personnel trained in cardiopulmonary resuscitation are present. The dose of lorazepam can be repeated every 20 minutes until the patient is sedated. Repeat dosing thereafter should be on an as-needed basis every 2 hours. Combinations of haloperidol and lorazepam may be quite useful in patients with marked hallucinations and delusions who remain hyperactive after large doses of haloperidol or who develop EPS on higher doses of haloperidol. In these patients, it is best to administer a fixed dose of haloperidol daily and then to titrate the level of sedation.

Neuroleptic-Induced Akathisia

Akathisia is an uncomfortable side effect of the typical neuroleptics described by patients as a subjective need to be in motion and characterized behaviorally by motor restlessness. Akathisia may produce severe agitation and lead to treatment refusal. (Treatment of akathisia is fully discussed in Chapter 2.) When a benzodiazepine is used, diazepam, 5 mg three times daily, or lorazepam, 1 mg three times daily, may be effective. When an effective dose is found, a response is seen within 1 to 2 days. The β blockers, such as propranolol, are more specifically efficacious in treating akathisia, however.

METHOD OF USE

Starting Therapy

Prior to starting a benzodiazepine, patients should be cautioned about possible sedation and warned not to drive vehicles or operate dangerous machinery until it is determined that their dose does not affect performance. Patients should be instructed to take their medication on an empty stomach and not concomitantly with antacids because meals and antacids may decrease absorption. No specific laboratory tests are required before beginning benzodiazepines. A prior history of alcohol or other substance abuse is a relative contraindication to the use of benzodiazepines; a compelling indication, lack of an effective alternative, and careful supervision are required in this population. An alternative for the detoxified alcoholic with GAD is buspirone or an antidepressant. Active alcoholics should not be treated for a putative anxiety disorder until they are detoxified.

For short-term treatment of situational anxiety, total doses of more than 30 mg of diazepam or the equivalent are almost never needed. Higher doses are occasionally needed in GAD. For sleep, 30 mg of flurazepam, 30 mg of temazepam, 5 mg of diazepam, 15 mg of quazepam, 1 mg of lorazepam, or 0.25 mg of triazolam is the average starting dose for healthy adults. In the elderly, lower doses and avoidance of long-acting drugs should be the rule.

When benzodiazepines are used as anxiolytics, lower doses (e.g., diazepam, 2–5 mg three times daily) should be used initially to assess patient sensitivity to the agent and to avoid initial oversedation. The dosage can be slowly increased until a therapeutic effect occurs. Dosage titration with long-acting drugs (e.g., diazepam, chlordiazepoxide, or clorazepate) should proceed more slowly because the drugs reach steady-state levels over a period of several days. Dosages of short-acting drugs (e.g., lorazepam or oxazepam) can be increased more rapidly (e.g., after 2 days).

In follow-up, patients should be asked not only about efficacy but also about side effects. Patients who complain of excessive sedation may do better with a temporary dosage reduction; over time, most individuals develop tolerance to sedative effects. Because the threshold plasma levels of benzodiazepines that result in sedation are higher than those that are anxiolytic, sedated patients being treated for anxiety may do better on multiple low doses during the day rather than fewer and larger doses. Patients on short-acting compounds such as alprazolam should be questioned about interdose rebound anxiety, which can also be addressed by increasing dosing frequency. Intolerance of or lack of efficacy of a benzodiazepine may result from pharmacokinetic factors, as with sedation or interdose rebound, and thus may improve with the switch to an agent with a different profile (e.g., alprazolam to clonazepam). An alternative approach is the switch to another class of drugs (e.g., buspirone or an antidepressant for GAD or an antidepressant for panic disorder).

Tolerance and Discontinuation Symptoms

The benzodiazepines may induce dependence, with a risk of clinically significant symptomatology on emerging discontinuation. Discontinuation symptoms can be conceptually divided into (a) recurrence of the original disorder, (b) rebound (a marked temporary return of original symptoms), and (c) withdrawal (recurrence of the original symptoms plus new symptoms such as tachycardia or hypertension). In clinical practice, these syndromes demonstrate a great deal of overlap and frequently coexist. The nature of the symptoms and their time course may help in making distinctions.

Recurrences reflect the loss of therapeutic benefit and typically do not subside with time; the symptoms are generally indistinguishable from those present prior to treatment. Recurrences are frequent in panic disorder. Generally, the response to recurrence of the original disorder is resumption of therapy.

Rebound symptoms occur soon after discontinuation and generally represent a return of original symptoms, such as anxiety or insomnia, but at a greater intensity than the original symptoms. The response to rebound symptoms is to observe to see if they defervesce quickly or to resume therapy and then taper the benzodiazepine more slowly. For some high-potency compounds with a short half-life, such as alprazolam and triazolam, rebound symptoms occasionally occur even during maintenance therapy as blood levels between doses reach their nadir. If interdose rebound symptoms or rebound occurring with attempts to decrease the dosage represents a serious clinical problem, a switch to a compound with a longer half-life may prove helpful.

The onset of **withdrawal** symptoms generally reflects the half-life of the drug used, usually 1 to 2 days after the last dose for short-acting drugs, 2 to 5 days for long-acting drugs (although symptoms beginning as late as 7–10 days have been reported). Withdrawal symptoms generally peak days after onset and slowly disappear over 1 to 3 weeks. In contrast to recurrence and rebound, withdrawal syndromes include symptoms that the patient has not previously experienced. Benzodiazepine withdrawal symptoms include anxiety, irritability, insomnia, tremulousness, sweating, anorexia, nausea, diarrhea, abdominal discomfort, lethargy, fatigue, tachycardia, systolic hypertension, delirium, and seizures.

The risk of developing dependence and thus rebound and withdrawal symptoms is higher with long-term treatment, higher doses, and higher potency drugs. The likelihood and severity of rebound and withdrawal symptoms also reflect the half-life of the compound; such symptoms occur more frequently and are generally more severe with compounds with a short half-life. In thinking about the risks of dependence and discontinuation syndromes, the benzodiazepines can be subdivided into four groups:

1. High potency and short duration of action: alprazolam, estazolam, midazolam, lorazepam, and triazolam
2. High potency and long duration of action: clonazepam
3. Low potency and short duration of action: oxazepam and temazepam
4. Low potency and long duration of action: chlordiazepoxide, clorazepate, diazepam, flurazepam, halazepam, and quazepam

No withdrawal syndrome has been detected for buspirone. Indeed, the lack of abuse, dependence, and withdrawal symptoms is the most appealing feature of buspirone's indication for the treatment of GAD.

Although dependence can be induced by any benzodiazepine, with low-potency, long-acting drugs, dependence is relatively uncommon in the therapeutic setting (although dependence readily occurs with very high doses). In addition, with this group of compounds, rebound and withdrawal symptoms are typically mild and self-limited when they occur. Dependence is most likely, and rebound and withdrawal symptoms are most severe with high-potency, short-acting benzodiazepines, such as alprazolam, lorazepam, and triazolam. These are the compounds that are most likely to produce delirium and seizures after abrupt discontinuation from high doses. In addition to the more common benzodiazepine withdrawal symptoms, severe dysphoria and psychotic-like symptoms have been reported in patients discontinuing alprazolam. Because they are atypical, these symptoms may be extremely confusing on presentation unless a history of alprazolam discontinuation is obtained.

For some patients, discontinuation of alprazolam may be easier via a switch to equipotent doses of a longer acting high-potency benzodiazepine such as clonazepam (see next section on Switching from Alprazolam to Clonazepam). A small number of reports also have suggested that carbamazepine may be a useful adjunct for alprazolam withdrawal. Although this strategy may aid an individual patient, a large controlled study failed to show evidence of efficacy.

Many sedative drugs share cross-tolerance with the benzodiazepines, including barbiturates, meprobamate, alcohols, propanediols, aldehydes, glutethimide, methyprylon, and methaqualone. Buspirone does not produce cross-tolerance with benzodiazepines, ethanol, or barbiturates and is not useful in withdrawal from these drugs.

Problems with benzodiazepine tolerance, rebound, and withdrawal can be minimized if low-potency, long-acting compounds are used whenever possible (e.g., in the treatment of GAD). If long-acting compounds are relatively contraindicated (e.g., in the elderly or in patients who develop excessive sedation with repeated dosing), use of low-potency, short-acting compounds may represent an alternative (e.g., temazepam for the treatment of insomnia). However, it must be recalled that at high doses, even low-potency compounds may cause discontinuation symptomatology. As with any drug that is being discontinued after a protracted period of use, gradual tapering of benzodiazepines is the most judicious approach. Probably the greatest dangers from benzodiazepine withdrawal occur when patients on short-acting drugs stop their medication suddenly without consulting their physician.

Switching from Alprazolam to Clonazepam

Despite the likely equal efficacy of alprazolam and clonazepam for panic disorder, there are clinical circumstances in which it is helpful to switch patients from alprazolam to clonazepam. These circumstances include significant interdose rebound anxiety (symptom recurrence after an increasingly short period and early morning anxiety prior to the first daily dose) or difficulty with tapering and discontinuing alprazolam. As described previously, both of these circumstances reflect the high potency and short half-life of alprazolam. Switching to clonazepam appears to address these clinical problems because clonazepam is potent enough to replace alprazolam but has a long half-life (2–4 days). One method is based on an open study of patients with panic disorder. The switch takes approximately 1 week (the minimum time to reach a steady-state level of clonazepam).

1. Clonazepam is given at half the total daily alprazolam dose, divided into an early morning and a mid-afternoon dose.
2. Regular alprazolam doses are stopped, but during the first 7 days, alprazolam can be taken as needed up to the full amount taken previously.
3. Alprazolam is stopped entirely after day 7.
4. If more medication is needed after day 7, clonazepam is increased by 0.25 to 0.5 mg every week until efficacy is reestablished.

Abuse

Contrary to public impressions, it appears that very few patients who have received benzodiazepines for valid indications become abusers (i.e., increase their dosage without medical supervision and take the drugs for nonmedical purposes). Most abusers of benzodiazepines also have abused other drugs. Serious abusers of CNS depressants may use the equivalent of hundreds of milligrams of diazepam per day. Serious CNS depressant abusers should be detoxified as inpatients using either phenobarbital or a long-acting benzodiazepine, such as diazepam, as the detoxification agent.

USE IN THE ELDERLY

Slowed hepatic metabolism and increased pharmacodynamic sensitivity mean that great care must be taken when prescribing benzodiazepines in the elderly. In general, short-acting benzodiazepines are safest, especially those metabolized by glucuronidation alone (lorazepam, temazepam, and oxazepam). In one study of patients over age 65, use of benzodiazepines with an elimination half-life of more than 24 hours, but not benzodiazepines with a short half-life, was associated with a 70% increase in the risk of hip fracture compared with individuals not using any psychotropic drugs. Accumulation of long-acting benzodiazepines must always be considered in the differential diagnosis of delirium or rapid cognitive decline in the elderly.

USE IN PREGNANCY

Earlier reports associating diazepam with both cleft lip and cleft palate have not been substantiated. On the other hand, there are no prospective studies to demonstrate that benzodiazepines are safe during pregnancy. One recent report described intra- and extrauterine growth restriction, dysmorphism, and CNS dysfunction as a result of intrauterine benzodiazepine exposure, but the study was compromised by biased patient selection and failure to control adequately for use of other psychotropic drugs. Although there is no convincing evidence that benzodiazepines are teratogenic, it would be wise to avoid benzodiazepines, especially early in pregnancy (oral cleft closure is usually complete by the 10th gestational week), unless there are compelling indications for their use.

SIDE EFFECTS AND TOXICITY

The benzodiazepines have little effect on autonomic function, unlike certain antipsychotic and antidepressant drugs. Thus, adverse effects on blood pressure, pulse, and cardiac rhythm are not typically seen. Benzodiazepines may produce slow-wave and low-voltage fast (β) activity on electroencephalographic testing that is without clinical consequence.

Sedation and Impairment of Performance

Fatigue and drowsiness are the most common side effects associated with benzodiazepine treatment. In addition, impairment of memory and recall, reduced motor coordination, and impairment of cognitive function may occur. The development of these side effects depends on dosage used, concomitant use of other medications, especially CNS depressants, and alcohol, and the sensitivity of the individual being treated. With repeated dosing, as would occur with the treatment of anxiety disorders, most patients develop tolerance to sedation. The suggestion that automobile accidents are more likely to occur among benzodiazepine users is complicated by the possibility that the condition being treated (e.g., anxiety, insomnia) may be a contributing factor. The interpretation of laboratory studies of attention, intellectual function, reflexes, cognitive function, and driving ability is difficult to generalize to real-life situations.

Effects on Memory

Acute dosages of benzodiazepines may produce transient anterograde amnesia. This effect appears to be independent of sedation; acquisition of new information is specifically impaired. The risk of anterograde amnesia appears to be worsened by concomitant ingestion of alcohol. Anterograde amnesia may be desirable when oral or parenteral benzodiazepines are given for preoperative sedation or potentially when used proximally to severe trauma; however, anterograde amnesia is undesirable in most other circumstances. Short-acting, high-potency agents (e.g., triazolam) appear to be the worst offenders; there have been reports of serious amnesia in travelers who have used triazolam to sleep during flights across time zones. Recall of distant memory may actually be enhanced by a benzodiazepine for anxious individuals in performance situations.

Disinhibition

Reports of paradoxical reactions to benzodiazepines (disinhibition), in particular describing rage outbursts or aggression in patients on chlordiazepoxide, diazepam, alprazolam, or clonazepam, have been published. Disinhibition can likely occur with any benzodiazepine, but the lower potency, slowly absorbed oxazepam may be less likely to trigger this effect. Many clinicians feel that the highest incidence of disinhibition occurs in personality disorder patients with prior histories of dyscontrol. When paradoxical excitement occurs in a patient given a benzodiazepine in an emergency room or inpatient ward, the administration of haloperidol, 5 mg intramuscularly, is often effective in reversing the state.

Depression

All benzodiazepines have been associated with the emergence or worsening of depression; whether they were causative or only failed to prevent the depression is unknown. Although it makes sense to lower the dosage or discontinue the benzodiazepine when depression occurs during the course of benzodiazepine treatment, the addition of an antidepressant is typically very effective. If the depression occurs during the course of treatment for panic disorder, the benzodiazepine can be combined with or possibly replaced by an antidepressant.

OVERDOSE

Benzodiazepines have proved to be remarkably safe in overdose. By themselves, only rarely have they been implicated in fatal overdoses, although when combined with other CNS depressants, such as alcohol, barbiturates, or narcotics, they may contribute to the lethality of the overdose. There have been some reports, however, of lethal overdoses with very high-potency benzodiazepines such as triazolam (e.g., Sunter et al., 1988). It is hard to interpret these reports because alcohol or concurrent medical illness was involved in some cases. The replacement of barbiturates and related compounds by benzodiazepines has markedly decreased the number of successful suicides associated with sleeping pills.

The treatment of benzodiazepine overdose includes induction of emesis or gastric lavage, when appropriate, and supportive care for patients who are stuporous or comatose. The benzodiazepine antagonist flumazenil is available for the treatment of benzodiazepine overdose. In tolerant patients, this drug may precipitate withdrawal symptoms in analogy with the actions of naloxone in opiate-dependent individuals.

Table 5.6.   Interactions of benzodiazepines with other drugs

Decrease absorption
  Antacids
Increase central nervous system depression
  Antihistamines
  Barbiturates and similarly acting drugs
  Cyclic antidepressants
  Ethanol
Increase benzodiazepine levels (compete for microsomal enzymes; probably little or no effect on lorazepam, oxazepam, temazepam)
  Cimetidine
  Disulfiram
  Erythromycin
  Estrogens
  Isoniazid
  SSRIs
Decrease benzodiazepine levels
  Carbamazepine (possibly other anticonvulsants)

INTERACTIONS WITH ALCOHOL AND OTHER DRUGS

Serious pharmacokinetic drug interactions are rare with benzodiazepines but may occur (Table 5.6).Benzodiazepines can cause a mild to moderate increase in CNS depression caused by coingested alcohol; when taken together in overdose, ethanol and benzodiazepines can result in death.

BIBLIOGRAPHY

Pharmacokinetics

Greenblatt DJ, Harmatz JS, Englehardt N, et al. Pharmacokinetic determinants of dynamic differences among three benzodiazepine hypnotics. *Arch Gen Psychiatry* 1989;46:326.

Greenblatt DJ, Shader RI, Koch-Weser J. Slow absorption of intramuscular chlordiazepoxide. *N Engl J Med* 1974;291:1116.

Salzman C, Shader RI, Greenblatt DJ, et al. Long vs. short half-life benzodiazepines in the elderly. *Arch Gen Psychiatry* 1983;40:293.

Scavone JM, Greenblatt DJ, Shader RI. Alprazolam kinetics following sublingual and oral administration. *J Clin Psychopharmacol* 1987;7:332.

Mechanism of Action

Levitan ES, Schofield PR, Burt DR, et al. Structural and functional basis for GABA$_A$ receptor heterogeneity. *Nature* 1988;335:76.

Pritchett DB, Sontheimer H, Shivers B, et al. Importance of a novel GABA$_A$ receptor subunit for benzodiazepine pharmacology. *Nature* 1989;338:582.

Disorders Treated

Anxiety

Davidson JRT, Potts N, Richichi E, et al. Treatment of social phobia with clonazepam and placebo. *J Clin Psychopharmacol* 1993;13:423.

Kahn RJ, McNair DM, Lipman RS, et al. Imipramine and chlor-diazepoxide in depressive and anxiety disorders: II. Efficacy in anxious outpatients. *Arch Gen Psychiatry* 1986;43:79.

Nagy LM, Krystal JH, Woods SW, et al. Clinical and medication outcome after short-term alprazolam and behavioral group treatment in panic disorder. *Arch Gen Psychiatry* 1989;46:993.

Rosenbaum JF, Moroz G, Bowden CL. Clonazepam in the treatment of panic disorder with or without agoraphobia: a dose-response study of efficacy, safety, and discontinuance. *J Clin Psychopharmacol* 1997;17:390.

Tesar GE, Rosenbaum JF, Pollack MH, et al. Double-blind, placebo-controlled comparison of clonazepam and alprazolam for panic disorder. *J Clin Psychiatry* 1991;52:69.

Depression

Lipman RS, Covi L, Rickels K, et al. Imipramine and chlordiazepoxide in depressive and anxiety disorders: I. Efficacy in depressed outpatients. *Arch Gen Psychiatry* 1986;43:68.

Rickels K, Chung HR, Csanalosi IB, et al. Alprazolam, diazepam, imipramine, and placebo in outpatients with major depression. *Arch Gen Psychiatry* 1987;44:862.

Insomnia

Dement WC. The proper use of sleeping pills in the primary care setting. *J Clin Psychiatry* 1992;53:50.

Gillin JC, Byerly WF. The diagnosis and management of insomnia. *N Engl J Med* 1990;332:239.

Gillin JC, Spinweber CL, Johnson LC. Rebound insomnia: a critical review. *J Clin Psychopharmacol* 1989;9:161.

Morin CM, Culbert JP, Schwartz SM. Nonpharmacological interventions for insomnia: a meta-analysis of treatment efficacy. *Am J Psychiatry* 1994;151:1172.

Nishino S, Dement WC. Neuropharmacology of sedative-hypnotics and central nervous system stimulants is sleep medicine. *Psychiatr Clin North Am Annu Drug Ther* 1998;5:85.

Alcohol Withdrawal

Saitz R, Mayo-Smith MF, Robert MS, et al. Individualized treatment for alcohol withdrawal: a randomized double-blind controlled trial. *JAMA* 1994;272:519.

Clonazepam for Mania

Aronson TA, Shukla S, Hirschkowitz J. Clonazepam treatment of five lithium-refractory patients with bipolar disorder. *Am J Psychiatry* 1989;146:77.

Sachs GA, Rosenbaum JF, Jones L. Adjunctive clonazepam for maintenance treatment of bipolar disorder. *J Clin Psychopharmacol* 1990;10:42.

Benzodiazepines in Psychotic Disorders

Modell JG, Lenox RH, Weiner S. Inpatient clinical trial of lorazepam for the management of manic agitation. *J Clin Psychopharmacol* 1985;5:109.

Wolkowitz OM, Pickar D. Benzodiazepines in the treatment of schizophrenia: a review and reappraisal. *Am J Psychiatry* 1991;148:714.

Catatonia

Salam SA, Pillai AK, Beresford TP. Lorazepam for psychogenic catatonia. *Am J Psychiatry* 1987;144:1082.

Therapeutic Use

Herman JB, Rosenbaum JF, Brotman AW. The alprazolam to clonazepam switch for the treatment of panic disorder. *J Clin Psychopharmacol* 1987;7:175.

Uhlenhuth EH, DeWit H, Balter MB, et al. Risks and benefits of long term benzodiazepine use. *J Clin Psychopharmacol* 1988;8:161.

Toxicity

Scharf MB, Khosla N, Brocker N, et al. Differential amnestic properties of short- and long-acting benzodiazepines. *J Clin Psychiatry* 1984;45:51.

Sunter JP, Bal TS, Cowan WK. Three cases of fatal triazolam poisoning. *BMJ* 1988;297:719.

Dependence and Abuse

American Psychiatric Association. *Benzodiazepine dependence, toxicity, and abuse.* Washington, DC: American Psychiatric Association, 1990.

Ciraulo DA, Sands BF, Shader RI. Critical review of liability for benzodiazepine abuse among alcoholics. *Am J Psychiatry* 1988;145:1501.

Sellers EM, Schneiderman JF, Romach MK, et al. Comparative drug effects and abuse liability of lorazepam, buspirone, and secobarbital in nondependent subjects. *J Clin Psychopharmacol* 1992;12:79.

Weintraub M, Singh S, Byrne L, et al. Consequences of the 1989 New York State triplicate benzodiazepine prescription regulations. *JAMA* 1991;266:2392.

Discontinuation

Fyer AJ, Liebowitz MR, Gorman JM, et al. Discontinuation of alprazolam treatment in panic patients. *Am J Psychiatry* 1987;144:303.

Rickels K, Case WG, Schweizer E, et al. Long-term benzodiazepine users 3 years after participation in a discontinuation program. *Am J Psychiatry* 1991;148:757.

Roy-Byrne PP, Dager SR, Cowley DS, et al. Relapse and rebound following discontinuation of benzodiazepine treatment of panic attacks: alprazolam versus diazepam. *Am J Psychiatry* 1989;146:860.

Use in the Elderly

Ray WA, Griffin MR, Downey W. Benzodiazepines of long and short elimination half-life and the risk of hip fracture. *JAMA* 1989;262:3303.

Use in Pregnancy

Laegrid L, Olegard R, Wahlstrom J, et al. Abnormalities in children exposed to benzodiazepines *in utero*. *Lancet* 1987;1:108.

Rosenberg L, Mitchell AA, Parsells JL, et al. Lack of relation of oral clefts to diazepam use during pregnancy. *N Engl J Med* 1983;309:1282.

Buspirone

Grady TA, Pigott TA, L'Heureux F, et al. Double-blind study of adjuvant buspirone for fluoxetine-treated patients with obsessive–compulsive disorder. *Am J Psychiatry* 1993;150:819.

Kranzler HR, Burleson JA, Del Boca FK, et al. Buspirone treatment of anxious alcoholics. *Arch Gen Psychiatry* 1994;51:720.

6

Other Drugs: Psychostimulants, β-Adrenergic Blockers, Clonidine, Disulfiram, Donepezil, and Tacrine

PSYCHOSTIMULANTS

A wide variety of compounds (e.g., caffeine and strychnine) can produce central nervous system (CNS) stimulation. However, the stimulant drugs that have found use in psychiatry are sympathomimetic amines, of which the prototype is amphetamine. Amphetamine was first used as a bronchodilator, respiratory stimulant, and analeptic during the 1930s. Psychostimulants were used in the treatment of depression until they were supplanted by tricyclic antidepressants and monoamine oxidase inhibitors (MAOIs) in the 1950s.

The clinical utility of stimulants had been limited by the perception of their risk to cause tolerance and psychological dependence and by their abuse potential. In 1970, the U.S. Food and Drug Administration (FDA) reclassified these drugs as schedule II, the most restrictive classification for drugs that are medically useful. They are currently approved only for the treatment of attention-deficit/hyperactivity disorder (ADHD) and for narcolepsy. The extensive experience with stimulant use in children, adolescents, and more recently in adults with ADHD has reassured the field about the efficacy and safety of these agents when prescribed in a thoughtful way for those without a prior history of substance abuse. Indeed, longitudinal data of ADHD children, comparing those treated or not treated with stimulants, show that treatment is protective against the later emergence of substance abuse difficulties in adolescence. They also have several other possible uses in psychiatric practice (Table 6.1). Those psychostimulants that are most widely used in clinical practice are dextroamphetamine, methylphenidate, and pemoline (Table 6.2).

Chemistry

Amphetamine is racemic β-phenylisopropanolamine; and dextroamphetamine is the D-isomer, which is three to four times more potent than the L-isomer as a CNS stimulant. Methylphenidate is a piperidine derivative that is structurally similar to amphetamine. Pemoline is structurally unrelated.

Pharmacology

Absorption and Metabolism

Amphetamine is well absorbed after oral administration. It has a short half-life (8–12 hours); thus, it is usually administered

210

Table 6.1. Indications for psychostimulants

Effective
  Narcolepsy
  Attention-deficit/hyperactivity disorder (in children)
Probably effective
  Treatment of apathy and withdrawal (in the medically ill and
    elderly)
  Potentiation of narcotic analgesics
Possibly effective
  Residual attention-deficit disorder (in adults)
  Antidepressant augmentation
  Treatment of SSRI-induced fatigue and apathy

two to three times daily. It crosses the blood–brain barrier easily
and develops high concentrations in the brain. Amphetamine is
partly metabolized in the liver and partly excreted unchanged in
the urine. Its excretion is hastened by acidification of the urine.

Methylphenidate is well absorbed after oral administration.
It has a very short biologic life; it reaches peak plasma concentrations in 1 to 2 hours and has an elimination half-life of 1 to 2
hours. Clinically, its effects last 3 to 4 hours, or even less in some
patients. Thus multiple doses (three to four) are required during
the day. Its concentrations in the brain appear to be higher than
those in the blood. Methylphenidate is metabolized by hepatic
microsomal enzymes.

Pemoline has a long half-life, permitting once daily dosing.
Its therapeutic actions in ADHD are usually delayed by 3 to 4

Table 6.2. Available preparations

Drug	Trade Name	Dosage Forms
Adderall (mixed salts of dextroamphetamine saccharate, dextroamphetamine sulfate, amphetamine aspartate, amphetamine sulfate)	Adderall	5-, 10-, 20-mg tablets
Dextroamphetamine	Dexedrine and generics	5-mg tablets 5 mg/5 mL elixir 5-, 10-, 15-mg SR tablets
Methylphenidate	Ritalin and generics	5-, 10-, 20-mg tablets 20-mg SR tablets
Pemoline	Cylert	18.75-, 37.5-, 75.0-mg tablets

SR, sustained release.

weeks. It is 60% metabolized by the liver and 40% excreted unchanged in the urine.

Adderall is the brand name for a single entity amphetamine product combining the neutral sulfate salts of dextroamphetamine and amphetamine, with the dextro isomer of amphetamine saccharate and d, l-amphetamine aspartate product.

All psychostimulant drugs can compete for hepatic enzymes and thus increase the levels of other drugs. Tolerance to the sympathomimetic effects and to the drug-induced euphoria of amphetamine and methylphenidate develops rapidly. Thus, chronic abusers often take very large doses that would be extremely toxic or lethal if taken by a nontolerant individual.

Mechanism of Action

Amphetamine and the similarly acting methylphenidate are often termed *indirectly acting amines*. This is because they act by causing release of norepinephrine, dopamine, and serotonin from presynaptic nerve terminals as opposed to having direct agonist effects on the postsynaptic receptors themselves. In addition, amphetamine inhibits both norepinephrine and dopamine reuptake and has very mild MAOI effects, thus prolonging and enhancing the effects of the amines it releases from presynaptic terminals.

Amphetamine and its derivatives probably increase alertness by stimulating monoamine release by the ascending reticular activating system. Hypothalamic effects are probably responsible for its appetite-suppressant properties. Its stimulatory effects on locomotion and its tendency to produce euphoria are largely a result of facilitation of dopaminergic neurotransmission in the striatum and limbic forebrain. It has been shown in animal models that dopamine lesions or dopamine receptor antagonists block the locomotor stimulant and reinforcing effects of amphetamine, whereas α- and β-adrenergic receptor antagonists do not. Amphetamine and its derivatives are potent stimulants of the sympathetic nervous system because they enhance noradrenergic neurotransmission. The peripheral effects of the amphetamine-like drugs at therapeutic doses include mild increases in both systolic and diastolic blood pressure and often a reflex slowing of the heart rate. With higher doses, the heart rate increases and there may be arrhythmias. Pemoline, which is structurally different, has fewer peripheral sympathetic effects than amphetamine.

The mechanism of action of psychostimulants in ADHD is unknown. In contrast to sympathomimetic effects and euphoria, tolerance to the therapeutic effects in ADHD appear to be quite rare. A prior hypothesis held that somehow the stimulants paradoxically sedated children with ADHD, but this appears not to be the case because the effects of amphetamine in children with ADHD differ only in degree, not in kind, from its effects in normal children.

Chronic use of high-dose amphetamines and related compounds may produce a psychotic syndrome with prominent paranoid ideation and stereotypic movements. It has been theorized that amphetamine-induced psychosis is caused primarily by the facilitation of dopaminergic neurotransmission in the forebrain.

Therapeutic Indications

Attention-Deficit/Hyperactivity Disorder

The symptoms of this childhood disorder include inattention, impulsiveness, and hyperactivity. Stimulant drugs are an effective treatment in 70% to 80% of children with ADHD but are best used as part of a comprehensive treatment program. Stimulant drugs improve attention and decrease impulsiveness and hyperactivity. However, they do not help with specific learning disabilities that are often associated with ADHD (e.g., dyslexia). Stimulants are not indicated for "problem children" who do not meet the diagnostic criteria for ADHD.

Methylphenidate is the most commonly used agent, although dextroamphetamine and related compounds are equally effective. Adderall was recently approved for the treatment of ADHD and also has been shown to be effective. The few studies published to date comparing methylphenidate with Adderall in ADHD found that Adderall was as effective as methylphenidate for children in a classroom setting with continued benefit into the evening home environment, suggesting minimal rebound. In addition, it was generally preferred by parents, counselors, and teachers over methylphenidate. That fewer dosings were required with Adderall is likely related to its longer half-life (6–10 hours) than that of methylphenidate (1–2 hours). Pemoline also appears to be effective, although its use is less well established. The dosage of dextroamphetamine and methylphenidate is 0.3 to 1.5 mg/kg/day in divided doses. Pemoline is given at 0.5 to 3.0 mg/kg/day in a single daily dose. The tricyclic antidepressant desipramine has been used as an alternative to psychostimulants for childhood ADHD, but rare reports of sudden death in children treated with desipramine clearly favor the use of psychostimulants as first-line drugs. The antidepressant bupropion, which has stimulant-like properties, and clonidine are currently under study for this indication.

Residual Attention-Deficit Disorder in Adults

DIAGNOSIS. Residual attention-deficit disorder in adulthood is an increasingly recognized condition, but offers challenges both diagnostically and therapeutically. The diagnosis requires an established diagnosis of attention-deficit disorder with or without hyperactivity in childhood, with residual inattention and impulsiveness in adulthood. The difficulty in diagnosing and studying this disorder reflects, in part, the difficulty of making a retrospective diagnosis of childhood ADHD based on the memories of the patient, the patient's parents, and teachers. As more children with well-documented ADHD reach adulthood, prospective studies should provide a clearer picture of this putative adult disorder. Another difficulty with the diagnosis is that adults with residual ADHD frequently suffer one or more comorbid psychiatric disorders, most frequently mood, substance abuse, and personality disorders, that may have significant symptom overlap with ADHD.

By themselves, the typical adult residual symptoms of ADHD are nonspecific, including restlessness, difficulty in concentrating, excitability, impulsiveness, and irritability. These symptoms often lead to poor job or academic performance, anxiety, temper outbursts, antisocial behavior, and substance abuse.

TREATMENT. In one of the early studies, Wender and associates (1985) studied 21 of 37 adults with residual ADHD and found moderate to marked symptomatic improvement on methylphenidate (average dosage 43.2 mg/day in divided doses, range 10–80), whereas only 4 of 37 adult patients responded to placebo. Pemoline found less clear benefits in a previous study. However, another study (Mattes et al., 1984) that compared both with and without a childhood history who had current symptoms consistent with ADHD found that methylphenidate (average dosage 48.2 mg/day) helped only a small number of patients (16 of 66) and that a childhood history of ADHD did not predict which of these phenomenologically similar patients would respond. More recent studies indicate response rates of 25% to 50% in adult ADHD with daily dosing limited to less than 0.7 mg/kg, but higher response rates were obtained when more robust doses (up to 1.0 mg/kg/day) were used, suggesting a dose–response relationship and a need for incremental increases to 1.0 mg/kg/day before assuming nonresponse. Diagnosis and treatment of adult ADHD must still be considered less well established than for children and adolescents. Methylphenidate might be administered to adults with ADHD-like symptoms as an empirical trial. The best candidates are patients with a childhood diagnosis of ADHD whose symptoms include difficulty in concentrating, irritability, impulsiveness, and restlessness. Patients with major depression, borderline or antisocial personality disorder, or a history of drug abuse are probably better treated with other modalities. The medication is begun at a low dosage and titrated upward as side effects permit until a therapeutic response is achieved. Anecdotal experience suggests that those who respond for this indication do not develop tolerance (Table 6.3).

Narcolepsy

Narcolepsy is a disorder of excessive daytime sleepiness combined with irresistible sleep attacks of short duration. In addition, patients may suffer from cataplexy, periods of partial or complete loss of motor tone (often precipitated by an episode of strong emotion), sleep paralysis, and/or hypnagogic hallucinations. The symptoms of daytime sleepiness and sleep attacks are most effectively treated with psychostimulants. Unlike use in ADHD, tolerance often develops with some narcoleptics using very high doses of stimulants. The range for both methylphenidate and dextroam-

Table 6.3. Dosage range (mg/day)

Drug	Usual Dosage Range	Extreme Dosage Range
Adderall	10–30	2.5–60
Dextroamphetamine	10–30	2.5–60
Methylphenidate	20–40	5.0–80
Pemoline	56.25–75.0	37.5–112.5

phetamine is 20 to 200 mg/day in divided doses. Alternatively, MAOIs (e.g., phenelzine, 30–75 mg/day) have been successful in treating sleep attacks. Cataplexy does not typically respond to psychostimulants or MAOIs, but it may respond to tricyclic antidepressants (e.g., imipramine, 75–150 mg/day). A recent addition to the options for treating narcolepsy and for excessive daytime sleepiness is modafinil. Of interest, although its mechanism of action is not well understood, it is not a stimulant and from animal studies does not appear to work through the dopaminergic system, but is thought to have wake-promoting effects by activity in the hypothalamus and brainstem. Available in 100- and 200-mg tablets, the recommended administration is a single 200-mg tablet in the morning. Adverse effects can include headache, nausea, nervousness, anxiety, anorexia and insomnia, but the drug is generally well tolerated. Drug interactions with other agents that induce, inhibit, or are metabolized by CYP450 3A4 isozymes are possible. An increased dose of 400 mg is reasonably well tolerated, but is not evidently more efficacious than the 200-mg tablet. Discontinuation has not been associated with withdrawal, and the medication is listed in the Controlled Substance Class of Schedule IV. It appears to have less abuse or dependence potential than stimulants.

Depressed and Apathetic States

MAJOR DEPRESSION. Despite multiple anecdotal reports and uncontrolled studies suggesting that dextroamphetamine, methylphenidate, or pemoline might be effective in the treatment of major depression, results of controlled studies have been largely negative or uninterpretable. Selective serotonin reuptake inhibitors (SSRIs), cyclic antidepressants, MAOIs, venlafaxine, and bupropion are all clearly preferable. Given the liabilities of the psychostimulants, including the development of tolerance, abuse potential in substance abusers, and side effects such as insomnia, anxiety, and agitation, there is little reason to prescribe these drugs as primary treatments for major depression. For patients who might benefit from stimulant-like effects during the treatment of depression or who have a history of serious weight gain on cyclic antidepressants, bupropion, reboxetine, or an SSRI is a better choice than one of the psychostimulants.

Psychostimulants have been used with some success as adjuncts to cyclic antidepressants in the treatment of major depression in situations in which an adequate therapeutic trial of a cyclic antidepressant has not produced a full therapeutic response. For example, methylphenidate, 10 to 30 mg/day in divided doses, has been added to cyclic antidepressant regimens. Psychostimulants produce a small increase in tricyclic serum levels, but there was not evidence to suggest that this is the mechanism by which patients improved. Stimulants have been added to SSRIs and other newer antidepressant treatments to augment response, with clinical reports suggesting improvement. Furthermore, they have been helpful in offsetting fatigue and apathy that can emerge with SSRI therapy. They must be considered dangerous in combination with MAOIs despite anecdotal reports of their successful combined use.

APATHETIC AND WITHDRAWN STATES IN MEDICALLY ILL PATIENTS. Medically ill patients (especially the elderly) may develop states of apathy, withdrawal, and a loss of appetite without the full manifestation of a major depressive episode. These states can compromise medical care by decreasing the patient's compliance with treatment and interest in life and diminishing adequate caloric intake. Although such patients might respond to antidepressant drugs, the time course of improvement (several weeks) is a definite disadvantage when medical treatment might be compromised. The judicious use of psychostimulants may improve the patient's mood, interest, compliance, and, in some cases, appetite. When effective, the stimulants work rapidly. They produce few side effects; and their cardiovascular side effect profile is relatively safe except for tachycardia. Their major limiting side effects are insomnia (usually controllable by giving doses early in the day), agitation (which requires a dosage decrease or discontinuation), and, very rarely, toxic psychoses.

Although there are many case series and retrospective reports in the literature, this indication for psychostimulants remains to be studied in well-designed trials. Use of psychostimulants should be avoided in patients with a history of stimulant abuse and perhaps in all drug abusers.

When prescribing stimulants to medically ill patients, generally only a short treatment course proves necessary (several days to several weeks) until the precipitating problem has passed. Patients are begun on low doses (5 mg twice daily in the elderly, 10 mg two or three times daily in younger patients) with gradual increases until a therapeutic effect is achieved.

Potentiation of Narcotic Analgesics

Oral dextroamphetamine can both reduce narcotic requirements in patients who are terminally ill and counteract excess sedation produced by high doses of narcotic drugs. This can be particularly useful in cancer patients who have severe pain requiring high narcotic doses but who object to excessive sedation. Dextroamphetamine, 5 to 20 mg, has been used successfully either as a single dose early in the day or in divided doses. When dextroamphetamine is added, the narcotic dosage should be decreased slightly.

Obesity

Although psychostimulants were previously used as appetite suppressants in the treatment of obesity, their effect was found to be too short lived to be of value in most weight reduction programs. Tolerance to the anorectic effect usually develops, severely limiting the usefulness of stimulants for this indication.

Therapeutic Use

Before Starting Psychostimulants

Prior to starting psychostimulants, patients should have a physical examination with attention directed to heart rate, rhythm, and blood pressure. Psychostimulants should be administered with caution in patients with hypertension, and follow-up monitoring is imperative. Psychostimulants should probably be withheld from patients with tachyarrhythmias. In children, an examination should be performed with attention to the presence of tics and dyskinetic movements (stimulants may precipitate or worsen Gilles de la Tourette syndrome and dyskinesias). In the case of pemoline, it is prudent to obtain baseline liver function tests because liver function abnormalities occasionally develop. Pemoline should be avoided in patients with preexisting liver disease; amphetamine and methylphenidate can be used, but in lower than usual dosages. For patients with renal disease, methylphenidate, which is metabolized by the liver, is the best choice.

Psychostimulant Use

Dextroamphetamine is usually begun at dosages of 5 to 10 mg twice daily in adults and at 5 mg once or twice daily in children and the elderly. For children under 6 and in debilitated elderly patients, a starting dosage of 2.5 mg once or twice daily is prudent. The dosage is increased until the desired therapeutic effects are achieved. In healthy adults, the usual dosage range is 20 to 30 mg/day, although dosages as high as 60 mg/day may be needed. The dosage for children is 0.3 to 1.5 mg/kg/day. Dextroamphetamine is usually given two to three times daily, with the last dose given by late afternoon to avoid insomnia (Table 6.3).

Methylphenidate is usually begun at 10 mg two to three times daily in adults; children and the elderly might be given a test dose of 10 mg and then begun, initially, on 5 to 10 mg twice daily. The dosage is slowly increased (10 mg every 2–4 days) until therapeutic results are achieved. The average daily adult dose is 30 to 40 mg, although doses as high as 80 mg may be used. Dosages for children are 0.3 to 1.5 mg/kg/day. Methylphenidate is usually given in three or four daily doses to maintain effectiveness and avoid rebound. The sustained-release form can be given once or twice daily, although some clinicians find its action not adequately prolonged.

The daily dose of Adderall in children is between 5 mg and 20 mg in split dosing, one in the early morning and the other around noon. The initial dosage can be 5 mg twice daily with increases over the course of the first week to 15 or 20 mg as needed or tolerated. In adult ADHD, the clinician needs to be thoughtful about substituting Adderall for methylphenidate. In adults, the dosing can start at 10 mg initially in the morning for several days, then 10 mg morning and noon for several days; the ultimate dose over the course of the first 2 weeks may be 20 mg twice daily.

Pemoline has little established use in adults. For children with ADHD, it is usually begun at 37.5 mg/day and increased weekly by 18.75 mg until a therapeutic effect is achieved. The usual dosage range is 0.5 to 3.0 mg/kg/day in a single daily dose. Patients given pemoline should have their liver function tests monitored periodically.

Use in Pregnancy

These drugs are lipophilic and thus cross the placental barrier. There appear to be no compelling reasons to use these drugs during pregnancy; thus, they should be avoided.

Use in the Elderly

These drugs are safe in elderly patients but should be used in lower dosages. Generally, dextroamphetamine or methylphenidate is used. Little information exists on the use of pemoline in the elderly.

Side Effects and Toxicity

CNS Side Effects

The major adverse effects of psychostimulants are central. These include anorexia, insomnia (which can often be minimized by administration early in the day), changes in arousal (either overstimulated and anxious or alternatively listless and lethargic), and changes in mood (either overly euphoric or occasionally tearful and oversensitive). Dysphoric reactions are more commonly reported in children. Rarely, patients develop toxic psychoses with therapeutic use. High doses, as may occur in some narcoleptics and drug abusers, may produce psychosis with marked paranoia.

Other Side Effects

Patients with underlying fixed or labile hypertension may have mild elevations in blood pressure; rarely, this is severe enough to require discontinuation of the drug. Sinus tachycardia and other tachyarrhythmias rarely occur at clinical doses. In general, these drugs have greater cardiovascular safety than tricyclic antidepressants. Other side effects include headaches and abdominal pain. Intravenous amphetamine abusers have developed necrotizing angiitis affecting the brain

In children, there has been concern about possible long-term growth and weight suppression, although this problem appears to be mild. Children given time off the drug (e.g., during summer vacation) appear to make up any weight loss. Pemoline produces liver function test abnormalities in some patients.

Abuse and Withdrawal

Stimulant Abuse

A major drawback to the use of psychostimulants is their potential for abuse, dependence, and addiction. Amphetamines are abused orally and intravenously, and methylphenidate is abused orally. Pemoline does not appear to be commonly abused. These drugs produce feelings of euphoria and enhanced self-confidence. In the high doses of abuse, there are often signs of adrenergic hyperactivity (i.e., increased pulse and blood pressure, dry mouth, and pupillary dilatation). High doses of amphetamine may result in stereotyped behaviors, bruxism, formication, irritability, restlessness, emotional lability, and paranoia. With chronic abuse, a paranoid psychosis may develop, characterized by paranoid delusions, ideas of reference, and auditory, visual, or tactile hallucinations.

Withdrawal

Although there are no physical withdrawal symptoms, patients who have used high doses for prolonged periods may experience a marked central syndrome, including fatigue, hypersomnia, hyperphagia, and severe depression in the short-term and anhedonia, dysphoria, and drug craving in the long-term. Currently, there is no proven pharmacologic treatment for psychostimulant dependence and withdrawal. Referral to a comprehensive treatment program is usually the best course. Patients should be observed for the emergence of a major depressive syndrome and suicidality or alternatively for recurrent drug abuse.

Overdose

Overdose with psychostimulants results in a syndrome of marked sympathetic hyperactivity (i.e., hypertension, tachycardia, hyperthermia) often accompanied by toxic psychosis or delirium. Patients may be irritable, paranoid, or violent. Grand mal seizures may occur. Death may result from hypertension, hyperthermia, arrhythmias, or uncontrollable seizures.

Treatment consists of supportive care and blockade of adrenergic receptors. If the patient is unconscious or seizing, the airway must be protected. High fevers should be treated with cooling blankets. Seizures can be controlled with an intravenous benzodiazepine, such as lorazepam (1–2 mg) or diazepam (5–10 mg), repeated as necessary.

Delirium or psychosis usually responds to an antipsychotic agent. If the patient is also hypertensive, chlorpromazine has the advantage of blocking both α-adrenergic and dopamine receptors. Dosages of 50 mg intramuscularly four times daily are usually adequate, although dosages up to 100 mg four times daily may be necessary. Otherwise, haloperidol might be a better choice; 5 mg twice daily will usually suffice. Additional sedation can be provided by benzodiazepines, such as lorazepam, 1 to 2 mg orally or 1 mg intramuscularly, or diazepam, 5 to 10 mg orally every 1 to 2 hours as needed. Delirium usually clears in 2 to 3 days, but paranoid psychoses due to long-term high-dose abuse may take longer to clear. Severe hypertension or tachyarrhythmias can usually be treated with propranolol, 1 mg intravenously every 5 to 10 minutes as needed up to a total of 8 mg.

β-ADRENERGIC BLOCKERS

Beta-adrenergic blockers have been used to treat a variety of psychiatric conditions (Table 6.4), although most of these uses

Table 6.4.   Psychiatric uses for β-adrenergic receptor antagonists

Effective
  Performance anxiety
  Lithium tremor
  Neuroleptic-induced akathisia
Probably effective
  Adjunct to benzodiazepines in ethanol withdrawal
Possibly effective
  Impulsive violence in patients with organic brain syndromes
  Alternative to benzodiazepines in generalized anxiety disorder

are not well studied and none is approved by the FDA. One or more of the β-adrenergic blockers is approved for the treatment of hypertension, angina, some tachyarrhythmias, symptoms of thyrotoxicosis, glaucoma, and migraine. Agents that have been reported on for psychiatric use in the United States include, propranolol, metoprolol, nadolol, atenolol, **and recently pindolol.**

Mechanism of Action

Beta-adrenergic blockers in clinical use are competitive antagonists of norepinephrine and epinephrine at β-adrenergic receptors. Thus, they are peripherally sympatholytic. A detailed understanding of their central actions awaits a more complete description of the functions of norepinephrine in the CNS.

Within the brain, norepinephrine is produced by a small number of neurons, all located in the brainstem tegmentum. The major noradrenergic nucleus is the locus ceruleus, found within the dorsal pons, which projects widely throughout the CNS. Functionally, noradrenergic systems in the brain appear to be involved in modulation of global vigilance, regulation of hormone release, modulation of pain perception, and central regulation of the sympathetic nervous system. It has been hypothesized that noradrenergic systems are involved in important aspects of anxiety and fear. Peripherally, norepinephrine is the major transmitter of postganglionic sympathetic neurons. Epinephrine has only a limited role in the CNS; it appears to be involved in blood pressure control. Peripherally, both epinephrine and norepinephrine are released as stress hormones from the adrenal medulla.

Norepinephrine and epinephrine share two types of receptors, called α and β, each of which has at least two subtypes. α_1 receptors are located postsynaptically in both the sympathetic nervous system and the brain. In the brain, α_1 receptors are found on both neurons and blood vessels. Stimulation of α_1 receptors produces vasoconstriction. Prazosin is a selective α_1 receptor antagonist used as an antihypertensive drug; specific α_1-receptor antagonists are not used in psychiatry at present. α_2 receptors are mostly presynaptic autoreceptors (in both sympathetic terminals and locus ceruleus neurons in the brain). Clonidine is a selective agonist at α_2-adrenergic receptors; yohimbine is a selective antagonist. Because α_2 receptors function, in large part, as inhibitory autoreceptors on noradrenergic neurons, clonidine decreases central noradrenergic neurotransmission, thereby producing centrally mediated hypotension and other effects.

Beta 1 receptors are found in the brain and heart. They stimulate the heart both chronotropically and inotropically. Metoprolol, atenolol, and practolol are selective β_1-receptor antagonists. β_2 receptors are found in the brain on glial cells more than on neurons; peripherally, they are found in the lung and blood vessels. Stimulation of β_2 receptors produces bronchodilation and vasodilation. Salbutamol and terbutaline are selective agonists used clinically in the treatment of asthma. No obvious clinical use for selective β_2-receptor antagonists exists. Pindolol, a β-adrenergic and presynaptic 5-HT$_{1vA}$ antagonist, has been reported to decrease the latency to response for SSRIs.

Pharmacology

Four major features differentiate the β blockers: their relative receptor selectivity, their relative lipophilicity, their route of metabolism, and their half-lives. The advent of relatively selective β-receptor antagonists (metoprolol and atenolol), with less effect at β_2 than β_1 receptors, has decreased the problem of bronchospasm induced by the older nonselective drugs. The selectivity is only relative, however; caution must still be exercised in treating patients with asthma. Both nonselective and β_1-selective compounds have been used for psychiatric disorders.

Beta-receptor blockers differ markedly in their lipophilicity. The least lipophilic drugs, nadolol and atenolol, cross the blood–brain barrier poorly and therefore have a higher ratio of peripheral to central effects, whereas the more lipophilic drugs, propranolol and metoprolol, have potent central as well as peripheral effects. Compounds of intermediate lipophilicity include acebutolol and timolol. Pindolol is also of intermediate lipophilicity; however, it differs from the other β blockers because it has intrinsic sympathomimetic activity also. Pindolol has no current use in psychiatry.

The drugs also vary markedly in elimination half-life. Nadolol and atenolol have relatively long half-lives, thus allowing once a day administration. In contrast, propranolol requires multiple daily dosing unless a sustained-release form is used. The major features of commonly used β-adrenergic blockers are given in Table 6.5.

The β blockers do not appear to induce tolerance to their psychiatric effects or to have abuse potential.

Psychiatric Use

Performance Anxiety

Performance anxiety, a well-known example of which is stage fright, is considered to be a form of social phobia. When severe, performance anxiety can interfere with life activities that are important to many individuals. It may lead to poor performance in or avoidance of such activities as interviews, speaking in class, public speaking, acting, or music. Symptoms include dry mouth, hoarse voice, pounding heart, difficulty in breathing, tremor, and, occasionally, weakness and dizziness. The anxiety may feed on itself, creating a vicious cycle of anticipatory anxiety leading up to the activity and worsening anxiety during the activity.

Table 6.5. Relevant pharmacologic properties of commonly used β-adrenergic blockers

Drug	Selectivity	Lipophilicity	Half-life (h)	Route of Elimination
Propranolol	None	High	3–6	Hepatic
Metoprolol	β_1	High	3–4	Hepatic
Atenolol	β_1	Low	6–9	Renal
Nadolol	None	Low	14–24	Renal

When this syndrome interferes with important activities, treatment is indicated. β blockers, used in optimal doses, have minimal central side effects and generally improve performance. Benzodiazepines, on the other hand, which may cause some sedation or disinhibition, are likely to worsen performance.

A single dose of propranolol, 10 to 40 mg or the equivalent, usually suffices. The dose can be given 20 to 30 minutes prior to the anxiogenic event. It is reasonable to administer a test dose on some anxiogenic occasion prior to an all-important engagement. Because most of the troublesome symptoms are peripheral, less lipophilic agents (e.g., nadolol or atenolol) are also effective. Cognitive and behavioral therapies are alternatives for individuals who do not wish to take or do not tolerate β blockers.

Lithium Tremor

Lithium may cause an action tremor even when used at therapeutic (nontoxic) blood levels. Although new onset or coarsening of tremor suggests lithium toxicity, a stable tremor occurring at therapeutic blood levels may be troublesome and merit treatment. Several interventions can be tried. First, it is important to establish that the patient is on the lowest dosage therapeutic for that individual. Second, it is helpful if the patient minimizes or eliminates caffeine consumption. Third, for some patients, dosing can be altered so that the entire dose is taken at bedtime (see Chapter 4); using such a dosage regimen, peak levels (which are most likely to cause tremor) occur during the night. Finally, if the patient is still bothered by tremor, especially if it interferes with daily activities, β blockers can be administered. Propranolol is often helpful in the range of 20 to 160 mg/day or the equivalent given in two or three divided doses. Less lipophilic drugs (i.e., atenolol or nadolol) also may be effective for this indication.

Neuroleptic-Induced Akathisia

This serious side effect of antipsychotic drugs is fully described in Chapter 2. Some clinicians believe that β-adrenergic blockers are the most effective treatment for neuroleptic-induced akathisia, and in at least one study, they were shown to be superior to benzodiazepines. For refractory akathisia, or akathisia occurring with parkinsonian symptoms, β blockers or benzodiazepines can be given in combination with an anticholinergic drug.

In case reports and small studies, patients have responded to both propranolol and nadolol. Dosages of propranolol were in the range of 30 to 80 mg/day in divided doses; dosages of nadolol ranged from 40 to 80 mg/day given as a single dose. Propranolol worked rapidly once an effective dosage was found; it had no effect on other extrapyramidal symptoms.

Adjunct to Benzodiazepines in Ethanol Withdrawal

In a randomized double-blind trial (Kraus et al., 1985), atenolol was found to be a useful adjunct to (not a replacement for) benzodiazepines in ethanol withdrawal. Sixty-one patients received atenolol, and 59 received placebo. Atenolol was administered as follows: no drug if the heart rate was less than 50 beats/min, 50 mg if it was 50 to 79 beats/min, and 100 mg for a heart rate of equal to or exceeding 80 beats/min. The drug was given once a day. Compared with those on placebo, the vital signs and tremors of patients on atenolol improved more rapidly from the first day, and shorter hospital stays and fewer benzodiazepines were required. Because β blockers do not cross-react with ethanol, they are probably not an adequate single agent for detoxification.

Violent Outbursts in Patients with Organic Brain Syndromes

Both case reports and small controlled trials have suggested utility for β-adrenergic blockers in the treatment of violent outbursts, especially in patients with organic brain syndromes. Patients who have been the subjects of reports have ranged in neurologic impairment from slight to very severe. Propranolol, in dosages of 40 to 520 mg/day in two to four divided doses, has been reported to be effective; nadolol, 120 mg, has been reported to be superior to placebo. In many case series, patients were being treated concomitantly with other drugs, including antipsychotics, carbamazepine, and lithium, which had not, by themselves, curbed the violent outbursts. Further study is needed, but a careful empirical clinical trial of a β-adrenergic blocker could reasonably be undertaken in patients with organic brain syndromes with episodic violence refractory to nonpharmacologic measures, so long as cardiovascular and respiratory status are well monitored and objective records of the frequency and severity of violent outbursts are maintained. Although doses of propranolol above 200 mg/day have been reported, they are not recommended.

Generalized Anxiety and Panic Disorder

Multiple controlled trials suggest that although the β-adrenergic blockers are effective in treating autonomic symptoms associated with generalized anxiety and panic attacks, they are less effective than other agents (e.g., benzodiazepines in generalized anxiety or antidepressants in panic disorder) in treating the psychological aspects of anxiety and in overall outcome. When used for generalized anxiety, variable success has been reported with propranolol in dosages of 40 to 320 mg/day given in two or three divided doses. The usefulness of β blockers in any given patient is empirical. It is important to watch for emergent signs of depression and to discontinue the β blocker if depression develops during the course of treatment.

Potentiation of Antidepressants

Although there is conflicting evidence for the potentiating effect of pindolol in the management of treatment-resistant depression, a trial in patients who have only partially responded to SSRIs or other antidepressants is reasonable when other efforts have failed.

Other Disorders

Very high doses of propranolol have been tried in **schizophrenia** without convincing benefit. β blockers also have been tried in the treatment of **tardive dyskinesia,** without sustained or reproducible benefit.

Therapeutic Use

Choice of Drug

For patients with asthma or other obstructive pulmonary disorders, a relatively selective β_1 antagonist (metoprolol or atenolol) is preferable. However, for such patients, the risk, even with selective agents, probably outweighs their established psychiatric benefits. β blockers should be used cautiously in diabetics prone to hypoglycemia, because they may interfere with the normal response to hypoglycemia.

For disorders in which a primarily peripheral effect is required and repetitive dosing is expected (lithium tremor), a less lipophilic agent might be chosen (nadolol or atenolol) to minimize potential central side effects (lassitude, depression, sleep disorder). For disorders in which a central effect is desired (e.g., control of violence), more lipophilic agents (propranolol, metoprolol) should be selected.

Use of β Blockers for Psychiatric Disorders

Beta blockers are begun at low doses, and side effects, such as bradycardia, hypotension, or bronchospasm, should be monitored. Doses are typically withheld if blood pressure is less than 90/60 mm Hg or heart rate is less than 55 beats/min. Bradycardia or hypotension also precludes dosage increases. If patients develop asthma during treatment for psychiatric symptoms, the dangers of drug therapy may outweigh the established benefits; thus, drug discontinuation should be considered.

Propranolol may be started at dosages of 10 mg three times daily or 10 to 20 mg twice daily and slowly increased (e.g., by no more than 20–30 mg/day at first) until therapeutic effects are achieved. It must be given in divided doses because of its short half-life. Metoprolol is usually begun at dosages of 50 mg twice daily. Nadolol and atenolol can be given in single daily doses.

Patients who have coronary artery disease or hypertension risk rebound worsening when β blockers are discontinued; in such patients, slow weaning with careful follow-up is the safest course.

Side Effects and Drug Interactions

Beta-adrenergic blockers have a variety of significant side effects (Table 6.6). β blockers have no apparent effect on memory. They may actually improve performance of tasks that require a mixture of perceptual motor, learning, and memory skills, perhaps because such tasks are sensitive to even low levels of anxiety. Several drug interactions have been reported, including increased levels of theophylline and thyroxine.

CLONIDINE

Although clonidine's primary use is as an antihypertensive drug, it also has properties that make it useful in psychiatric drug therapy. Its principal mechanism of action appears to be as an agonist at α_2-adrenergic receptors in the CNS. Because the predominant role of central α_2 receptors is to act as autoreceptors with a negative feedback function, the major effect of clonidine is to decrease the activity of central noradrenergic neurons.

Table 6.6. Side effects and toxicity of β blockers

Cardiovascular
  Hypotension
  Bradycardia
  Dizziness
  Congestive failure (in patients with compromised myocardial
    function)
Respiratory
  Asthma (less risk with β₁-selective drugs)
Metabolic
  Worsened hypoglycemia in diabetics on insulin or oral agents
Gastrointestinal
  Nausea
  Diarrhea
  Abdominal pain
Sexual function
  Impotence
Neuropsychiatric
  Lassitude
  Fatigue
  Dysphoria
  Insomnia
  Vivid nightmares
  Depression
  Psychosis (rare)
Other (rare)
  Raynaud's phenomenon
  Peyronie's disease
Withdrawal syndrome
  Rebound worsening of preexisting angina pectoris when
    β blockers are discontinued

This has complex effects, including decreased sympathetic outflow.

The psychiatric uses of clonidine (Table 6.7) are currently experimental. The similarly acting agents guanabenz and guanfacine have rarely been reported on for psychiatric indications. Clonidine is available for oral use only under the trade name Catapres. Tablets are available in 0.1-, 0.2-, and 0.3-mg strengths.

Pharmacology

Clonidine is almost completely absorbed after oral administration; it achieves peak plasma concentrations in 1 to 3 hours. The drug is very lipophilic, easily penetrating the blood–brain barrier. Approximately half is metabolized in the liver, and the rest is excreted unchanged by the kidney. It has no known active metabolites. It has an elimination half-life of 9 hours; thus, it is usually given in two daily doses.

Table 6.7.   Uses of clonidine in psychiatry

Probably effective
   Opioid withdrawal
   Gilles de la Tourette syndrome
Investigational
   Mania
   Anxiety disorders
   Neuroleptic-induced akathisia
   Attention deficit hyperactivity disorder

Psychiatric Use

Opioid Withdrawal

Several controlled trials have demonstrated the usefulness of clonidine during withdrawal from narcotics. Clonidine may suppress many signs and symptoms of withdrawal, thus enhancing patient comfort and compliance. It is particularly effective in suppressing autonomic symptoms, having proved more effective than morphine or placebo. It is less effective than morphine, however, in treating subjective symptoms of abstinence such as drug craving. Sedation and hypotension limit its usefulness in outpatients.

The mainstay of opiate detoxification is the long-acting opiate methadone. In typical detoxification protocols, the requirement for methadone is determined using objective criteria (hypertension or tachycardia above baseline, dilated pupils, sweating, gooseflesh, rhinorrhea, or lacrimation) rather than subjective complaints. Methadone is administered in dosages of 10 mg orally every 4 hours when at least two objective criteria for withdrawal are met. The total dose of methadone given on day 1 is given the next day in two divided doses. Methadone is then withdrawn by 5 mg/day. During the withdrawal of methadone, clonidine may be administered beginning at low dosages, such as 0.1 mg two or three times daily, and increased as needed and tolerated. Dosages above 0.3 mg three times daily are rarely necessary. With completion of withdrawal, clonidine can be rapidly tapered. In neonates with narcotic abstinence syndrome, dosages of 3 to 4 μg/kg/day have been reported to be quite effective without toxicity.

Withdrawal from Other Drugs

In one small but well-designed study, clonidine was ineffective in treating withdrawal from either long or short half-life benzodiazepines. After an initial report claimed that clonidine aided in cessation of tobacco smoking, a well-designed study found it to be of no benefit.

Gilles de la Tourette Syndrome

This disorder is characterized by multiple motor and phonic tics, which develop during childhood and are chronic in duration. The nature and severity of the symptoms vary markedly among individuals and for any given patient over time. In addition to their motor and phonic symptoms, patients may have difficulty in concentrating, impulsiveness, and obsessions and compulsions.

When severe, this disorder is socially disabling and merits a trial of drug treatment. Although antipsychotic drugs (especially haloperidol and more recently pimozide) have traditionally been used to treat Gilles de la Tourette syndrome (see Chapter 2), clonidine appears to be useful as an alternative. The mechanism by which clonidine is effective in this disorder is unknown. When effective, it may take 2 to 3 months for its beneficial effects to manifest. In one randomized trial, clonidine, 3 to 5 µg/kg/day, was superior to placebo in decreasing tic severity. When given for this disorder, clonidine is begun at very low dosages, typically 0.05 mg/day, and slowly titrated upward over several weeks to the range of 0.15 to 0.3 mg/day given in two divided doses. Dosages above 0.5 mg/day often have more side effects than patients are willing to tolerate for the amount of benefit.

Mania

There are case reports and uncontrolled trials suggesting possible efficacy for clonidine in acute mania. Patients in these reports were treated with clonidine alone or in combination with lithium or carbamazepine. The reported dosages of clonidine were 0.2 to 0.4 mg twice daily. Patients were reported to improve within 2 to 3 days after an effective dosage of clonidine was reached. However, in a double-blind crossover study of 24 patients with mania, lithium was found to be clearly more effective than clonidine. Evidence for the effectiveness of clonidine in mania or bipolar prophylaxis is unconvincing

Anxiety Disorders

There have been sporadic reports of effectiveness in panic disorder and generalized anxiety. Although some individuals may benefit, clonidine does not appear to be generally effective.

Neuroleptic-Induced Akathisia

Akathisia, a serious side effect of antipsychotic drugs, is fully discussed in Chapter 2. Clonidine has been reported to help some patients. In both open- and single-blind studies, clonidine in dosages of 0.15 to 2.0 mg/day (extreme range reported as 0.1–0.8 mg/day) in divided doses has a significant effect on both subjective symptoms and objective signs of akathisia. Therapy is limited, however, by sedation and hypotension. Hypotensive side effects may be exacerbated with concomitant administration of low-potency neuroleptics. Because its efficacy has been less well studied than other drugs and because of these side effects, it is reasonable to reserve the use of clonidine for patients whose akathisia does not respond to antipsychotic dosage reduction and treatment with anticholinergic drugs, β blockers, or benzodiazepines.

Therapeutic Use

Clonidine is begun at low dosages to minimize side effects such as sedation and hypotension. Typically 0.1 mg twice daily is safe, although in children with Gilles de la Tourette syndrome, the starting dosage may be as low as 0.05 mg/day. The dosage is increased slowly, by no more than 0.1 mg/day, until the desired therapeutic effects are achieved. For most psychiatric uses, optimal dosages are unknown. One group reports that dosages of 5 µg/kg/day in divided doses is effective in opiate withdrawal. Clonidine's maximal effect on blood pressure appears to be at dosages in the range of 0.3 mg twice daily. In a minority of cases in which clonidine is used as an antihypertensive agent, tolerance occurs; the occurrence of tolerance for psychiatric indications is unknown. Long-term uses in which tolerance might be a problem are in the treatment of akathisia and Gilles de la Tourette syndrome.

Drug Discontinuation

In treating hypertensive patients, sudden withdrawal of clonidine occasionally precipitates a hypertensive crisis that may be life threatening. This has usually been reported after use of higher dosages, although dosages as low as 0.6 mg/day have been implicated. This hypertensive rebound begins 18 to 20 hours after the last dose. When rebound hypertension is severe, treatment includes combined α- and β-adrenergic blockers or sodium nitroprusside. Because of this possibility, clonidine should be used with care in hypertensive patients, even if the indications for use are psychiatric. It is prudent to wean the drug rather than discontinue it at once in all patients who have received high doses for more than 2 to 3 weeks.

Side Effects and Toxicity

Almost all of the experience with clonidine comes from patients using it for hypertension, but the side effects in psychiatric patients are likely to be similar. About 50% of patients report dry mouth and some degree of sedation during the first 2 to 4 weeks of therapy. Tolerance to these effects usually occurs. About 10% of patients discontinue this agent because of persistent side effects, including sedation, postural dizziness, dry mouth or dry eyes, nausea, and impotence. Fluid retention may occur, but this effect is correctable with diuretics.

Central nervous system side effects are particularly important in psychiatric patients because they may be confused with the underlying disorder for which the agent was prescribed. They include:

Sedation, drowsiness
Vivid dreams or nightmares
Insomnia
Restlessness
Anxiety
Depression
Visual or auditory hallucinations (rare)

Rare **idiosyncratic side effects** include rash, pruritus, alopecia, hyperglycemia, gynecomastia, and increased sensitivity to alcohol.

Drug interactions are uncommon, but concurrent use with a tricyclic antidepressant may reduce the antihypertensive effect of clonidine.

Overdoses may result in decreased blood pressure, heart rate, and respiratory rate. Patients may be stuporous or comatose with small pupils, thus mimicking an opioid overdose. Treatment consists of ventilatory support, intravenous fluids or pressors for hypotension, and atropine for bradycardia.

DISULFIRAM

One strategy in the treatment of alcoholism is the use of sensitizing agents that produce a feeling of sickness when the patient consumes ethanol. The rationale behind their use is that the threat of an aversive reaction will deter alcohol consumption. Disulfiram is one of several compounds that can cause sensitization to alcohol, but it is the only one commonly used in the United States. Although controlled clinical trials do not favor the use of sensitizing agents as effective treatments for alcoholism, disulfiram continues to be prescribed in the United States.

Controlled trials (Fuller and Roth, 1979; Fuller et al., 1986) do not indicate any advantage of disulfiram over placebo in achieving total abstinence, in delaying resumption of drinking, or in improving employment status or social stability. At dosages of 250 mg/day, however, the drug appears to increase the proportion of days in which no alcohol is consumed. This modest benefit may decrease the medical complications of alcoholism in the long run, but this has not been proved definitively.

Although disulfiram has only limited value in the general population, some clinicians believe that the drug is useful for selected individuals who remain employed and socially stable. Because these patients have the best outcomes in any case, it is unclear that disulfiram actually contributes to therapeutic success.

Pharmacology and Mechanism of Action

Disulfiram is 80% to 90% absorbed after an oral dose. Although it has a short half-life (because it is rapidly metabolized by the liver), its biologic effect is long-lived because it is an irreversible inhibitor of certain enzymes, most importantly, aldehyde dehydrogenase. This is a hepatic enzyme involved in the intermediary metabolism of ethanol. In normal ethanol metabolism, acetaldehyde is produced but does not accumulate because it is rapidly oxidized by aldehyde dehydrogenase. However, when this enzyme has been inhibited by disulfiram, acetaldehyde levels accumulate to 5 to 10 times higher than usual. It is acetaldehyde that is responsible for most of the resulting symptoms.

Disulfiram inhibits enzymes other than aldehyde dehydrogenase. It inhibits hepatic microsomal enzymes, thus interfering with the metabolism of a variety of drugs, including:

Phenytoin
Isoniazid
Warfarin
Rifampin
Barbiturates
Long-acting benzodiazepines (e.g., diazepam, chlordiazepoxide)

Disulfiram also inhibits dopamine β-hydroxylase, thus potentially decreasing the concentrations of norepinephrine and epinephrine in the sympathetic nervous system. This may be partly responsible for the severity of hypotension observed in the disulfiram–alcohol reaction.

The Disulfiram–Alcohol Reaction

Five to ten minutes after consuming alcohol, the patient on disulfiram develops a feeling of heat in the face, followed by facial and then whole-body flushing due to vasodilation. This is accompanied by throbbing in the head and neck and a severe headache. Sweating, dry mouth, nausea, vomiting, dizziness, and weakness usually occur. In more severe reactions, there may be chest pain, dyspnea, severe hypotension, and confusion. Death has been reported, usually in patients who have taken more than 500 mg of disulfiram, but occasionally with lower doses. After the symptoms pass, the patient is usually exhausted and often sleeps, after which the patient usually recovers entirely. The symptoms last from 30 minutes to 2 hours. The length and severity depend both on the dose of disulfiram and the amount of ethanol consumed. The threshold for the reaction is approximately 7 mL of 100% ethanol or its equivalent. After a dose of disulfiram, sensitization to ethanol lasts for 6 to 14 days, the time required to synthesize an adequate number of new molecules of aldehyde dehydrogenase.

Diphenhydramine, 50 mg intramuscularly or intravenously, has been reported to be symptomatically helpful. Severe reactions may require emergency supportive treatment, most often with intravenous fluids for hypotension and dehydration. Shock, requiring pressors, may occur, as may arrhythmias. Respiratory distress often improves with the administration of oxygen.

Therapeutic Use

Disulfiram should only be prescribed to alcoholics who seek total abstinence, agree to use the drug, and appear able to comply with its use. Its use is therefore not recommended in severely impulsive, psychotic, or suicidal patients. In addition, patients should have no medical contraindications to its use. These contraindications include:

Pregnancy
Moderate to severe hepatic dysfunction
Renal failure
Peripheral neuropathies
Cardiac disease

Patients must be made to understand the dangers of drinking alcohol while on the drug. They should be warned to avoid ethanol in any form, including such disguised forms as sauces, cough syrups, and even topical preparations such as aftershave.

There is no evidence that disulfiram or any alcohol-sensitizing agent is effective long-term (months to years). In individual patients, the agent may be useful as an adjunct to a comprehensive psychosocial treatment plan in which the maintenance of complete abstinence is sought.

Patients should be thoroughly detoxified before starting the drug. The usual dosage is 250 mg/day, usually taken in the morning, when the resolve to remain abstinent is often greatest. Patients who feel drowsy on the drug may prefer to take their dose at bedtime. An optimal dosage that is both safe and effective is not known. Doses above 250 mg are associated with more severe side effects and do not appear to be warranted. Doses as low as 100 mg have been used when side effects do not permit higher doses.

Once therapy is established, it is important to assess compliance at regular intervals. A complete blood count and liver function test should be checked every 3 to 6 months. Disulfiram may be teratogenic and should not be used by pregnant women.

Side Effects and Toxicity

The most common adverse effects are fatigue and drowsiness, which can be managed by taking the dose at bedtime or reducing the dosage. Some patients complain of body odor or halitosis, which also may improve with dosage reduction. Other reported side effects include tremor, headache, impotence, dizziness, and a foul taste in the mouth. Rare but severe side effects include hepatotoxicity and neuropathies. Psychiatric side effects appear to be rare, although psychosis and catatonic-like reactions have been reported.

A reported overdose of disulfiram alone caused delirium with prominent hallucinations, tachycardia, and hypertension. The patient recovered in 7 days with supportive care plus haloperidol to control delirium.

Drug Interactions

Because hepatic microsomal enzymes are inhibited by disulfiram, levels of several drugs (i.e., vasodilators, α- or β-adrenergic antagonists, antidepressants, antipsychotic agents) may be increased with a risk of toxicity. Hepatic glucuronic acid conjugation is not affected; thus the metabolism of such drugs as oxazepam and lorazepam is not affected.

Certain drugs increase the severity of the disulfiram–alcohol reaction, and their use should be considered as a relative contraindication for disulfiram. The following drugs may worsen the disulfiram–alcohol reaction:

MAOIs
Vasodilators
α- or β-adrenergic antagonists
Tricyclic antidepressants
Antipsychotic drugs

DONEPEZIL

Donepezil is a reversible inhibitor of acetylcholinesterase that has become the available drug of choice for mild to moderate Alzheimer's disease, and its development was based on the observed deficiency in cholinergic transmission in that condition. Alzheimer's disease produces widespread death of neurons in the brain. Cholinergic neurons in the basal forebrain that innervate the cerebral cortex and hippocampus are thought to play critical roles in memory function. In Alzheimer's disease, these cholinergic neurons are often particularly seriously affected. By inhibiting the metabolism of acetylcholine in the brain, tacrine is thought to ameliorate the partial depletion of this neurotransmitter brought about by the dropout of cholinergic neurons. Because Alzheimer's disease is a progressive disease of cell death, tacrine is meant only as a palliative symptomatic treatment for the earlier stages of illness. Because acetylcholine is only one of many neurotransmitters affected, donepezil is only partially palliative. The drug has been shown to improve cognitive performance and enhance activities of daily living in Alzheimer's patients, compared with placebo. The drug is well tolerated at both a 5- and 10-mg dose per day. Possible adverse effects include nausea, diarrhea, insomnia, muscle cramps, fatigue, and anorexia, but these are typically mild and time limited. Both 5- and 10-mg doses were efficacious, but treatment is begun with 5 mg for 4 to 6 months. Although 10 mg is not proven to be more efficacious than 5 mg, an increase to 10 mg can be considered at that point. The tablets are usually given in the evening. Donepezil is a substrate for metabolism by CYP450 2D6 and 3A4. Although follow-up studies suggest sustained benefit for close to 2 years, there is not clear evidence that the drug alters the course of the disease, and with progression of the illness, the efficacy of the drug could diminish. Because the drug lacks hepatotoxicity, has a log elimination half-life that permits single daily dosing, is well absorbed without significant influence of food, and is relatively selective for brain (versus gastrointestinal) acetylcholinesterase, donepezil has replaced tacrine as the treatment of first choice for Alzheimer's disease.

Based on the hypothesis of cholinergic influences in bipolar disorder, donepezil is an experimental agent in the treatment of that condition.

TACRINE

Tacrine is an acridinamine derivative for the treatment of cognitive deficits due to Alzheimer's disease. It is a noncompetitive, reversible inhibitor of acetylcholinesterase.

Tacrine is highly lipid soluble, unlike many acetylcholinesterase inhibitors; thus, it produces high levels in the brain. Oral absorption produces highly variable plasma levels, which peak at approximately 2 hours after administration. The drug is extensively metabolized in the liver; its half-life is prolonged in the elderly and in individuals with liver disease. In healthy volunteers the elimination half-life is 2 hours; in the elderly it is approximately 3.5 hours.

Double-blind placebo-controlled trials of tacrine have demonstrated benefit in a minority of mildly to moderately impaired patients with probable Alzheimer's disease. The study reporting the greatest benefit used high dosages of 160 mg/day, but not all patients in the study could tolerate that dosage. Even for those who respond to tacrine, the benefit is modest, consisting of slower decline or some improvement in cognitive and living skills test scores. There are no data to suggest that tacrine produces clinically significant functional improvement.

Tacrine is usually begun at a dosage of 10 mg four times daily and is slowly increased as side effects allow. The maximum dosage is 40 mg four times daily. Because of hepatic toxicity, aminotransferase activity should be monitored throughout treatment; the manufacturer recommends monitoring weekly.

Approximately 50% of patients on tacrine develop elevations in hepatic aminotransferase activity. In short-term studies of tacrine, these elevations have usually returned to normal within

6 weeks of drug discontinuation. Approximately 25% of patients studied have had marked abnormalities (at least three times the upper limit of normal). Several patients on dosages of 100 to 200 mg/day have had biopsy-proven hepatitis, which resolved clinically upon drug discontinuation. Other side effects include nausea, vomiting, diarrhea, headache, and ataxia.

Tacrine may interact with drugs metabolized by the hepatic P450 pathway; it has been shown to increase levels of theophylline.

BIBLIOGRAPHY

Psychostimulants

Review

Chiarello RJ, Cole JO. The use of psychostimulants in general psychiatry. *Arch Gen Psychiatry* 1987;44:286.

Therapeutic Indications

Forrest WH Jr, Brown BW Jr, Brown CR, et al. Dextroamphetamine with morphine for the treatment of postoperative pain. *N Engl J Med* 1977;296:712.

Katon W, Raskind M. Treatment of depression in the medically ill elderly with methylphenidate. *Am J Psychiatry* 1980;137:963.

Kaufmann MW, Marray GB, Cassem NH. Use of psychostimulants in medically ill depressed patients. *Psychosomatics* 1982;23:817.

Mannuzza S, Klein RG, Bessler A, et al. Adult outcome of hyperactive boys: educational achievement, occupational rank, and psychiatric status. *Arch Gen Psychiatry* 1993;50:885, 1993.

Mattes JA, Boswell L, Oliver H. Methylphenidate effects on symptoms of attention deficit disorder in adults. *Arch Gen Psychiatry* 1984;41:1059.

Spencer T, Wilens TE, Biederman J, et al. A double-blind, cross-over comparison of methylphenidate and placebo in adults with childhood onset attention deficit hyperactivity disorder. *Arch Gen Psychiatry* 1995;52:434.

Spencer T, Biederman J, Wilens TE, et al. Is attention deficit hyperactivity disorder in adults a valid diagnosis? *Harvard Rev Psychiatry* 1994;1:326.

Wender PH, Reimherr FW, Wood DR. Attention deficit disorder ("minimal brain dysfunction") in adults. *Arch Gen Psychiatry* 1981;38:449.

Wender PH, Reimherr FW, Wood D, Ward M. A controlled study of methylphenidate in the treatment of attention deficit disorder, residual type, in adults. *Am J Psychiatry* 1985;142:547.

Wilens TE, Biederman J, Spencer TJ, et al. Controlled trial of high doses of pemoline for adults with attention-deficit/hyperactivity disorder. *J Clin Psychopharmacol* 1999;19:257.

Wood DR, Reimherr FW, Wender PH, et al. Diagnosis and treatment of minimal brain dysfunction in adults: a preliminary report. *Arch Gen Psychiatry* 1976;33:1453.

β-adrenergic Blockers

Treatment of Anxiety

James I, Pearson R, Griffith D, et al. Effect of oxprenolol on stage fright in musicians. *Lancet* 1977;2:952.

Kathol R, Noyes R Jr, Slymen DJ, et al. Propranolol in chronic anxiety disorders: a controlled study. *Arch Gen Psychiatry* 1981;37:1361.

Treatment of Aggressive Outbursts

Greendyke RM, Schuster DB, Wooton JA. Propranolol in the treatment of assaultive patients with organic brain disease. *J Clin Psychopharmacol* 1984;4:282.

Mattes JA. Metoprolol for intermittent explosive disorder. *Am J Psychiatry* 1985;142:1108.

Ratey JJ, Morrill R, Oxenkrug G. Use of propranolol for provoked and unprovoked episodes of rage. *Am J Psychiatry* 1983;140:1356.

Ratey JJ, Sorgi P, O'Driscoll GA, et al. Nadolol to treat aggression and psychiatric symptomatology in chronic psychiatric inpatients: a double-blind, placebo-controlled study. *J Clin Psychiatry* 1992; 53:41.

Treatment of Akathisia

Lipinski JF, Zubenko GS, Cohen BM, et al. Propranolol in the treatment of neuroleptic-induced akathisia. *Am J Psychiatry* 1984;141: 412.

Ratey JJ, Sorgi P, Polakoff S. Nadolol as a treatment for akathisia. *Am J Psychiatry* 1985;142:640.

Treatment of Ethanol Withdrawal

Kraus ML, Gottlieb LD, Horwitz RI, et al. Randomized clinical trial of atenolol in patients with alcohol withdrawal. *N Engl J Med* 1985;313:905.

Adverse Effects

Dimsdale JE, Newton RP, Joist T. Neuropsychological side effects of beta-blockers. *Arch Intern Med* 1989;149:514.

Griffin SJ, Friedman MJ. Depressive symptoms in propranolol users. *J Clin Psychiatry* 1986;47:453.

Clonidine

Adler LA, Angrist B, Peselow E, et al. Clonidine in neuroleptic-induced akathisia. *Am J Psychiatry* 1987;144:235.

Bond WS. Psychiatric indications for clonidine: the neuropharmacologic and clinical basis. *J Clin Psychopharmacol* 1986;6:81.

Cohen DJ, Detlor J, Young JG, et al. Clonidine ameliorates Gilles de la Tourette syndrome. *Arch Gen Psychiatry* 1980;37:1350.

Franks P, Harp J, Bell B. Randomized, controlled trial of clonidine for smoking cessation in a primary care setting. *JAMA* 1989;262:3011.

Giannini AJ, Pascarzi GA, Loiselle RH, et al. Comparison of clonidine and lithium in the treatment of mania. *Am J Psychiatry* 1986;143:1608.

Goodman WK, Charney DS, Price LH, et al. Ineffectiveness of clonidine in the treatment of the benzodiazepine withdrawal syndrome: report of three cases. *Am J Psychiatry* 1986;143:900.

Hardy MC, Lecrubier Y, Widlocher D. Efficacy of clonidine in 24 patients with acute mania. *Am J Psychiatry* 1986;143:1450.

Jouvent R, Lecrubier Y, Puech AJ, et al. Antimanic effect of clonidine. *Am J Psychiatry* 1980;137:1275.

Leckman JF, Hardin MT, Riddle MA. Clonidine treatment of Gilles de la Tourette's Syndrome. *Arch Gen Psychiatry* 1991;48:324.

San L, Cami J, Peir JM, et al. Efficacy of clonidine, guanfacine and methadone is the rapid detoxification of heroin addicts: a controlled clinical trial. *Br J Addict* 1990;85:141.

Zubenko GS, Cohen BM, Lipinski JF, et al. Use of clonidine in treating neuroleptic-induced akathisia. *Psychiatry Res* 1984;13:253.

Zubenko GS, Cohen BM, Lipinski JF, et al. Clonidine in the treatment of mania and mixed bipolar disorder. *Am J Psychiatry* 1984;141:1617.

Verapamil

Barton BM, Gitlin MJ. Verapamil in treatment-resistant mania: an open trial. *J Clin Psychopharmacol* 1987;7:101.

Dubovsky SL, Franks RD, Lifschitz M, et al. Effectiveness of verapamil in the treatment of a manic patient. *Am J Psychiatry* 1982;139:502.

Dubovsky SL, Franks RD, Allen S, et al. Calcium antagonists in mania: a double-blind study of verapamil. *Psychiatry Res* 1986;18:309.

Giannini AJ, Houser WL, Loiselle RH, et al. Antimanic effects of verapamil. *Am J Psychiatry* 1984;141:1602.

Gitlin M, Weiss J. Verapamil as maintenance treatment in bipolar illness: a case report. *J Clin Psychopharmacol* 1984;4:341.

Disulfiram

Branchey L, Davis W, Lee KK, et al. Psychiatric complications of disulfiram treatment. *Am J Psychiatry* 1987;14:1310.

Eneanya DL, Bianchine JR, Duran DO, et al. The actions and metabolic fate of disulfiram. *Ann Rev Pharmacol Toxicol* 1981;21:575.

Fisher CM. Catatonia due to disulfiram toxicity. *Arch Neurol* 1989;46:798.

Fuller RK, Branchey L, Brightwell DR, et al. Disulfiram treatment of alcoholism: a Veterans Administration cooperative study. *JAMA* 1986;256:1449.

Fuller RK, Roth HP. Disulfiram for the treatment of alcoholism. *Ann Intern Med* 1979;90:901.

Kirubakaran V, Liskow B, Mayfield D, et al. Case report of acute disulfiram overdose. *Am J Psychiatry* 1983;140:1513.

Sellers EM, Naranjo CA, Peachey JE. Drugs to decrease alcohol consumption. *N Engl J Med* 1981;305:1255.

Donepezil

Roger SL, Friedhoff LT. The efficacy and safety of donepezilin patients with Alzheimer's disease: result of a multicentre, randomized, double-blind, placebo-controlled trial. The Donepezil Study Group. *Dementia* 1996;7:293.

Tacrine

Knapp MJ, Knopman DS, Solomon PR, et al. A 30-week randomized controlled trial of high-dose tacrine in patients with Alzheimer's disease. *JAMA* 1994;271:985.

Watkins PB, Zimmerman HJ, Knapp MJ, et al. Hepatotoxic effects of tacrine administration in patients with Alzheimer's disease. *JAMA* 1994;271:992.

Adderall

Pelham WE, Aronoff HR, Midlam JK, et al. A comparison of ritalin and Adderall: efficacy and time course in children with attention-deficit/hyperactivity disorder. *Pediatrics* 1999;103:43.

Pliszka SR. The use of psychostimulants in the pediatric patient. *Pediatr Clin North Am* 1998;45:1085.

Swanson J, Wigal S, Greenhill L, et al. Objective and subjective measures of the pharmacodynamic effects of Adderall in the treatment of children with ADHD in a controlled laboratory classroom setting. *Psychopharmacol Bull* 1998;34:55.

Subject Index

Note: Page numbers followed by f indicate figures; those followed by t indicate tables.